ISCCM
Manual of
Obstetric Critical Care

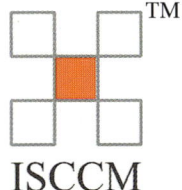

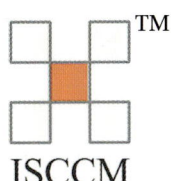
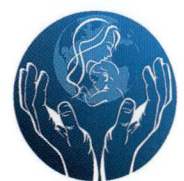

ISCCM Manual of Obstetric Critical Care

Chief Editors

Rajesh Mishra
MBBS MD (Medicine) FNB (CCM)
EDICM FCCP FCCM FICCM FICP
Consultant Intensivist and Internist
Khyati Multispecialty Hospitals and
Shaibya Comprehensive Care Clinic
Ahmedabad, Gujarat, India
President ISCCM Chancellor, ICCM
National Representative India, ESICM

Srinivas Samavedam
MD DNB FRCP FNB EDIC FICCM DMLE MBA
Chief Intensivist
Ramdev Rao Hospital
Hyderabad, Telangana, India
Associate Editor, IJCCM

Associate Editors

Tarakeswari Surapaneni MBBS MD (Obs & Gyne)
Consultant Obstetrician
Fernandez Hospital
Hyderabad, Telangana, India

Sharmili Sinha MD DNB EDIC FICCM PGDHM
Associate Professor
Department of Critical Care
Apollo Hospitals Educational and Research Foundation (AHERF)
Senior Consultant
Department of Critical Care Medicine
Apollo Hospitals
Bhubaneswar, Odisha, India

Forewords
PC Mahapatra, Jorge Hidalgo

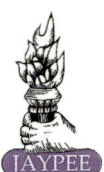

JAYPEE BROTHERS MEDICAL PUBLISHERS
The Health Sciences Publisher
New Delhi | London

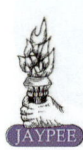 **Jaypee Brothers Medical Publishers (P) Ltd**

Headquarters
Jaypee Brothers Medical Publishers (P) Ltd
EMCA House, 23/23-B
Ansari Road, Daryaganj
New Delhi 110 002, India
Landline: +91-11-23272143, +91-11-23272703
+91-11-23282021, +91-11-23245672
Email: jaypee@jaypeebrothers.com

Corporate Office
Jaypee Brothers Medical Publishers (P) Ltd
4838/24, Ansari Road, Daryaganj
New Delhi 110 002, India
Phone: +91-11-43574357
Fax: +91-11-43574314
Email: jaypee@jaypeebrothers.com

Overseas Office
JP Medical Ltd
83 Victoria Street, London
SW1H 0HW (UK)
Phone: +44 20 3170 8910
Fax: +44 (0)20 3008 6180
Email: info@jpmedpub.com

Website: www.jaypeebrothers.com
Website: www.jaypeedigital.com

© 2024, Jaypee Brothers Medical Publishers

The views and opinions expressed in this book are solely those of the original contributor(s)/author(s) and do not necessarily represent those of editor(s) or publisher of the book.

All rights reserved. No part of this publication may be reproduced, stored or transmitted in any form or by any means, electronic, mechanical, photocopying, recording or otherwise, without the prior permission in writing of the publishers.

All brand names and product names used in this book are trade names, service marks, trademarks or registered trademarks of their respective owners. The publisher is not associated with any product or vendor mentioned in this book.

Medical knowledge and practice change constantly. This book is designed to provide accurate, authoritative information about the subject matter in question. However, readers are advised to check the most current information available on procedures included and check information from the manufacturer of each product to be administered, to verify the recommended dose, formula, method and duration of administration, adverse effects and contraindications. It is the responsibility of the practitioner to take all appropriate safety precautions. Neither the publisher nor the author(s)/editor(s) assume any liability for any injury and/or damage to persons or property arising from or related to use of material in this book.

This book is sold on the understanding that the publisher is not engaged in providing professional medical services. If such advice or services are required, the services of a competent medical professional should be sought.

Every effort has been made where necessary to contact holders of copyright to obtain permission to reproduce copyright material. If any have been inadvertently overlooked, the publisher will be pleased to make the necessary arrangements at the first opportunity.

Inquiries for bulk sales may be solicited at: jaypee@jaypeebrothers.com

ISCCM Manual of Obstetric Critical Care

First Edition: **2024**

ISBN: 978-93-5696-192-0

Printed at: Samrat Offset Pvt. Ltd.

Contributors

Ahsan Ahmed MBBS DA DNB MNAMS IFCCM EDIC
Assistant Professor and Chief
Department of Critical Care and
Emergency Services
KPC Medical College and Hospital
Kolkata, West Bengal, India

Ahsina Jahan Lopa MBBS FICM
Consultant and Incharge
Department of ICU and Emergency
Shahabuddin Medical College Hospital
Dhaka, Bangladesh

Ajay Singh MD
Assistant Professor
Department of Anesthesiology and Intensive Care
Postgraduate Institute of Medical Education and Research
Chandigarh, India

Ajith Kumar AK MD DNB EDIC
Lead Consultant
Department of Critical Care Medicine
Aster Whitefield Hospital
Bengaluru, Karnataka, India

Aklesh Tandekar MD EDIC IDCCM FIMSA FCPS CPS
Head
Department of Critical Care
Wockhardt Hospitals
Mumbai, Maharashtra, India

Amrita Patel MBBS MD (Obs & Gyne)
Assistant Professor
Department of Obstetrics and Gynecology
BJ Medical College
Ahmedabad, Gujarat, India

Amrita Shah MD (Anes) IDCCM
DrNB Trainee
Department of Critical Care Medicine
Manipal Hospital
Bengaluru, Karnataka, India

Anirban Bose MBBS DNB FNB
Consultant
Department of Critical Care
Dr Malay's Hospital and Neurosciences Centre
Thalamus Institute of Medical Sciences
Siliguri, West Bengal, India

Anirban Hom Choudhuri
MBBS MD FICCM PGDMLE FIAMLE
Director Professor and Critical Care Expert
GB Pant Institute of Postgraduate Medical Education and Research
New Delhi, India

Anisha Gala Shah
MBBS DGO/DNB (Obs & Gyne)
Postdoc Fellowship (Obstetric Medicine)
Consultant
Department of Obstetrics
Fernandez Hospital
Hyderabad, Telangana, India

Anjan Trikha MD
Visiting Professor
Department of Anesthesia and
Perioperative Medicine
School of Medicine
University of California
San Francisco, CA, USA
Former Professor
Department of Anesthesiology, Pain Medicine and Critical Care
All India Institute of Medical Sciences
New Delhi, India

Anuj Clerk MD IDCCM EDIC FNB FIECMO
Head
Department of Intensive Care Services
Sunshine Global Hospital
Surat, Gujarat, India

Contributors

Arindam Kar MD DNB FNBE EDICM FCCP FCCM FICCM
Chief Intensivist
Department of Critical Care Medicine
Sir HN Reliance Foundation Hospital
Mumbai, Maharashtra, India
National General Secretary (2021–2022)
Indian Society of Critical Care Medicine
Former Asia-Pacific Representative, European Society of Intensive Care Medicine (2015–2018)
Center Director, EDIC Examination Part 1
India Chapter

Arun Kumar MD (Anesthesiology) PGDMLE CCEPC
Director
Department of Critical Care, Palliation, and ICU Rehabilitation
Fortis Hospital
Mohali, Punjab, India

Asish Kumar Sahoo MD DM
Consultant
Institute of Critical Care Medicine
Sir Ganga Ram Hospital
New Delhi, India

Beena Daniel MBBS DA
Consultant Intensivist
Medicover Hospital
Aurangabad, Maharashtra, India

Bhagyesh Shah MBBS DA IDCCM MBA (Healthcare Mgt)
Incharge ICU and Consultant
Department of Critical Care Medicine
Marengo CIMS Hospital
Ahmedabad, Gujarat, India

Bhawesh Upreti MBBS MD PDCC
Senior Resident (Academics)
Indira Gandhi Institute of Medical Sciences
Patna, Bihar, India

Bhumika Sambyal
MBBS FCCCM FICM Fellowship in Ventilation (ACE, Jaipur)
Associate Consultant
Department of Critical Care Medicine
PSRI Hospital
New Delhi, India
FCCS Instructor
FCCS OBS Instructor

Bhuvna Ahuja MD (Anesthesiology)
Assistant Professor
Department of Neurosurgery (Neuroanesthesia)
Lok Nayak Hospital
Maulana Azad Medical College
New Delhi, India

Deepika Jain
MBBS MD DNB EDAIC IDRA Fellow IAPA
Consultant (Anesthesia)
BLK-Max Superspecialty Hospital
New Delhi, India

Devang Patel
MD (Obs & Gyne Gold Medalist)
FNB (High Risk Pregnancy & Perinatology)
Consultant
Department of Obstetrics and Gynecology
Marengo CIMS Hospital
Ahmedabad
Director
Divine Women's Hospital
Gujarat Fetal Medicine Center
Ahmedabad, Gujarat, India

Durgesh Makwana
MBBS DA DNB (Anesthesiology)
FNB Critical Care Medicine IDCCM
Senior Consultant
Ruby Hall Clinic
Pune, Maharashtra, India

Ganshyam Jagathkar MD FNB FICCM
Director (Critical Care)
Medicover Hospital
Hyderabad, Telangana, India

Gaurav Mittal MD
Senior Resident (Academics)
Critical Care Medicine
Department of Anesthesiology
Pain Medicine and Critical Care
All India Institute of Medical Sciences
New Delhi, India

Hetal Patolia
MD (Obs & Gyne) PGDMLS PGHHM PGDCR PGDART
Consultant Gynecologist
Khyati Multispecialty Hospital and
SGVP Holistic Hospital
Ahmedabad, Gujarat, India

Contributors

Ipe Jacob MBBS CTCCM IDCCM
ICU Registrar
Manipal Hospital
Bengaluru, Karnataka, India

Jay Prakash MBBS MD (Gold Medal) FCCS
Assistant Professor
Department of Critical Care Medicine
Rajendra Institute of Medical Sciences
Ranchi, Jharkhand, India

Jitin Sharma MD IDCCM IFCCM
Consultant
Department of Critical Care Medicine
BLK-Max Superspecialty Hospital
New Delhi, India

Kallur Sailaja Devi MBBS DGO/DNB (Obs & Gyne)
Medical Director (Unit 2) and Senior Consultant
Department of Obstetrics
Fernandez Hospital
Hyderabad, Telangana, India

Kalpesh Parekh MBBS DA DNB (Anesthesia) FCCM
Assistant Professor
SMBT IMS & RC (Institute of Medical Sciences and Research Centre)
Nashik, Maharashtra, India

Kanwalpreet Sodhi DA DNB IDCCM EDIC FICCM
Director and Head
Department of Critical Care
Deep Hospital
Ludhiana, Punjab, India

Kesari Masaipeta
MD (Anesthesiology) PDCC (Critical Care-AIIMS)
DNB Resident
Sir HN Reliance Foundation Hospital
Mumbai, Maharashtra, India

Lalita Gouri Mitra DA MD DNB MNAMS FICCM
Professor and Officer Incharge
Department of Anesthesia, Critical Care and Pain
Homi Bhabha Cancer Hospital and Research Centre
Medicity, New Chandigarh
All India Institute of Medical Sciences, Bhopal, Madhya Pradesh
Homi Bhabha Cancer Hospital
(A Unit of Tata Memorial Centre Mumbai and Department of Atomic Energy Govt. of India)
Sangrur, Punjab, India

Maimoona Ahmed
MS (Obs & Gyne) FNB (High Risk Pregnancy and Perinatology)
Consultant
Department of Obstetrics
Fernandez Hospital
Hyderabad, Telangana, India

Maitree Pandey MD
Director Professor and Head
Department of Anesthesiology and Critical Care
Lady Hardinge Medical College
New Delhi, India

Malini Sukayogula
MS (Obs & Gyne) FNB (High Risk Pregnancy and Perinatology)
Consultant Maternal and Fetal Medicine Labor Ward Lead
Fernandez Hospital
Hyderabad, Telangana, India

Maneendra Singarapu MD FNB EDIC DHQM
Consultant and Head
Department of Critical Care
Global Hospital
Hyderabad, Telangana, India

Manisha Pradhan
MBBS DGO/DNB (Obs & Gyne) FNB (High Risk Pregnancy and Perinatology)
Consultant
Department of Obstetrics and Fetal Medicine
Fernandez Hospital
Hyderabad, Telangana, India

Mithilesh Raut MBBS DA DNB EDIC
Consultant Intensivist
Department of Critical Care Medicine
Medicover Hospital
Hyderabad, Telangana, India

Mohd Saif Khan
MBBS MD DNB DM (Critical Care Medicine) Postdoc Fellowship (Critical Care) MNAMS
Consultant ICU
Department of Critical Care Medicine
King Hamad University Hospital
Kingdom of Bahrain

Mukta Seth MD (Obs & Gyne)
Senior Consultant
Department of Obstetrics and Gynecology
Jeevan Anmol Hospital
New Delhi, India

Neeraj Kumar
MBBS (Hons) MD (Anesthesiology) FCCS
Associate Professor
Department of Anesthesia
All India Institute of Medical Sciences
Patna, Bihar, India

Nidhi Bhatia MD DNB MAMS
Professor
Core Faculty (DM-Trauma Anesthesia and Acute Care)
Department of Anesthesia and Intensive Care
Postgraduate Institute of Medical Education and Research
Chandigarh, India

Nilashree Das MD (Internal Medicine)
Associate Consultant
Mission Multispeciality Hospital
Durgapur, West Bengal, India

Nithya CA
MD IDCCM FNB (Critical Care Medicine) EDIC
Consultant
Department of Critical Care Medicine
Manipal Hospitals
Bengaluru, Karnataka, India

Pallavi Chandra Ravula MS (Obs & Gyne)
Consultant and Head
Department of Obstetrics
Fernandez Hospital
Hyderabad, Telangana, India

Prachee Sathe MD FRCP FCCCM
Founder Director
ICU Ruby Hall Clinic, Pune
Professor
(Critical Care Medicine)
DY Patil Medical College
Pune, Maharashtra, India

Pradeep Rangappa
DNB (Int Med) FJFICM EDIC FCICM PGDipEcho
MBA (HCS) FICCM PGDMLE (NLSUI)
Consultant
Department of Intensive Care Physician
Manipal Hospitals
Bengaluru, Karnataka, India

Pradip Kumar Bhattacharya
MD ACME FICCM FCCCM FCCM
Professor and Head
Department of Critical Care Medicine
Incharge New Trauma and Emergency Center
Dean Research
Rajendra Institute of Medical Sciences
Ranchi, Jharkhand, India

Prashant Kumar
MD IDCCM FNB (Critical Care) EDIC ADHA DOA
Head
Department of Critical Care
Kailash Hospital and Neuro Institute
Noida, Uttar Pradesh, India

Priteema Chanana
DNB (Anesthesiology) IDCCM ECMO Specialist (ELSO Certified) FICCN
Consultant
Associate Consultant
Department of Critical Care Medicine
Fortis Memorial Research Institute
Gurugram, Haryana, India

Priyanka H Chhabra MBBS MD DNB
Associate Professor
Department of Anesthesia
Vardhman Mahavir Medical College and Safdarjung Hospital
New Delhi, India

Rachit Sinha MD (Anesthesiology)
Attending Consultant
Department of Critical Care
Medanta Hospital
Ranchi, Jharkhand, India

Rahul Kumar MD IFCCM
Consultant
Department of Critical Care Medicine
Sir Ganga Ram Hospital
New Delhi, India

Rajesh Mishra
MBBS MD (Medicine) FNB (CCM)
EDICM FCCP FCCM FICCM FICP
Consultant Intensivist and Internist
Khyati Multispecialty Hospitals and
Shaibya Comprehensive Care Clinic
Ahmedabad, Gujarat, India
President ISCCM Chancellor, ICCM
National Representative India, ESICM

Rajesh Pande MD PDCC FICCM FCCM
Senior Director and Head
Department of Critical Care Medicine
BLK-Max Superspecialty Hospital
New Delhi, India

Ranajit Chatterjee
MBBS MRCP FRCP EDIC DA (Gold Medal) FIACM
Head, Critical Care
Department of Anesthesia
Intensive Care and Perioperative Medicine
Swami Dayanand Hospital
New Delhi, India

Ranjan Joshi
MBBS MD DNB FCICM Grad Dip in Clin Ultrasound
Director, Obstetric Intensive Care
Senior Consultant
Paediatric Intensive Care Unit
Women's and Children's Hospital
Adelaide, Australia

Raymond Dominic Savio MD DM EDIC FICCM
Consultant
Department of Critical Care
Apollo Proton Cancer Centre
Chennai, Tamil Nadu, India

Ritesh Shah MD IDCCM FICCM FIECMO
Critical Care Consultant
Director, Critical Care Unit
Sterling Hospital
Vadodara, Gujarat, India

Ritu Singh MD PDCC EDIC
Associate Professor
Department of Critical Care Medicine
Indira Gandhi Institute of Medical Sciences
Patna, Bihar, India

Ruchira Khasne MBBS DA DNB IDCCM EDAIC EDIC
Consultant and Head
Department of Critical Care Medicine
SMBT Institute of Medical Sciences and
Research Centre
Nashik, Maharashtra, India

Sabina Regmi
MBBS MD DM DrNB (Neuroanesthesia)
Consultant (Anesthesiologist)
Neo Multispeciality Hospital
Noida, Uttar Pradesh, India

Sachin Narayan Rathore MD (Anesthesia)
Physician Specialist Anesthesia
Sheikh Shakhbout Medical City
Abu Dhabi, UAE

Sai Saran MD DM EDIC
Assistant Professor
Department of Critical Care Medicine
King George's Medical University
Lucknow, Uttar Pradesh, India

Sameer Bhuwania MD DNB (Nephrology)
Consultant Nephrologist
NHS Hospital
Jalandhar, Punjab, India

Sanjeev Kumar MD FICCM
Professor and Head
Department of Critical Care Medicine
Indira Gandhi Institute of Medical Sciences
Patna, Bihar, India

Sanmay Chowdhury
MBBS FCPS (Internal Medicine) DNB IDCCM
Physician and Intensivist
Department of Medicine
Ruby Hall Clinic
Pune, Maharashtra, India

Santanu Bagchi FNB (CCM)
Consultant
Department of Critical Care Medicine
Tata Medical Center
Kolkata, West Bengal, India

Contributors

Saurabh Debnath MBBS DNB FNB IDCCM FCCM
Senior Consultant
Department of Critical Care Medicine
Peerless Hospitex Hospital
Kolkata, West Bengal, India

Saurabh Taneja MD FNB EDIC
Senior Consultant
Institute of Critical Care Medicine
Sir Ganga Ram Hospital
New Delhi, India

Sauren Panja
MBBS MD (Internal Medicine)
FNB (Critical Care Medicine) EDIC
Head and Senior Consultant
Department of Critical Care Medicine and
Internal Medicine
Administrative Lead
(Critical Care Services) NH Eastern Region
NH-Rabindranath Tagore International Institute
of Cardiac Sciences
Kolkata, West Bengal, India

Sharmili Sinha MD DNB EDIC FICCM PGDI IM
Associate Professor
Department of Critical Care
Apollo Hospitals Educational and Research
Foundation (AHERF)
Senior Consultant
Department of Critical Care Medicine
Apollo Hospitals
Bhubaneswar, Odisha, India

Shibba Takkar Chhabra
DM (Cardiology) FACC FCSI
Professor
Department of Cardiology
Hero DMC Heart Institute
Dayanand Medical College and Hospital
Ludhiana, Punjab, India

Shrikant Sahasrabudhe
MD (Chest) IDCCM
Director and Head
Department of Pulmonology and
Critical Care Medicine
Medicover Hospitals
Aurangabad, Maharashtra, India

Shweta Bhatt Dave
MBBS DGO DNB FRM
Reproductive Endocrinologist and
Infertility Specialist
Milann Hospital
Bengaluru, Karnataka, India

Simant Kumar Jha
DA DNB PGDHM PDCR FIPM Certificate Course in Medical
Law and Ethics ATLS Faculty FCCS
Consultant
FCCS Course Director
FCCS Surgical Instructor
Senior Consultant
Department of Critical Care Medicine
Pushpawati Singhania Hospital and
Research Institute
New Delhi, India

Siri Yerubandi
MBBS DNB (Obs & Gyne)
Consultant Obstetrics
Fernandez Hospital
Hyderabad, Telangana, India

Soumya Sharma MBBS DA DNB
Senior Resident
Department of Critical Care Medicine
King George's Medical University
Lucknow, Uttar Pradesh, India

Souvik Maitra MD DNB EDIC
Associate Professor
Department of Anesthesiology, Pain Medicine
and Critical Care
All India Institute of Medical Sciences
New Delhi, India

Srinivas Samavedam
MD DNB FRCP FNB EDIC FICCM DMLE MBA
Chief Intensivist
Ramdev Rao Hospital
Hyderabad, Telangana, India
Associate Editor, IJCCM

Sulagna Bhattacharjee
MD DNB DM (Critical Care Med)
Assistant Professor
Department of Anesthesiology, Pain Medicine
and Critical Care
All India Institute of Medical Sciences
New Delhi, India

Sunaina Tejpal Karna MBBS MD
Additional Professor
Department of Anesthesiology
All India Institute of Medical Sciences
Bhopal, Madhya Pradesh, India

Suresh Kumar Sundaramurthy
MD DNB EDAIC IDCCM
Consultant
Department of Critical Care
Apollo Proton Cancer Centre
Chennai, Tamil Nadu, India

Suruchi Ambasta MD
Assistant Professor
Department of Anesthesiology
Sanjay Gandhi Institute of Medical Sciences
Lucknow, Uttar Pradesh, India

Susruta Bandyopadhyay
MD Dip in Cardiology
Director (Critical Care)
Intensivist and Cardiologist
AMRI Hospitals
Kolkata, West Bengal, India

Suvadeep Sen MD FNB EDIC
Consultant Intensivist
Department of Critical Care
Apollo Hospital
Navi Mumbai, Maharashtra, India

Tanima Baronia MD (Anesthesia) IDCCM
Deputy Director
Department of Critical Care Medicine
Ruby Hall Clinic
Pune, Maharashtra, India

Tapas Kumar Sahoo
MD FNB FICCM FCCP EDIC MBA Canadian Critical Care Fellowship
Associate Director and Head
Department of Critical Care
Medanta Hospital
Ranchi, Jharkhand, India

Tarakeswari Surapaneni MBBS MD (Obs & Gyne)
Consultant Obstetrician
Fernandez Hospital
Hyderabad, Telangana, India

Tushar Kumar MBBS DA DNB PDCC
Assistant Professor
Department of Anesthesiology
Rajendra Institute of Medical Sciences
Ranchi, Jharkhand, India

Venigalla Rama
MBBS DGO/DNB (Obs & Gyne) Postdoc Fellowship (Obstetric Medicine)
Consultant Obstetrician
Fernandez Hospital
Hyderabad, Telangana, India

Vinay Singhal MD (Anesthesiology) IDCCM FICCM
Senior Consultant and Head
Department of Critical Care
MM College of Medical Sciences and Research
Ambala, Haryana, India

Vinod K Singh MD FRCP EDIC
Senior Consultant
Department of Critical Care Medicine
Sir Ganga Ram Hospital
New Delhi, India

Vivek Gupta
DA DNB (Anesthesia) FIACTA FICCM FIDSA MNAMS
Consultant
Department of Cardiac Anesthesia and Intensive Care
Coordinator ECMO Program
Hero DMC Heart Institute
Ludhiana, Punjab, India

Y Subhashini
MBBS DNB (Obs & Gyne)
Consultant Obstetrician
Department of Obstetrics and Gynecology
Fernandez Hospital
Hyderabad, Telangana, India

Foreword

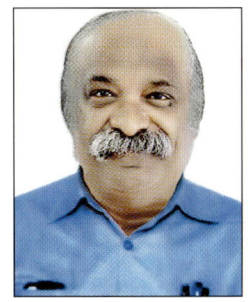

The physiological changes in various systems brought about during pregnancy begins right from the first trimester of pregnancy till delivery and the changes are considered as physiological adaptation in pregnancy for the benefit of fetal as well as maternal environment.

At the same time, newer specific entities emerge during pregnancy such as pregnancy-induced hypertension (PIH), gestational diabetes mellitus (GDM), anemia, thromboembolic episodes, and others which need special focus as regards diagnosis and treatment. However, preexisting medical or surgical diseases are also going to affect the course of pregnancy to a considerable extent.

With the advancing wisdom and conceptual advances to reduce maternal and perinatal mortalities and morbidities, critical care obstetrics has emerged as a distinct subspecialty by itself and therefore the confluence of obstetricians and critical care specialists is the need of the hour.

Viewed in these contexts Dr Sharmili Sinha, a renowned critical care specialist and intensivist has toiled hard in bringing out this focused *Manual of Obstetric Critical Care*. The five different sections as well as the different subsections are designed in such a way that the clinicians will get latest knowledge and practical skills in various aspects of fetomaternal medicine with special emphasis in managing the spectrum of illness.

I am sure this manuscript will really be a boon to the obstetricians not only in updating their knowledge but also help to acquire skill to manage the critically ill obstetric patients.

PC Mahapatra MD FICMCH
Ex-Professor and Head
Department of Obstetrics and Gynecology
SCB Medical College
Cuttack, Odisha, India

Foreword

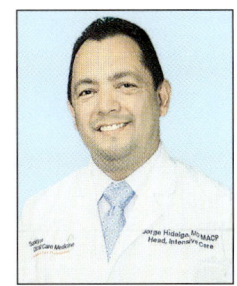

Obstetric Critical Care has grown and gained its space as a relatively new medical field. In the modern world, whether at home, in our office, or while driving, we can access our patient's vital signs, imaging, and laboratory results electronically at the click of a mouse. We can access the literature of the world. Having critical obstetric care as a textbook in the modern era? A textbook that allows us to understand the common mechanisms in the critically ill pregnant patient and provide an in-depth, specific discussion of the essential mechanism of the diseases and an understanding of different procedures.

Our clinical practice fundamentally drives how we approach our patients, teaching, and critical care investigation. In turn, our practice is informed, animated, and balanced by the information and environment arising around learning and research. Careful history taking, detailed physical examination, and support by laboratory testing are essential to achieve clinical excellence. These data raise questions concerning the patient's disease mechanisms, upon which a complete, prioritized differential diagnosis is formulated and a treatment plan initiated. The intensive care units (ICUs) reality, complexity, and limitations drive our search for a better understanding of critical care's pathophysiology and new, effective therapies. This textbook reflects the interweaving and mutually supporting threads of critical care practice, teaching, and research. The chapters reflect the growing scope of critical care obstetrics and the increasing importance and recognition of the hospital structure's field. Furthermore, most hospitals today contain ICUs mixed by intention or by overflow, and multidisciplinary trained intensivists equipped to recognize and manage the wide range of acute care problems, promoting and keeping the team approach and multiprofessional nature of critical care delivery. Regardless of primary discipline, all intensivists must possess a core set of critical care skills that allow them to manage critically ill patients.

This textbook, in addition to the practicing critical care physicians and fellows in training, is designed to be a valuable resource for all critical care providers, hospitalists, subspecialty physicians, residents, nurses, physician assistants, nurse practitioners, nutritionists, pharmacists, respiratory therapists, and medical students involved in the care of critically ill obstetric patients.

Jorge Hidalgo MD MACP MCCM FCCP
Head of the Intensive Care and COVID-19
Belize Healthcare Partners Limited
Belize City, Belize
President-Elect
World Federation of Intensive and Critical Care

Preface

Critical care has evolved as a dynamic specialty and the understanding of the pathophysiology of critical illness is improving continuously. Subspecialty areas of critical care are also gaining in attention and popularity. One of the key areas where critical care plays a crucial and effective role is obstetric critical care. Obstetric physiology is unique and deals with maternal and fetal units with distinct implications. While most pregnancies go to completion uneventfully, a small proportion do get complicated with maternal and fetal compromise. A thorough understanding of the intricacies of obstetrics and intensive care is needed among all specialists handling these complex patients.

The Indian Society of Critical Care Medicine (ISCCM) is in the forefront of education and training in the field of critical care. Society aims to have an inclusive approach in expanding the horizons of the specialty. As part of this endeavor, the President, Dr Rajesh Mishra, envisaged a training module which deals with the basic understanding of the intricacies involved in the management of a critically ill obstetric patient. The core group constituted by him designed a training platform and set about compiling a course manual which gives a comprehensive view of the problems of critical nature occurring in a pregnant lady.

The core team enlisted the expertise of key opinion leaders in the field to write up the gist of issues and solutions for the clinical problems identified. These write ups have been compiled as a *Manual of Obstetric Critical Care*. This is by no means a textbook on the topic but is more of a practical knowledge resource for day-to-day problems. This manual will serve as the template for the online course and the practical hands-on session linked to this academic exercise.

The editorial board wishes to place on record its genuine gratitude to all authors and editors who stuck to timelines and made this publication possible. The board also thanks M/s Jaypee Brothers Medical Publishers (P) Ltd, New Delhi, India, for constant support and streamlining. Lastly, thanks are also due to the office staff of ISCCM who have diligently followed the timelines and ensured smooth execution of this activity.

This manual is dedicated to all the patients who have suffered from critical illness, to teach us more about the problems and their solutions.

Rajesh Mishra
Srinivas Samavedam
Tarakeswari Surapaneni
Sharmili Sinha

Preface

Critical care has evolved as a dynamic specialty after understanding of the pathophysiology of critical illness is improving continuously. Subspecialty areas of critical care are also gaining in stature and popularity. One of the key areas where critical care plays a crucial and effective role is obstetric critical care. Obstetric phenomenon is unique and deals with maternal-fetal dyad following innate actions. While most pregnancies go to completion uneventful, a small population do get complicated with maternal, fetal and fetal compromise. A thorough understanding of obstetric physiology of obese and non-obese conditions can prevent complications leading these events to crisis.

Acknowledgments

This *Manual of Obstetric Critical Care* is the brainchild of the President of the ISCCM—Dr Rajesh Mishra. The editorial board wishes to acknowledge his immense contribution and guidance in making this possible. One of the doyens of obstetric critical care, Dr PC Mahapatra, has been a consistent guide in the execution of this ambitious project. The editorial board is indebted to him and thanks him for writing the foreword.

This manual is a compilation of the professional and clinical knowledge and experience of the best practitioners in obstetrics and critical care. The fact that they could spare time and put their thoughts on paper and match the timelines is worthy of appreciation. The editorial board is eternally indebted to all the authors who have lent a helping shoulder for this unique attempt. The output from the authors also needs to be edited by equally competent editors and each of the section editors deserves special praise for completing this task effortlessly.

A project of this magnitude needs a committed and professional publisher who can coordinate with the editorial board and the authors and bring out the finished product in a timely and elegant manner. Shri Jitendar P Vij (Group Chairman), Mr Ankit Vij (Managing Director), Mr MS Mani (Group President), Ms Chetna Malhotra (Senior Director—Professional Publishing, Marketing, and Business Development), Ms Pooja Bhandari (Director—Production), Ms Suchita Gera (Development Editor), and Ms Kritika Dua (Senior Development Editor) of M/s Jaypee Brothers Medical Publishers (P) Ltd, New Delhi, India, has fulfilled this requirement and more, and the editorial board is grateful to them for this.

This manual needed a lot of compiling, communication, and liaising. This was achieved by the Indian Society of Critical Care Medicine (ISCCM) team of Dhawal and Ninad. The editorial board places its appreciation for both, on record.

Finally, this kind of work needs a lot of time to write and edit. This invariably happens at the expense of time allocated to family and personal life. The editorial board thanks the family members of all the authors, editors, publishers, and office staff for facilitating that to accomplish this humane initiative.

Contents

SECTION 1: Basic Physiology and Epidemiology

1. **Spectrum of Critical Illness in Pregnancy: Epidemiology and Outcomes** 3
   Anjan Trikha, Ajay Singh

2. **Physiological Changes Induced by Pregnancy** 8
   Tanima Baronia, Durgesh Makwana

3. **Acid–Base Physiology** 14
   Tapas Kumar Sahoo, Rachit Sinha

SECTION 2: Principles of Fetomaternal Monitoring

4. **Monitoring of Critically Ill Expectant Mother and Parturient** 23
   Ranjan Joshi

5. **Monitoring of Fetus in a Critically Ill Mother** 32
   Devang Patel, Amrita Patel

SECTION 3: Systemic Disorders

Respiratory Disorders

6. **Asthma in Pregnancy** 41
   Prachee Sathe, Sanmay Chowdhury

7. **Community Acquired Pneumonia in Pregnancy** 46
   Ruchira Khasne, Kalpesh Parekh

8. **Acute Respiratory Distress Syndrome in Pregnancy** 53
   Sauren Panja, Nilashree Das

9. **Pulmonary Thromboembolism: Preexistent and Concurrent** 62
   Vivek Gupta, Shibba Takkar Chhabra

10. **Nonthrombotic Pulmonary Embolism** 70
    Ahsan Ahmed, Anirban Bose

Cardiovascular Disorders

11. **Hypertensive Emergencies** 76
    Siri Yerubandi

12. **Valvular Heart Diseases in Pregnancy** 88
    Anisha Gala Shah

13. **Heart Failure in Pregnancy** 97
    Susruta Bandyopadhyay

Renal Disorders and Drug Dosing

14. **Acute Kidney Injury including Hemolytic Uremic Syndrome in Pregnancy** 104
    Ranajit Chatterjee, Priyanka H Chhabra

15. **Chronic Kidney Disease and Pregnancy** 114
    Manisha Pradhan

16. **Urinary Tract Infections in Pregnancy** 124
    Kallur Sailaja Devi

17. **Drug Dosing in Renal Failure** 129
    Shrikant Sahasrabudhe, Beena Daniel

Metabolic Conditions

18. **Hyperosmolar State in Pregnancy: Diabetic Ketoacidosis and
    Hyperosmolar Hyperglycemic Syndrome** 135
    Ritesh Shah, Anuj Clerk

19. **Thyroid Disorders in Critically Ill Pregnant Lady** 145
    Bhagyesh Shah

Electrolyte Disorders

20. **Disorders of Sodium Homeostasis and Fluid Balance in Pregnancy** 152
    Santanu Bagchi, Saurabh Debnath

21. **Disorders of Potassium Homeostasis** 158
    Soumya Sharma, Sai Saran

22. **Disorders of Calcium, Magnesium, and Phosphorus Homeostasis** 169
    Prashant Kumar, Mukta Seth

Neurological Disorders

23. **Severe Preeclampsia and Eclampsia** 177
    Pallavi Chandra Ravula, Tarakeswari Surapaneni

24. **Central Venous Sinus Thrombosis** 187
    Sulagna Bhattacharjee, Gaurav Mittal, Souvik Maitra

Rheumatological Disorders

25. **Systemic Lupus Erythematosus Flare during Pregnancy** 196
    Ritu Singh, Suruchi Ambasta, Sanjeev Kumar

26. **Catastrophic Antiphospholipid Antibodies Syndrome** 203
    Hetal Patolia, Shweta Bhatt Dave

Trauma

27. **Polytrauma in a Pregnant Lady** 210
    Amrita Shah, Pradeep Rangappa, Ipe Jacob

Hematological Disorders

28. **Sickle Cell Crisis** 219
    Maimoona Ahmed, Tarakeswari Surapaneni

29. **Thalassemia in Pregnancy** 226
    Y Subhashini

30. **Thrombocytopenia in Pregnancy** 233
    Venigalla Rama

Transplant Medicine

31. **Transplant Recipients** 239
    Malini Sukayogula

SECTION 4: Procedures and Transport

32. **Cardiopulmonary Resuscitation in Obstetric Patients** 249
    Pradip Kumar Bhattacharya, Mohd Saif Khan

33. **Renal Replacement Therapy and Extracorporeal Membrane Oxygenation in Pregnancy** 257
    Kanwalpreet Sodhi, Nidhi Bhatia

34. Transport of Critically Ill Pregnant Patients 268
    Vinod K Singh, Rahul Kumar

35. Vascular Access 272
    Vinay Singhal, Arun Kumar

SECTION 5: Syndromic Approach

36. Hypoxia in Pregnancy 281
    Priteema Chanana, Kesari Masaipeta, Arindam Kar

37. Altered Sensorium in Pregnancy 291
    Mithilesh Raut, Ganshyam Jagathkar

38. Fulminant Hepatic Failure in Pregnancy 303
    Lalita Gouri Mitra, Sunaina Tejpal Karna

39. Sepsis in Full Term Pregnancy 318
    Rajesh Mishra, Maneendra Singarapu

40. Noncardiogenic Pulmonary Edema in Pregnancy 329
    Sharmili Sinha, Neeraj Kumar

41. Acute Disseminated Encephalomyelitis 334
    Simant Kumar Jha, Sameer Bhuwania, Bhumika Sambyal

42. Neuromuscular Disorders in Pregnancy 340
    Saurabh Taneja, Asish Kumar Sahoo

43. Posterior Reversible Encephalopathy Syndrome 348
    Nithya CA, Ajith Kumar AK

44. Management of Obstetric Shock with Emphasis on Fluids and Vasopressors 352
    Rajesh Pande, Maitree Pandey, Jitin Sharma

45. Hematological Cancers in Pregnancy 360
    Suresh Kumar Sundaramurthy, Raymond Dominic Savio

46. Airway Management in Critically Ill Obstetric Patients 368
    Anirban Hom Choudhuri, Deepika Jain

47. Status Epilepticus in Pregnancy 374
    Bhuvna Ahuja, Ahsina Jahan Lopa, Sabina Regmi

48. Pyrexia of Unknown Origin during Pregnancy 380
    Jay Prakash, Tushar Kumar, Bhawesh Upreti

49. Anaphylaxis in Pregnancy 386
    Aklesh Tandekar, Suvadeep Sen, Sachin Narayan Rathore

Index *389*

SECTION 1

Basic Physiology and Epidemiology

1. Spectrum of Critical Illness in Pregnancy: Epidemiology and Outcomes
   Anjan Trikha, Ajay Singh

2. Physiological Changes Induced by Pregnancy
   Tanima Baronia, Durgesh Makwana

3. Acid–Base Physiology
   Tapas Kumar Sahoo, Rachit Sinha

CHAPTER 1

Spectrum of Critical Illness in Pregnancy: Epidemiology and Outcomes

Anjan Trikha, Ajay Singh

■ INTRODUCTION

The advances in obstetric medicine around the world have led to decrease in maternal mortality rate and better pregnancy outcomes. However, some proportion of complicated pregnancies requires intensive care. Since pregnant patients are uniformly excluded from all trials due to harms and risk to both mother and fetus, the obstetric critical care is challenging as there is a lack of evidence-based guidelines for management. The maternal morbidity and mortality of critically ill pregnant patients vary greatly between high and low income countries. Most causes of maternal morbidity are preventable. Therefore, developing well equipped critical care units exclusively for pregnant patients and implementation of patient safety bundles can significantly impact the health of the mother and the fetus.

■ EPIDEMIOLOGY AND MAGNITUDE OF PROBLEM

According to a 2017 World Health Organization (WHO) report, 800 pregnant women die all over the world each day.[1] Maternal death is defined as death of a patient while pregnant or within 42 days of termination of pregnancy, irrespective of the duration or site of pregnancy, from any cause related to or aggravated by pregnancy or its management, but not from accidental or incidental causes. *Maternal mortality ratio* is steadily declining globally (211 deaths per 100,000 live births in 2017) with significant differences between low and high income countries with obstetric hemorrhage being the most common cause.[2] However, in countries such as the United States, deaths due to cardiovascular conditions in pregnant mothers are the highest. The rise in obesity, age at pregnancy, and metabolic disorders may be contributory factors.

In high income countries, where maternal mortality rate is very low, maternal morbidity is being considered as a new outcome variable of complicated pregnancies. *Severe maternal morbidity* may be defined as unintended outcomes of the process of labor and delivery that result in significant short-term or long-term consequences to a woman's health. Mortality may be considered as one of the outcomes of severe morbidity. Like mortality, morbidity is preventable if timely treatment is given to the mother. Morbidity can be identified by need of intensive care unit (ICU)/high dependency units (HDU) admissions as well as transfusion of more than 4 units of blood for the purpose of uniformity. The Department of Health in the UK in the year 2000 suggested that the terms high dependency and intensive care should be replaced with "critical care".[3] It focuses on the levels or intensity of care that a patient needs regardless of the location. The level of care required by the pregnant woman is classified from level 0 (normal ward care) to level 3 (support of two or more organ systems). This organ support is usually in the form of respiratory support (basic and advanced), cardiovascular support with inotropic agents, renal replacement therapy, or other systems such as gastrointestinal, metabolic, hematological or neurological. Level 3 support would include ventilation, or basic respiratory support plus support of at least two other organ systems. In high-income countries up to 1% of the total deliveries get admitted to ICU with median length of stay of 1–2 days.[4] The most common causes of critical care admission are hemorrhage and hypertension.[5] The various indications for admission to ICU are similar in developed and developing countries and are summarized in **Table 1**.

The number of ICU beds is eightfold in high-income countries (up to 30/100,000 of population) as compared to low-income countries (1–3/100,000 of population). Due to lack of resources, the care model of developing countries is a hybrid one with combined ICU and HDU beds for critically ill mothers.

CRITICAL ILLNESS IN PARTURIENTS: OUTCOMES

Mortality in parturients admitted in an ICU varies from 0 to 4.9% of critical care unit admissions in high income countries and from 2 to 43.6% in low-income countries.[6] There is a high risk of long-term psychiatric morbidity and substance use disorder in critically ill mother. Many maternal risk factors such as teenage or pregnancy in later age, lower socioeconomic status, and medical comorbidities are linked to higher morbidity. The maternal outcomes in resource limited countries may be worse because of lack of

TABLE 1: Indications for admission in maternal critical care units.

Obstetric causes	*Non-obstetric causes*	*Others*
Hemorrhage	Congenital heart diseases	Trauma
Hypertensive disorders of pregnancy	Valvular heart diseases	Drug abuse
Ovarian hyperstimulation syndrome	Pulmonary hypertension	Deep vein thrombosis
Acute fatty liver of pregnancy	Autoimmune diseases (SLE, myasthenia gravis)	
Aspiration syndromes	Asthma	
Postpartum cardiomyopathy	Infectious diseases (severe COVID-19, hepatitis E)	
Diabetes	Post renal transplant graft failure	
Retained products	Epilepsy	
Sepsis	Intracranial neoplasms	
Amniotic fluid embolism	*Hematological:* Sickle cell disease	

(COVID-19: coronavirus disease; SLE: systemic lupus erythematosus)

trained staff and physicians, delay in referral to higher centers, poor resources, and non-availability of transport facilities for sick patients.

The outcomes can be improved by early identification of high risk patients, improving patient care and implementation of various bundles to manage specific emergencies and conditions.

The various assessment tools to identify critical illness such as sequential organ failure assessment (SOFA), quick SOFA, acute physiological and chronic health evaluation (APACHE) scoring may not be accurate for parturients because many parameters noted in these scoring tools may be normal in this subgroup of patients due to the physiological changes of pregnancy. Further, many times, the termination of pregnancy can drastically improve the outcomes while score may suggest otherwise. Hence it is advisable to use the maternal early warning systems (MEWS).[7] It tracks physiological parameters and evolving morbidity and once a threshold is reached, it triggers intense evaluation or may be escalated treatment. The various modifications to MEWS are in use such as maternal obstetric early warning system (MOEWS) and maternal early warning trigger tool (MEWT).

The various disease-related obstetric scoring systems such as shock index (SI) for hypovolemia in major obstetric hemorrhage, miniPIERS (preeclampsia integrated estimation of risk) for patients at risk of complications of preeclampsia are also used.[8,9] The early warning systems have advantages that tools are based on vital signs so quick assessment can be made. The virtual obstetric ICU is another proposal to manage problems of scarce number of trained personnel and physicians.

■ IMPLICATIONS ON FETAL HEALTH

Maternal critical illness can have adverse effects on the fetus.[10] Uteroplacental circulation has high blood flow, no capillary microcirculation, low resistance of spiral arteries, and absent autoregulation. The vasculature has an alpha-adrenergic receptor system and blood flow can decrease markedly by endogenous and exogenous stimulation. Maternal shock, maternal hypoxia, and use of vasopressors can lead to significant decrease of fetal oxygenation and uterine blood flow. The effects of ICU management on fetus are summarized in **Table 2**.

Prediction of fetal risk factors and outcomes in critically ill mothers is difficult.

TABLE 2: Effect of critical care management on fetus.

S. no.	ICU management	Effect on fetus
1.	Drug therapy antibiotics, analgesics	Risk of teratogenicity (1–3%) and highest in first trimester, NSAIDs can cause early closure of PDA
2.	Radiological investigations	• Oncogenicity at exposure of 2–5 rads • Teratogenicity at exposure of 5–10 rads
3.	Sedation and neuromuscular blocking agents	All drugs cross placenta and can cause neonatal respiratory depression during delivery, decrease uteroplacental blood flow by hypotension due to propofol and thiopentone, neuromuscular agents do not cross placenta
4.	Vasopressors, inotropes	Decreased uteroplacental blood flow by alpha adrenergic stimulation

(ICU: intensive care unit; NSAIDs: non-steroidal anti-inflammatory drugs)

TABLE 3: General care of pregnant patient in ICU.		
S. no.	*General care*	*Special concerns*
1.	Monitoring	Fetal monitoring after 24 weeks, the choice of invasive and non-invasive monitors on patient to patient basis
2.	Ventilator strategies	Low threshold of intubation due to high risk of aspiration, modes of ventilation based on severity and type of respiratory failure, early use of ECMO in refractory hypoxemia
3.	Drugs	Be aware of FDA category of the prescribed medicine
4.	Nutrition	Extra 350–450 kcal/day in late trimesters. Protein requirement and iron content doubles as compared to non-obstetric population, use anti-aspiration prophylaxis
5.	Thromboprophylaxis	Higher risk of thrombosis, pharmacological, and mechanical thromboprophylaxis
6.	Cardiopulmonary arrest	After 20 weeks, bedside arrangement of perimortem cesarean section for critically ill patient and manual left uterine displacement during CPR should be considered
7.	Sedation	All ICU sedatives cross placenta, inform pediatrician before delivery

(CPR: cardiopulmonary resuscitation; ECMO: extracorporeal membrane oxygenation; FDA: Food and Drug Administration; ICU: intensive care unit)

Maternal shock—due to any cause—and low gestational age are the most important risk factures in this regard and perinatal mortality in these mothers is high. Fetal monitoring—continuous or intermittent is recommended in critically ill pregnant patients admitted in an ICU. A poor cardiotocography trace may indicate compromised maternal physiology and requirement of further optimization. The physicians may encounter ethical dilemmas of termination of pregnancy for maternal well being at expense of the fetus versus early delivery for the benefit of the fetus. The decisions should be taken by a multidisciplinary team.

■ MANAGEMENT ALGORITHM

These are mentioned in detail in the later chapters, a few are summarized in **Table 3**.

As mentioned earlier the maternal mortality rate varies between the developed and the developing countries. The death rates reported in various published studies range between 0 and 41.67%.[11-13] The latter figure has been reported from North India. In another study from South India this figure was 9.9%.[14] In the Indian perspective there is no uniform registry where ICU deaths in this subgroup of patients are recorded so maternal mortality continues to be the best possible indicator of the outcome. The outcome in India would also vary between the rural and the urban area and further would vary between bigger cities and the small towns. The important causes of mortality among parturients admitted in an ICU are sepsis, complications of hemorrhage, massive blood transfusions, renal failure, respiratory failure, and acute respiratory distress syndrome.

■ CONCLUSION

- Maternal mortality and severe maternal morbidity are both indicators of women's health and vary greatly between high-income and low income countries.
- Obstetric hemorrhage, sepsis, and hypertensive disorders are the most

common causes of morbidity and mortality in parturients.
- The outcome data of such parturients admitted in a critical unit in India are varied due to the difference in health care availability in rural and urban India.

TAKE HOME MESSAGES

- Development of maternal critical care units, use of tools for early identification of high-risk patients and implementation of care bundles can improve maternal and fetal outcomes.
- Managing obstetric emergencies in ICU requires a complete understanding of the changed physiology, pharmacokinetics as well as pathology of the disease.
- Critically ill obstetric patients should be managed by a multidisciplinary team of obstetricians, intensivists, pediatricians, nurses and physiotherapists.

■ REFERENCES

1. World Health Organization. (2019). Maternal Mortality. [online] Available from: http://www.who.int/news-room/fact-sheets/detail/maternal-mortality [Last accessed February, 2023].
2. Alkema L, Chou D, Hogan D, Zhang S, Moller AB, Gemmill A, et al. Global, regional, and national levels and trends in maternal mortality between 1990 and 2015, with scenario-based projections to 2030: a systematic analysis by the UN Maternal Mortality Estimation Inter-Agency Group. Lancet. 2016;387(10017):462-74.
3. UK Government Web Archive. Department of Health. Comprehensive critical care: a review of adult critical care services. [online] Available from: http://webarchive.nationalarchives.gov.uk/20121014090959/http://www.dh.gov.uk/prod_consum_dh/groups/dh_digitalassets/@dh/@en/documents/digitalasset/dh_4082872.pdf [Last accessed February, 2023].
4. Chantry AA, Deneux-Tharaux C, Bonnet MP, Bouvier-Colle MH. Pregnancy-related ICU admissions in France: trends in rate and severity, 2006-2009. Crit Care Med. 2015; 43(1):78-86.
5. Pollock W, Rose L, Dennis CL. Pregnant and postpartum admissions to the intensive care unit: a systematic review. Intensive Care Med. 2010;36(9):1465-74.
6. Creanga AA. Maternal Mortality in the United States: A Review of Contemporary Data and Their Limitations. Clin Obstet Gynecol. 2018; 61(2):296-306.
7. Friedman AM. Maternal early warning systems. Obstet Gynecol Clin North Am. 2015;42(2):289-98.
8. El Ayadi AM, Nathan HL, Seed PT, Butrick EA, Hezelgrave NL, Shennan AH, et al. Vital sign prediction of adverse maternal outcomes in women with hypovolemic shock: the role of shock index. PLoS One. 2016;11(2):e0148729.
9. Payne BA, Hutcheon JA, Ansermino JM, Hall DR, Bhutta ZA, Bhutta SZ, et al. A risk prediction model for the assessment and triage of women with hypertensive disorders of pregnancy in low-resourced settings: the miniPIERS (Pre-eclampsia Integrated Estimate of RiSk) multi-country prospective cohort study. PLoS Med. 2014; 11(1):e1001589.
10. Aoyama K, Seaward PG, Lapinsky SE. Fetal outcome in the critically ill pregnant woman. Crit Care. 2014;18:307.
11. Zwart JJ, Dupuis JR, Richters A, Ory F, van Roosmalen J. Obstetric intensive care unit admission: a 2-year nationwide population-based cohort study. Intensive Care Med. 2010;36(2):256-63.
12. Vasquez DN, Neves AV, Vidal L, Moseinco M, Lapadula J, Zakalik G, et al. Characteristics, outcomes, and predictability of critically ill obstetric patients: a multicenter prospective cohort study. Critical Care Med. 2015; 43(9):1887-97.
13. Gupta S, Naithani U, Doshi V, Bhargava V, Vijay BS. Obstetric critical care: a prospective analysis of clinical characteristics, predictability, and fetomaternal outcome in a new dedicated obstetric intensive care unit. Indian J Anaesth. 2011;55(2):146-53.
14. Sailaja B, Renuka MK. Critically Ill obstetric admissions to an intensive care unit: a prospective analysis from a tertiary care university hospital in South India. Indian J Crit Care Med. 2019;23(2):78-82.

CHAPTER 2

Physiological Changes Induced by Pregnancy

Tanima Baronia, Durgesh Makwana

■ INTRODUCTION

Pregnancy causes significant anatomical and physiological changes to accommodate and cater to the needs of the developing fetus.

These changes are a result of:
- Changes in hormonal activity
- Biochemical changes
- Increased metabolic needs of the growing fetus, placenta, and uterus
- Mechanical displacement by an enlarging uterus.

The changes begin at conception and affect every organ system in the body, resolving gradually in the postpartum period (6 weeks).

The clinical manifestations of these changes and their implications for the mother and fetus, should be considered while treating obstetric patients. Their understanding may help differentiate normal obstetric physiology from abnormal adaptations. Further, physiological changes impact drug metabolism and efficacy. Standard dosing regimens may lead to either decreased efficacy or increased side effects.

■ CARDIOVASCULAR CHANGES

The cardiovascular system undergoes significant anatomic and physiologic remodeling as a result of pregnancy. Myocardial contractility and cardiac compliance increase along with an increase in ventricular wall mass.[1] Cardiac output also increases by 30–50% during pregnancy. Most of this increase occurs by the end of the first trimester along with an increase in the heart rate and stroke volume.[2] The increased cardiac output preferentially increases the uterine blood flow tenfold and renal blood flow by 50%.[3] The increase in cardiac output plateaus between 28 and 32 weeks of gestation. During labor, with each uterine contraction, cardiac output increases as a result of increased blood volume (300–500 mL). In the immediate postpartum period, blood is redirected from the uteroplacental circulation to the maternal circulation (autotransfusion) with a resultant increase in cardiac output.[3]

The systemic and pulmonary vascular resistances decrease significantly secondary to the vasodilatory effects of progesterone, nitric oxide, and prostaglandins. These changes reach their lowest around 20–24 weeks, leading to physiologic hypotension.[2] The vascular resistances along with blood pressure, begin rising again, approaching prepregnancy values by term.

The maternal blood volume increases by 40–50% above non-pregnant volumes, starting at 6–8 weeks of gestation and peaking at 32 weeks. The mechanism, though not fully understood, may be through nitric oxide mediated vasodilation, increased arginine and vasopressin production and mineralocorticoid activity, causing water and sodium retention, leading to hypervolemia.[2] At term, the plasma volume increases 45% above non-pregnant state while erythrocyte volume increases about 20%.[2] This results in the "relative anemia" of pregnancy. The decrease in total plasma protein is also a result of the dilutional effect of the increased intravascular fluid volume.

Aortocaval Compression

In the supine position, the gravid uterus compresses the aorta and inferior vena cava (IVC). Compression of the IVC can decrease the preload, the cardiac output, and subsequently, the systolic blood pressure. This is known as supine hypotension. At term, there can be an almost full occlusion of the IVC in the supine position. The epidural, azygous, and vertebral veins accommodate the veinous return from the lower extremities, leading to engorgement of these veins.[2]

Clinical Implications

Decompensation of the myocardial function can develop at 24 weeks of gestation, during labor and immediately after delivery, especially with valvular heart disease (e.g., mitral stenosis) or coronary disease. The risk of pulmonary edema is high due to increased blood volume and reduced oncotic pressure.

Return of the blood pressures and the systemic and pulmonary vascular resistances to normal toward term is very important in patients with pre-existing hypertension on antihypertensive drugs. Monitoring of blood pressure beyond 20 weeks is key to effective management and for diagnosis of pregnancy-induced hypertension (PIH).

The hypervolemia and physiologic anemia are advantageous to both, the mother and the fetus, in that the less viscous blood improves uterine and placental perfusion, while the increased red blood cell mass coupled with increased uterine blood flow optimizes oxygen transport to the fetus. The expanded volume of 1–1.5 L helps offset the 300–500 mL blood loss accompanying vaginal delivery, and the average 800 mL–1 L loss seen with cesarean section.

The supine hypotension occurring as a result of aortocaval compression causes a reduction in uterine blood flow with resultant fetal acidosis and hypoxia if the hypotension persists for >10–15 minutes. This can be mitigated by a lateral tilt or elevation of the right hip by 10–15 cm with a wedge.

■ RESPIRATORY CHANGES

Respiratory system undergoes changes starting as early as the 4th week of pregnancy.

The most significant changes include alterations in:
- Upper airway
- Minute ventilation
- Arterial oxygenation
- Lung volumes.

The increased vascularity due to the rise in estrogen concentration causes edema of the upper respiratory mucosa.[4] There is an increase in the tidal volume (40%) along with an increase in the respiratory rate (15%). This leads to an increase in the minute ventilation by approximately 50%. Increased circulating levels of progesterone and increased CO_2 production act as the stimulus for the increased minute ventilation. Oxygen consumption is increased by 20%.[5]

Resting $PaCO_2$ decreases from 40 to 30–32 mm Hg during the first trimester as a result of the increased minute ventilation.

Arterial pH, however, is only mildly alkalotic (7.42–7.44) because of increased renal excretion of bicarbonate ions. This leads to reduced sodium bicarbonate levels (18–21 mEq/L) and reduced buffering capacity.[6]

Early in gestation, maternal PaO_2 while breathing room air remains above 100 as a result of the decrease in alveolar CO_2. This normalizes in the later stages of pregnancy. The increase in PaO_2 facilitates transfer of oxygen from mother to fetus and the lower $PaCO_2$ facilitates transfer of CO_2 from fetus to mother, where it can be eliminated through maternal lungs.[5]

The cephalad displacement of the diaphragm by the gravid uterus leads to a decrease in functional residual capacity up to 20%. The expiratory reserve volume and the residual volume decrease by equal measure. Vital capacity, however, remains unchanged.

Respiratory parameters return to non-pregnant values within 6–12 weeks postpartum.[5]

Clinical Implications

Airway edema can make intubation difficult and smaller sized endotracheal tube may be required to prevent worsening of edema. The capillary engorgement leads to increased tissue friability and requires careful handling to avoid the risk of obstruction due to tissue edema and bleeding during instrumentation of the airway.

Decreased oxygen reserve due to reduced FRC along with increased oxygen consumption predisposes this population of patients to hypoxia with adverse maternal and fetal outcomes.

In critically ill pregnant women requiring mechanical ventilation, lung protective ventilation should be avoided to reduce the likelihood of fetal acidosis.

The cephalad movement of the diaphragm demands placement of chest drains higher than normal.

■ RENAL CHANGES

The effect of progesterone and relaxin on smooth muscles causes dilation of the urinary collecting system with consequent urinary stasis. Renal blood flow and glomerular filtration rate (GFR) increase by 50% as early as 14 weeks of pregnancy. Glycosuria and aminoaciduria may develop in normal gestation. Water and sodium osmoregulation is also affected. The dilutional effect due to significant water and sodium retention leads to mild reduction of serum sodium.

Serum osmolarity is also mildly reduced.[7]

Clinical Implications of Genitourinary Changes

Urinary stasis predisposes pregnant women to urinary tract infection.

Increased GFR leads to decreased serum creatinine, urea, and uric acid so that if serum creatinine is found to be above 0.8 mg/dL it may indicate underlying renal dysfunction.[7]

At 12 weeks the bladder becomes an abdominal structure and is thus, susceptible to blunt trauma.

At 20 weeks, the fundus is at the umbilicus, thus making it susceptible to both blunt or penetrating trauma.

■ GASTROINTESTINAL CHANGES

The rise in progesterone leads to delayed gastric emptying and prolonged small bowel transit time by 30–50%.[8] Delayed emptying along with compression by the gravid uterus results in increased gastric pressure. Furthermore, there is cephalad displacement of the stomach and pylorus by the enlarged uterus beyond 20 weeks. This, along with decrease in the competence of the lower esophageal sphincter sets the stage for aspiration.[8,9]

Slight increase in the hepatic transaminases, bilirubin, and lactate dehydrogenase (LDH) may be seen in pregnancy. Serum cholinesterase activity is reduced by 24%. Alkaline phosphatase is, however, increased 2–4-fold as it is also produced by the placenta. This limits its utility when liver function or enzymes are assayed.[6]

Clinical Implications

The gastrointestinal changes beyond 20 weeks predispose women to regurgitation, aspiration of gastric content, and development of aspiration pneumonia or Mendelson syndrome. This makes airway protection in susceptible individuals a necessity.

Reduced serum cholinesterase results in an exaggerated and prolonged response to succinylcholine and must be kept in mind during rapid sequence intubation.

▌HEMATOLOGIC AND COAGULATION SYSTEM CHANGES

White blood cells (WBC) and red blood cells (RBC) count increases in pregnancy. The former is believed to be due to bone marrow granulopoieses, while the latter is driven by an increase in erythropoietin production.[6]

Pregnancy is a hypercoagulable state. This is due to blood stasis along with changes in the coagulation and fibrinolytic pathway. Pregnancy-induced changes in coagulation include an increase in factors I, VII, VIII, IX, X, and XII and a decrease in factors XI, XIII, and antithrombin III. A 20% decrease in prothrombin time and partial thromboplastin time is seen. Plasminogen activator levels are decreased, and plasminogen activator inhibitor (PAI)-levels are increased 2–3-fold leading to a suppressed fibrinolytic state. Protein S levels decrease while protein C levels remain unchanged. Thus, protein C levels may be assayed if needed in pregnancy.[6]

Clinical Implications

Higher WBC count can sometimes make diagnosis of infections challenging.

However, this rise in WBC is not associated with a significant increase in bands or other immature forms.

Increased RBC mass is accompanied by an increased maternal demand for iron.

The hypercoagulable state may offer a survival benefit by minimizing blood loss after delivery, but also predisposes to a five-fold increase in the risk of venous thromboembolism. Venous thromboembolism (VTE) prophylaxis must be kept in mind.

▌ENDOCRINE CHANGES

Due to increase in maternal clearance of iodide along with fetal use, plasma iodide concentration decreases in pregnancy. In almost 15% women, the thyroid gland tends to increase in volume. The production of thyroid hormone is also increased due to stimulation by human chorionic gonadotropin (hCG) and an upregulation of thyroid binding globulin. While the total tetraiodotyronine and tri-iodothyronine levels increase, the free forms of the hormone (fT4 and fT3) remain within normal range. Thyroid-stimulating hormone (TSH) levels decrease during first half of pregnancy due to the negative feedback from peripheral T3 and T4.[10]

Clinical Implications

The use of total T4 (TT4), total T3 (TT3), and resin tri-iodothyronine uptake (rT3U) is not recommended to monitor the status of the thyroid hormone in pregnancy as the TT4 and TT3 will be increased and rT3U will be decreased.[10]

For hypothyroid pregnant patients on thyroxine replacement, a 30% increase in dosage is recommended early in pregnancy with adequate monitoring along with a decrease in the dose in the postpartum period.[10]

■ NERVOUS SYSTEM CHANGES

Progesterone is known to have a sedative activity. Requirement of sedatives and volatile anesthetic agents is decreased. Sensitivity to local anesthetic agents is increased. Wider dermatomal spread of regional anesthesia is seen due to reduction in the epidural space. There is also an increased risk of epidural catheter becoming intravascular. This is because of the engorged epidural venous plexus as a result of aortocaval syndrome.[2,11]

■ PHYSIOLOGY OF UTEROPLACENTAL BLOOD FLOW AND PLACENTAL EXCHANGE

The placenta functions as an interface between maternal and fetal tissue for the purpose of physiologic exchange.

Uterine Blood Flow

A total of 80% of the uterine blood flow goes to the placenta while 20% perfuses the myometrium. Decrease in the uterine blood flow decreases blood supply to the fetus causing fetal hypoxemia and acidosis **(Flowchart 1)**.[3]

Under normal conditions, the fetal oxygen dissociation curve is shifted to the left (greater affinity to oxygen) while maternal curve is shifted to right (decreased O_2 affinity). This facilitates oxygen transport to the fetus (*see* **Flowchart 1**).[3]

■ PHARMACOLOGICAL IMPLICATIONS[12]

Changes in maternal physiology affect the pharmacodynamics and pharmacokinetics of different therapeutic agents.

The increase in total body water, blood volume, and capillary hydrostatic pressure increases the volume of distribution of hydrophilic drugs. This necessitates higher initial and maintenance doses to obtain therapeutic plasma concentrations.

Decreased serum albumin levels along with other drug binding proteins results in free levels of the highly protein bound drugs with higher bioactivity. Digoxin, midazolam, phenytoin, etc., are examples of drugs highly bound to albumin.[6]

Flowchart 1: Factors affecting fetal perfusion.

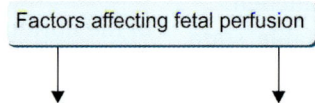

Reduction in uterine blood flow
- Reduced perfusion pressure secondary to systemic hypotension
  - Aortocaval compression
  - Hypovolemia
- Extreme hypocapnia ($PaCO_2$ < 20 mm Hg), commonly associated with hyperventilation secondary to labor pains
- Vasoconstriction as seen due to both endogenous catecholamines induced by stress or pain and exogenous vasopressors

Factors reducing placental exchange:
Alterations in
- Ratio of maternal uterine blood flow to fetal umbilical blood flow
- Oxygen partial pressure gradient
- Maternal and fetal hemoglobin concentrations and affinities
- Transplacental diffusion capacity
- Maternal and fetal acid base status

The partially compensated respiratory alkalosis though improves oxygen transport across the placenta, it may affect the protein binding of drugs.

Increase in renal clearance may significantly increase elimination rates of renally cleared medications leading to shorter half-lives. Drugs eliminated by the kidneys include ampicillin, cefuroxime, cefazolin, piperacillin, atenolol, digoxin among others.

The delayed gastric emptying may alter peak serum concentrations (C_{max}) and time to maximum concentration (T_{max}) of orally administered medications. Drug absorption is also decreased by vomiting early in pregnancy.

Increase in gastric pH may increase ionization of weak acids. This reduces absorption of such drugs.

Drug metabolism is also altered as a result of changes in metabolizing enzymes.

TAKE HOME MESSAGES

- Aortocaval compression by the gravid uterus must be countered with a lateral tilt or a wedge.
- Airway management of a pregnant woman requires meticulous planning, keeping a difficult intubation trolley ready, bearing in mind mucosal edema, tissue friability, decreased oxygen reserves, and increased oxygen consumption.
- The gastrointestinal changes predispose a pregnant woman to aspiration, hence rapid sequence intubation must be considered.
- Pregnancy being a hypercoagulable state, it increases the risk of thromboembolism. Thromboprophylaxis must be prioritized wherever necessary.
- Fetal outcomes largely depend upon maintenance of maternal uterine blood flow and acid base status.

■ REFERENCES

1. Rubler S, Damani PM, Pinto ER. Cardiac size and performance during pregnancy estimated with echocardiography. Am J Cardiol. 1977;40(4):534-40.
2. Clark SL, Cotton DB, Lee W, Bishop C, Hill T, Southwick J, et al. Central hemodynamic assessment of normal term pregnancy. Am J Obstet. Gynecol. 1989;161 (6 Pt 1):1439-42.
3. Robson SC, Hunter S, Moore M, Dunlop W. Haemodynamic changes during the puerperium: a Doppler and M-mode echocardiographic study. Br J Obstet Gynaecol. 1987;94(11):1028-39.
4. Crosby ET. The difficult airway in obstetric anaesthesia. In: Benumof JL (Ed). Airway Management Principles and Practice. St. Louis, MO: Mosby Year Book; 1996. pp. 638-65.
5. Prowse CM, Gaensler EA. Respiratory and acid-base changes during pregnancy. Anesthesiology. 1965;26:381-92.
6. Pacheco L, Constantine MM, Hankins GDV. "Physiologic changes during pregnancy" in Clinical Pharmacology during pregnancy. In: Mattison DR (Ed). San Diego: Academic Press; 2013. pp. 5-14.
7. Jeyabalan A, Conrad KP. Renal function during normal pregnancy and preeclampsia. Front Biosci. 2007;12:2425-37.
8. Whitehead EM, Smith M, Dean Y, O'Sullivan G. An evaluation of gastric emptying times in pregnancy and the puerperium. Anaesthesia. 1993;48(1):53-7.
9. Fisher RS, Roberts GS, Grabowski CJ, Cohen S. Altered lower esophageal sphincter function during early pregnancy. Gastroenterology. 1978;74(6):1233-7.
10. Glinoer D. The regulation of thyroid function in pregnancy: pathways of endocrine adaptation from physiology to pathology. Endocr Rev. 1997;18(3):404-33.
11. Bromage PR. Continuous lumbar epidural analgesia for obstetrics. Can Med Assoc J. 1961;85:1136-40.
12. Costantine MM. Physiologic and pharmacokinetic changes in pregnancy. Front Pharmacol. 2014;5:65.

CHAPTER 3

Acid–Base Physiology

Tapas Kumar Sahoo, Rachit Sinha

■ INTRODUCTION

A through clinical assessment of critically ill obstetric patient is the best step forward but a quick aid like arterial blood gas (ABG) can work wonders. The acid–base assessment is one of the most powerful tools in the hand of the clinician, owing to its rapid analysis, wide range of parameters, easy accessibility at most centers. A weapon is as strong as the wielder, and so a mere ABG without a proper interpretation is weapon underused! The mother and the fetus both are going to get benefited with a rapid, accurate assessment in those critical times.

▍EPIDEMIOLOGY AND MAGNITUDE OF THE PROBLEM

The maternal mortality rate in India is declining at 98–99/10,000 live birth in 2020.[1] There has been some breakthrough by numerous health programs being run by the government of India, but the problem persists. The leading cause is being the obstetric hemorrhage and pregnancy related infection and hypertensive disorders of pregnancy.[1] Numerous families continue to suffer due to limited facilities and lack of knowledge at different level.

▍IMPLICATIONS FOR MATERNAL HEALTH AND FETAL WELL-BEING

Many of these can be averted by a simplest tool like an ABG. An accurate and rapid assessment can save lives, not one but two. ABG has been suggested to predict multiple organ dysfunction syndrome (MODS), preeclampsia.[2] ABG has other baseline parameters such as electrolyte, hemoglobin as well which can further the cause of emergency management of obstetric patients, thereby changing the outcome of the care.

Maternal and fetal physiology is a different ball game and the minute changes are the ones which turn out to be the game changer. The physiological changes begin early in pregnancy and extend into postpartum. Understanding key changes during pregnancy will aid to better interpretation of ABG **(Table 1)**.

Fetal oxygen level depends on three important factors namely, maternal oxygen level, uterine artery perfusion, maternal Hb, concession in any of the factor can have delirious effect such as fetal hypoxia and acidosis.[3]

■ BASIC CONCEPTS

The pH of the body is maintained through a delicate balance between acid and bases. The body produces 15,000 mEq volatile acids and 1–1.5 mEq/kg/day of fixed acids respectively. These acids are kept in balance by the renal and respiratory buffer system. The most important buffer system is the carbonic acid bicarbonate.

$$H^+ \text{ (removed via kidney)} = H^+ + HCO_3 = H_2CO_3$$
$$= H_2O + CO_2 = CO_2 \text{ (removed via lungs)}$$

TABLE 1: Physiological changes in pregnancy and its implication in arterial blood gas.

Parameter	Change	Implication
Minute ventilation	Increases 30–40%	
pCO_2	Decreases to 26–32 mm Hg	Decreased level aids in clearing fetal pCO_2, which is 10 mm Hg higher than maternal
Hemoglobin (Hb)	Reduced Hb concentration and arterial oxygen content	O_2 content maintained by an increase of 50% in cardiac output
pO_2	Increased to 100–106 mm Hg	Increases to cover the additional requirement during pregnancy
HCO_3	Decreases to 18–21 mEq/L	To compensate for decreased pCO_2
pH	Increased 7.40–7.46	

TABLE 2: Common sampling errors of arterial blood gas and their precaution.

Variable	Effect	Precaution
Excess heparin	↓ pCO_2 and HCO_3	Discard extra heparin and obtain 3 mL of blood sample
Air bubble	Can ↑/↓ pO_2, as the air bubble has a pO_2 of 150 mm Hg and pCO_2 ↓	Discard all the air bubble, following sampling
Arterial catheter	Dilutional error due to contamination with fluid	Discard 3–5 mL of volume, prior to sample
Temperature	pO_2 and pH ↓, while pO_2 ↑ if there is delay in analysis	Syringe should be placed in ice water bath, for up to 1 hour
Leukocytosis	pO_2 ↓ due to consumption by the leukocyte	Effect decreased by placing the sample ice immediately
General anesthesia with halothane	Halothane molecule mimics the O_2, thus pO_2 ↑	Wait for the halothane to wash out prior to sampling

The pH of the blood is determined by Henderson-Hasselbalch equation. It illustrates that pH is determined not by the concentration of pCO_2 and HCO_3 but by the ratio of the two.

■ SAMPLING FOR ABG

The ABG analysis can be misleading, if appropriate precautions are not taken and standard guidelines not followed. Some of the common factors are listed in the **Table 2**.

■ MANAGEMENT

A stepwise approach is recommended for solving the mystery of ABG.
- A thorough *history* and *examination* is the first step in the interpretation of ABG, many a time this gives us clues to the underlying disorder.
- We need to check the internal validity of the ABG, this is done by a simple calculation. The H^+ concentration can be checked from **Table 3**, while HCO_3 pCO_2 levels are available from ABG.

$$\frac{H^+ \times HCO_3}{pCO_2} = 24$$

- Assess the pH, if it is acidosis or alkalosis (**Flowchart 1**).
- Assess the disturbance by looking at pCO_2 and HCO_3.

A simple acid–base disorder can be easily deduced with the help of algorithm in **Flowchart 1** and **Table 4**.

If the primary defect is respiratory, we need to assess if it is acute or chronic. As the renal compensation is slower, the change in bicarbonate is different depending on time.

In case the primary defect is metabolic acidosis, we need to assess the anion gap (AG). If the primary defect is metabolic alkalosis we need to check if the pCO_2 is adequately compensating for the change.

TABLE 3: H^+ concentration at different pH.

pH	(H^+) nmol/L	pH	(H^+) nmol/L
7.7	20	7.2	60
7.6	25	7.1	80
7.5	30	7.0	100
7.4	40	6.9	120
7.3	50	6.8	140

Mixed Acid–Base Disorders

- Simple acid–base disorders are easier to calculate and assess, but owing to the complex physiological response the patient presents with mixed disorders. So a careful assessment of the primary defect and the secondary response is required.

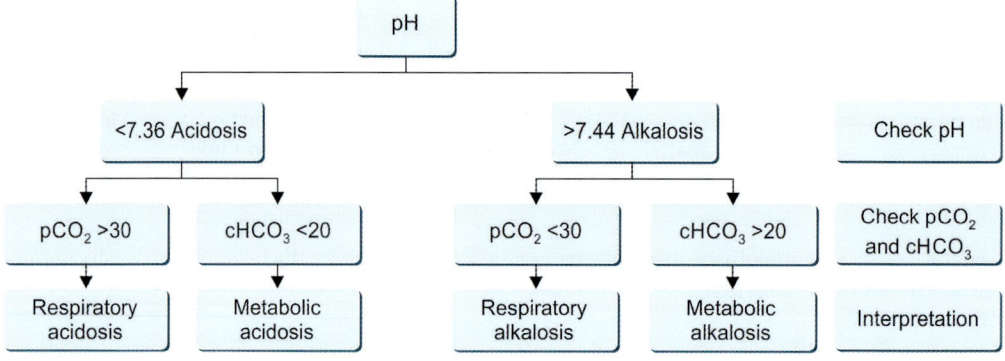

Flowchart 1: Basic approach to interpretation of arterial blood gas.

TABLE 4: The secondary response and expected change in acid–base disorder.[4]

Primary disorder	Primary disturbance	Secondary response	Expected change
Respiratory acidosis	↑ pCO_2	↑ $cHCO_3$	Acute $\Delta HCO_3 = 0.1 \times \Delta pCO_2$ Chronic $\Delta HCO_3 = 0.35 \times \Delta pCO_2$
Respiratory alkalosis	↓ pCO_2	↓ $cHCO_3$	Acute $\Delta HCO_3 = 0.2 \times \Delta pCO_2$ Chronic $\Delta HCO_3 = 0.5 \times \Delta pCO_2$
Metabolic acidosis	↓ $cHCO_3$	↓ pCO_2	$\Delta pCO_2 = 1.2 \times \Delta HCO_3$
Metabolic alkalosis	↑ $cHCO_3$	↑ pCO_2	$\Delta pCO_2 = 0.6 \times \Delta HCO_3$

- Calculate the AG in metabolic acidosis, and

  $AG = ([Na^+]+[K^+])-([Cl^-]+[HCO_3^-])$,
  (normal value = 12–20 mEq/L)

  The causes are mentioned for raised and normal AG in **Table 5**.

  Raised AG is due to accumulation of H^+ ion with unmeasured anions, while in normal AG the H^+ and Cl^- ion is accumulated which has no effect on AG.

  Calculate other GAPS, in high AG metabolic acidosis:[6]
- If $\Delta AG/\Delta HCO_3 = 1$, acidosis is pure non-anion gap metabolic acidosis
- If $\Delta AG/\Delta HCO_3 \geq 1$ (decrease in AG is more than decrease in HCO_3), the acidosis is due to HCO_3 loss. This disorder may be (i) metabolic alkalosis with high AG metabolic acidosis OR (ii) mixed high AG acidosis with chronic respiratory acidosis.
- If $\Delta AG/\Delta HCO_3 \leq 0.7$ (decrease in AG is less than the fall in HCO_3), this suggests the presence of a coexistent metabolic alkalosis. The disorder can be (i) high AG acidosis with respiratory alkalosis or (ii) high AG with normal or low anion gaps.

DIFFERENT ACID–BASE DISORDERS

Metabolic Acidosis

The disorder is primarily diagnosed with low pH and decreased HCO_3 levels. The basic pathophysiology is loss of HCO_3 or overproduction/decreased clearance of acids, which in turn can be due to multiple reasons (*see* **Table 5**).

Clinically: There are no specific signs/symptoms but we can see the tachycardia, bradycardia (as the acidosis worsens), poor

TABLE 5: Major causes of metabolic acidosis.[5]

Mechanism of acidosis	Increased AG	Normal AG
Increased acid production	• Lactic acidosis • Ketoacidosis—diabetes mellitus, starvation, alcohol • Ingestions—methanol, ethylene glycol, aspirin, toluene (if early or if kidney function is impaired), diethylene glycol, propylene glycol	Ingestions—toluene ingestion (if late and if kidney function is preserved)
Loss of bicarbonate or bicarbonate precursors		• Diarrhea or other intestinal losses (e.g., tube drainage) • Type 2 (proximal) RTA • Post-treatment of ketoacidosis • Carbonic anhydrase inhibitors • Ureteral diversion (e.g., ileal loop)
Decreased renal acid excretion	Severe kidney dysfunction (eGFR <15 to 20 mL/min/1.73 m²)	• Moderate kidney dysfunction (eGFR >15–20 mL/min/1.73 m²) • Type 1 (distal) RTA (hypokalemia) • Hyperkalemia RTA • Type 4 RTA (hypoaldosteronism) • Voltage defect
Large volume infusion of normal saline		Diffusion acidosis

(AG: anion gap; eGFR: estimated glomerular filtration rate; RTA: renal tubular acidosis)

cardiac contractility, with reduced cardiac output. Maternal acidosis worsens the fetal pH as well, which in turn can have multiple complications. The compensatory response is to decrease pCO_2 with tachypnea in a bid to bring pH within normal range.

The secondary response of lowering the pCO_2 may be achieved; however in certain situation the same may not be possible. Thus giving us mixed acid–base disorder. If the actual pCO_2 is greater than expected pCO_2, we have an additional respiratory acidosis. If the actual pCO_2 is less than expected pCO_2 we have additional respiratory alkalosis.

The next step in mixed metabolic acidosis is to calculate the GAPs which have been previously discussed which aids to find the hidden 3rd acid–base disorder.

Treatment: The mainstay of treatment of any ABG disorder is treating the cause rather than the symptom. So alkali therapy is indicated only when the pH <7.1, the aim is to maintain the pH >7.1 until the main pathology is reversed. The dose of sodium bicarbonate therapy to start with is 50 mL and then ABG is rechecked if more doses are required. Sodium bicarbonate (available in 50 mEq/mL solution) is commonly used in India, others include tris-hydroxymethyl aminomethane (THAM). THAM has the benefit of not producing pCO_2 and not increasing sodium load.[5]

Metabolic Alkalosis

An increased pH with an elevated $cHCO_3$ is said to be a metabolic alkalosis.

Clinically: We may find the patient to have neurological signs and symptoms, which may manifest as confusion, lethargy, tetany, muscle cramps. Other symptoms such as cardiac arrhythmia, hypotension, and hypoventilation may also present.

Mechanism: The loss of acid or gain of alkali is the main reason for this disorder. Kidney may not be able to remove the additional HCO_3. Once the metabolic alkalosis is set, it is worsened by volume depletion, hypercapnia, and hypokalemia.

TABLE 6: Causes of metabolic alkalosis.[7]

Measure urinary chloride	
>20 mEq (chloride resistant)	<10 mEq (chloride responsive)
With hypertension: • Primary and secondary hyperaldosteronism • Liddle's syndrome • Cushing disease • Apparent mineralocorticoid excess • Conn's syndrome	• Diuretics • Gastric volume loss • Posthypercapnia
Without hypertension: • Bartter syndrome • Gitelman syndrome • Excessive bicarbonate administration	

Causes: See **Table 6**.

Treatment: The treatment is aimed at removal of excess bicarbonate and treating the main pathology for alkalosis. Chloride responsive metabolic alkalosis responds well to saline infusion, while in the chloride resistant, focus is more on treating the cause.

Respiratory Acidosis

A decreased pH and elevated pCO_2 is seen in respiratory acidosis. The main reason is failure to remove the CO_2 from the body, in a background of normal or increased production.

Clinically: The pCO_2 crosses the blood brain barrier, lowering the pH of the brain. It causes decreased cerebral vascular resistance, increased blood flow, thus leading to increased intracranial pressure (ICP).

Mechanism: The increased pCO_2 may or may not be accompanied with hypoxemia but it has delirious effect on uterine perfusion, leading to fetal hypoxemia. So a prompt intubation and ventilatory support is indicated in such scenario to protect the maternal and fetal well-being.

It can be acute or chronic depending on the degree of secondary response achieved. The renal compensation is slower and requires more time. Therefore the expected $cHCO_3$ levels are different in acute and chronic (see **Table 4**).

Causes: Refer to **Table 7**.

Treatment: Adequate and urgent respiratory support to increase ventilation in form of noninvasive ventilation (NIV) or invasive mechanical ventilation. At the same time we should also avoid hypoxemia which may or may not be concurrently there.

Respiratory Alkalosis

An increased pH and decreased pCO_2 is seen in respiratory alkalosis.

Mechanism: The main pathophysiology is hyperventilation, which decreased the pCO_2 levels thus increasing the pH. The hyperventilation in turn may be caused by brainstem stimulation or the peripheral chemoreceptor stimulation. The compensation by renal is again slower and so we have an acute or chronic respiratory alkalosis. The duration determines the degree of secondary response achieved by $cHCO_3$.

Clinically: Paresthesia, circumoral numbness, confusion, tachycardia, with decreased cerebral blood flow.

Causes: Refer to **Table 8**.

Treatment: Aimed at treating the inciting cause. Patients on ventilator require proper adjustment of setting, drugs need to be reassessed, and any psychological causes of hyperventilation might require attention.

TABLE 7: Causes of respiratory acidosis.[8]

Airway obstruction	Aspiration, laryngospasm, severe bronchospasm
Impaired ventilation	Pneumothorax, hemothorax, severe pneumonia, acute respiratory distress syndrome, pulmonary edema
Circulatory collapse	Massive pulmonary embolism, cardiac arrest
Central nervous system depression	Medication (sedation, narcotic), cerebral infarct, obesity
Neuromuscular disease	Myasthenic crisis, severe hypokalemia, Guillain–Barré syndrome

TABLE 8: Causes of respiratory alkalosis.[8]

Pulmonary disease	Pneumonia, pulmonary embolism, pulmonary congestion, asthma
Drugs	Salicylates, xanthines, nicotine
Central nervous system disorders	Voluntary hyperventilation, anxiety, neurological (infection, trauma, stroke)
Others	Pregnancy, pain, sepsis, hepatic failure, iatrogenic mechanical ventilation

CONCLUSION

- A good clinical history, examination is the very first step of the ABG.
- ABG is a gold standard tool to clinician, but without a proper interpretation it is rather futile.
- A proper sampling is highly essential as it very much changes the values.
- Attention toward the need of maternal and fetal well-being should always be kept in mind, as those precious few minutes can very well change the course of two lives.

- For understanding arterial blood gas changes in pregnancy well, we need to understand maternal physiology changes and disease state alternations in clarity.

REFERENCES

1. Meh C, Sharma A, Ram U, Fadel S, Correa N, Snelgrove JW, et al. Trends in maternal mortality in India over two decades in nationally representative surveys. BJOG. 2022;129(4):550-61.
2. Eliana M, Carrizosa J, Castro A, Sanchez A, Nino R. Blood gas analysis utility predicting multiple organ dysfunction syndrome in obstetric patients [38E]. Obstet Gynecol. 2017;129(5):61S-62S.
3. Novy MJ, Edwards MJ. Respiratory problems in pregnancy. Am J Obstet Gynecol. 1967;99(7):1024-45.
4. Vincent JL, Abraham E, Kochanek P, Moore FA, Fink MP. Arterial Blood Gas Interpretation. In: Textbook of Critical Care. 7th edition. Amsterdam: Elsevier; 2017. pp. 167-74.
5. UpToDate. (2022). Approach to the adult with metabolic acidosis. [online] Available from: https://www.uptodate.com/contents/approach-to-the-adult-with-metabolic-acidosis?search=metabolic%20acidosis&source=search_result&selectedTitle=1~150&usage_type=default&display_rank=1#H1145637971 [Last accessed February, 2023].
6. Salem MM, Mujais SK. Gaps in the anion gap. Arch Intern Med. 1992;152(8):1625-9.
7. UpToDate. (2022). Causes of metabolic alkalosis. [online] Available from: https://www.uptodate.com/contents/causes-of-metabolic-alkalosis?search=ABG&topicRef=2330&source=see_link#H3160990 [Last accessed February, 2023].
8. Phelan JP, Pacheco LD, Foley MR, Saade GR, Dildy GA, Belfort MA. Maternal Blood Gas Physiology. In: Critical Care Obstetrics, 6th edition. Hoboken, New Jersey: Wiley-Blackwell; 2018. pp. 69-86.

SECTION 2

Principles of Fetomaternal Monitoring

4. Monitoring of Critically Ill Expectant Mother and Parturient
   Ranjan Joshi

5. Monitoring of Fetus in a Critically Ill Mother
   Devang Patel, Amrita Patel

CHAPTER 4

Monitoring of Critically Ill Expectant Mother and Parturient

Ranjan Joshi

INTRODUCTION

Pregnancy-related complications contribute significantly to fetomaternal morbidity and mortality. The prevalence rate of obstetric patients who may require intensive care unit (ICU) admission during pregnancy ranges from 1 to 9 in 1,000 gestations.[1] The most important function of any intensive care is to closely monitor the patient and interpret the objective data provided by the monitors and make decision in the best interest of the patient. Collection of data over time allows dynamic assessment of trends of the physiologic state of the patient. The monitoring of patients in ICU is done mostly in two ways—noninvasive and invasive.

NONINVASIVE MONITORING

Electrocardiography

Monitoring of electrocardiography (ECG) of obstetric patients is very important and commonly done in the ICU. It is inexpensive, noninvasive, and relatively easy to interpret. Continuous ECG monitoring in ICU is used mostly to detect arrhythmias and ischemia.

Normal findings on ECG in pregnancy that may partly relate to changes in the position of the heart include:[2]

- Atrial and ventricular ectopic
- Q wave (small) and inverted T wave in lead III
- ST-segment depression and T-wave inversion in the inferior and lateral leads
- Left-axis shift of QRS.

The ECG criteria used to diagnose ST-elevation myocardial infarction (STEMI) and non-ST-elevation myocardial infarction (NSTEMI) in nonpregnant patients should also apply to pregnant patients. Furthermore, although large-scale studies examining cardiac biomarkers in pregnancy are lacking, elevated serum troponin levels during pregnancy suggest underlying myocardial ischemia and should be evaluated further.[2]

The dilated cardiac chambers due to blood volume expansion in pregnancy and increased resting heart rates favor the development of rhythm disturbances. There is an increase in the prevalence of both benign arrhythmias and arrhythmias with potential danger during peripartum period, which contributes to the morbidity and mortality of parturient women and the fetus. Obstetric patients with underlying cardiac conditions or congenital cardiac anomalies may develop medical complications in 5–15% of pregnancies. A total of 20–44% of obstetric patients with a prior history of arrhythmia will present with symptomatic recurrences, including palpitations, dizziness, or syncope.[3]

Noninvasive Blood Pressure Monitoring

Automated blood pressure cuffs are used for noninvasive blood pressure monitoring in most of the ICUs. The validity of most of the automated blood pressure units is questionable in pregnancy, and they have been found to underestimate blood pressure in women with preeclampsia compared with invasive intra-arterial measurements.[4] Hence, caution should be advised in patients with preeclampsia and eclampsia while measuring blood pressure with noninvasive technique.

Urine Output

The urine output of 0.5 mL/kg/hour is often felt to be adequate to excrete the daily production of nitrogenous waste product in a normal adult. However, following factors will influence adequacy of urine output in critically ill obstetric patients:
- Nitrogen production is increased in pregnancy due to increased metabolism
- Maximal concentration of the urine is decreased during pregnancy
- Nitrogenous load may increase or decrease in critically ill patient
- Capillary leak syndrome and redistribution of renal blood flow in critically ill obstetric patient can decrease the urine output
- Presence of syndrome of inappropriate antidiuretic hormone secretion (SIADH) due to the critical illness and medications, etc.

Pulse Oximetry

Pulse oximetry is probably the most useful monitor in any obstetric patient receiving supplemental oxygen in ICU. Dyshemoglobinemia, low cardiac output (CO) state, dark skin tone, and nail polish will affect the readings of SpO_2. However, the accuracy of SpO_2 measurement is not affected by anemia in pregnancy. The advantages of pulse oximeter are:
- Less expensive
- Noninvasive
- Better tolerated
- Able to instantaneously detect significant hypoxic episodes
- Virtually has no potential for harm.

End-tidal Carbon Dioxide

The end-tidal carbon dioxide ($ETCO_2$) measurement is a key monitor to assess the patient's ventilatory status and confirm the appropriate placement of endotracheal tube. $ETCO_2$ functions as a surrogate for $PaCO_2$. The gradient between $PaCO_2$ and $ETCO_2$ reflects the amount of dead space and is typically <5. Minute ventilation increases by 40% in the second trimester of pregnancy due to the progesterone effect which results in a baseline $PaCO_2$ of 27–32 mm Hg. The development of respiratory alkalosis during third trimester of pregnancy is countered by a compensatory decrease in serum bicarbonate. Changes in end-tidal partial pressure of CO_2 have been correlated to changes in CO and may be used as a means of monitoring the efficacy of resuscitation in obstetric patients.

Point-of-Care Ultrasound

Point-of-care ultrasound (POCUS) is defined as ultrasonography performed at the bedside by the clinician looking after the patient. Presently, there are no recommendations regarding the use of ultrasound in critically ill patients in the peripartum period. It seems POCUS is not used commonly in obstetric ICUs, despite its many advantages for obstetric anesthesia and maternal critical care.[5]

Nonetheless, the critically ill obstetric patients represent an ideal group where application for POCUS should be commonly used for following reasons:
- Point-of-care ultrasound is noninvasive and decrease exposure to ionizing radiation
- POCUS can provide information regarding the physiological changes related to pregnancy
- POCUS has a high diagnostic and therapeutic value.

Cardiovascular POCUS

Cardiac output can be calculated by using two echocardiographic variables:
1. The velocity time integral (VTI)
2. The cross-sectional area of left ventricular (LV) outflow tract (LVOT).

Transthoracic echocardiography (TTE) measurement of CO has been validated against pulmonary artery catheter hemodynamic measurements in critically ill obstetric patients.[6] Hence, cardiac ultrasound is the gold standard for measurement of CO in critically ill pregnant and postpartum women. LV function in echocardiography can be assessed by following methods **(Fig. 1)**.
- Visual semiquantitative estimations performed from parasternal long axis, parasternal short axis, and four-chamber view
- Teichholtz method using M-mode
- The Simpson biplane method
- Speckle tracking echocardiography.

Peripartum cardiomyopathy presents with systolic dysfunction with reduced left ventricular ejection fraction (LVEF). Global reduction of LV function and low CO with significant mitral regurgitation (MR) on echocardiography proves the diagnosis of cardiomyopathy on symptomatic obstetric patients **(Fig. 2)**.

Heart failure in preeclampsia presents with diastolic dysfunction due to cardiac structural changes such as LV hypertrophy and interstitial fibrosis secondary to hypertension.[7] Patients with severe diastolic dysfunction with elevated LV filling pressure have E/A ratio >2 and an average E/Ea ratio >13 on echocardiography.[8]

Most pregnancy-associated acute myocardial infarction (AMI) occurs in the 6 weeks postpartum. It is mostly related to acute coronary dissection rather than coronary occlusive disease due to the hormonal effect on vasculature. TTE of obstetric patients with AMI shows regional wall motion abnormalities (hypokinesia or akinesia) with impaired thickening of the affected myocardium.

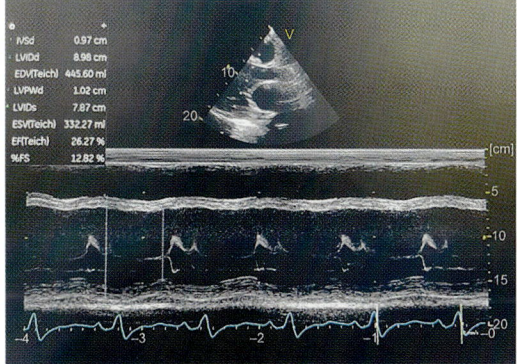 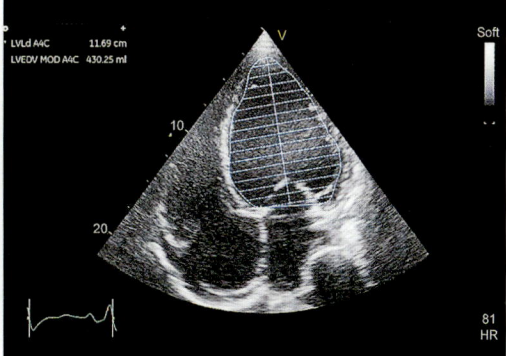

Fig. 1: Measurement of fractional shortening and ejection fraction by bedside transthoracic echocardiography.

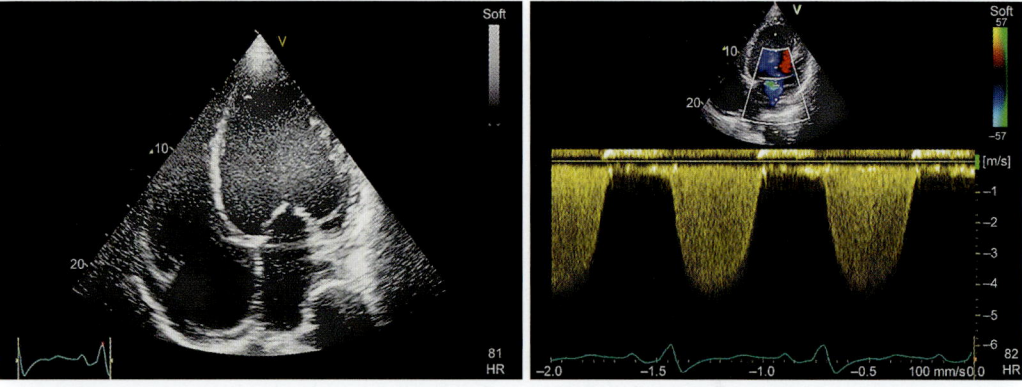

Fig. 2: Postpartum patient with dilated cardiomyopathy and moderate mitral regurgitation.

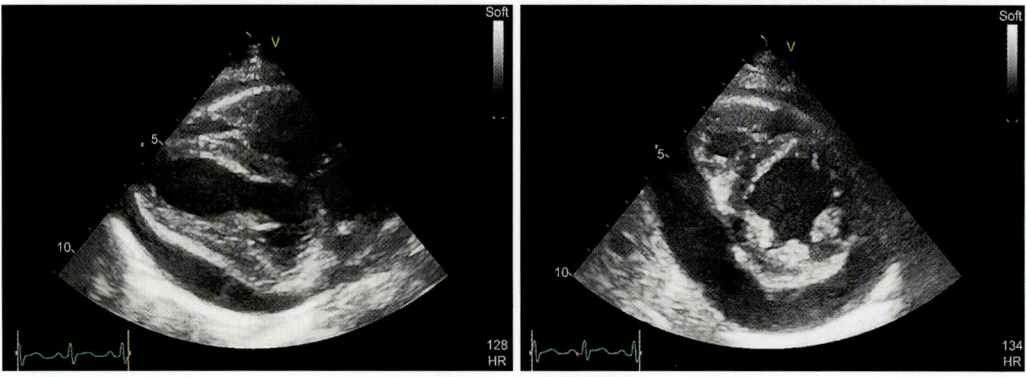

Fig. 3: Postpartum patient with pericardial effusion.

Aortic dissection is a significant cardiovascular cause of maternal death. Pregnant patients are at higher risk of dissection due to structural changes of aortic wall secondary to progesterone effect. Almost 50% of the cases of pregnancy associated AMIs and severe aortic regurgitation (AR) are associated with or complication of aortic dissection. Cardiac tamponade is the most common cause of cardiac arrest in peripartum patients with Type A aortic dissection.

Emergency TTE is the quickest way to diagnose aortic dissection in peripartum period. TTE can also be very helpful in diagnosing acute AR and pericardial effusion. Acute AR is characterized by abrupt overload of LV with normal size with high filling pressure, whereas chronic AR is associated with dilated LV.

Pericardial effusion and cardiac tamponade are easy to diagnose from subcostal and parasternal long axis views with TTE. Typical TTE findings of pericardial tamponade include right atrial and ventricular collapse with a circumferential pericardial effusion >1 cm. Collapse of cardiac chambers first occurs during diastole (mild tamponade) and only later occurs during systole (severe tamponade) **(Fig. 3)**.

Thromboembolic diseases (pulmonary embolism and amniotic fluid embolism) are the most common cause of maternal death in western countries. POCUS can help in diagnosis of a thromboembolic

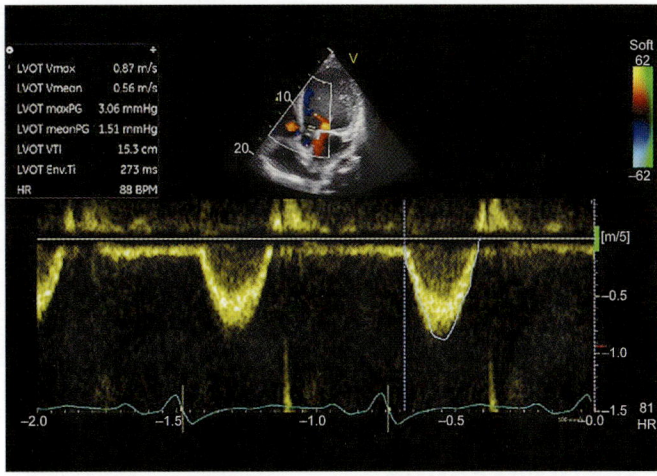

Fig. 4: Left ventricular outflow tract velocity time integral measurement in a postpartum cardiomyopathy patient.

event during peripartum period. Cardiac ultrasound combining with lung ultrasound and an assessment for deep vein thrombosis can provide very valuable information required for the diagnosis and management of thromboembolism in pregnancy and postpartum period.

Acute circulatory failure in peripartum period is either due to severe bleeding or sepsis. The echocardiographic findings for severe hypovolemia include decreased LV diastolic volume and direct contact between the mitral pillars at the end of systole called "kissing heart". Serial measurement of LVOT VTI dynamics can predict fluid responsiveness in acute circulatory failure in peripartum period **(Fig. 4)**.

Point-of-care ultrasound is also being used during management of maternal collapse to identify and treat reversible causes of arrest. The FEEL (focused echocardiography evaluation in life support) protocol is getting increasingly popular in resuscitation of obstetric patients. Interruptions to chest compression should not be >10 seconds to perform POCUS. POCUS should ideally be performed between the chest compression cycles.

FOCUSED ABDOMINAL SONOGRAPHY FOR TRAUMA DURING PREGNANCY

Trauma during pregnancy is one of the leading causes of death. The pregnant woman with an abdominal trauma is always difficult to manage. Fast scan demonstrating >4 mm of intraperitoneal free fluid or parenchymal abnormality in the abdominal viscera is considered as positive focused abdominal sonography for trauma (FAST) scan regardless of gestational age.[9]

The specificity of FAST in pregnant patients is similar to that in nonpregnant women. Moreover, the accuracy of FAST for detecting abdominal injury is reported to be similar to CT scan. Ultrasound also helps in diagnosing placental injury including placental disruption and rare fetal injury. Integration of FAST scan into the trauma assessment does not delay diagnosis and prevent fetal and maternal exposure to radiation **(Fig. 5)**.

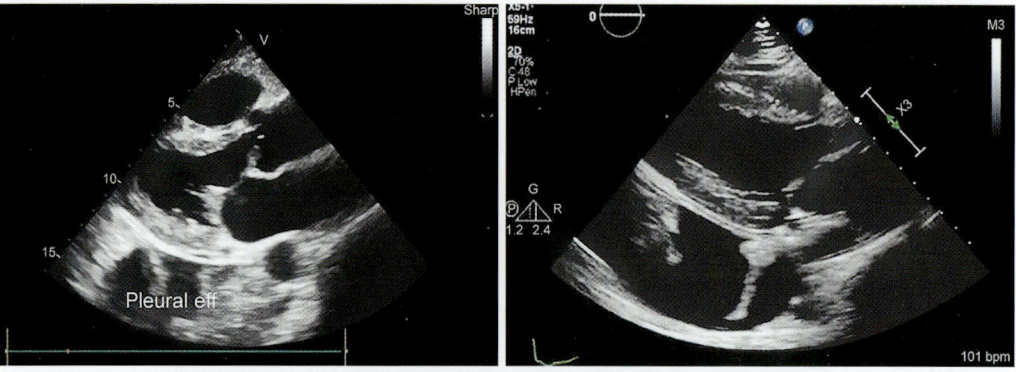

Fig. 5: Bedside echocardiography demonstrating a large left hemothorax in a 36 weeks pregnant patient with trauma.

POINT-OF-CARE ULTRASOUND FOR OBSTETRIC COMPLICATIONS

In hemodynamically unstable obstetric patients, pelvic view with ultrasonography should be followed by right and left upper quadrant views and a pericardial view to evaluate right heart strain.[10] The pelvic view quickly detects the presence or absence of intrauterine or ectopic pregnancy. Both intrauterine and ectopic pregnancy presenting with free abdominal fluid raise the possibility of hemorrhage.

In patients diagnosed with HELLP (hemolysis, elevated liver enzymes, and low platelets) syndrome, POCUS is helpful in diagnosing subcapsular or intraparenchymal hemorrhage in liver, hepatic rupture, hepatic parenchymal infarction, placental disruption, and retroplacental hematoma.

In hemodynamically unstable postpartum patients with no per-vaginal bleeding, POCUS is used to detect unusual or rare causes such as rupture of uterine artery aneurysm, subcapsular hemorrhage in the liver, spontaneous rupture of utero-ovarian vessels, etc.

INVASIVE MONITORING

The potential indications for invasive hemodynamic monitoring in critically ill obstetric patients are:

- *Cardiac indications:*
  - Cardiomyopathy with EF <15–20%
  - Severe valvular heart disease (aortic stenosis or mitral stenosis associated with pulmonary hypertension)
  - Sudden cardiovascular collapse (suspected amniotic fluid embolism or pulmonary embolism)
- *Pulmonary indications:*
  - Acute respiratory distress syndrome
  - Severe pulmonary disease with secondary pulmonary hypertension
  - Pulmonary edema associated with preeclampsia
- *Renal indications:* Persistent oliguria despite fluid resuscitation (e.g., severe preeclampsia)
- *Miscellaneous:* Septic shock refractory to fluid resuscitation and vasopressor therapy.

Arterial Pressure Monitoring

Arterial pressure monitoring system consists of an indwelling arterial catheter connected to an external transducer, which converts the pressure to an electrical signal, which gets interpreted and displayed on a monitor. It permits continuous monitoring of systolic, diastolic, and mean blood pressures and provides access for sampling of blood.

Hence, it helps the clinicians in titrating the vasopressor medications required by the patient. Radial artery is always the preferred site. However ulnar, brachial and femoral arteries are also used for access for arterial line. The incidence of catheter related blood stream infection from arterial line is similar to central venous line.

Central Venous Pressure Monitoring

Central venous monitoring needs a catheter inserted from internal jugular, subclavian or femoral vein whose tip is placed at the junction of superior vena cava and right atrium. As right heart filling pressure may not accurately reflect the filling pressure of LV in critically ill obstetric patients. Hence, use of central venous pressure (CVP) as a parameter to diagnose and/or treat LV pathology is controversial. However, the trend of CVP will definitely be helpful in guiding therapy particularly fluid resuscitation and vasopressor therapy. Central venous line in obstetric patients can be used in following purposes:
- Monitoring of CVP
- Rapid administration of large volumes of fluids
- Administration of medications
- Parenteral nutrition
- Monitoring of central venous oxygen saturation ($ScvO_2$)
- Sampling of blood.

The waveform of CVP is directly related to the cardiac cycle, and hence, to the ECG (Fig. 6).

Complications associated with CVC cannulation are carotid artery puncture, hemorrhage, pneumothorax, thrombosis, and catheter-related infection. The rate of catheter-related infection has decreased quite significantly due to the institutions of guidelines to the ICUs for the prevention of catheter-related infections.

Pulmonary Artery Catheter

The pulmonary artery catheter (PAC) has been in use since the early 1970s for management of patients receiving critical care in ICU. The PAC is inserted mostly via internal jugular or subclavian vein and directed by an inflated balloon present at its tip of the PAC

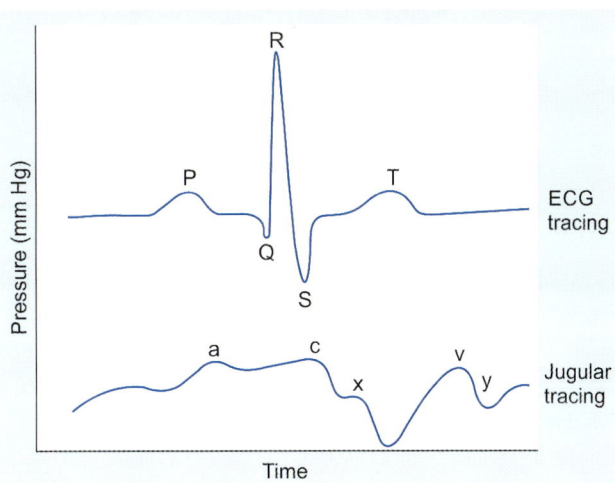

Fig. 6: Relationship of central venous pressure waveforms and electrocardiography (ECG).

through the right ventricular outflow tract (RVOT) and placed at the pulmonary artery. A transducer distal to the inflated balloon measures the pressure in the pulmonary artery called the pulmonary capillary wedge pressure (PCWP) or pulmonary artery occlusion pressure (PAOP). PACs equipped with thermistor allow measurement and calculation of RV stroke volume, CO, SVRI, etc., by using thermodilution method. Use of PAC has been reported to be of benefit in the management of obstetric patient with severe eclampsia.[11] The PACs help in differentiating hypovolemia from vasodilatation (due to sepsis) and primary cardiogenic shock. The hemodynamics in pregnant patient particularly in the third trimester has increased CO and decreased systemic and pulmonary vascular resistance resembling that of sepsis **(Table 1)**.[12]

The potential indications of insertion of PAC in obstetric patients are:
- Refractory sepsis and septic shock
- Refractory pulmonary edema, oliguria, or heart failure
- Severe pregnancy-induced hypertension with pulmonary edema
- Low CO state or cardiogenic shock
- Massive hemorrhage
- Peripartum unstable angina or myocardial infarction.

Common complications of PAC insertion and use are:
- Pneumothorax
- Arterial puncture
- Hemorrhage
- Transient dysrhythmia
- Ventricular fibrillation
- Mural thrombus
- Infection
- Pulmonary infarction
- Pulmonary artery rupture.

Although the PAC has been used in obstetric patients particularly with severe preeclampsia, the overall use of pulmonary artery catheter has been declining. This is

TABLE 1: Hemodynamic parameters of antepartum and postpartum women.

Hemodynamic variable	Antepartum (36–38 weeks of gestation)	Postpartum (11–13 weeks after delivery)
Cardiac output (L/min ± SD)	6.2 ± 1.0	4.3 ± 0.9
Heart rate (beats/min ± SD)	83 ± 10	71 ± 10
Mean arterial pressure (mm Hg ± SD)	90 ± 6	86 ± 7
Systemic vascular resistance (dyne/cm^5 ± SD)	1210 ± 266	1530 ± 520
Pulmonary vascular resistance (dyne/cm^5 ± SD)	78 ± 22	119 ± 47.0
Colloid osmotic pressure (mm Hg ± SD)	18.0 ± 1.5	20.8 ± 1.0
Pulmonary capillary wedge pressure (mm Hg ± SD)	7.5 ± 1.8	6.3 ± 2.1

probably because of the increasing use of echocardiography in ICU and as a reflection of the general rate of decline in use in recent years.[13]

TAKE HOME MESSAGES

- Monitoring of physiological variables in ICU is very important component of critical care obstetrics and is required to manage obstetric emergencies optimally.
- Data obtained from noninvasive and invasive monitoring of obstetric patients should be interpreted in the context of physiological changes in pregnancy.
- Use of bedside ultrasound has reduced the requirement of invasive monitoring in obstetric patients in ICU.
- FAST scan is validated to use in obstetric patients in the setting of trauma and provides very valuable information.
- Hemodynamic monitoring is needed in three subsets of patients with preeclampsia: (1) Those with refractory oliguria, (2) pulmonary edema, and (3) refractory hypertension.

■ REFERENCES

1. Baskett TF, Sternadel J. Maternal intensive care and near-miss mortality in obstetrics. Br J Obstet Gynaecol. 1998;105(9):981-4.
2. Shade GH Jr, Ross G, Bever FN, Uddin Z, Devireddy L, Gardin JM. Troponin I in the diagnosis of acute myocardial infarction in pregnancy, labor, and post partum. Am J Obstet Gynecol. 2002;187(6):1719-20.
3. Shotan A, Ostrzega E, Mehra A, Johnson JV, Elkayam U. Incidence of arrhythmias in normal pregnancy and relation to palpitations, dizziness, and syncope. Am J Cardiol. 1997;79(8):1061-4.
4. Shennan AH, Halligan AWF. Measuring blood pressure in normal and hypertensive pregnancy. Balliere Clin Obstet Gynecol. 1999;13:1-26.
5. Bernier-Jean A, Albert M, Shiloh AL, Eisen LA, Williamson D, Beaulieu Y. The diagnostic and therapeutic impact of point-of-care ultrasonography in the intensive care unit. J Intensive Care Med. 2017;32(3):197-203.
6. Cornette J, Laker S, Jeffery B, Lombaard H, Alberts A, Rizopoulos D. Validation of maternal cardiac output assessed by transthoracic echocardiography against pulmonary artery catheterization in severely ill pregnant women: prospective comparative study and systematic review. Ultrasound Obstet Gynecol. 2017;49(1):25-31.
7. Dennis AT, Castro JM. Echocardiographic differences between preeclampsia and peripartum cardiomyopathy. Int J Obstet Anesth. 2014;23(3):260-6.
8. Nagueh SF, Smiseth OA, Appleton CP, Byrd BF 3rd, Dokainish H, Edvardsen T, et al. Recommendations for the evaluation of left ventricular diastolic function by echocardiography: an update from the American Society of Echocardiography and the European Association of Cardiovascular Imaging. J Am Soc Echocardiogr. 2016;29(4): 277-314.
9. Hussain ZJ, Figueroa R, Budorick NE. How much free fluid can a pregnant patient have? Assessment of pelvic free fluid in pregnant patients without antecedent trauma. J Trauma. 2011;70(6):1420-3.
10. Jackson HT, Diaconu SC, Maluso PJ, Abell B, Lee J. Ruptured splenic artery aneurysms and the use of an adapted fast protocol in reproductive age women with hemodynamic collapse: case series. Case Rep Emerg Med. 2014;2014:454923.
11. Benedetti TJ, Kates R, Williams V. Hemodynamic observations in severe pre-eclampsia complicated by pulmonary edema. Am J Obstet Gynecol. 1985;152(3):330-4.
12. Clark SL, Cotton DB, Lee W, Bishop C, Hill T, Southwick J, et al. Central Haemodynamic assessment of normal term pregnancy. Am J Obstet Gynaecol. 1989;161(6 Pt 1): 1439-42.
13. Koo KY, Sun JCJ, Zhou Q, Guyatt G, Cook DJ, Walter SD, et al. Pulmonary artery catheters: evolving rates and reasons for use. Crit Care Med. 2011;39:1613-8.

CHAPTER 5

Monitoring of Fetus in a Critically Ill Mother

Devang Patel, Amrita Patel

■ INTRODUCTION

Fetus is completely dependent on maternal circulation for the survival. Whenever maternal condition is compromised, there are enough chances that fetus will be at risk of hypoxia and hypoxia related injury. To reduce the perinatal morbidity and mortality associated with critical illness in mother, it is of utmost importance to monitor the fetus. The goal of fetal monitoring is to identify the fetus at risk and deliver the at risk fetus if age of viability is achieved.

Monitoring of fetoplacental system should be a part of evaluation of critically ill mother. Consider fetoplacental as an organ system such as brain, heart, lungs, blood, gastrointestinal, and liver. All these systems require systematic investigation to reach to a diagnosis and subsequent monitoring of the condition. A direct recognition of ill fetus warrants complete evaluation of mother to determine whether condition of fetus is secondarily to maternal compromise or a primary fetal disorder. Maternal condition and medicines used in critical care which can hinder in accurate interpretation of surveillance test. Accurate knowledge of this can help in preventing unwanted interventions.

■ TIMING

Basic fetal evaluation is mandatory in all patients at the time of admission. Continuous fetal monitoring is warranted if age of viability is achieved and patient shows sign of true labor.

■ MODALITIES

Critically ill mothers require intense monitoring in view of compromised organ system, circulatory collapse, or disturbed acid base homeostasis. Standard of care should be followed in all patient with nuchal translucency (NT) scan (first trimester scan), Anomaly scan and fetal well-being scan depending on the gestational age (GA) of presentation.

Before Labor

Daily Fetal Kick Count

Patients are advised to monitor perception of fetal movements with various different cut offs such as 10 counts in 12 hours, 3–4 counts in 1 hour after each meal. This data originated from study involving high risk patients. Physiological reduction in intensity or count may occur in late pregnancy due to variation in amniotic fluid, intrauterine space, and neurological maturity. Decrease in fetal movements in acute hypoxemic condition is mainly due to mechanism of fetus to

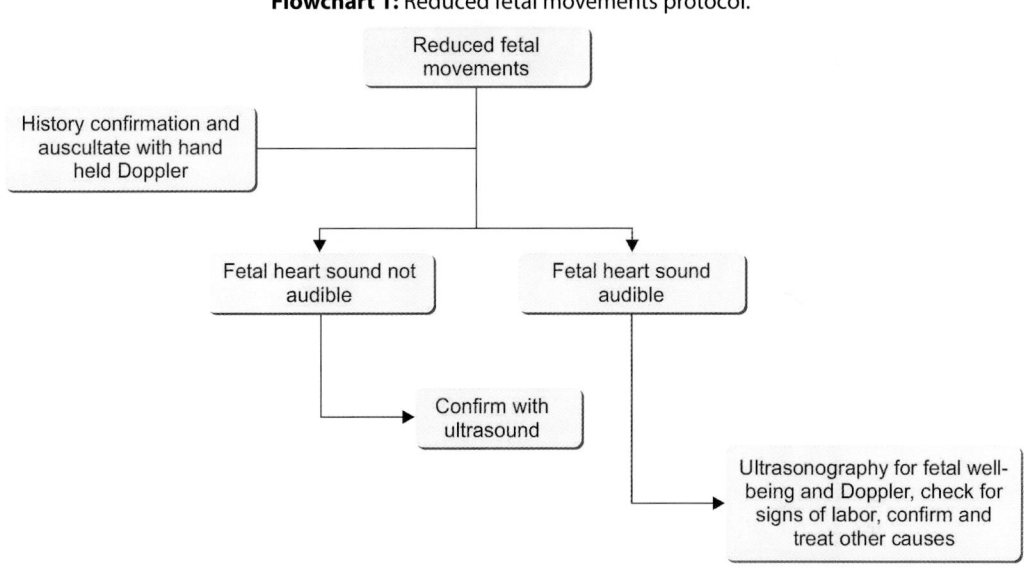

Flowchart 1: Reduced fetal movements protocol.[2]

conserve energy and redistribute oxygenated blood to vital organs.[1] It has been observed that there was no such difference in outcome of groups counting versus not counting fetal movements.

Clinicians should be aware (and should advise women) that although fetal movements tend to plateau at 32 weeks of gestation, there is no reduction in the frequency of fetal movements in the late third trimester. Reduced fetal movement **(Flowchart 1)** should never be ignored and subsequent fetal well-being test should be done. Potential association of decreased fetal movements with key risk factors such as fetal growth restriction (FGR), small for gestational age (SGA) fetus, placental insufficiency and congenital malformations should be kept in mind.

Ultrasonography: Fetal Growth/Structural Abnormalities/Amniotic Fluid/Fetal Doppler Study

Due to compromised fetoplacental circulation there could be lag in growth. FGR is failure to achieve growth potential. It is important to follow such fetus with serial growth scan and multivessel fetoplacental Doppler.

Fetal growth: Fetal growth has to be assessed after confirming correct dates and plotting the ultrasound parameters (biparietal diameter, head circumference, abdominal circumference, femur length, estimated fetal weight) in appropriate graph. Serial growth assessment at interval of 14 days is a good tool for differentiating fetal growth restricted fetus and SGA fetus.

Structural abnormalities: Lethal structural abnormalities or non-lethal structural abnormalities with poor prognosis should be identified to decide for continuation or termination of pregnancy for fetal indication.

Amniotic fluid: Amniotic fluid level is maintained by inflow and outflow by various routes, with fetal urination and fetal swallowing being the major mode. Any disturbance in fetal physiology will affect these parameters and subsequent increase or decrease in fluids level may occur. Objective

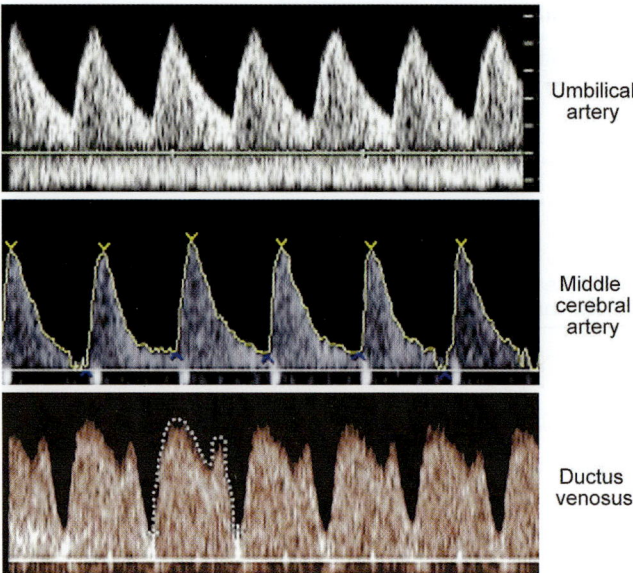

Fig. 1: Doppler waveform.

evaluation of amniotic fluid is done by measuring deepest vertical cord free amniotic fluid pockets in all four quadrants formed by imaginary horizontal and vertical line at the umbilicus. Normal value of amniotic fluid index (AFI) is from 8 to 20.

Oligohydramnios (AFI <5th centile) is commonly seen in uteroplacental insufficiency and amniotic membrane rupture. Oligohydramnios in a common finding in case of persistent maternal fever commonly seen in critically ill mother. Polyhydramnios (AFI >95th centile) is commonly seen in maternal diabetes mellitus, fetal structural abnormalities such as esophageal atresia, duodenal atresia, congenital diaphragmatic hernia, etc.

Uteroplacental Doppler study: Doppler study involves the waveform **(Fig. 1)** analysis of blood flow velocity by pulsatility index (PI), resistive index (RI), S/D ratio, and peak systolic velocity (PSV). Indices are kept in gestational age dependent graphs for interpretation. Each vessel has a signature waveform and changes in them may help to recognize pathology.

Point of care ultrasound—"5 Ps" of pregnancy:[4]
- Parity (number)
- Pulse (fetal heartbeat)
- Pocket (fluid)
- Placenta (location)
- Presentation (cephalic vs breech).

Nonstress Test

Nonstress test (NST) is usually performed after 28 weeks of gestation. It involves recording of fetal heart rate (FHR) over a period of 30 minutes and subjective interpretation of FHR pattern. A reactive NST shows at least two acceleration (15 beats per minute, sustained for at least 15 seconds) in association of fetal movements with normal baseline heart rate, baseline variability, and absence of deceleration. A reactive test is highly predictive of healthy fetus. A nonreactive test does not always indicate fetal

TABLE 1: Stage based classification and management of fetal growth restriction.[3]

Stage	Pathophysiological correlate	Criteria (any of)	Monitoring*	GA/mode of delivery
I	Severe smallness or mild placental insufficiency	• EFW <3rd centile • CPR <p5 • UA PI >p95 • MCA PI <p5 • UtA PI >p95	Weekly	37 weeks LI
II	Severe placental insufficiency	• UA AEDV • Reverse AoI	Biweekly	34 weeks CS
III	Low-suspicion fetal acidosis	• UA REDV • DV-PI >p95	1–2 days	30 weeks CS
IV	High-suspicion fetal acidosis	• DV reverse a flow • cCTG <3 ms • FHR decelerations	12 hours	26 weeks** CS

All Doppler signs described above should be confirmed at least twice, ideally at least 12 hours apart. (AEDV: absent end-diastolic velocity; AoI: aortic isthmus; CPR: rebroplacental ratio; CS: cesarean section; CTG: cardiotocography; DV: ductus venosus; FHR: fetal heart rate; GA: gestational age; LI: labor induction; MCA: middle cerebral artery; PI: pulsatility index; REDV: reversed end-diastolic velocity; UA: umbilical artery; UtA: umbilical artery)

*Recommended intervals in the absence of severe preeclampsia. If fetal growth restriction is accompanied by this complication, strict fetal monitoring is warranted regardless of the stage.

**Lower GA threshold recommended according to current literature figures reporting at least 50% intact survival. Threshold could be tailored according to parents' wishes or adjusted according to local statistics of intact survival.

compromise. A non-reactive NST requires repeat NST or supplemented by other tests.

■ BIOPHYSICAL PROFILE

Components of biophysical profile (BPP) involve fetal breathing movements, gross body movement, fetal tone, amniotic fluid volume, and reactive FHR. Modified BPP involves amniotic fluid volume assessment by ultrasound and recording of antenatal cardiotocography (CTG) (NST). The negative predictive value of BPP/modified BPP is 99.9% and positive predictive value is only 50%. An abnormal score does not necessarily indicate need for immediate delivery. But it requires close monitoring and decision based on assessment of both maternal and fetal condition.

During Labor
Continuous Electronic Fetal Monitoring
Terminology[5]
- *Baseline heart rate:* The mean of the stable FHR is determined in the absence of uterine activity, fetal movements (accelerations or decelerations) over 5–10 minutes, expressed in beats per minute (bpm), and calculated on resting heart rate, NOT sleeping heart rate. It is expected that the FHR of preterm fetuses may be in the upper range.
  • Normal: 110–160 bpm
  • Baseline tachycardia: FHR >160 bpm
  • Baseline bradycardia: FHR <110 bpm
- *Baseline variability:* The minor baseline FHR fluctuations measured by estimating

	Normal	Suspicious	Pathological
Baseline	110–160 bpm	Lacking at least one characteristic of normality, but with no pathological features	<100 bpm
Variability	5–25 bpm		Reduced variability for >50 minutes, increased variability for >30 minutes, or sinusoidal pattern for >30 minutes
Decelerations	No repetitive* decelerations		Repetitive* late or prolonged decelerations during >30 minutes or 20 minutes if reduced variability, or one prolonged deceleration with >5 minutes
Interpretation	Fetus with no hypoxia/acidosis	Fetus with a low probability of having hypoxia/acidosis	Fetus with a high probability of having hypoxia/acidosis
Clinical management	No intervention necessary to improve fetal oxygenation state	Action to correct reversible causes if identified, close monitoring or additional methods to evaluate fetal oxygenation (Chapter 4)	Immediate action to correct reversible causes, addition al methods to evaluate fetal oxygenation (Chapter 4), or if this is not possible expedite delivery. In acute situations (cord prolapse, uterine rupture or placental abruption) immediate delivery should be accomplished

TABLE 2: Classification.

The presence of accelerations denotes a fetus that does not have hypoxia/acidosis, but their absence during labor is of uncertain significance.

*Decelerations are repetitive in nature when they are associated with >50% of uterine contractions.[6]

the difference in bpm between the highest peak and lowest trough of fluctuation in 1 minute segments of the CTG trace between contractions.
- Normal baseline variability: FHR fluctuates 6–25 bpm between contractions
- Reduced baseline variability: FHR fluctuates 3–5 bpm for >30 minutes
- Absent baseline variability: FHR fluctuates <3 bpm
- Increased baseline variability: FHR fluctuates >25 bpm

- *Accelerations:* Transient increases in FHR of 15 bpm or more above the baseline and lasting 15 seconds.
- *Decelerations:* Transient episodes of decrease of FHR below the baseline lasting at least 15 seconds and conforming to one of the patterns below:
  - *Early decelerations:* Uniform, repetitive decrease of FHR where there is a slow onset early in contraction with a slow return to baseline prior to the end of the contraction.
  - *Variable decelerations:* Repetitive or intermittent decrease in FHR with rapid descent and rapid recovery. Timing may be variable but usually simultaneous with contractions.
  - *Late decelerations:* Uniform, repetitive decreasing of FHR usually with slow onset mid-to-end of the contraction with nadir >20 seconds after the peak of the contraction and ending after the contraction.

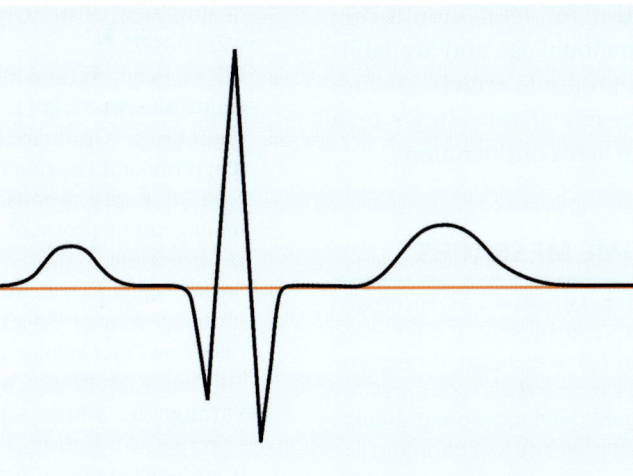

Fig. 2: Normal electrocardiogram wave.

Computerized Cardiotocography and Electrocardiogram Analysis in Labor (Fig. 2)

Computerized CTG:[7] Computerized CTG is an objective analysis of CTG. Computerized CTG is reproducible and consistent, making it superior to subjective visual analysis of CTG. It uses the computerized numerical analysis known as Dawes–Redman CTG analysis.

Short-term variability (STV) is measured over a much smaller interval of just 3.75s (typically 7–10 beats). It is based on the difference between average beat intervals in each 3.75s segment. It cannot be assessed from visual inspection of trace and it is independent of baseline rate.

Thresholds for management (only valid when measured over the full 60 minutes):
- <4 ms low
- <3 ms abnormal
- <2 ms highly abnormal.

ST analysis (STAN)[8] is intended for fetal monitoring during labor.

Prerequisites:
- Singleton pregnancy
- >36 weeks gestational age
- Cephalic presentation
- Rupture of membranes.

It is not recommended to start STAN in second stage of labor, however if started in first stage can be continued in second stage of labor.

Contraindications: Maternal blood borne viruses or suspicion of a fetal bleeding disorder.

Rationale: Anaerobic metabolism by cardiac myocytes in oxygen deficiency causes breakdown of glycogen and release of potassium ions which increases the height of T wave. Similar to adult ECG, cardiac hypoxia and ischemia cause ST depression and inversion of the T wave.

The interpretation of STAN is in terms of episodic T/QRS rise, baseline T/QRS rise, and biphasic ST.

Any acute event in mother (such as hypoxia, eclampsia, shock, drug administration, cardiac arrest, fever) may give abnormal results in fetal monitoring tests. It is important to correct maternal condition and resuscitate so that fetal condition improves, rather than delivering the fetus prematurely. Always identify proper test for fetal monitoring depending on gestational age and availability of tools with appropriate exercise. Before acting upon the result of test always take maternal condition in to consideration.

TAKE HOME MESSAGES

- Consider fetoplacental system as an organ system and have specific tests.
- NST and modified BPP are choice of tests for fetal monitoring in antenatal period.
- Continuous electronic fetal monitoring should be used in all maternal critical conditions in labor.
- Ultrasonography in expert hands can guide in better management of fetus and improve outcome.
- Before acting on any abnormal result, take maternal condition into consideration and rectify the correctable maternal condition.

■ REFERENCES

1. Lai J, Nowlan NC, Vaidyanathan R, Shaw CJ, Lees CC. Fetal movements as a predictor of health. Acta Obstet Gynecol Scand. 2016; 95(9):968-75.
2. RCOG. Reduced Fetal Movement. Green top Guidelines No. 57; 2011.
3. Figueras F, Gratacós E. Update on the diagnosis and classification of fetal growth restriction and proposal of a stage-based management protocol. Fetal Diagn Ther. 2014;36:86-98.
4. Shen-Wagner J, Deutchman M. Point-of-care ultrasound: a practical guide for primary care. Fam Pract Manag. 2020;27(6):33-40.
5. Tilbrook V, Smith R, Chenia F, Coomblas J, Parange A. South Australian Perinatal Practice Guideline Fetal Surveillance (Cardiotocography); 2019.
6. Ayres-de-Campos D, Spong CY, Chandraharan E; FIGO Intrapartum Fetal Monitoring Expert Consensus Panel. FIGO consensus guidelines on intrapartum fetal monitoring: Cardiotocography. Int J Gynaecol Obstet. 2015;131(1):13-24.
7. Blackwell S, Roy C. Antenatal Cardiotocography Obstetric UHL Guideline; 2021.
8. Sacco A, Muglu J, Navaratnarajah R, Hogg M. ST analysis for intrapartum fetal monitoring. Obstet Gynaecol. 2015;17:5-12.

SECTION 3

Systemic Disorders

Respiratory Disorders

6. **Asthma in Pregnancy**
   Prachee Sathe, Sanmay Chowdhury

7. **Community Acquired Pneumonia in Pregnancy**
   Ruchira Khasne, Kalpesh Parekh

8. **Acute Respiratory Distress Syndrome in Pregnancy**
   Sauren Panja, Nilashree Das

9. **Pulmonary Thromboembolism: Preexistent and Concurrent**
   Vivek Gupta, Shibba Takkar Chhabra

10. **Nonthrombotic Pulmonary Embolism**
    Ahsan Ahmed, Anirban Bose

Cardiovascular Disorders

11. **Hypertensive Emergencies**
    Siri Yerubandi

12. **Valvular Heart Diseases in Pregnancy**
    Anisha Gala Shah

13. **Heart Failure in Pregnancy**
    Susruta Bandyopadhyay

Renal Disorders and Drug Dosing

14. **Acute Kidney Injury including Hemolytic Uremic Syndrome in Pregnancy**
    Ranajit Chatterjee, Priyanka H Chhabra

15. **Chronic Kidney Disease and Pregnancy**
    Manisha Pradhan

16. **Urinary Tract Infections in Pregnancy**
    Kallur Sailaja Devi

17. **Drug Dosing in Renal Failure**
    Shrikant Sahasrabudhe, Beena Daniel

Metabolic Conditions

18. **Hyperosmolar State in Pregnancy: Diabetic Ketoacidosis and Hyperosmolar Hyperglycemic Syndrome**
    Ritesh Shah, Anuj Clerk

19. **Thyroid Disorders in Critically Ill Pregnant Lady**
    Bhagyesh Shah

Electrolyte Disorders

20. **Disorders of Sodium Homeostasis and Fluid Balance in Pregnancy**
    Santanu Bagchi, Saurabh Debnath

21. **Disorders of Potassium Homeostasis**
    Soumya Sharma, Sai Saran

22. **Disorders of Calcium, Magnesium, and Phosphorus Homeostasis**
    Prashant Kumar, Mukta Seth

Neurological Disorders

23. **Severe Preeclampsia and Eclampsia**
    Pallavi Chandra Ravula, Tarakeswari Surapaneni

24. **Central Venous Sinus Thrombosis**
    Sulagna Bhattacharjee, Gaurav Mittal, Souvik Maitra

Rheumatological Disorders

25. Systemic Lupus Erythematosus Flare during Pregnancy
    Ritu Singh, Suruchi Ambasta, Sanjeev Kumar

26. Catastrophic Antiphospholipid Antibodies Syndrome
    Hetal Patolia, Shweta Bhatt Dave

Trauma

27. Polytrauma in a Pregnant Lady
    Amrita Shah, Pradeep Rangappa, Ipe Jacob

Hematological Disorders

28. Sickle Cell Crisis
    Maimoona Ahmed, Tarakeswari Surapaneni

29. Thalassemia in Pregnancy
    Y Subhashini

30. Thrombocytopenia in Pregnancy
    Venigalla Rama

Transplant Medicine

31. Transplant Recipients
    Malini Sukayogula

Respiratory Disorders

CHAPTER 6

Asthma in Pregnancy

Prachee Sathe, Sanmay Chowdhury

INTRODUCTION

Why it is important to understand the early diagnosis, proper assessment of severity of bronchial asthma in a pregnant lady is for the safety of both, the mother and the child. It could be preexisting asthma in most of the cases; de novo diagnosis of bronchial reactivity is rare. It is important to note that the physiology of pregnancy may affect different patients and react differently during asthmatic attack.

EPIDEMIOLOGY AND MAGNITUDE OF PROBLEM

Asthma, a common problem, has poor outcome for mother and babies and is associated with increased maternal morbidity. It is associated with preeclampsia gestational diabetes and results in fetal hypoxia leading to preterm deliveries, malformations such as cleft lip or palate or some delayed complications in babies.

PREGNACY-RELATED PHYSIOLOGICAL CHANGES AND ITS IMPLICATIONS FOR MATERNAL HEALTH DURING ASTHMA

Physiological changes in respiratory system in a pregnant mother occur because of enlarged uterus affecting the diaphragmatic anatomy (pushed up by up to 5 cm) affecting lung function by 5% decrease in the volume and 20% decrease in functional residual capacity (FRC), associated with increased oxygen demands and dilutional anemia leading to dyspnea in pregnancy. During pregnancy due to hypercortisolism the placenta is known to excrete high levels of corticotrophin-releasing hormone (CRH) and adrenocorticotrophin hormone (ACTH).

Increased beta adrenoreceptor causes increased free cortisol levels which provoke increased incidence of bronchiectasis.

Prostaglandins have a beneficial effect on smooth muscle cell profile especially prostaglandin E2 levels which are high and help in bronchial relaxation. Progesterone changes smooth muscle wall tension and causes bronchiectasis.[1]

Respiratory cycle is influenced by both progesterone and estrogen by increasing sensitivity to carbon dioxide. There is no change in respiratory rate although there is increase in minute ventilation by 30–50% which is due to rise in tidal volume by 40%. The minute ventilation increases by 30–50% which is due to a 40% increase in tidal volume, while there is no significant change in respiratory rate. The parameters which are unchanged include TLC (total lung capacity),

VC (vital capacity), lung compliance, and DLCO (diffusing capacity of the lungs for carbon monoxide), forced expiratory volume 1 (FEV1)/forced vital capacity (FVC) and peak expiratory flow rate (PEFR). Hence spirometry for FEV1 with its diurnal variations can be used for early diagnosis and treatment response during pregnancy.[2]

High progesterone leads vasodilatation and congestion of mucosa in upper respiratory tract leading to rhinitis and stimulates the respiratory center. Women are in the state of hypercortisonism during pregnancy; meanwhile, the placenta secretes both CRH and ACTH, which results in the increase of free cortisol secreted by placenta and conjugated cortisol during pregnancy. The increased free cortisol mediates the increase of beta-adrenoceptor and the enhancement of bronchiectasis. Increased secretion causes high levels of prostaglandin E2 (PGE2) during pregnancy. Through its anti-inflammatory effects and inhibition of smooth muscle cell proliferation, bronchial relaxation, and other mechanisms, prostaglandins have the effects that can be protective for the mother with bronchial asthma. In addition, progesterone also has the effect of changing the airway smooth muscle tension and causing bronchiectasis. These factors are associated with asthmatic remission during pregnancy.

Severe attacks get triggered by viral infections, non-adherence to inhaled corticosteroids and gastrointestinal reflux disease (GERD) which should be prevented.

Guidelines include review prior to conception and managing asthma actively during pregnancy with regular 4 weekly reviews along with management of comorbid condition like rhinitis and GERD.

The basic aim of asthma treatment in pregnancy includes control of asthma, prevents exacerbation and birth of healthy babies aim of control includes day and nights exposure of exacerbation and improving function and having normal activity concerns of pharmacological agents on developing fetus and the risk benefit ratios for maternal health are considered in global initiative for asthma (GINA) guidelines extensively and suggest that poor asthma control and acute exacerbations during pregnancy are more risky than taking asthma medications.

Stepwise Approach for Using Drugs for Asthma in Pregnancy

Groups of Drugs for Treatment of Asthma during Pregnancy Based on the Severity

Currently, the most commonly used and safe drugs during pregnancy include glucocorticoids, beta 2-agonist, anticholinergics, theophylline, omalizumab, and allergen immunotherapy (AIT).

- *Glucocorticoids:* Inhaled corticosteroids are used for prevention as well as management of acute attacks either by MDI (metered dose inhalers), Rotahalers or nebulizers (ultrasonic nebulizers preferential for deliveries up to the tertiary bronchi). The molecules recommended are Budesonide mainly.

    Oral corticosteroids/systemic corticosteroids are reserved for severe cases. Drugs used in asthma such as corticosteroids are considered to have no bad effect on uterus or fetus but some observational studies raise the concerns that steroids may be associated with infant cleft palate, gestational diabetes, and adrenal problems in fetus.

    There should be quarterly and weekly review in patients with asthma to rule out comorbid conditions such as rhinitis and GERD as per GINA guidelines there is increased incidence of acute exacerbation and poor asthma control can have a high risk profile than taking asthma medication itself.

Drugs that can be safely used in pregnancy include glucocorticoids, anticholinergics, theophylline, omalizumab, and allergen immunotherapy. Role of oral corticosteroids has been proven beneficial in poorly controlled asthma.

- *Beta-2 agonists:* SABA (short-acting like salbutamol) and LABA (long-acting, salmeterol and formoterol) have been shown to be safe for the use during pregnancy.

  While SABA can be used in small doses more frequently during acute phases LABA are more for long-term management.

  It is notable that more women on inhaled corticosteroids have improved fetal respiratory health at the 12 months of age.

  Doses: Salbutamol: 2.5–5 mg 4 times a day by nebulization (maximum 40 mg/day in hospital settings under supervision) watch for tachycardia and hypokalemia Salmeterol: 50 µg puffs twice a day.

  Formoterol: 12–20 µg puffs twice a day.

  Albuterol is known to get distributed in breast milk and known to affect uterine contractility.[3]

  Albuterol use should be limited as it causes fetal and maternal tachycardia and hyperglycemia. Prolonged usage in excess can lead to tetralogy of Fallot.

- *Anticholinergics:* Anticholinergics are of two types: 1. Short-acting muscarinic antagonist (SAMAS)—ipratropium bromide. 2. Long-acting muscarinic antagonists (LAMAS)—tiotropium bromide. For acute asthma attacks, GINA guidelines suggest combination of formoterol and SABA.

- *Theophylline:* It is safe for the fetus and does cross through the placental barrier; it is used as an added therapy for bronchospasm and is useful for treating moderate asthma.

- *Leukotriene receptor antagonists (LTRAs):* It is used in prevention mild persistent asthma and severe asthmatic attacks during pregnancy and can be used instead of injectable corticosteroids (ICS).

- *Omalizumab and allergen immunotherapy:* Rarely used in pregnancy as monoclonal antibody against IL-5 because of its adverse and unknown effects on mother and fetus.

Drug treatment with high dose magnesium as an adjunctive therapy in severe asthma in pregnancy beyond standard drugs described above.

Intravenous magnesium sulfate administered as 4 g loading dose followed by 2 g/hour continuous infusion until successful tocolysis or failure of treatment can be useful to break the bronchospasm without side-effects on the mother or the baby.[3]

Alternatively high dose regimen 4 g loading dose followed by 5 g/hour continuous infusion and increased by 1 g/hour until successful tocolysis OR failure of treatment.

Considerations for Asthma during Pregnancy Needing ICU Care

Emergency department visits or unscheduled doctor's visits should be treated with alertness. Normal physiological washout of CO_2 during pregnancy may mask the assessment of severity. Watch pulse oximetry closely and inability to speak a full sentence in single breath, patient complaining of exhaustion and tiredness, inability to eat or drink due to severe tachypnea should prompt the admission for close observation, oxygen therapy with nebulized, and systemic appropriate drug administration in high dependency units.[4]

State-of-the-art strategies for extracorporeal membrane oxygenation (ECMO) in acute asthma with respiratory failure despite all life saving measures venovenous ECMO have been found to be helpful without any side effects.[5]

Identify the Patient at Risk

- Silent chest with disappearing wheezes is an ominous sign
- Low minute ventilation with rapid shallow breathing index with rising pCO_2
- pH <7.0
- Patient getting exhausted and fatigued despite maximal therapy
- Worsening mental status
- Refractory hypoxia, rising lactate
- Worsening hypercapnia
- Hemodynamic instability
- Impending coma
- In such cases intubation may become mandatory. Sedation with propofol or ketamine has bronchodilator properties and is preferred over benzodiazepines during and after intubation if needed.

Oxygen Therapy Modalities

Venturi devices for high flow humidified oxygen with attachments for nebulizers are preferred.

If it is inadequate, 100% rebreathing mask can be used till the effects of inhaled bronchodilator drugs on bronchospasm are awaited.

In current times HFNO (high flow nasal oxygen) or non-invasive bilevel positive end expiratory pressure (BiPAP) ventilation to tide over the crisis till the effect of inhaled and systemic drugs can be used.[4]

Need and Risks of Intubation and Invasive Ventilation

Invasive ventilation would be the last resort, with risks of intubation in a pregnant patient and its algorithms kept in mind. It mandates expert help.

Ventilating a severely asthmatic patient is a domain of expert intensivists. Nevertheless each one dealing with such situations at remote or resource poor settings should be aware of the objectives of ventilation, which are as follows:[6]

- Adequate gas exchange with acceptable oxygenation and avoiding ventilator-induced lung damage with lung-protective ventilation.
- Protective principles for lungs include low ventilator rates and accepting more acidic pH and high pCO_2 levels with permissive hypercapnia.
- Avoiding auto positive end expiratory pressure is a major goal to avoid hemodynamic instability and barotrauma.

■ CONCLUSION

Asthma has been a common respiratory ailment in our country post-covid and due to increasing population. Hence early recognition and treatment in pregnacy helps reduce post pregnancy complications due to asthma in maternal and fetal side with better outcomes.

TAKE HOME MESSAGES

- Inhaled steroids are the primary controller for bronchial asthma in pregnancy. Among inhaled steroids, budesonide is classified in pregnancy category B while the rest, including fluticasone and beclomethasone, are in pregnancy category C. Budesonide is, therefore, the preferred agent to initiate therapy unless the patient has already been on another inhaled steroid.
- It is safe to use inhaled corticosteroids, theophylline, and montelukast during pregnancy.

- Systemic steroids may be indicated in cases of bronchial asthma exacerbation during pregnancy. However, they are not to be tried before the initiation of inhaled corticosteroids.
- The goals of bronchial asthma treatment in pregnancy are to control asthma symptoms, maintain optimal lung function, and avoid bronchial asthma exacerbation. In addition, maintaining fetal oxygenation by avoiding attacks of maternal hypoxia is crucial.

REFERENCES

1. Wang H, Li N, Huang H. Asthma in Pregnancy: Pathophysiology, Diagnosis, Whole-Course Management, and Medication Safety. Can Respir J. 2020. https://doi.org/10.1155/2020/9046842.
2. Chan AL, Juarez MM, Gidwani N, Albertson TE. Management of critical asthma syndrome during pregnancy. Clin Rev Allergy Immunol. 2015;48(1):45-53.
3. 2022 GINA Report, Global Strategy for Asthma Management and Prevention. (2022) 2022 GINA Report, Global Strategy for Asthma Management and Prevention. [online] Available from: https://ginasthma.org/gina-reports/#:~:text=2022%20GINA%20Report%2C%20Global%20Strategy,on%20the%20GINA%20Science%20Committee [Last accessed February, 2023].
4. Cochrane database systematic review in ERS guidelines 2019.
5. ELSO support group for use of extracorporeal support like venovenousecmo.
6. National heart lung and blood institure working group 2004 update.

CHAPTER 7

Community Acquired Pneumonia in Pregnancy

Ruchira Khasne, Kalpesh Parekh

■ INTRODUCTION

Community acquired pneumonia (CAP) is one of the most common infectious diseases and an important cause of mortality and morbidity worldwide. Any inflammation and consolidation of lung tissue due to infectious agent which develops outside the hospital is defined as CAP.[1] Clinical manifestations and diagnostic evaluation with suspected pneumonia are similar to those in nonpregnant individuals. But pregnancy-related alterations in cell-mediated immunity and associated physiological changes may increase the risk and severity of infection. Besides that, there are associated concerns of health of the fetus as well.[2]

Causative agents: The pathogens responsible for CAP are similar in pregnant and nonpregnant patients. Bacterial infections such as *Streptococcus pneumoniae, Haemophilus influenzae, Staphylococcus aureus, Mycoplasma pneumoniae,* viruses such as influenza virus, respiratory syncytial virus (RSV), coronavirus [severe acute respiratory syndrome coronavirus disease-2019 (SARS COVID-19)], rhinovirus, and varicella are common causative agents.[2-4] Varicella can cause severe maternal infection leading to congenital abnormalities with devastating consequences. The clinical course is unpredictable and may rapidly progress to hypoxia and respiratory failure, with high rates of mortality if untreated.

■ EPIDEMIOLOGY AND MAGNITUDE OF THE PROBLEM

In a pregnant patient, pneumonia is the most common cause of fatal nonobstetric infection. The incidence of pneumonia has varied widely as per number of published surveys. Historically there was increased incidence, morbidity and mortality of pneumonia in pregnancy, however now with advanced antibiotics, good obstetric care, preventive measures and vaccines the incidence and mortality has reduced significantly.[5,6] The rate of hospitalization for pneumonia has been found to be similar in pregnant and non-pregnant population with reported incidence of 1.51/1,000 deliveries versus 1.47/1,000 in nonpregnant controls.[7] The Centers for Disease Control and Prevention (CDC) reported that hospitalization with coronavirus disease-2019 (COVID-19) occurred in 31.5% of pregnant women compared with 5.8% of nonpregnant women.[8]

■ IMPLICATIONS FOR MATERNAL HEALTH

Pregnant women can predispose to various respiratory infections irrespective of the period of gestation, with the mean gestational age from 24.4 ± 9.2 weeks.[9]

Following are the factors, which predispose pregnant patients to infections:

Maternal physiological changes: Elevation of the diaphragm by up to 4 cm, decrease in functional residual capacity, increase in oxygen consumption, and increase in lung water may predispose pregnant patient to tachypnea and hypoxia, which might cause respiratory alkalosis leading to reduced uterine blood flow.

Immunological changes: Reduced lymphocyte proliferative response, diminished cell-mediated cytotoxicity, reduced number of helper T cells, reduced lymphokine response to alloantigens makes this group of patients more vulnerable to catch infections.

Additional risk factors: Presence of comorbid illness, maternal diseases, smoking, anemia, alcohol, on steroids therapy or maternal administration of steroids for fetal lung maturity, and tocolytic therapy lead to poor perinatal outcome.

Detailed evaluation of these patients with prior identification of risk factors and careful review of various differential diagnosis is of vital importance. In current antibiotic era, maternal prognosis of bacterial pneumonia is often better and it does not affect fetus directly.[7] Viruses such as varicella may cause disseminated disease and are fatal with maternal mortality ~14%.[10]

Symptoms: Symptoms such as dyspnea, productive cough, purulent sputum, excessive fatigue, fever, chills, rigors, pleuritic chest pain, loss of appetite, and localized inspiratory crackles are common.

Severity of illness: Severity is more if patients present with respiratory rate >30 breaths/min, PaO_2/FiO_2 ratio <250, multilobar infiltrates, confusion/disorientation, uremia (blood urea nitrogen level >20 mg/dL), leukopenia (white blood cell count <4,000 cells/mm^3), thrombocytopenia (platelet count <100,000 cells/mm^3), hypothermia (core temperature <36°C), hypotension requiring aggressive fluid resuscitation, hypoglycemia (in nondiabetic patients), hyponatremia, or unexplained metabolic acidosis or elevated lactate level.

Complications: Pleural effusions, necrotizing pneumonia—abscess formation with lung cavitation, empyema, pneumothorax, acute respiratory distress syndrome, renal, hepatic failure, coagulopathy, meningitis, encephalopathy, multiorgan dysfunction syndrome (MODS), cardiac complications—arrhythmias, cardiac failure, pericardial tamponade and placental abruption are seen especially if associated with comorbidity.[11]

IMPLICATIONS FOR FETAL WELL-BEING

Fetal death has been reported as a complication of CAP in earlier series, but mortality has reduced due to advanced care. Fetal health is routinely not affected in bacterial pneumonia but association of maternal risk factors may compromise the fetal well-being. Any factor causing compromised uteroplacental blood flow can lead to miscarriage, preterm labor, prematurity, low birth weight baby, and fetal respiratory failure.

In influenza pneumonia there is a paucity of data, which supports increased incidence of fetal death or malformations.[5] The major concern is about varicella infections. If mother acquires varicella infection during the early gestational period (8–20 weeks), the fetus is at risk for developing congenital varicella syndrome such as limb hypoplasia, skin lesions, neurologic abnormalities, and structural eye damage. The risk of transplacental infection and embryopathy particularly in first half month of the pregnancy is 1–2%.[10] If the mother acquires varicella immediately before or after delivery; the baby is at risk for neonatal varicella, which may present with mild rash to fatal disseminated infection.

■ MANAGEMENT STEPS

Management comprises initial assessment of severity based on scoring system, diagnostic testing, antimicrobial therapy, immunoprophylaxis, and supportive measures.

Initial assessment of severity: Routine physiological changes occurring in pregnancy may bring limitations to scoring systems. For example, hematocrit of 30 considered as anemia in normal population is accepted as normal in pregnancy, similarly elevated white cell count may be accepted as normal in pregnancy. These parameters may underscore the scoring systems to predict the disease severity. Pneumonia severity index (PSI) is the most widely used score to define severity of illness in patients with CAP, but it may underestimate the need for hospital admission in pregnant patients compared to nonpregnant patients. Thus, clinician should keep a low threshold for hospital admissions. Additionally, one has to give special attention to potential fetomaternal risk of hypoxia, which can prove to be detrimental to both the lives.

Diagnostic testing: According to the American Thoracic Society/Infectious Diseases Society of America (ATS/IDSA)[12] guidelines for the management of adults with CAP, all patients with suspected CAP should have a chest radiograph, which remains the gold standard. The indications for chest radiograph are the same as in nonpregnant patients. It is estimated that radiation doses to the mother from a posteroanterior chest radiograph, performed with a shield covering abdomen is equal to 1 day's background radiation. There should not be any hesitation to perform chest radiography in pregnant patients.[10] Recently lung ultrasound is emerging as a valuable diagnostic bedside tool, with no radiation exposure risk. But currently, there are no recommended guidelines for its use.

Additionally, assessment of gas exchange by arterial blood gas, routine blood chemistry, blood counts, quantitative C-reactive protein, two sets of blood cultures (before initiation of antibiotics), sputum Gram stain culture (if resistance to routine drug is suspected) should be routinely done. For patients with severe CAP, *Legionella* urinary antigen, and pneumococcal urinary antigen should be measured. Establishing an etiologic diagnosis should be given priority in case of pneumonia not responding to routine treatment, including consideration of bronchoscopy.[12]

Treatment: Before prescribing antimicrobials therapy for pneumonia in pregnancy, their safety should be confirmed first. Current guidelines for CAP recommend to use combined therapy to cover *Pneumococcus* and atypical pathogens and should be continued for 10–14 days[12] **(Table 1)**. Due to increased renal clearance in pregnancy upper range of recommended doses should be used.

Antivirals: Antiviral agents should be considered if influenza viral pneumonia is likely, especially early in the course of illness. Antiviral agents such as amantadine and rimantadine have activity against influenza A pneumonia and reduce the duration of symptoms if given within 48 hours of the onset of illness. As a chemoprophylaxis

TABLE 1: Empirical antibiotic therapy in community-acquired pneumonia.

Category of patient	Associated risk factors	Treatment

Outpatients	• No comorbid illness
	• No recent antibiotics
	• No drug resistance
	• Drug-resistant *Streptococcus pneumoniae* (DRSP) risks
	• Coexisting cardiopulmonary disease
	• Recent antibiotic therapy, or DRSP risk factors
		• *Oral macrolide:*
		  – Azithromycin (or erythromycin)
		
		• *Macrolide plus beta-lactam:*
		  – Azithromycin (or erythromycin) + (high dose amoxicillin 3 g/day, cefuroxime 500 BD, or cefpodoxime)
		  – For those with a type-I allergy to beta-lactams, clindamycin can be substituted for the beta-lactam

Inpatient, not in ICU	• No comorbid illness or DRSP risks
	• Coexisting cardiopulmonary disease or DRSP risk factors
		• *Intravenous macrolide:*
		  – Azithromycin or erythromycin
		• *Intravenous beta-lactam plus intravenous macrolide* (cefotaxime, ceftriaxone) plus azithromycin (or erythromycin):
		  – Those with past allergic reactions to cephalosporins can be treated with clindamycin plus aztreonam

Inpatient in ICU	• No pseudomonal risks • Pseudomonal risks present (include bronchiectasis, prolonged corticosteroid therapy, and cystic fibrosis)	• *Intravenous beta-lactam* (cefotaxime, ceftriaxone) *PLUS intravenous macrolide* azithromycin (or erythromycin) • *Intravenous antipseudomonal beta-lactam* (cefepime, imipenem, meropenem, piperacillin/tazobactam) *PLUS an aminoglycoside* (amikacin, gentamycin, tobramycin) *PLUS intravenous macrolide* azithromycin (or erythromycin)

(ICU: intensive care unit)

these agents are 70–90% effective[5] but the primary method of influenza prevention is vaccination.

Acyclovir should be administered intravenously in all patients with complicated varicella pneumonia at 10 mg/kg every 8-hourly dose.[10]

There is little experience in pregnancy with the newer neuraminidase inhibitors, zanamivir, and oseltamivir, which can also be effective for treatment and prophylaxis, if started within 48 hours of the onset of symptoms.

Pneumocystis pneumonia (PCP) prophylaxis should be given in pregnant patients with human immunodeficiency virus (HIV) infection having low CD4 counts.

At present vaccination against influenza and to some extent *Streptococcus pneumoniae* have definitive role in preventing pneumonia.

Inactivated influenza vaccine can be safely given in any trimester of pregnancy and so should be recommended to all pregnant women who have not yet been vaccinated.[13]

Pneumococcal vaccine should be given to all pregnant women with comorbidities such as sickle cell disease, immunodeficiency, prior splenectomy, and HIV.[14]

Varicella virus immunization should be preplanned prior to pregnancy as it is live-attenuated vaccine particularly in those who had no evidence of immunity against this virus. Due to associated risk of primary varicella causing pneumonia varicella zoster immune globulin (VZIG) should be administered within 96 hours in an attempt to prevent maternal infection.

Supportive therapy: Supportive treatment comprises hydration, antipyretic therapy with acetaminophen, and supplemental oxygen same as nonpregnant patients.

Hypoxemia is less well tolerated in the pregnant female. The goal of oxygen therapy is to maintain the saturation level >94%. Continuous monitoring of saturation levels is recommended. Arterial oxygen tension should be kept well above 70 mm Hg to maintain a favorable maternofetal oxygen diffusion. In case of worsening O_2 therapy should be escalated to noninvasive ventilation (NIV) or invasive ventilation to reduce work of breathing.[15] Respiratory alkalosis causes reduction in uterine blood flow and ongoing respiratory acidosis is suggestive of impending respiratory failure.

- Vigilant monitoring is required to anticipate intubation well in advance. Difficult airway cart and experienced personnel should be readily available.
- Position the patient on left lateral so that the gravid uterus does not obstruct venous return.
- Due to associated risk of preterm labor, assessment fetal well-being with continuous fetal heart rate monitoring, and frequent obstetric ultrasound is essential.

TABLE 2: Antimicrobials to be avoided in pregnancy.

Drug to be avoided	Considerations/side effects
Clarithromycin	• Not recommended for use in pregnancy • Teratogenic in animal model
Fluoroquinolones	• Commonly used for community acquired pneumonia in nonpregnant patients, but avoided during pregnancy • Risk of malformations, arthropathy, and carcinogenic • Some reports suggested they can be used if absolutely necessary
Chloramphenicol	Can cause bone marrow suppression and "gray baby syndrome" (gray facies, flaccidity, and cardiovascular collapse)
Tetracyclines	• Should be avoided in pregnancy • The mother is at risk for fulminant hepatitis • Can cause staining in fetal bone and teeth • Doxycycline can be considered if its use is warranted, e.g., Rocky Mountain spotted fever
Sulfa compounds	Can cause fetal kernicterus
Aminoglycosides	Risk of ototoxicity to the fetus, to be used only if strong clinical indication of serious gram-negative infection
Vancomycin	Risk of fetal nephrotoxicity and ototoxicity so used only if absolutely necessary
Linezolid	Belongs to pregnancy category C, and there is limited experience in pregnancy but it is a protein synthesis inhibitor, so it should also be avoided unless no other alternative therapy is available

- Fluids should be judiciously used as these patients have risk of developing pulmonary edema.
- If patient is in shock early use of vasopressors is recommended after optimizing fluid status.
- Further management of sepsis should be done as per surviving sepsis campaign guidelines.[16]
- Nutritional support, chest physiotherapy, stress ulcer prophylaxis, and other supportive care are equally important.
- Due to high risk of deep vein thrombosis (DVT), pharmacological prophylaxis is recommended for bedridden patients.

PHARMACOLOGICAL CONSIDERATIONS

Maternal-fetal side effects and safety of the antimicrobials should be taken into consideration before giving any drug to pregnant patient. Following are the antimicrobials to be avoided in pregnancy as mentioned in **Table 2**.

CONCLUSION

Community acquired pneumonia during pregnancy is associated with significant maternal complications and neonatal morbidity especially preterm labor. Certain physiological changes in pregnancy predisposes this state to various infections and makes it less sustainable. Thus, pregnant patients require a higher level of surveillance, early intervention, and the prognostic scoring systems compared to nonpregnant patients. Early diagnosis and treatment play a key role to reduce morbidity and mortality in pregnancy. Additionally there has been a safety concerns of antimicrobials while treating a pregnant patient for pneumonia which one must take in to an account.

TAKE HOME MESSAGES

- Identify pregnant patients with additional risk factors, keep a close watch, and hospitalize early if in doubt.
- Preterm delivery is common in pneumonia in pregnancy but mortality is rare due to advancement in treatment.
- Chest radiography should be done in all pregnant patients with pneumonia as per recommendations with proper shielding.
- While selecting antibiotics safety and efficacy should always be considered.
- Vaccination should be done in pregnancy as per CDC recommendations. Pneumococcal and influenza vaccine can be given in any trimester.

REFERENCES

1. Fishman JA, Grippi MA, Elias JA. Fishman's Pulmonary Diseases and Disorders, 5th edition. New York: McGraw-Hill Education; 2015. pp. 4181-211.
2. Lim WS, Macfarlane JT, Colthorpe CL. Pneumonia and pregnancy. Thorax. 2001;56(5): 398-405.
3. Rodrigues J, Niederman MS. Pneumonia complicating Pregnancy. Clin Chest Med. 1992;13:679-91.
4. Goodnight WH, Soper DE. Pneumonia in pregnancy. Crit Care Med. 2005;33:S390-7.
5. Laibl VR, Sheffield JS. Influenza and pneumonia in pregnancy. Clin Perinatol. 2005;32:727-38.
6. Madinger NE, Greenspoon JS, Elrodt AG. Pneumonia during pregnancy: has modern technology improved maternal and fetal outcome? Am J Obstet Gynecol. 1989;161:657-62.
7. Jin Y, Carriere KC, Marrie TJ, Predy G, Johnson DH. The effects of community acquired pneumonia during pregnancy ending in a live birth. Am J Obst Gynecol. 2003;18: 800-6.
8. Ellington S, Strid P, Tong VT, Woodworth K, Galang RR, Zambrano LD, et al. Characteristics of women of reproductive age with laboratory-confirmed SARS-CoV-2 infection by pregnancy status—United States, January

22-June 7, 2020. MMWR Morb Mortal Wkly Rep. 2020;69(25):769-75.
9. Yost NP, Bloom SL, Richey SD, Ramin SM, Cunningham FG. An appraisal of treatment guidelines for antepartum community acquired pneumonia. Am J Obstet Gynecol. 2000;183:131-5.
10. James D, Steer P, Weiner CP, Gonik B, Crowther CA, Robson SC (Eds). In: Chapter 37 respiratory disease. High Risk Pregnancy Management Options, 4th edition. Saunders, St Louis, MO, USA: Elsevier; 2011. pp. 657-82.
11. Ramsey PS, Ramin KD. Pneumonia in pregnancy: medical complications of pregnancy. Obstet Gynecol Clin North Am. 2001; 28:553-69.
12. Mandell LA, Wunderink RG, Anzueto A, Bartlett JG, Campbell GD, Dean NC, et al. Infectious Diseases Society of America/American Thoracic Society consensus guidelines on the management of community-acquired pneumonia in adults. Clin Infect Dis. 2007;44(Suppl 2):S27-72.
13. ACOG Committee Opinion No. 732: Influenza vaccination during pregnancy. Obstet Gynecol. 2018;131:e109-14.
14. Centers for Disease Control and Prevention. Use of 13-valent pneumococcal conjugate vaccine and 23-valent pneumococcal polysaccharide vaccine for adults with immunocompromising conditions: recommendations of the Advisory Committee on Immunization Practices (ACIP). MMWR Morb Mortal Wkly Rep. 2012;61(40):816-9.
15. Carrillo A, Gonzalez-Diaz G, Ferrer M, Martinez-Quintana ME, Lopez-Martinez A, Llamas N, et al. Non-invasive ventilation in community acquired pneumonia and severe acute respiratory failure. Intensive Care Med. 2012;38(3):458-66.
16. Rhodes A, Evans Le, Alhazzani W, Levy MM, Antonelli MM, Ferrer R, et al. Surviving Sepsis Campaign: International Guidelines for Management of Sepsis and Septic Shock: 2016. Intensive Care Med. 2017; 43(3):304-77.

CHAPTER 8

Acute Respiratory Distress Syndrome in Pregnancy

Sauren Panja, Nilashree Das

■ INTRODUCTION

Acute respiratory distress syndrome (ARDS) is characterized by the presence of non-cardiogenic pulmonary edema along with hypoxemia as a result of injury to the lung parenchyma.

The Berlin definition (2012) proposed by the European Society of Intensive Care Medicine defines ARDS as a new or worsening respiratory symptom that includes a combination of acute hypoxemia ($PaO_2/FiO_2 \leq 300$ mm Hg), in a ventilated patient with a positive end-expiratory pressure (PEEP)/continuous positive airway pressure (CPAP) of at least 5 cmH_2O, and bilateral opacities not fully explained by effusion, lung collapse, or nodules that occurs within 7 days of a clinical insult. Further, the respiratory failure is not fully explained by volume overload or cardiac failure. The levels of PaO_2/FiO_2 ratio are used to categorize ARDS as mild (200–≤300 mm Hg), moderate (100–≤200 mm Hg), and severe (≤100 mm Hg) on CPAP/PEEP of ≥5 cmH_2O.[1]

The Kigali modification of the Berlin definition uses alternate criteria, including peripheral oxygen saturation (SpO_2) to FiO_2 ratio and chest ultrasound, which is a convenient adaptation in the low-resource setting. The Kigali modification considers a $SpO_2/FiO_2 \leq 315$ corresponding to a P/F ratio of 300 and $SpO_2/FiO_2 \leq 235$ to a P/F ratio of 200.[2]

Acute respiratory distress syndrome and respiratory failure can complicate 0.1–0.2% of all pregnant patients.[3] Pregnancy has been an exclusion criterion in the previously conducted major trials on ARDS; thereby the management of pregnant patients with ARDS depends mainly on clinical experience or extrapolation of the existing data from other studies, case reports, and pathophysiological understanding of the disease.

▌ PHYSIOLOGICAL CHANGES IN THE RESPIRATORY SYSTEM OF PREGNANT WOMEN

Respiratory changes occurring during pregnancy are as a result of hormonal changes, mechanical effects of the enlarging uterus and increased metabolic demands of the fetoplacental unit.[4,5] Chest wall compliance reduces by approximately 30% along with reduction of functional residual capacity (FRC).[6] The increase in tidal volume and respiratory rate results in low partial pressure of carbon dioxide ($PaCO_2$) and higher PaO_2. Due to an increased respiratory drive owing to high progesterone level, a respiratory alkalosis state develops resulting in the $PaCO_2$ falling to 27–34 mm Hg.[7] The partial pressure of oxygen (PaO_2) ranges

BOX 1: Respiratory changes in pregnancy.	
• Functional residual capacity	• Reduced by 20%
• Residual volume	• Reduced by 15%
• Inspiratory reserve volume	• Increased by 5%
• Inspiratory capacity	• Increased by 15%
• Expiratory reserve volume	• Reduced by 25%
• Total lung capacity	• Reduced by 5%
• Tidal volume	• Increased by 45%
• Respiratory rate	• Increased to 15–17/min
• Vital capacity	• No change
• Closing capacity	• No change

BOX 2: Causes of respiratory failure in pregnancy.

Pregnancy related:
- Sepsis—pyelonephritis, chorioamnionitis, puerperal infection, septic abortion, preeclampsia
- Amniotic fluid embolism, trophoblastic embolism
- Hemorrhagic shock, massive transfusion, TRALI (transfusion-related acute lung injury)
- Tocolytic therapy
- Placental abruption
- Peripartum cardiomyopathy-induced pulmonary edema

Increased risk in pregnancy:
- Pneumonia—bacteria, viral, aspiration
- Asthma
- Venous thromboembolism and pulmonary embolism
- Gastric acid aspiration

Other conditions:
- Pancreatitis
- Trauma
- Acute respiratory distress syndrome due to sepsis
- Drugs/toxins

between 90 and 110 mm Hg in pregnant women.[4,5]

An increase in the oxygen consumption and decrease in FRC causes rapid desaturation in pregnancy.[8] Fetoplacental oxygen transfer is reduced by low pressure in the uterine artery and also during uterine contractions. Fetoplacental blood flow depends upon hemoglobin concentration, saturation, uteroplacental blood flow, and maternal hypotension. A maternal PaO_2 >75 mm Hg is required to prevent hypoxic injury in a fetus. A fetal $PaCO_2$ of ≥65 mm Hg and pH > 7.48 causes reduced fetal perfusion **(Boxes 1 and 2)**.[9,10]

■ INITIAL WORKUP

The initial workup should include proper history, clinical features, the routine laboratory investigations, chest X-ray, arterial blood gas, and electrocardiography (ECG) **(Table 1)**.

■ MANAGEMENT

The general management of ARDS is treatment of the precipitating cause along with respiratory support. The primary objective is to optimize the maternal and placental gas exchange and prevent further lung injury.

Prompt identification of the predisposing factor and cause specific treatment (e.g., early source control, appropriate antibiotic therapy in sepsis, adequate blood pressure control in preeclampsia, prophylaxis with H_2 receptor blockers against gastric aspiration, etc.) has shown better outcome.

The various supportive therapies aim to provide adequate gas exchange and minimize further lung injury.

Supportive Therapies in Acute Respiratory Distress Syndrome

- Noninvasive ventilation (NIV)/high-flow nasal cannula (HFNC)

TABLE 1: Initial workup in pregnant patients with ARDS.

History and clinical features	• Proper history is important (drugs, new onset hypertension with end organ dysfunction, hemorrhage and massive blood transfusion, fever, new onset calf pain, abdominal pain) • Clinical features include tachypnea, dyspnea, respiratory distress, confusion, agitation, and diaphoresis. Patients have more of a rapid shallow breathing pattern. On auscultation there may be crepitations, rhonchi, wheeze depending upon the cause of respiratory failure
Laboratory investigations	• A complete blood count reveals a fall of hemoglobin (owing to anemia of pregnancy), leukocytosis or leukopenia due to infectious etiology • Abnormalities in electrolytes may aggravate respiratory failure. Hepatic and renal function tests help to assess the presence of multiorgan failure • Site specific cultures (respiratory, blood, urine) if infection is the precipitating cause
Arterial blood gas	Blood gas reveals respiratory alkalosis with compensatory renal excretion of bicarbonate. $PaCO_2$ reduced to 27–34 mm Hg with plasma bicarbonate level of 18–21 mEq/L. Hypoxia depends on severity of ARDS and also increased oxygen consumption during pregnancy. Presence of hypercapnic respiratory acidosis is an ominous sign and may represent severe ARDS with impending respiratory failure
ECG	Look out for cardiac dysfunction, arrhythmias, ST segment changes
Imaging	• Radiological investigations like chest X-ray needed for evaluation can be achieved through abdominal shields and properly collimated X-ray beams. CT chest may show widespread patchy opacities, though the risk of ionizing radiation increases • Furthermore, findings on lung ultrasound [e.g., nonhomogeneous B lines, presence of consolidation (shred sign), coarse pleural line, absent lung slide] and absence of cardiac failure on echocardiography can help in corroboration of the diagnosis

(ARDS: acute respiratory distress syndrome; ECG: electrocardiography; $PaCO_2$: partial pressure of carbon dioxide)

- Invasive ventilation with lower tidal volume (lung protective strategy)
- PEEP titration
- Prone position
- Recruitment maneuvers
- Corticosteroids
- Negative fluid balance
- Neuromuscular blocking agents
- Inhaled nitric oxide
- High frequency oscillation
- ECMO (extracorporeal membrane oxygenation)
- $ECCO_2R$ (extracorporeal carbon dioxide removal).

Noninvasive Ventilation/High-flow Nasal Cannula

Noninvasive ventilation reduces the work of breathing, improves oxygenation, circumvents the complications of intubation, and mechanical ventilation; hence can be used for the management of mild ARDS in pregnancy.[11] However, a gravida is considered to be a "full stomach" as there is an increased risk of gastric aspiration due to a combination of increased intragastric pressure and reduced tone of the lower esophageal sphincter.[4] NIV under supervision can be applied early only in patients who have mild ARDS, those who are alert and conscious with a patent airway and are hemodynamically stable without severe acid–base disturbances.[4] Delaying tracheal intubation leads to worsened outcome and higher hospital mortality in patients with ARDS who failed NIV support.[12]

High-flow nasal cannula delivers warm, humidified high-flow oxygen through nose, which is comfortable to the patient.[13] It improves oxygenation, improves CO_2 clearance, improves mucociliary clearance and reduces work of breathing. The posthoc analysis of FLORALI trial showed intubation rates to be lower in HFNC group with P/F ratio of <200 when compared to NIV and standard face mask group.[14] However, further trials are required in pregnant patient to compare the efficacy of both the modalities.

Mechanical Ventilation

Pregnancy is associated with capillary engorgement and mucosal edema of the upper airway. Also, increase in chest diameter and breast size in pregnant women makes intubation difficult. Adequate preoxygenation is essential to prevent rapid desaturation. Smaller size endotracheal tubes and airway adjuncts should be readily available in anticipation of difficult intubation **(Box 3)**.[4]

Lung-protective ventilation strategies include low tidal volume, plateau pressure limited ventilation. ARMA trial has reported a mortality benefit when patients received lower tidal volumes.[15] A lung protective ventilation strategy reduces ventilator-induced lung injury (VILI) by avoiding both alveolar overdistension and repetitive cyclical opening and closing of atelectatic alveoli, therefore, reducing the pulmonary and systemic cytokine response.[16] Open lung ventilation strategy is aimed to achieve an open and homogeneously ventilated lung by combining recruitment maneuver for opening up the collapsed lung and high PEEP for alveolar stability.[17] Lung open ventilation study trial showed open lung ventilation strategy improved oxygenation with no mortality benefit over standard ventilation strategy.[18]

Positive end-expiratory pressure benefits patients by preventing the cyclic opening and closing of alveoli and decreases shunt by recruitment of collapsed alveoli at the end of exhalation. ALVEOLI trial concluded no mortality benefit of high PEEP over low PEEP when low tidal volumes and limitations of plateau pressure are considered.[19] Levels of 5–15 mm Hg, is considered safe, but at higher levels of PEEP, venous return might be impaired leading to a fall in cardiac output with decreased uteroplacental perfusion, alveolar overdistension, and barotrauma.[20]

A higher plateau pressure target can be considered due to the presence of gravid uterus. However, the major determining factor of total respiratory compliance is the

> **BOX 3:** Lung protective ventilation goals in pregnant patients with ARDS.
> - *Tidal volume:* 6–8 mL/kg ideal body weight higher respiratory rate
> - Peak inspiratory pressure ≤35 cmH_2O
> - Plateau pressure ≤30 cmH_2O may be exceeded due to the presence of gravid uterus
> - Driving pressure ≤14 cmH_2O
> - PEEP 5–15 cmH_2O
> - PaO_2 > 70 mm Hg
> - $PaCO_2$: 45–55 mm Hg, pregnant patients poorly tolerate permissive hypercapnia
> - SpO_2: 94–98% in obstetric patients
>
> (ARDS: acute respiratory distress syndrome; $PaCO_2$: partial pressure of carbon dioxide; PEEP: positive end-expiratory pressure)

lung compliance rather than the effect of pregnancy on chest wall compliance.[21]

Adequate fetal oxygenation requires a maternal PaO_2 of 70 mm Hg, which corresponds to SpO_2 of 95%.[9] A gradient of approximately 10 mm Hg is required for the adequate clearance of fetal $PaCO_2$ by the placenta.[9] Pregnant patients cannot tolerate permissive hypercapnia as there is increased risk of fetal acidosis. With increase in $PaCO_2$, affinity of fetal hemoglobin for oxygen will decrease. Target $PaCO_2$ levels of 45–55 mm Hg are reasonable in the latter part of pregnancy.[10] Similarly, maternal hyperventilation and hypocapnia should also be avoided while in pregnancy as it is associated with uteroplacental vasoconstriction and reduction in uteroplacental blood flow leading to fetal hypoxia.[22]

Unfortunately, pregnancy has been an excluded from the various randomized controlled trials on ARDS. The general consensus to mechanical ventilation in pregnant patients with ARDS is the same as the general population while preventing ventilator-induced lung injury.

Negative Fluid Balance

Attaining "the dry lungs" may help in improvement of oxygenation and outcome. As the hallmark in ARDS is pulmonary edema, restricting fluid intake and keeping negative fluid balance once circulatory shock is over is beneficial for the patients. Though the FACTT trial had not shown any mortality benefit with the conservative fluid therapy, it resulted in more ventilation free days.[23]

Neuromuscular Blocking Agents

Neuromuscular blocking agents (NMBA) might improve the pulmonary compliance by abolition in spontaneous ventilatory activity, promoting better ventilator patient synchrony. However, prolonged use of NMBA increases the risk of critical illness neuromyopathy. ACURASYS study reported improved outcomes with the early use of NMBA in ARDS patients.[24] However, the ROSE trial found no mortality benefit with NMBA when compared with light sedation targets without NMBA.[25] Unfortunately, this study had a loss of significant patients at screening as they had already received an NMBA prior to randomization.

Prone Position

Prone ventilation has been found effective in pregnant patients with severe ARDS. However, prone ventilation is relatively difficult and has several limitations in parturients. These include the lack of experienced manpower, difficulty to prone term patients, and possibility of hemodynamically instability along with the risk of aortocaval compression. Highly dedicated staff and continuous fetal monitoring is essential during prone ventilation.

Placing patients in the prone position has physiologic benefits that include improved oxygenation attributable to the recruitment and improved ventilation of previously dependent dorsal lung and better perfusion toward the previously better ventilated ventral lung. This results in recruitment of collapsed lung units and more homogeneous distribution of perfusion.[26] The PROSEVA trial showed a mortality benefit in patients who were placed in the prone position within 48 hours after ARDS onset and those who were maintained in the prone position for up to 17 hours/day until the gas exchange significantly improved.[27] A few case-series reports a duration of 8–20 hours of prone positioning in pregnant population.[28] Further studies are necessary to determine the feasibility of prone positioning in pregnant patients.

Corticosteroids

Steroids when used in early ARDS causes downregulation of systemic inflammation, increases ventilator free days, shock-free days along with improvement in oxygenation. The study performed by Annane D et al. recommended the early use of systemic corticosteroids in moderate to severe ARDS (i.e., 14 days of onset).[29] Also, the trial concluded that there was increased rate of death in ARDS, if steroids were initiated after 14 days of diagnosis of ARDS. These principles might be applied to pregnant patients with ARDS as well. However, further trials are required in this group of population.

Extracorporeal Membrane Oxygenation

Extracorporeal membrane oxygenation should be initiated early if the patient has refractory hypoxemia although it exposes the fetus to the complications of systemic heparinization and extracorporeal circulation.[4] The associated bleeding and the risk of thrombosis may influence the decision on cesarean sections. ECMO can be considered if there is a mortality risk ≥50% which can be identified by a PaO_2/FiO_2 < 150, an FiO_2 > 90%, and/or a Murray score of 2-3. ECMO is indicated if the mortality risk is ≥80% which can be identified by a PaO_2/FiO_2 < 100 on FiO_2 > 90%, and/or a Murray score of 3-4.[30]

Sharma et al. reported cases of ECLS during pregnancy and postpartum period, with the conclusion that the maternal survival and fetal survival rates were 80% and 70% respectively.[31] Also, studies done by Moore et al. on ECMO during pregnancy showed that ECMO during pregnancy had reduced maternal and perinatal mortality rates.[30] However, Nair et al. reported that ECMO in pregnancy was technically challenging, bleeding was common requiring large volumes of blood transfusion, which contributed to increased mortality rates.[32]

Extracorporeal Carbon Dioxide Removal

This is a relatively new technology, which mainly targets the removal of CO_2 only. In that sense the application of this technique will be of limited value in severe ARDS patients.

■ SUPPORTIVE CARE

Other supportive care includes sedation, analgesia, nutritional support, deep venous thromboprophylaxis, and stress ulcer prophylaxis.

Imaging in Pregnancy

The various maternal imaging should not be withheld if deemed necessary for the diagnosis and assessment of ARDS. However, the ionizing radiation depending upon the gestation period and the strength of the radiation can have adverse effects on fetus, which includes teratogenicity, increased risk of leukemia and neurological developmental defects **(Table 2)**.

Fetal Monitoring

Daily fetal heart rate monitoring and a weekly fetal Doppler test are important for assessment of fetal growth. However, the stabilization of maternal health is the primary focus and decisions should not be solely based on the fetal monitoring status.

TABLE 2: Risk of radiation from common radiologic investigations.[33,34]

Investigation	Maternal breast exposure (m Gy)	Fetal radiation exposure (m Gy)	Maternal and fetal risk
Chest radiograph	0.2	0.010	Low risk for fetus
Ventilation—perfusion scan	<1.5	0.20–1	Avoid ventilation scan if perfusion is normal
CT chest/angiogram	10–18	0.1–0.8	More exposure on a large fetus

Childbirth

The timing and mode of delivery depends on the progression of ARDS along with maternal and fetal risks and benefits. A multidisciplinary team decision is generally required. Fetal monitoring can help assessment of fetal health till fetal maturity is achieved. Delivery is usually planned after fetal maturity is achieved; however, an urgent delivery might be required in the scenario of deteriorating maternal health. It is important that the ICU should be well equipped for urgent delivery and neonatal resuscitation in the event of spontaneous labor or sudden maternal or fetal deterioration.

Weaning and Rehabilitation

Patients requiring long-term mechanical ventilation or ECMO support may require delivery while on ventilatory support or while on ECMO. Postdelivery, weaning can be expedited by facilitated extubation with NIV support.

Outcome

Mortality of severe ARDS in pregnancy is reported to be 9%, the risk factors being prolonged mechanical ventilation, multiorgan failure, and amniotic fluid embolism.[35]

■ CONCLUSION

Acute respiratory distress syndrome in pregnancy may develop because of disorders specific to the pregnancy such as eclampsia, preeclampsia, amniotic fluid embolism, etc., or generalized disorders such as sepsis from any sources, pancreatitis, trauma, etc.

The clinical diagnosis may be based on the Berlin definition. The management varies depending on the clinical presentation, severity of the disease and response to the specific modalities. As almost all clinical trials on ARDS till date excluded patients with pregnancy from trial enrolment, the evidence in favor of any ventilatory modalities or specific modes and settings are lacking. Most of the intensivists manage ARDS in pregnancy on the basis of their own experience, trial results from case series, pathophysiologic understanding or extrapolation of the study results for different published trials. We need more trials specifically performed in pregnancy with ARDS for better understanding and evidence for optimal outcomes in this group of patients.

■ REFERENCES

1. Ranieri VM, Rubenfeld GD, Thompson BT, Ferguson ND, Caldwell E, Fan E, et al. Acute respiratory distress syndrome: the Berlin definition. JAMA. 2012;307(23):2526-33.
2. Riviello ED, Buregeya E, Twagirumugabe T. Diagnosing acute respiratory distress syndrome in resource limited settings: the Kigali modification of the Berlin definition. Curr Opin Crit Care. 2017;23(1):18-23.
3. Pollock W, Rose L, Dennis CL. Pregnant and postpartum admissions to the intensive care

4. Bhatia PK, Biyani G, Mohammed S, Sethi P, Bihani P. Acute respiratory failure and mechanical ventilation in pregnant patient: a narrative review of literature. J Anaesthesiol Clin Pharmacol. 2016;32(4):431-9.
5. Hegewald MJ, Crapo RO. Respiratory physiology in pregnancy. Clin Chest Med. 2011;32(1):1-13.
6. Bobrowski RA. Pulmonary physiology in pregnancy. Clin Obstet Gynecol. 2010;53(2):285-300.
7. Crapo RO. Normal cardiopulmonary physiology during pregnancy. Clin Obstet Gynecol. 1996;39(1):3-16.
8. Templeton A, Kelman GR. Maternal blood-gases (PaO_2-PaO_2), Hysiological shunt and VD/VT in normal pregnancy. Br J Anaesth. 1976;48(10):1001-4.
9. Catanzarite V, Williams D, Wong D, Landers C, Cousins L, Schrimmer D. Acute respiratory distress syndrome in pregnancy and the puerperium: Causes, courses, and outcomes. Obstet Gynecol. 2001;97(5 Pt1):760-4.
10. Al-Ansari MA, Hameed AA, Al-jawder SE, Saeed HM. Use of noninvasive positive pressure ventilation during pregnancy: case series. Ann Thorac Med. 2007;2(1):23-5.
11. Banga A, Khilnani GC. Use of non-invasive ventilation in a pregnant woman with acute respiratory distress syndrome due to pneumonia. Indian J Chest Dis Allied Sci. 2009;51(2):115-7.
12. Schettino G, Altobelli N, Kacmarek RM. Noninvasive positive-pressure ventilation in acute respiratory failure outside clinical trials: experience at the Massachusetts General Hospital. Crit Care Med. 2008;36(2):441-7.
13. Lee JH, Rehder KJ, Williford L, Cheifetz IM, Turner DA. Use of high flow nasal cannula in critically ill infants, children, and adults: a critical review of the literature. Intensive Care Med. 2013;39(2):247-57.
14. Frat JP, Thille AW, Mercat A, Girault C, Ragot S, Perbet S, et al. High-flow oxygen through nasal cannula in acute hypoxemic respiratory failure. N Engl J Med. 2015;372(23):2185-96.
15. Acute Respiratory Distress Syndrome Network, Brower RG, Matthay MA, Morris A, Schoenfeld D, Thompson BT, et al. Ventilation with lower tidal volumes as compared with traditional tidal volumes for acute lung injury and the acute respiratory distress syndrome. N Engl J Med. 2000;342(18):1301-08.
16. Ware LB, Matthay MA. The acute respiratory syndrome. N Engl J Med. 2000;342(18):1334-49.
17. Kacmarek RM, Villar J, Sulemanji D, Montiel R, Ferrando C, Blanco J, et al. Open lung approach for the acute respiratory distress syndrome: a pilot, randomized controlled trial. Crit Care Med. 2016;44(1):32-42.
18. Meade MO, Cook DJ, Guyatt GH, Slutsky AS, Arabi YM, Cooper DJ, et al. Ventilation strategy using low tidal volumes, recruitment maneuvers, and high positive end-expiratory pressure for acute lung injury and acute respiratory distress syndrome: a randomized controlled trial. JAMA. 2008;299(6):637-45.
19. Brower RG, Lanken PN, MacIntyre N, Matthay MA, Morris A, Ancukiewicz M, et al. Higher versus lower positive end-expiratory pressures in patients with the acute respiratory distress syndrome. N Engl J Med. 2004;351(4):327-36.
20. Mendelson C. The aspiration of stomach contents into lungs during obstetric anesthesia. AM J Obstet Gynecol. 1946;52:191-205.
21. Campbell LA, Klocke RA. Implications for the pregnant patient. Am J Respir Crit Care Med. 2001;163(5):1051-4.
22. Corton M, Leveno K, Bloom S, Spong C, Dashe J. Williams Obstetrics. In: Chapter 47 Critical Care and Trauma, Acute Respiratory Distress Syndrome, 24th edition. New York: McGraw-Hill Education; 2014. pp. 943-6.
23. National Heart, Lung, and Blood Institute Acute Respiratory Distress Syndrome (ARDS) Clinical Trials Network, Wiedemann HP, Wheeler AP, Bernard GR, Thompson BT, Hayden D, et al. Comparison of two fluid-management strategies in acute lung injury. N Engl J Med. 2006;354:2564-75.

24. Bourenne J, Hraiech S, Roch A, Gainnier M, Papazian L, Forel JM. Sedation and neuromuscular blocking agents in acute respiratory distress syndrome. Ann Transl Med. 2017;5:291.
25. The National Heart, Lung, and Blood Institute PETAL Clinical Trials Network. Early neuromuscular blockade in acute respiratory distress syndrome. NEJM. 2019;380:1997-2008.
26. Peck TJ, Hibbert KA. Recent advances in the understanding and management of ARDS. F1000Res 2019;8:F1000 Faculty Rev-1959.
27. Guérin C, Reignier J, Richard JC, Beuret P, Gacouin A, Boulain T, et al. Prone positioning in severe acute respiratory distress syndrome. N Engl J Med. 2013;368(23):2159-68.
28. Samanta S, Samanta S, Wig J, Baronia AK. How safe is the prone position in acute respiratory distress syndrome at late pregnancy? Am J Emerg Med. 2014;32(6):687.e1-3.
29. Annane D, Pastores SM, Rochwerg B, Arlt W, Balk RA, Beishuizen A, et al. Guidelines for the diagnosis and management of critical illness-related corticosteroid insufficiency (CIRCI) in critically ill patients (Part I): Society of Critical Care Medicine (SCCM) and European Society of Intensive Care Medicine (ESICM) 2017. Intensive Care Med. 2017;43:1751-63.
30. Moore SA, Dietl CA, Coleman DM. Extracorporeal life support during pregnancy. J Thorac Cardiovasc Surg. 2016;151(4):1154-60.
31. Sharma NS, Wille KM, Bellot SC, Diaz-Guzman E. Modern use of extracorporeal life support in pregnancy and postpartum. ASAIO J. 2015;61:110-4.
32. Nair P, Davies AR, Beca J, Bellomo R, Ellwood D, Forrest P, et al. Extracorporeal membrane oxygenation for severe ARDS in pregnant and postpartum women during the 2009 H1N1 pandemic. Intensive Care Med. 2011;37:648-54.
33. Parker MS, Hui FK, Camacho MA, Chung JK, Broga DW, Sethi NN. Female breast radiation exposure during CT pulmonary angiography. Am J Roentgenol. 2005;185:1228-33.
34. Burns SK, Haramati LB. Diagnostic imaging and risk stratification of patients with acute pulmonary embolism. Cardiol Rev. 2012;20:15-24.
35. Rush B, Martinka P, Kilb B, McDermid RC, Boyd JH, Celi LA. Acute respiratory distress syndrome in pregnant women. Obstet Gynecol. 2017;129:530-5.

CHAPTER 9

Pulmonary Thromboembolism: Preexistent and Concurrent

Vivek Gupta, Shibba Takkar Chhabra

■ INTRODUCTION

Pregnancy-associated pulmonary thromboembolism (PTE) is difficult to diagnose due to close similarity of physiological changes of pregnancy and clinical presentation of PTE. There is always a risk of radiation exposure for diagnosing pulmonary embolism to both mother and fetus. However, PTE is associated with direct maternal mortality.[1]

Pregnant women have a 5–10 times higher risk of developing thromboembolic event as compared to nonpregnant women of similar age group. The postpartum period poses a higher risk and almost 50% cases occur 3–6 weeks after the delivery. However the PTE risk may persist up to 12 weeks after delivery.[2] Most women with pregnancy-associated PTE usually have one or more identifiable risk factors, more prevalent risk factors include obesity, increasing age, multiple pregnancy, etc., making them high risk for thromboembolic events during peripartum period[3] **(Box 1)**. The high degree of suspicion is key to diagnose and initiate early management since the majority of deaths occur in the initial few hours.

Clinician must be careful in managing these pregnant women for prophylaxis as well as for treatment of pregnancy-associated venous thromboembolism due to potential for complication to both mother and fetus.

■ ETIOLOGY

The incidence of nonfatal PTE and deep vein thrombosis (DVT) is about 1:1,000 in pregnant women in developed world. The hypercoagulability due to pregnancy is primarily due to increase in clotting factors VIII, IX, X, and fibrinogen levels, and a fall in protein S and antithrombin (AT) III level. These physiological alterations in coagulation parameters predispose a pregnant woman to thromboembolic event.[4] The other factors include venous stasis in the lower limbs due to the gravid uterus and immobility during puerperium. Due to venous stasis, there is thrombi formation usually in deep venous system. These thrombi may migrate along with blood to the right atrium, right ventricle, pulmonary artery, and its branches. The hemodynamic instability usually occurs with large embolus and depends upon its location. The small emboli can travel to the distal part and occlude the smaller vessels in the peripheral part of the lungs. The emboli mostly are multiple and are often to the upper lobes of the lungs.[5]

■ DIAGNOSIS

An early suspicion and thorough evaluation of PTE in pregnant women is very important at early stage because most of the deaths occur in the early hours.

> **BOX 1:** Risk factors for pulmonary thromboembolism.
>
> **Peripartum**
>
> *General:*
> - Surgical procedures (e.g., ERPC, postpartum sterilization)
> - Immobility
> - Dehydration
> - Sepsis
> - Travel >4 h
>
> *Antenatal:*
> - Multiple gestation
> - IVF pregnancy
> - Preeclampsia
>
> *Natal:*
> - Emergency cesarean section
> - Prolonged labor
> - Midcavity rotational forceps delivery
>
> *Postnatal:*
> - Postpartum hemorrhage (>1 L)
> - Need of blood transfusion
>
> **Preexisting:**
> - Age >35 years
> - Obesity (BMI >30 kg/m^2)
> - Multiparity
> - Pelvic veins injury
> - Previous history of thromboembolic event
> - Comorbid conditions such as inflammatory diseases, thrombophilia, systemic lupus erythematosus, etc.
> - Varicose veins
> - Smoking
> - Malignancy
> - Immobilization/bed rest
>
> (BMI: body mass index; ERPC: endoscopic retrograde cholangiopancreatogaraphy; IVF: in vitro fertilization)

The PTE may be *acute or chronic*. The acute thrombus can be diagnosed if it is present centrally in the vascular lumen and occluding the diameter of vessel leading to distension of occluded vessel. The chronic pulmonary embolism is characterized by eccentric thrombus, which is contiguous to the vessel wall leading to reduction in vessel diameter >50%, there may be recanalization within the embolus.

The location of thrombus in pulmonary arterial system helps to label as *central or peripheral*. Involvement of main pulmonary artery or its bifurcation or trunk or the lobar arteries is considered as central pulmonary embolism whereas segmental or subsegmental arterial occlusion is considered as peripheral involvement.

If the embolus in present in both pulmonary arteries and a pregnant woman is hemodynamically unstable this is labelled as *massive pulmonary embolism* and is associated with sudden cardiac death. The usual clinical presentation is shock including hypotension, tachypnea, tachycardia and poor peripheral perfusion, pulmonary hypertension, altered sensorium, and decreased urine output.

The diagnoses of pulmonary embolism in the pregnant patient require specific diagnostic tests because the routine investigations may not be specific for confirming the diagnosis.

■ CLINICAL PRESENTATION

The most common symptoms include breathlessness, pleuritic chest pain along with hypoxia along with cough, and occasionally hemoptysis. There may be sudden hemodynamic instability. Pleuritic chest pain at presentation suggests smaller thrombus with peripheral obstruction.

The physical findings depend on the extent of occlusion and are categorized as—massive, acute lung infarction, acute thrombosis without infarction, and multiple lung thrombi.

In *massive event*, the presentation to the hospital is shock, hypotension, sign of poor perfusion, tachycardia, and tachypnea. Pulmonary hypertension may also be evident.

Patients with *acute lung infarction*, present with acute pleuritic chest pain, shortness of breath and hemoptysis. It is difficulty to differentiate the chest pain from pain from myocardial origin. Pleural effusion may also be present. In *acute thrombosis without infarction* nonspecific physical findings such as tachycardia, tachypnea, pleuritic pain crackles, and local wheeze make the diagnosis difficult.[5]

When there is *multiple pulmonary thrombi*, the patient may demonstrate increased venous pressure, thrill over the second left intercostal space, loud P2, right ventricular S3 gallop, systolic murmur at left sternal border, hepatomegaly, ascites, and edema, which is suggestive of pulmonary hypertension and cor pulmonale.[5]

The presentations of acute pulmonary embolism may mimic with other clinical conditions and may be difficult to differentiate **(Table 1 and Box 2)**.

TABLE 1: Acute pulmonary embolism presentations.[6-9]

Presentation	Possible mechanism	Remarks
Sudden cardiac arrest (SCA)	• Acute pulmonary obstruction with embolus • PE with underlying CAD	• Usually with massive PE there is PEA • VT/VF if underlying CAD
ARDS picture	• Release of vasoactive substances from clots • Maldistribution of blood flow	Non-cardiogenic pulmonary edema
Respiratory failure	Ventilation perfusion mismatch	Hypoxia and hypocapnia
Asthmatic crisis	Release of pharmacologically active substances such as histamine	• No previous history of bronchial asthma • No trigger for bronchial asthma
Fever syndrome with or without pseudo-pneumonia and pleural effusion	• Fever • Evidence of pulmonary infiltrates at X-ray	PTE is more sudden onset, and the dyspnea is more prominent than cough and expectoration
Acute right heart failure/shock/hypotension	• A pulmonary vascular obstruction of >30% • Physiologic reaction to the vasoactive substances • Size of embolus	Signs of RV dysfunction ratio of RV to LV end-diastolic diameter >1, or an RV end-diastolic diameter >30 mm and/or loss of inspiratory collapse of the inferior vena cava
Left heart failure with possible pulmonary congestion	• Occlusion of PA branch causing increased flow in the other branches thus increasing lung capillary pressure • Compression of LV by dilated RV	Long-standing dyspnea, bilateral pulmonary congestion dilated RV (D sign)
Chest pain similar to pleuritic syndrome with or without hemoptysis	Pulmonary infarction due to small emboli	
Similar to ACS (with or without chest pain)	• Diffuse subendocardial ischemia, • Subsequent poor coronary blood flow as well as acute RV overload and possible RV infarct	• Chest pain, hypotension, tachycardia, hypoxia; ECG with ST elevation • Coronary angiography revealing nonobstructive coronary arteries

Contd...

Contd...

Presentation	Possible mechanism	Remarks
PE with paradoxical embolism	PTE migrating through an intracardiac or pulmonary shunt into the systemic circulation	• Clinical picture depend on site of embolization • Acute MI • Stroke • Mesenteric ischemia • Lower limb ischemia
Syncope	• Thrombosis of >50% of the lung arterial system leading to hypotension and cerebral hypoperfusion • Activation of the vasovagal reflex • Arrhythmias and conduction disturbances due to RV distension	
• Persistent or paroxysm • Atrial fibrillation (AF), atrial flutter, atrial tachycardia, paroxysmal supraventricular tachycardia (PSVT)	Pulmonary artery stretching	Underdiagnosed because asymptomatic, diagnosis is made only when the patient presents with an arrhythmia

(ACS: acute coronary syndrome; ARDS: adult respiratory distress syndrome; CAD: coronary artery disease; ECG: electrocardiography; LV: left ventricular; MI: myocardial infarction; PA: pulmonary artery; PE: pulmonary embolism; PEA: pulseless electrical activity; PTE: pulmonary thromboembolism; RV: right ventricular; VT/VF: ventricular fibrillation/ventricular tachycardia)

> **BOX 2:** Life-threatening complications of pulmonary embolism.
>
> • Obstructive shock
> • Severe hypoxemia
> • Pulseless electrical activity (cardiac arrest)
> • Atrial or ventricular arrhythmias
> • Paradoxical embolism
> • Acute cor pulmonale

■ INVESTIGATIONS

Blood Test

The routine blood test may not be helpful in diagnosing pulmonary embolism during pregnancy however imaging techniques have the major concern for radiation exposure during pregnancy.

If the detailed history does not reveal any obvious cause for embolic disease, one must look for the deficiency of antithrombin III, protein C or protein S, lupus anticoagulant, occult neoplasm, homocystinuria or connective tissue disorders.

D-dimer Testing

Negative results of D-dimer exclude the diagnosis of pulmonary embolism.[10] However, during pregnancy, D-dimer level increases gradually and falls in the immediate postpartum period and returns to normal after 4–6 weeks making the diagnosis of pulmonary embolism difficult.

Ischemia-modified albumin level (IMA): It has been suggested as a sensitive biomarker as an additional investigation for pulmonary embolism,[11] is still not used widely.

White blood cell counts may be normal or increased but are nonspecific.

The higher levels of serum troponin[12] and brain natriuretic peptide (BNP) are associated with more complications and higher mortality in pulmonary embolism.

Imaging Modalities

The radiation exposure to fetus is relatively low with ventilation–perfusion (around

TABLE 2: Imaging techniques for pulmonary embolism: Pros and cons.[13,14]

Imaging modality	Pros	Cons
X-ray chest		Nonspecific radiation exposure
Echocardiography	• Noninvasive • Central pulmonary embolism can be detected	Smaller emboli may be missed
Ventilation perfusion scan	Low radiation exposure to fetus and breast	• Does not offer alternative diagnosis • Accuracy studies in pregnancy not available
CT pulmonary angiography	• Safe in all trimester of pregnancy • Help in making other diagnosis • Fetal radiation exposure is low • Better availability • Cost effective	*Radiation exposure to breast (reduced with shields):* • Modification required due to pregnancy in imaging and injection protocol • Identification of subsegmental emboli • Impact of iodinated dye on fetal thyroid
Magnetic resonance imaging	• High sensitivity and specificity • No radiation risk • Subsegmental emboli not detected	• Insufficient accuracy or outcome data • Fetal safety due to use of gadolinium

0.32–0.64 mGy) scan and computed tomographic (CT) angiography. The selection of the imaging modality will also depend on availability and expertise **(Table 2 and Box 3)**.

■ MANAGEMENT

An empirical anticoagulation therapy should be started until contraindicated if a pregnant woman is presenting with symptoms and signs strongly suggestive of acute PTE even before the final diagnosis. Once the diagnosis of PTE or DVT is confirmed, therapeutic dose of anticoagulation should be initiated immediately. The use of heparin has reduced mortality from 30 to 10%.[15]

The therapeutic anticoagulation in pregnancy is achieved with heparins (both unfractionated and low molecular weight). Heparin is considered safe since it does not cross the placenta and does not produce teratogenic effects. However the heparin administration is associated with maternal risks such as uteroplacental bleeding hemorrhage, thrombocytopenia, and osteopenia.[16] Once the acute PTE is diagnosed, blood test including complete blood count, liver and renal function tests, electrolytes, and coagulation profile should be performed before initiating anticoagulant therapy.

BOX 3: Confirm diagnosis of pulmonary embolism.

- Intraluminal filling defect on pulmonary angiography or on spiral CTPA
- High probability scan and moderate/high clinical probability
- Evidence of acute DVT with non-diagnostic scan or spiral CTPA

(CTPA: computerized tomography pulmonary angiogram)

The mainstay of treatment of PTE during pregnancy includes low molecular weight heparin (LMWH) throughout the pregnancy after the diagnosis and around 6 weeks in postnatal period. The warfarin crosses the placental barrier and is associated with teratogenic effect to fetus during pregnancy, though it can be safely used in the postpartum period in breastfeeding women.

The direct thrombin inhibitors such as dabigatran, rivaroxaban, apixaban, etc., may cross the placenta and should be avoided in pregnant women. Direct thrombin inhibitors may be administered in women who are not breastfeeding.

Low molecular weight heparin may be administered as single daily or twice daily dose of enoxaparin (1 mg/kg) or dalteparin (100 units/kg) and is usually safe not requiring regular monitoring of coagulation parameters and platelets. The reason for administering twice-daily dose is due to increased renal clearance of LMWH during pregnancy. Lower doses of LMWH should be prescribed in pregnant women with renal impairment, and enoxaparin is a preferred option. Though fondaparinux has been used in pregnancy safely but the use is restricted for cases having heparin allergy or heparin induced thrombocytopenia.[16]

Anti-Xa levels monitoring may be required in patients with morbid obesity, renal dysfunction, and recurrent thromboembolic event. The unfractionated heparin (UFH) is preferred in acute massive pulmonary embolism due to its rapid onset of action and dose adjustment if thrombolytic therapy administered simultaneously. The intravenous administration of UFH includes a loading dose of 80 units/kg, followed by infusion of 18 units/kg/hour. This dose should be titrated on the basis of activated partial thromboplastin time (aPTT) monitoring every 6 hours with target aPTT 46–70 seconds.

The role of thrombolytic therapy in high-risk pulmonary embolism case is not yet defined in pregnant patients, however in the nonobstetric patients, it is used in hemodynamically unstable patients with low risk of bleeding. This may be lifesaving in pregnant patients with massive PTE who are hemodynamic unstable.[17]

A balance between the risk of postpartum hemorrhage and thromboembolic event is paramount during induction and progression of labor in a woman on therapeutic anticoagulation. Spontaneous labor can be considered as an appropriate option if not contraindicated otherwise. The use of LWMH in patients who have been given neuraxial blockade may be a concern due to risk of spinal hematoma. The LMWH should be stopped 24 hours prior, if neuraxial technique is planned for cesarean section. The anticoagulation should be restarted at least 4 hours after subarachnoid block or epidural catheter removal. The therapeutic anti-coagulation should be restarted 6–12 hours after uncomplicated vaginal delivery and 12–24 hours after cesarean section.

Supportive Therapies

Graduated elastic compression stockings reduce pain and swelling in patients with acute DVT, with no increased risk of clot progression and subsequent pulmonary embolism. The use of compression hosiery with predetermined pressure for reducing post thrombotic syndrome has been debated and is not recommended.

Inferior Vena Cava Filters

The role of inferior vena cava (IVC) filters is limited during pregnancy due the risks and complications associated with placement and removal, which include migration of filter, fracture, IVC perforation, and even death. Whenever required a temporary retrievable caval filter may be appropriate in women who are delivering or expected to deliver in <2 weeks of anticoagulation or in women where anticoagulation is contraindicated.

TAKE HOME MESSAGES

- Pregnancy-associated PTE is difficult to diagnose due to close similarity of physiological changes of pregnancy and clinical presentation of PTE.
- Strong degree of suspicion is key to diagnose PTE in pregnancy because many deaths in pregnant patients occur due to either delay in diagnosis or misdiagnosis of pulmonary embolism in spite of advancement in diagnostic modalities.
- The radiation risk to the fetus is minimal with diagnostic imaging for confirmation of diagnosis of pulmonary embolism.
- An early administration of anticoagulation (LMWH or heparin) reduces the severity of disease and risk of death and facilitates normal delivery.
- Management with anticoagulation has improved the survival in PTE. Mortality is low in the first 6 month (<5%) in submassive pulmonary embolism. However there is risk of recurrence.

■ REFERENCES

1. Knight M, Kenyon S, Brocklehurst P, Neilson J, Shakespeare J, Kurinczuk JJ, et al. (Eds). On behalf of MBRRACE-UK. Saving Lives, Improving Mothers' Care: Lessons learned to inform future maternity care from the UK and Ireland Confidential Enquiries into Maternal Deaths and Morbidity 2009-12. Oxford, University of Oxford; 2014.
2. Jacobsen AF, Skjeldestad FE, Sandset PM. Incidence and risk patterns of venous thromboembolism in pregnancy and puerperium: a register-based case-control study. Am J Obstet Gynecol. 2008;198:233. e1-e7.
3. Knight M, UKOSS. Antenatal pulmonary embolism: risk factors, management and outcomes. BJOG. 2008;115:453-61.
4. Gherman RB, Goodwin TM, Leung B, Byrne JD, Hethumumi R, Montoro M. Incidence, clinical characteristics, and timing of objectively diagnosed venous thromboembolism during pregnancy. Obstet Gynecol. 1999;94(5 Pt 1):730-4.
5. Ouellette DR, Harrington A, Kamangar N. Pulmonary Embolism. In: Mosenifar Z (Ed). 2018.
6. Bougouin W, Marijon E, Planquette B, Karam N, Dumas F, Celermajer DS, et al. Factors associated with pulmonary embolism-related sudden cardiac arrest. Circulation. 2016;134(25):2125-7.
7. Wood KE. Major pulmonary embolism: review of a pathophysiologic approach to the golden hour of hemodynamically significant pulmonary embolism. Chest. 2002;121:877-905.
8. Omar HR. ST-segment elevation in V1-V4 in acute pulmonary embolism: a case presentation and review of literature. Eur Heart J Acute Cardiovasc Care. 2016;5: 579-86.
9. Duplyakov D, Kurakina E, Pavlova T, Khokhlunov S, Surkova E. Value of syncope in patients with high-to-intermediate risk pulmonary artery embolism. Eur Heart J Acute Cardiovasc Care. 2015;4(4):353-8.
10. Tapson VF. Acute pulmonary embolism. N Engl J Med. 2008;358(10):1037-53.
11. Turedi S, Gunduz A, Mentese A, Topbas M, Karahan SC, Yeniocak S, et al. The value of ischemia-modified albumin compared with d-dimer in the diagnosis of pulmonary embolism. Respir Res. 2008;9:49.
12. El-Menyar A, Sathian B, Al-Thani H. Elevated serum cardiac troponin and mortality in acute pulmonary embolism: systematic review and meta-analysis. Respir Med. 2019;157:26-35.
13. Chan WS, Ray JG, Murray S, Coady GE, Coates G, Ginsberg JS. Suspected pulmonary embolism in pregnancy: clinical presentation, results of lung scanning, and subsequent maternal and pediatric outcomes. Arch Intern Med. 2002;162(10):1170-5.
14. Shahir K, Goodman LR, Tali A, Thorsen KM, Hellman RS. Pulmonary embolism in pregnancy: CT pulmonary angiography versus perfusion scanning. Am J Roentgenol. 2010;195:W214-20.

15. Royal College of Obstetricians and Gynaecologists. (2015). Thromboembolic Disease in Pregnancy and the Puerperium: Acute Management Greentop Guideline No. 37b. [online] Available from: https://www.rcog.org.uk/en/guidelines-research-services/guidelines/gtg37b/ [Last accessed February, 2023].
16. Bates SM, Ginsberg JS. How we manage venous thromboembolism during pregnancy? Blood. 2002;100(10):3470-8.
17. Konstantinides SV, Meyer G, Becattini C, Bueno H, Geersing GJ, Harjola VP, et al. ESC Scientific Document Group, 2019. ESC Guidelines for the diagnosis and management of acute pulmonary embolism developed in collaboration with the European Respiratory Society (ERS): The Task Force for the diagnosis and management of acute pulmonary embolism of the European Society of Cardiology (ESC). Eur Heart J. 2020;41(4):543-603.

CHAPTER 10

Nonthrombotic Pulmonary Embolism

Ahsan Ahmed, Anirban Bose

■ INTRODUCTION

Nonthrombotic pulmonary embolism is a rare but life-threatening condition due to embolization to the pulmonary circulation by various cells/tissues, organisms, foreign materials, or gas. The purpose of this review is to describe the different subtypes of nonthrombotic pulmonary embolism observed in obstetric patients.

■ AMNIOTIC FLUID EMBOLISM

Introduction: Amniotic fluid embolism is a rare but catastrophic syndrome usually occurring during labor, delivery or in the postpartum period. The first case was reported in 1926 but it was recognized widely in 1941.

Epidemiology and magnitude of the problem: The incidence of amniotic fluid embolism varies from one in 12,000 to one in 50,000. Although it is rare, it is common in the population of women who died during pregnancy. Actual incidence and mortality due to amniotic fluid embolism is confounded by many factors such as variable clinical definition, overlapping symptoms, and an absence of gold standard diagnostic tests. It is usually a diagnosis of exclusion.[1]

Implications for maternal health: This life-threatening condition is initiated by the entry of amniotic fluid, fetal cells, hair, and other debris in maternal circulation. Usual risk factors are cesarean section, instrumental delivery, cervical trauma, placenta previa and abruption, eclampsia, polyhydramnios, multiple gestation, maternal age and parity, and male fetus.[1]

Clinical presentation is not uniform, although it classically presents as sudden onset hypotension and hypoxemia, followed by coagulopathy.[2] The mechanism of hemodynamic alteration is poorly understood. The mechanical obstruction theory is losing popularity as recent evidence shows activation of systemic inflammatory response syndrome (SIRS) like inflammatory responses causing transient pulmonary and systemic vasoconstriction, leading to myocardial depression and circulatory collapse. Hypoxemia occurs due to profound shunting followed by pulmonary edema and/or lung injury such as acute respiratory distress syndrome. Amniotic fluid activates platelet factor III, factor X, complement factors as well as the coagulation cascade leading to diffuse intravascular coagulation and hemorrhage. Neurological symptoms ranging from altered mentation to tonic-clonic seizures are due to injury to the central nervous system by inflammatory mediators, hypotension, and hypoxemia.[1-3]

Management: Diagnosis of amniotic fluid embolism is largely clinical with classical triad of hypoxemia, hypotension, and coagulopathy along with onset during labor and delivery or within first 30 minutes of postpartum period.[2] Differential diagnoses such as pulmonary thromboembolism, air embolism, anaphylaxis, high spinal anesthesia, peripartum cardiomyopathy, myocardial infarction, septic shock, transfusion reaction, hemorrhage, eclampsia, placental abruption, and uterine rupture should also be kept in mind.[1]

The mainstay of treatment is cardiopulmonary stabilization. The initial phase consists of right ventricular failure, which should be treated with preload optimization, vasopressors, and mechanical ventilatory support with emphasis on avoidance of hypoxemia, hypercarbia, and acidosis to prevent increase in pulmonary vascular resistance. Dobutamine and milrinone are used to improve right ventricular output while sildenafil, inhaled, or intravenous prostacyclin and inhaled nitric oxide are used to reduce pulmonary vascular resistance. However, the data is not promising. Gradually, the left ventricle fails and causes further hemodynamic alteration.[1] At this stage patient may need intra- aortic balloon pump (IABP) or extracorporeal membrane oxygenation (ECMO) support but severe coagulopathy restricts its use.[2,4]

Coagulopathy and bleeding should be managed by blood component therapy as per standard guidelines. Massive blood transfusion protocol may need to be initiated.[1,3] Use of activated recombinant factor VIIa has been reported but significant adverse effects limit its use.[4]

In case of cardiac arrest, resuscitation and post-resuscitation care should be done as per advanced cardiovascular life support (ACLS) guidelines. Removal of fetal monitor during defibrillation to prevent formation of electrical arch has theoretical benefits. If an undelivered viable fetus is present, expeditious delivery by operative vaginal delivery if patient is on labor, or cesarean section otherwise, is indicated. Perimortem cesarean section is indicated if spontaneous circulation is not restored within 4 minutes of cardiac arrest. Preparation for perimortem cesarean section should be started along with cardiopulmonary resuscitation.[2]

■ FAT EMBOLISM

Introduction: Fat embolism was first described way back in 1861. Fat embolism is defined as the release of fat into the circulation but fat embolism syndrome is a rare clinical consequence, characterized by respiratory distress, altered mental status, and petechial rash.

Epidemiology and magnitude of the problem: Fat embolism occurs in nearly all patients with pelvic or long bone fractures undergoing endomedullary procedure or joint prosthesis placement, due to disruption of sinusoids, but fortunately, fat embolism syndrome is rarely observed.

Fat embolism is also common after blast injury without skeletal injury where the soft tissue is likely to be the source. Fat embolism can also occur in patients receiving intraosseous transfusions, bone marrow infarcts due to sickle cell anemia and prolonged steroids therapy. Acute pancreatitis, mobilization of fat in viral hepatitis in preexisting fatty liver, liquefying hematoma, liposome-embedded drugs, total parenteral nutrition are very unusual causes of fat embolism. In rare circumstances, fat embolism has been reported after normal delivery and cesarean section and in acute fatty liver of pregnancy.[4,5]

Implications for maternal health: Pathophysiology of fat embolism syndrome remains unclear. Two theories have been proposed, the mechanical theory and the biochemical theory. In the mechanical theory, small fat globules obstruct the pulmonary capillary causing interstitial hemorrhage and edema as well as hypoxic pulmonary vasoconstriction while large fat globules obstruct a major pulmonary artery causing major hemodynamic instability. Some fat globules enter the systemic circulation via a pulmonary capillary or any arteriovenous shunt. They may get deposited in the brain and can cause petechial hemorrhage. They are also deposited in the skin, causing petechial rash. In the biochemical theory, the release of high concentration of glycerol and toxic free fatty acids in circulation initiates the inflammatory cascade leading to end-organ damage, causing pulmonary hemorrhage and edema, acute renal injury and disseminated intravascular coagulation.[4,6]

Patients usually present with hypoxemia, altered neurological status (encephalopathy, focal neurodeficit, seizure, and coma) and petechial rash. Other associated findings are fever, anemia, thrombocytopenia, altered renal and liver function and retinopathy. In severe cases, patients may have right ventricular followed by biventricular dysfunction, acute respiratory distress syndrome, coagulopathy, and shock.[4,6]

Management: Diagnosis is usually clinical and supported by imaging and laboratory values. The Gurd and Wilson's criteria are widely used for diagnosis. One of the three major criteria (respiratory distress, petechial rash, cerebral symptoms in nonhead injury patient) and four of the eight minor criteria (tachycardia, fever, jaundice, renal changes, retinal changes, acute anemia, acute thrombocytopenia, elevated erythrocyte sedimentation rate and fat macroglobulinemia) are required to diagnose the case. Investigations such as complete blood picture, inflammatory markers, blood culture, liver, and renal function, chest radiograph, echocardiography, and magnetic resonance imaging (MRI) brain should be carried out.[4,6]

Differential diagnosis should include pulmonary thromboembolism, amniotic fluid embolism, air embolism, and acute myocardial infarction. Sepsis must also be kept in mind.

Treatment is largely supportive as fat embolism is self-limiting. Cardiopulmonary support along with usual critical care management is all that is needed. Severe cases may need ECMO support. Cardiac arrest and post-resuscitation care should be done as per ACLS protocol.[4,6]

TROPHOBLASTIC MATERIAL EMBOLISM

Introduction: Gestational trophoblastic disease is a group of lesion originating from abnormal proliferation of placental trophoblastic epithelium. It includes hydatidiform mole (partial or complete) and malignancies (invasive mole, choriocarcinoma, and placental site trophoblastic tumors). It was first described way back in 1893.

Epidemiology and magnitude of the problem: In both normal and abnormal pregnancies, a good amount of trophoblastic material enters into the maternal circulation but trophoblastic embolism is usually seen in gestational trophoblastic disease and rarely in eclampsia and placental side. The actual incidence of trophoblastic material embolism is unknown. A total of 3–25% molar evacuation patients become symptomatic.[4]

Implications for maternal health: The most common symptom is shortness of breath, which is rarely severe and self-limited.

Trophoblastic tissue in circulation and in the lung presents in majority of the patients but severe symptoms such as circulatory collapse and cardiac arrest are rarely reported. Severe symptoms are most likely due to pulmonary edema due to accompanying hyperthyroidism, dilutional anemia, preeclampsia, fluid overload, or any combination of these.[4,7,8]

Implications for Fetal Well-being

Management: Diagnosis is usually clinical in view of background history. Radiographic features include alveolar, nodular and miliary patterns and signs of pulmonary artery occlusion.

Treatment is largely symptomatic and supportive. Oxygen therapy and diuretics are the mainstay of treatment. In severe cases, patients need ventilatory and vasopressor support. Patients with cardiac arrest need resuscitation and post-resuscitation care as per ACLS protocol. Emergency pulmonary embolectomy was also reported in a case.[4,7,8]

■ SEPTIC EMBOLISM

Introduction: Septic pulmonary embolism is a rare but life-threatening condition usually associated with right-sided infective endocarditis, infected deep venous thrombosis, infected vascular catheter, periodontal disease, infection elsewhere with septal defect, and immunodeficiency.

Epidemiology and magnitude of the problem: The reported incidence of infective endocarditis in pregnant women is 0.006% and septic embolism is even rarer. Early recognition of infection and use of appropriate antimicrobial therapy has reduced the incidence significantly but a little increase is seen recently due to increased number of intravenous drugs users.[9]

Implications for maternal health: Staphylococcus aureus (S. aureus) is the most commonly involved organism. Staphylococcus infection has a rising trend due to an increasing number of drug users. Fungal emboli are usually found in malignancy patients. Anaerobic organisms are commonly involved in oropharyngeal and maxillofacial infections.[4,9]

Clinical features include features of extra pulmonary infections along with cough, hemoptysis, chest pain, and shortness of breath.

Management: Investigations include complete hemogram, infection markers, blood cultures, renal and liver function tests, urine analysis, echocardiography (transesophageal is superior to transthoracic to see vegetation, abscess, and leaflet perforation), CT chest with angiography and other investigations according to the source. Chest radiograph may show patchy pneumonia, feeding vessel sign, cavities, or abscess formation.[4,9]

The mainstay of treatment is management of sepsis with appropriate antibiotics and other supportive care. Inferior vena cava filter has theoretical benefit in proximal deep venous thrombosis with sepsis but the efficacy and safety is questionable. Although surgery is indicated in some severe cases, it should be balanced with the high risk of mortality.[4,9]

■ GAS EMBOLISM

Introduction: Gas embolism is a well-recognized phenomenon in obstetric population. It was first reported in the obstetric population in 1850. Two types of gas embolism can occur, arterial, and venous. Among these, venous air embolism is more common and is usually iatrogenic.

Epidemiology and magnitude of the problem: Venous air embolism is the most common embolism in obstetric population but fortunately, the amount of air entering is not significant to cause symptoms. Most commonly, air enters during cesarean section due to exteriorization of the uterus. Oral sex by insufflating large amount of air in vagina during pregnancy or puerperium can cause air embolism. Other infrequent causes are placenta previa, manual extraction of placenta, uterine rupture, criminal abortion, manipulation of central venous catheter, and hemodialysis catheter, infusion through peripheral venous cannula, and invasive and non-invasive ventilation.[10]

Implications for maternal health: Usually, the pulmonary capillaries prevent entry of air into the systemic and coronary circulations. Large accumulation of air in the pulmonary circulation can cause right ventricle outflow obstruction leading to right ventricular failure. Adhered and absorbed air bubbles can activate the inflammatory cascade leading to lung edema, microthrombi formation, and coagulopathy. Rarely, air bubble can enter the systemic circulation via an arteriovenous shunt or by overwhelming the pulmonary capillary trapping mechanism causing end organ infarcts such as cerebral or cardiac infarcts.[10,11]

Cough, dyspnea, tachypnea, chest pain are common symptoms and acute cardiorespiratory failure can occur in severe cases. Paradoxical embolism can cause neurological symptoms such as focal neurodeficit, visual disturbance, headache, seizure, and acute coronary syndrome like symptoms. Cyanosis, pallor, mottled skin, pallor of mucous membranes, pallor in tongue, air in retinal vessels, and a "mill-wheel" murmur can be found.[10,11]

Management: Diagnosis is largely done by history of the event and clinical scenario. End-tidal carbon dioxide ($EtCO_2$) monitor can facilitate early detection. Intracardiac air can be detected by precordial Doppler, transthoracic Doppler, and trans-esophageal Doppler (most sensitive). A computed tomography scan of the chest may show pulmonary edema, dilatation of pulmonary artery, and air in the pulmonary artery or right heart. An MRI brain can pick up a cerebral infarct and electrocardiogram (ECG), echocardiography, and cardiac enzymes can detect coronary insufficiency.

The first step of treatment for venous air embolism is to stop further entry of air. Semi-Fowler position with leftward tilt is advisable to prevent further air entry and promote movement of air from right ventricle to pulmonary capillary. Maintaining adequate preload, providing 100% oxygen, and vasopressor support is an absolute necessity. If the patient is under general anesthesia, Nitrous oxide should be stopped and ventilation should be adequate. Suction of the air from right ventricle by multiple orifice central venous or pulmonary artery catheter, keeping it's tip 2 cm below the junction of right ventricle and superior vena cava is recommended as it can suck out up to 50% of entrained air. Arterial air embolism is managed by flat position, hyperbaric oxygen therapy and management of cerebral and coronary infarct. Nitric oxide can be used and role of fluorocarbon is under investigation.[4,10,11]

IMPLICATIONS FOR FETAL WELL-BEING

Non-thrombotic pulmonary embolism causes cardiopulmonary issues in various degrees. The fetus can suffer from hypoxic and hypotensive insult in severe cases and prognosis is usually guarded. There are no consensus recommendations for the delivery of the fetus. In case of severe cardiorespiratory instability and fetal age more than 23 weeks, prompt delivery is usually indicated. If the fetal age is <23 weeks and maternal condition is not life-threatening, decision should be taken on a case-to-case basis.

TAKE HOME MESSAGES

- Nonthrombotic pulmonary embolism is a rare but life-threatening condition.
- Nonthrombotic pulmonary embolism should be suspected along with other causes, if a patient has cardiorespiratory symptoms in the peripartum period.
- There is no gold standard test for diagnosis.
- Diagnosis, in a majority of cases, is done by exclusion.
- Treatment is usually supportive, along with good critical care practice.

■ REFERENCES

1. Shamshirsaz AA, Clark SL. Amniotic fluid embolism. Obstet Gynecol Clin N Am. 2016;43:779-90.
2. Society for Maternal-Fetal Medicine (SMFM). Pacheco LD, Saade G, Hankins GD, Clark SL. Amniotic fluid embolism: diagnosis and management. Am J Obstet Gynecol. 2016;215:B16-24.
3. Kaur K, Bhardwaj M, Kumar P, Singhal S, Singh T, Hooda S. Amniotic fluid embolism. J Anaesthesiol Clin Pharmacol. 2016;32(2):153-9.
4. Jorens PG, Van Marck E, Snoeckx A, Parizel PM. Nonthrombotic pulmonary embolism. Eur Respir J. 2009;34:452-74.
5. Schrufer-Poland T, Singh P, Jodicke C, Reynolds S, Maulik D. Nontraumatic fat embolism found following maternal death after cesarean delivery. AJP Rep. 2015;5(1):e1-e5.
6. Kosova E, Bergmark B, Piazza G. Fat embolism syndrome. Circulation. 2015;131:317-20.
7. Smith JC, Alsuleiman SA, Bishop H, Kassar NS, Jonas HS. Trophoblastic pulmonary embolism. South Med J. 1981;74(8):916-9.
8. Delmis J, Pfeifer D, Ivanisevic M, Forko JI, Hlupic L. Sudden death from trophoblastic embolism in pregnancy. Gynecol Reprod Biol. 2000;92(2):225-7.
9. English N, Weston P. Multivalvular infective endocarditis in pregnancy presenting with septic pulmonary emboli. BMJ Case Rep. 2015;2015:bcr2014209131.
10. Gei AF, Vadhera RB, Hankins GD. Embolism during pregnancy: thrombus, air, and amniotic fluid. Anesthesiol Clin N Am. 2003;21(1):165-82.
11. Mushkat Y, Luxman D, Nachum Z, David MP, Melamed Y. Gas embolism complicating obstetric or gynecologic procedures: case reports and review of the literature. Eur J Obstet Gynecol Reprod Biol. 1995;63(1):97-103.

Cardiovascular Disorders

CHAPTER 11

Hypertensive Emergencies

Siri Yerubandi

■ INTRODUCTION

Hypertensive emergency in obstetrics is defined as acute-onset, severe hypertension with a blood pressure of more than or equal to 160/110 mm Hg, which is persistent over 15 minutes during pregnancy and the postpartum period.[1] It is often associated with end-organ damage, which includes the brain, the eyes, the heart, the liver, the kidneys, and central and peripheral arteries.[2] Irrespective of the underlying cause, this condition requires immediate intervention and intensive care as markedly elevated blood pressure if not treated promptly can lead to hypertension-mediated end-organ damage like cerebral hemorrhage, pulmonary edema, myocardial infarction, and eclampsia.[3]

■ EPIDEMIOLOGY

Hypertensive disorders of pregnancy affect one out of every 10 women and are one of the leading causes of maternal mortality worldwide and the incidence is much higher in low and middle-income countries.[4] Hypertensive emergencies affect 1% of women with hypertensive disorders of pregnancy with a significantly higher mortality rate if not treated immediately and women with preexisting hypertension, cardiovascular, and renal diseases are more vulnerable. Though hypertensive disorders of pregnancy rank after postpartum hemorrhage in causing maternal deaths, verbal autopsies from low- and middle-income countries have inferred those women who presented with bleeding had premonitory symptoms of eclampsia indicating that they might have had complications such as abruption and disseminated intravascular coagulation, which was masked by low blood pressure at the time of presentation due to significant bleeding. This indicates that the mortality rate due to hypertensive disorders during pregnancy is higher than reported and this can be brought down by reducing delay in transport and initiation of treatment.[5]

■ MATERNAL COMPLICATIONS

Women with acute uncontrolled hypertension can present with stroke (25%), pulmonary edema (23%), congestive heart failure (12%), acute kidney injury, and intracranial hemorrhage, aortic dissection, eclampsia, and retinal involvement.[6] Among these, the cerebral injury was found to be the most common cause of maternal death.[7]

Stroke

Stroke during pregnancy can be either hemorrhagic or ischemic and systolic blood pressure of more than or equal to 160 mm Hg is a more important determinant compared to diastolic blood pressure.[8] With an incidence of 30/100,000 pregnancies, the risk of stroke in pregnancy is 3 times higher than in the nonpregnant state.[9] Hemorrhagic stroke is more prevalent in women with advanced maternal age and preeclampsia when compared to ischemic stroke. In the presence of preeclampsia, the incidence of stroke is 4 times higher and in the absence of preeclampsia, the incidence of stroke was almost nil, and this is attributable to disrupted blood-brain barrier due to failure of cerebral autoregulation and endothelial dysfunction, which are associated with preeclampsia and eclampsia. The risk of stroke is higher in the postpartum period emphasizing the importance to follow-up on women with pregnancies complicated by preeclampsia.

Respiratory Failure

Pulmonary edema is another life-threatening condition caused by elevated systolic blood pressure above 160 mm Hg more commonly when complicated by preeclampsia or eclampsia with an incidence ranging from 0.6 to 5%.[10] Increased hydrostatic pressure in capillaries caused by a rise in afterload, reduced oncotic pressure in plasma, and endothelial dysfunction, which are consequences of preeclampsia altogether lead to pulmonary edema.

Congestive Heart Failure

Increased peripheral vascular resistance due to high blood pressure increases afterload leading to congestive heart failure. The risk of heart failure is increased by twofold in pregnancies complicated by severe hypertension in the immediate and later part of life.

Renal Failure

Acute kidney injury is commonly associated with HELLP (hemolysis, elevated liver enzymes, low platelet count) syndrome with an incidence of 1–5% and is due to endotheliosis of the glomerular capillary bed. The maternal and fetal mortality rate associated with acute kidney injury is as high as 30–60% and the morbidity leading to renal dialysis and transplantation is also significantly high.

Eclampsia

This is a result of uncontrolled blood pressure causing failure of cerebral autoregulation in women with preeclampsia, which presents as generalized tonic-clonic seizures in the absence of other cerebral diseases and the incidence is around 5%.

Severe Maternal Morbidity

One of the strategies to reduce maternal mortality is to investigate factors leading to severe maternal morbidity, which precedes death. The grave circumstance that is faced by a woman due to severe morbidity is like those just before death. Hypertensive disorders of pregnancy along with hemorrhage are the common causes of severe maternal morbidity and mortality in both high- and low-income countries. The incidence of severe maternal morbidity in hypertensive emergencies is as high as 10%.[11]

■ FETAL COMPLICATIONS

The pathophysiology of hypertensive disorders of pregnancy resulting in uteroplacental and fetoplacental insufficiency contributes to fetal growth restriction, preterm delivery and stillbirth, respiratory distress, intensive care unit admission, and neonatal deaths. The risk of fetal growth restriction and stillbirth is one and a half times higher in pregnancies affected with hypertension.[12] The end-organ damage that is caused by an acute rise in blood pressure also involves the placenta leading to abruption, resulting in stillbirth within no time if not intervened immediately.

■ DIAGNOSIS

Blood Pressure

Hypertensive emergency in pregnancy is diagnosed when a woman presents with either of the following:
1. A systolic blood pressure of 160 mm Hg or more and diastolic blood pressure of 110 mm Hg or more are recorded twice at an interval of 15 minutes.
2. A single record of systolic blood pressure equal to 160 mm Hg or more and diastolic blood pressure equal to 110 mm Hg or more in the presence of symptoms related to end-organ damage.

Signs and Symptoms

The clinical manifestation depends on the organ involved and triaging immediately based on the symptoms at arrival is an essential step. Around 22% of women present with shortness of breath, 27% with chest pain, and 21% with neurological symptoms such as headache, visual disturbances, and altered consciousness, which indicate hypertension mediated end-organ damage. The woman should be admitted into a high dependency unit and treated immediately to prevent progression to permanent damage.

■ MATERNAL EVALUATION

A complete history of drug usage, past medical history, and present medications should be noted. The physical examination directed towards evaluating for end-organ damage should be undertaken. Oxygen saturation of <93%, respiratory rate above 24/min, and grunting or gurgling sounds on auscultation indicate pulmonary edema.

Laboratory evaluation should include the following:
1. Hemogram to look for hemolysis and thrombocytopenia indicating endothelial damage.
2. Serum creatinine, 24-hour urine protein, or urinary spot protein creatinine ratio to rule out renal involvement.
3. Liver function tests wherein if the liver enzymes are elevated twice the normal range are considered as significant.
4. Serum electrolytes and lactate dehydrogenase.
5. Electrocardiogram (ECG) and chest X-ray when suspecting pulmonary edema.
6. Imaging in the presence of neurological symptoms to rule out intracranial hemorrhage, cerebral thrombosis, and posterior reversible encephalopathy syndrome.
7. Ultrasound abdomen if there is abdominal pain to look for hepatic hematoma and rupture.

■ FETAL EVALUATION

If the fetus is viable, fetal evaluation should include:
- Fetal heart rate monitoring during maternal stabilization.
- Ultrasound to rule out fetal growth restriction and amniotic fluid assessment.
- Doppler study to look for uteroplacental or fetoplacental insufficiency.

■ MANAGEMENT

The adverse maternal and fetal outcomes in a hypertensive emergency can be prevented by early identification and initiation of the treatment. Maternal early warning trigger (MEWT) tool is one of the clinical tools, which is designed to identify women with abnormal physiology and addresses four major causes of maternal morbidity and mortality. The hypertension pathway is one among them and overlaps with the cardiovascular dysfunction pathway.[13] The pathway is activated when the blood pressure is persistently elevated to 160/110 mm Hg and above or in the presence of headache, visual disturbances, vomiting, and abdominal pain. Antihypertensive drugs should be administered within 1 hour, maternal and fetal evaluation to be done and magnesium sulfate infusion to be given if blood pressure remains constantly elevated or in the presence of clinical symptoms despite well-controlled blood pressures. Pulmonary edema is suspected if a woman with severe hypertension presents with a low oxygen saturation of <93% or a respiratory rate of >24/min. In the presence of signs indicating respiratory failure, overlap with the cardiopulmonary pathway to rule out other cardiac causes to be thought out and evaluated accordingly **(Flowchart 1)**.

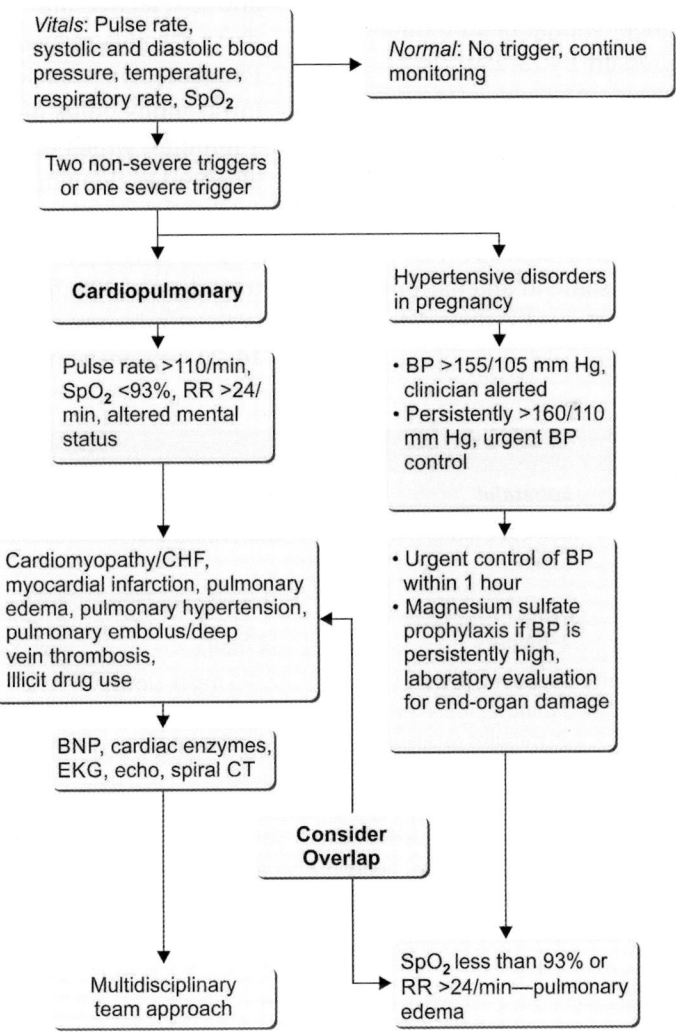

Flowchart 1: MEWT hypertension pathway.

(BNP: brain natriuretic peptide; BP: blood pressure; CHF: congestive heart failure; CT: computed tomography; EKG: electrocardiogram; MEWT: maternal early warning trigger; RR: respiratory rate)

Reducing blood pressure expeditiously is the primary goal in the management of hypertensive emergency. Antihypertensive treatment should be initiated immediately to reduce systolic blood pressure to <160 mm Hg maintaining at 140–150 mm Hg and diastolic blood pressure to be maintained at 90–100 mm Hg. Sudden fall in blood pressure results in ischemia, infarction, and uteroplacental hypoperfusion leading to adverse maternal and fetal outcomes. Considering the adverse effects of sudden hypotension, the aim of initiating treatment should be to reduce the mean arterial pressure by 15–25%.

ANTIHYPERTENSIVE DRUGS FOR HYPERTENSIVE EMERGENCY IN PREGNANCY

The antihypertensive therapy for acute hypertension is the same in antepartum and postpartum (up to 6 weeks after delivery) period.

Labetalol and hydralazine are administered intravenously and immediate release nifedipine is administered orally. No significant difference was found among these three drugs concerning safety and efficacy and any of these drugs can be used based on the clinical situation.[14] In the absence of intravenous access immediate-release oral nifedipine is the preferred choice of drug **(Table 1)**.[1]

- Labetalol is a non-selective beta-blocker and a selective alpha-1 blocker. It is a direct vasodilator metabolized in the liver. For acute hypertension, it is given as an intravenous bolus of 20 mg slowly over 2 minutes, which can be repeated every 20 minutes, doubling the bolus dose to a maximum of 80 mg/bolus based on the response, not exceeding the maximum total dose of 300 mg. The onset of action is 5–10 minutes with a peak action at 10–20 minutes and a half-life of 6 hours.

TABLE 1: First line antihypertensive drugs used in a hypertensive emergency.

	Labetalol	Hydralazine	Nifedipine
Mechanism of action	Selective alpha-1 and beta-blocker	Direct vasodilator	Calcium channel blocker
Onset of action	5–10 minutes	10 minutes	5–10 minutes
Duration of action	2–6 hours	12 hours	2–4 hours
Dose	10–20 mg IV bolus over 2 minutes repeated every 20 minutes escalating the bolus up to 80 mg maximum of 300 mg	2.5–5 mg IV slowly repeated every 20–40 minutes	10–20 mg oral repeated every 30 minutes maximum of 50 mg
Contraindications	Asthma, bradycardia, heart block, congestive heart failure, cardiogenic shock	Mitral valve rheumatic heart disease, coronary artery disease, stroke	Aortic stenosis, coronary artery disease, severe hypotension, acute myocardial infarction, cardiogenic shock
Pregnancy category	C	C	C

American College of Obstetricians and Gynaecologists Taskforce on Hypertension in Pregnancy. Hypertension in pregnancy.

Labetalol reduces blood pressure by causing vasodilatation due to alpha-blockade without the side-effect of tachycardia due to beta-blockade action. It can be given as a single drug in the coarctation of the aorta. It is contraindicated in asthmatics, acute congestive heart failure, bradycardia, and heart blocks.

- Hydralazine is a hydrazine-derived vasodilator that reduces systemic vascular resistance by its direct effect on arterioles. It directly relaxes the smooth muscle in the precapillary resistance vessels with the least effect on the postcapillary venous capacitance vessels. Hydralazine is metabolized in the liver and 15% of it is excreted unchanged by the kidneys. The onset of action is slower compared to labetalol which occurs at around 5–30 minutes after administration and the effect lasts up to 2–6 hours. The dose is 2.5–5 mg intravenous bolus, which is repeated every 20 minutes until the desired blood pressure control. Hydralazine can cause hypotension and reduced urine output when given to women who are already volume depleted. Its side effects are headache, dizziness, nausea, tremors, and reflex tachycardia. It should be given with caution to women with raised intracranial pressures as it causes cerebral vasodilatation and consequently cerebral edema.
- Nifedipine belongs to the dihydropyridine class of calcium-channel blockers, which act by reducing the entry of calcium ions into the muscle cells in the heart and blood vessels resulting in vasodilation. It is available as oral preparations available in different formulations. For hypertensive emergency, immediate-release oral nifedipine is given in doses of 10–20 mg repeated every 30 minutes until the target blood pressure is achieved to a maximum of 50 mg. The most common side effects are headache, nausea, dizziness, flushing, and tachycardia.

The algorithms for drug dosage and escalation according to the response for the first-line antihypertensive drugs are depicted in **Flowcharts 2 to 4**.

In case of resistant hypertension wherein the first-line drugs have failed to reduce blood pressure, the second-line antihypertensive drugs to be considered are nicardipine, esmolol, nitroglycerine, sodium nitroprusside.

- Nicardipine is a second-line antihypertensive agent, which is administered intravenously in a hypertensive emergency. This is another calcium-channel blocker belonging to the dihydropyridine class, which acts on the smooth muscle of blood vessels reducing peripheral vascular resistance. It has a rapid onset of action within 5–15 minutes and a short half-life, which allows for easy titration. It brings about general arterial dilatation with selective action on cerebrovascular and coronary arteries and thus is a good option in preventing cerebral and cardiac ischemia. It increases the stroke volume without affecting uteroplacental or fetal circulation.[15] It is given as an infusion of 2.5–5 mg/hour up to a maximum of 15 mg/hour until the desired response. Its side effects are headache, flushing, and dizziness and are contraindicated in severe aortic stenosis.
- Nitroglycerine is an antihypertensive drug that is administered intravenously and is particularly useful in the presence of pulmonary edema. It is given as an infusion of 1–10 mg/hour.
- Esmolol is a short-acting cardioselective beta-1 blocker with an onset of action

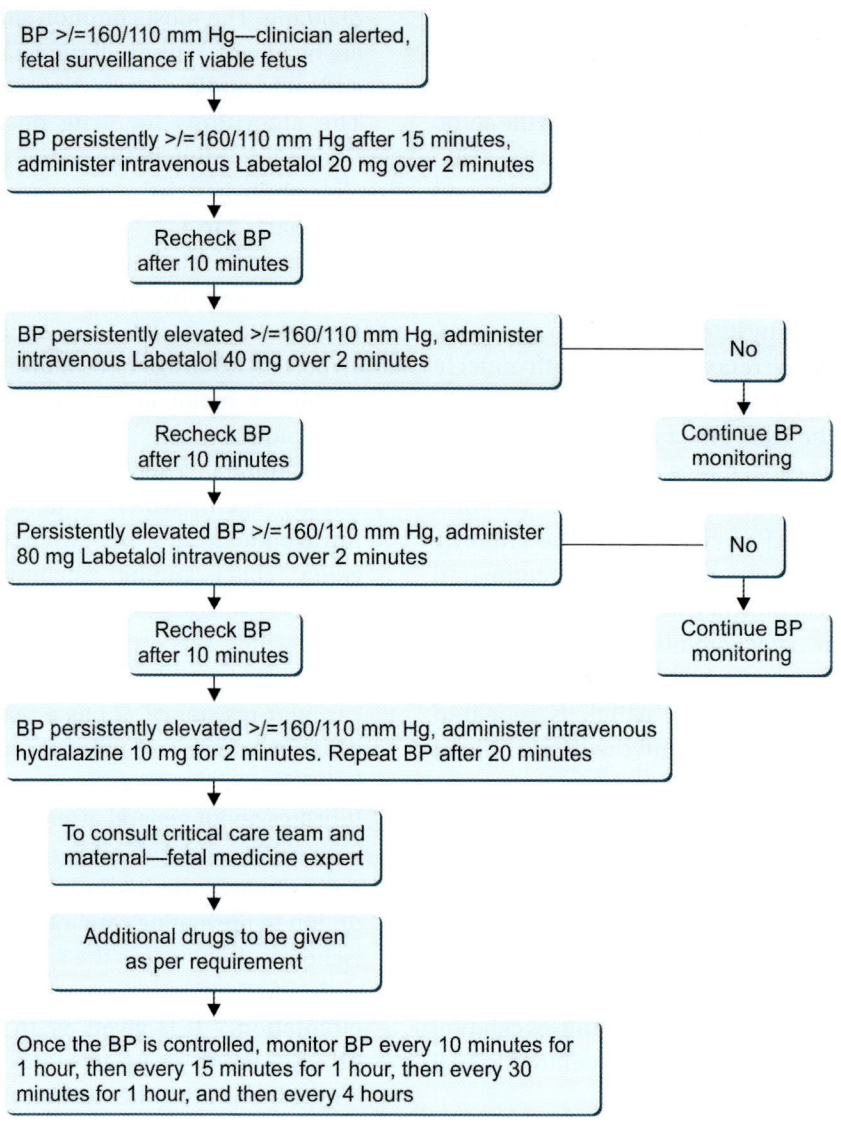

Flowchart 2: Labetalol algorithm.

(BP: blood pressure)

within 60 seconds, which lasts for 15–30 minutes. It is given as an intravenous bolus of 500 µg/kg, with a maintenance dose of 50 µg/kg/min. It is increased by 50 µg/kg/min every 4 minutes to a maximum dose of 300 µg/kg/min. It is a preferred drug in acute myocardial infarction and aortic dissection and is contraindicated in congestive heart failure, first-degree heart block, bronchospasm, and maternal bradycardia. It can also cross the placenta and cause fetal bradycardia.

- Sodium nitroprusside is a fast-acting drug with a short period of action that acts by releasing nitric oxide. It is given

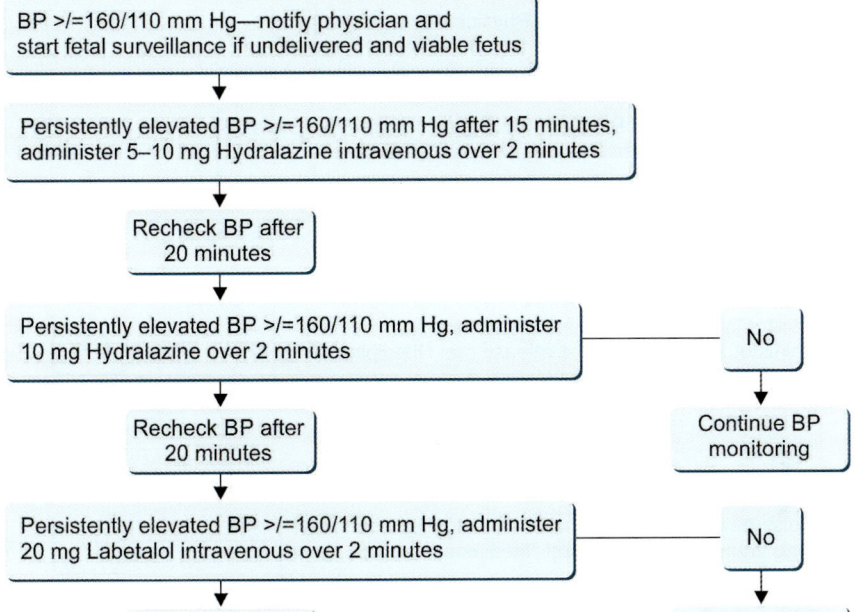

Flowchart 3: Hydralazine algorithm.

(BP: blood pressure)

as an intravenous infusion of 0.25 µg/kg/min and increased by 0.25–0.5 µg/kg/min every 2–3 minutes with the onset of action within 1 minute lasting for 2–3 minutes. It is indicated in aortic dissection, left ventricular dysfunction, and pulmonary edema. When given for a prolonged duration or in the presence of renal insufficiency, cyanide toxicity is an important concern and hence should be considered as a last resort when the hypertension is not controlled by other agents.

The choice of the antihypertensive drug also depends on the organ involved as shown in **Table 2**.[2]

Seizure Prophylaxis

In addition to immediate control of severe hypertension in women with preeclampsia, simultaneous administration of magnesium

Flowchart 4: Nifedipine algorithm.

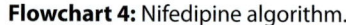

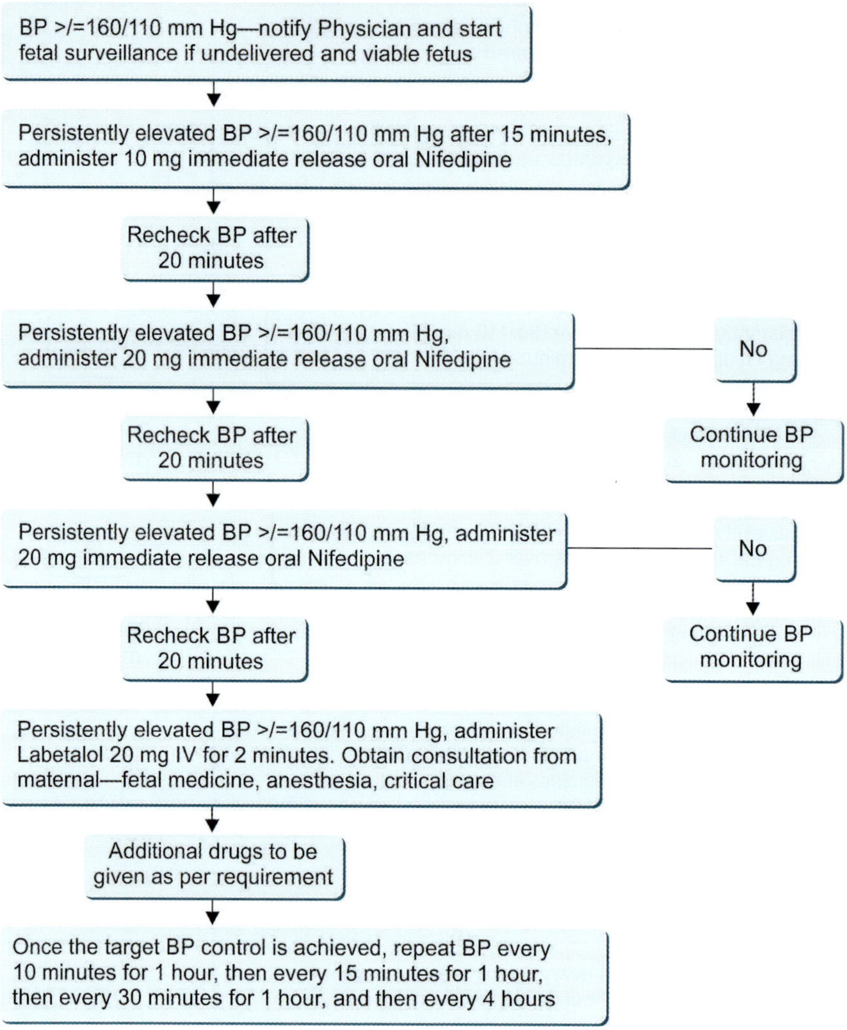

(BP: blood pressure; IV: intravenous)

sulfate has proven to significantly reduce the incidence of eclampsia halving the rate in both antenatal and postpartum periods.[16]

Fetal Assessment

This depends on the gestational age at presentation wherein the fetal monitoring commences after the period of viability and all women with a hypertensive emergency should be delivered after 34 weeks after steroid cover if she is stable and blood pressure is under control.

Acute and severe hypertension is an emergency that needs a systematic approach to diagnosing and implementing the treatment regime. Hence, it is detrimental that all the healthcare workers are aware of the management protocol. Implementation of treatment algorithms has been shown to reduce the time taken for initiating therapy **(Flowchart 5)**.

TABLE 2: Hypertensive emergencies requiring immediate blood pressure control.

Clinical presentation	Timeline and target BP	First-line treatment
Malignant hypertension with or without TMA or acute renal failure	Several hours, MAP −20% to −25%	Labetalol Nicardipine
Hypertensive encephalopathy	Immediate, MAP −20% to −25%	Labetalol Nicardipine
Acute ischemic stroke and SBP >220 mm Hg or DBP >120 mm Hg	1 hour, MAP −15%	Labetalol Nicardipine
Acute ischemic stroke with an indication for thrombolytic therapy and SBP >185 mm Hg or DBP >110 mm Hg	1 hour, MAP −15%	Labetalol Nicardipine
Acute hemorrhagic stroke and SBP >180 mm Hg	Immediate, 130 <SBP <180 mm Hg	Labetalol Nicardipine
Acute coronary event	Immediate, SBP <140 mm Hg	Nitroglycerine Labetalol
Acute cardiogenic pulmonary edema	Immediate, SBP <140 mm Hg	Nitroprusside or nitroglycerine (with loop diuretic)
Acute aortic disease	Immediate, SBP <120 mm Hg and heart rate <60 bpm	Esmolol and nitroprusside or nitroglycerine or nicardipine
Eclampsia and severe preeclampsia/HELLP	Immediate, SBP <160 mm Hg and DBP <105 mm Hg	Labetalol or nicardipine and magnesium sulfate

(DBP: diastolic blood pressure; HELLP: hemolysis, elevated liver enzymes, low platelet count; MAP: mean arterial pressure; SBP: systolic blood pressure; TMA: thrombotic microangiopathy)

Source: van den Born BH, Lip GYH, Brguljan-Hitij J, Cremer A, Segura J, Morales E, et al. ESC Council on Hypertension Position Document on the Management of Hypertensive Emergencies. Eur Heart J Cardiovasc Pharmacother. 2019;5(1):37-46. Erratum in: Eur Heart J Cardiovasc Pharmacother. 2019;5(1):46.

TAKE HOME MESSAGES

- Acute-onset, severe hypertension with a blood pressure of more than or equal to 160/110 mm Hg, which is persistent over 15 minutes during pregnancy and postpartum is treated as a hypertensive emergency.
- Antihypertensive drugs should be administered within 60 minutes of recording a blood pressure of more than or equal to 160/110 mm Hg to avoid end-organ damage.
- Intravenous labetalol and hydralazine, immediate-release oral nifedipine are the first line of antihypertensive drugs that are used to treat the hypertensive emergency.
- The target of blood pressure control is to maintain systolic blood pressure at 140–150 mm Hg and a diastolic blood pressure at 90–100 mm Hg reducing the mean arterial pressure by 15–25% to prevent hypotension.
- Setting up treatment algorithms for quick reference in emergency conditions helps in reducing delays in initiating treatment and improving the quality of care.

Flowchart 5: Treatment algorithm for hypertensive emergency.

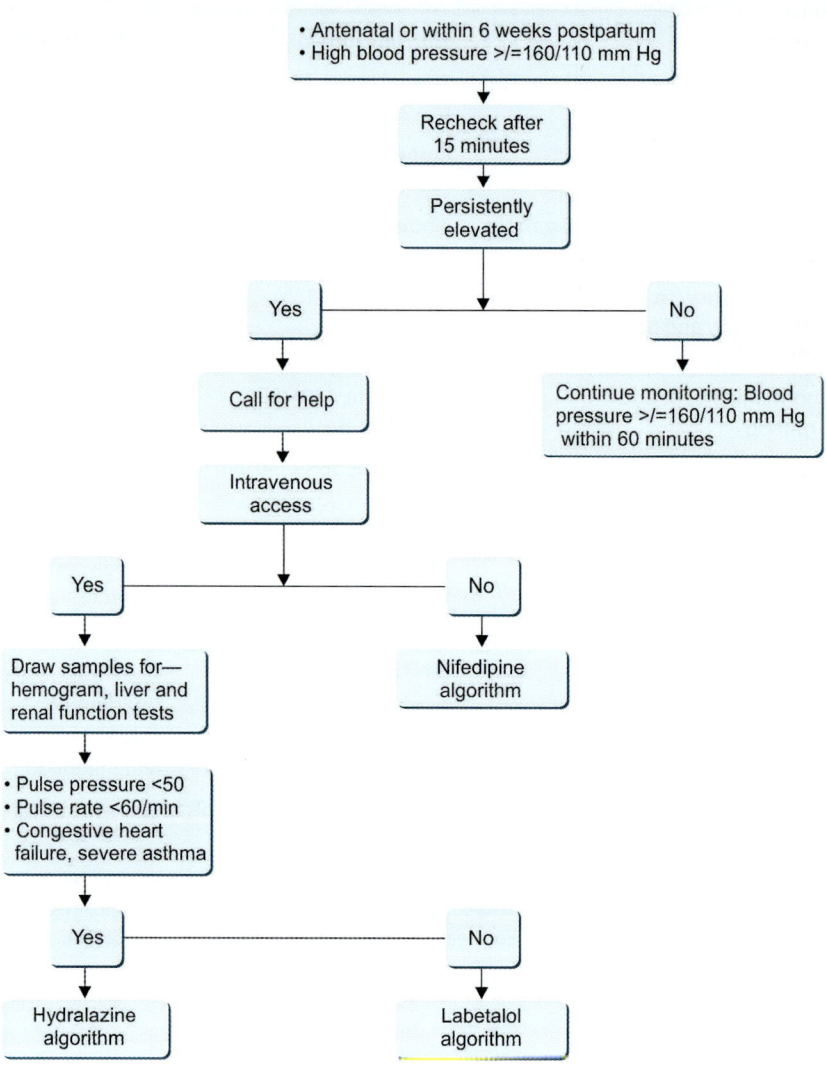

REFERENCES

1. ACOG Committee Opinion No. 767. Emergent therapy for acute-onset, severe hypertension during pregnancy and the postpartum period. Obstet Gynecol. 2019;133(2): e174-80.
2. van den Born BH, Lip GYH, Brguljan-Hitij J, Cremer A, Segura J, Morales E, et al. ESC Council on Hypertension Position Document on the Management of Hypertensive Emergencies. Eur Heart J Cardiovasc Pharmacother. 2019;5(1):37-46. Erratum in: Eur Heart J Cardiovasc Pharmacother. 2019;5(1):46.
3. Cantwell R, Clutton-Brock T, Cooper G, Dawson A, Drife J, Garrod D, et al. Saving mothers' lives: reviewing maternal deaths to make motherhood safer: 2006–2008. The eighth report of the confidential enquiries into maternal deaths in the United Kingdom. BJOG. 2011;118(suppl 1):1-203.

4. Firoz T, Sanghvi H, Merialdi M, von Dadelszen P. Pre-eclampsia in low- and middle-income countries. Best Pract Res Clin Obstet Gynaecol. 2011;25:537-48.
5. Hutcheon JA, Lisonkova S, Joseph KS. Epidemiology of pre-eclampsia and the other hypertensive disorders of pregnancy. Best Pract Res Clin Obstet Gynaecol. 2011;25(4):391e403.
6. Dhadke SV, Dhadke VN, Batra DS. Clinical profile of hypertensive emergencies in an intensive care unit. J Assoc Physicians India. 2017;65(5):18-22.
7. Martin JN Jr, Thigpen BD, Moore RC, Rose CH, Cushman J, May W. Stroke and severe preeclampsia and eclampsia: a paradigm shift focusing on systolic blood pressure. Obstet Gynecol. 2005;105:246-54.
8. Swartz RH, Cayley ML, Foley N, Ladhani NNN, Leffert L, Bushnell C, et al. The incidence of pregnancy-related stroke: a systematic review and meta-analysis. Int J Stroke. 2017;12:687-97.
9. Liu S, Chan W-S, Ray JG, Kramer MS, Joseph KS. Stroke and cerebrovascular disease in pregnancy: incidence, temporal trends, and risk factors. Stroke. 2019;50:13-20.
10. Pordeus ACB, Katz L, Soares MC, Maia SB, Amorim MMR. Acute pulmonary edema in an obstetric intensive care unit: a case series study. Medicine (Baltimore). 2018; 97(28):e11508.
11. Kilpatrick SJ, Abreo A, Greene N, Melsop K, Peterson N, Shields LE, et al. Severe maternal morbidity in a large cohort of women with acute severe intrapartum hypertension. Am J Obstet Gynecol. 2016; 215(1):91.e1-7.
12. Allen VM, Joseph K, Murphy KE, Magee LA, Ohlsson A. The effect of hypertensive disorders in pregnancy on small for gestational age and stillbirth: a population-based study. BMC Pregnancy Childbirth. 2004;4(1):17.
13. Shields LE, Wiesner S, Klein C, Pelletreau B, Hedriana HL. Use of Maternal Early Warning Trigger tool reduces maternal morbidity. Am J Obstet Gynecol. 2016; 214(4): 527.e1-527.e6.
14. Duley L, Meher S, Jones L. Drugs for treatment of very high blood pressure during pregnancy. Cochrane Database Syst Rev. 2013;2013(7):CD001449.
15. Cornette J, Buijs EA, Duvekot JJ, Herzog E, Roos-Hesselink JW, Rizopoulos D, et al. Hemodynamic effects of intravenous nicardipine in severely pre-eclamptic women with a hypertensive crisis. Ultrasound Obstet Gynecol. 2016;47(1):89-95.
16. Altman D, Carroli G, Duley L, Farrell B, Moodley J, Neilson J, et al. Do women with pre-eclampsia, and their babies, benefit from magnesium sulfate? The Magpie Trial: a randomized placebo-controlled trial. Lancet. 2002;359:1877-90.

CHAPTER 12

Valvular Heart Diseases in Pregnancy

Anisha Gala Shah

■ INTRODUCTION

Maternal mortality ratio (MMR) in India declined by 17 points in 2016-2018 as compared to years 2014-2016. In the years 2016-2018 it was reported to be 113/100,000 births[1] and in the year 2020 MMR was 99/100,000.[2] This was for the first time that MMR had reached double digit number for India. The commonest causes noted for maternal death were hemorrhage, sepsis, hypertensive diseases, and complications of illegal abortion.[2] Cardiac diseases amount to indirect cause of maternal death.

■ EPIDEMIOLOGY AND MAGNITUDE OF THE PROBLEM

In the United States, cardiovascular diseases are the commonest cause of maternal death.[3,4] The incidence has risen from 7.2/100,000 in 1987 to 17.2/100,000 in 2015.[3,4] This is because a greater number of women with advanced age and those with comorbidities are planning pregnancy. Also, women with congenital heart conditions are surviving to reproductive age. In India, cardiac diseases complicate 1-4% of pregnancies.[5] Of these, rheumatic heart diseases (RHD) is a major (69%) contributor.[5] Most of the conditions are mixed mitral valve diseases.[5] Mitral valve is the commonest single valve involved.[5,6] In one study, the incidence of combined mitral stenosis (MS) and mitral regurgitation (MR) was 52.7%, isolated MS 27.7%, and multiple valve lesions 12.9%.[5] Another study found incidence of MS as 69%, MR 35.2%, aortic stenosis (AS) 9.8%, aortic regurgitation (AR) 17%, and bicuspid aortic valve 2.8%.[6] Maternal mortality is seen in 0.5-7% of these women.[5]

■ IMPLICATIONS ON MATERNAL HEALTH

This subset of women is at high risk for maternal mortality and morbidity. The ability of a woman to carry her pregnancy depends on factors such as functional class [New York Heart Association (NYHA)] **(Table 1)**, hemodynamic implications of the underlying lesion, presence of pulmonary hypertension (of any cause), and presence of cyanosis (arterial oxygen saturation <80%).[7,8] History of arrhythmias, transient ischemic attack or cardiac failure is a predictor of poor outcome. Echocardiographic findings such as left heart obstruction (mitral valve area <2 cm^2 or aortic valve area <1.5 cm^2) and myocardial dysfunction [left ventricular ejection fraction (LVEF) <40%] pose a serious threat to maternal life. Regardless of lesion, NYHA functional class III and IV have poor outcome.

Taking above points into account, various risk scoring systems to assess risks of

TABLE 1: New York Heart Association (NYHA) functional class.

Class I	No limitation of physical activity. Ordinary physical activity does not cause undue fatigue, palpitation, and dyspnea
Class II	Slight limitation of physical activity. Comfortable at rest. Ordinary physical activity results in fatigue, palpitation, and dyspnea
Class III	Marked limitation of physical activity. Comfortable at rest. Less than ordinary activity causes fatigue, palpitation, or dyspnea
Class IV	Unable to carry on any physical activity without discomfort. Symptoms of heart failure at rest. If any physical activity is undertaken, discomfort increases

TABLE 2: CARPREG risk score (each carries 1 point).

- *Prior cardiac event:*
  - Cardiac insufficiency
  - Transient ischemic attack
  - Arrhythmia
  - Stroke
- NYHA class >II or cyanosis
- *Left ventricular obstruction:*
  - Mitral valve area <2 cm^2
  - Aortic valve area <1.5 cm^2
  - Peak left outflow gradient >30 mm Hg
- Reduced systemic ventricular function (LVEF <40%)

Score	Risk of complications
0	5%
1	27%
2	75%

(CARPREG: cardiac disease in pregnancy; LVEF: left ventricular ejection fraction; NYHA: New York Heart Association)

pregnancy in cardiac disease have been developed (CARPREG, CARPREG II, ZAHARA) as depicted in **Tables 2, 3** and **4** respectively.[9-11] The modified World Health Organization (mWHO) risk scoring system is disease specific and most widely used **(Table 5)**.[8] Ideally, all women planning pregnancy must undergo lesion-specific risk estimation based on mWHO scoring system. The risk must be revaluated once the pregnancy is confirmed and also be done as morbidities add on (example—preeclampsia). This is best done by a specialized team (pregnancy heart team or cardio-obstetric team) geared to care for these women.[8]

Ideally, a compromised valvular condition must be treated before conception. If valve replacement is needed, a bioprosthetic valve must be considered over mechanical one in women of reproductive age to avoid complications of thromboembolism and anticoagulant drugs in pregnancy. However, each case must be individualised.[4] Women with left sided stenotic lesions, mechanical prosthetic valves, moderate or severe regurgitant lesions, ventricular dysfunction, and those with pulmonary hypertension are at highest risk of adverse outcomes. Hence, these women must ideally be evaluated, treated, and counseled before conception.[4]

IMPLICATIONS ON FETAL WELL-BEING

The risks to fetus are miscarriage, growth restriction, preterm birth, low birth weight, and stillbirth. In women with mechanical valves, apart from the risk of fetal loss, there is also a risk of warfarin embryopathy owing to anticoagulation regimens.[8]

Implications on maternal and fetal well-being due to specific lesions are covered in the discussion that follows.

TABLE 3: CARPREG II risk score.

Predictor	Score
Prior cardiac events or arrhythmia	3
Baseline NYHA III/IV or cyanosis	3
Mechanical valve	3
LVEF <55%	2
High risk valve disease or left ventricular outflow tract obstruction (mitral valve area <2 cm^2, aortic valve area <1.2 cm^2 or gradient across aortic valve >30 mm Hg)	2
Pulmonary arterial hypertension (RVSP >49 mm Hg)	2
High risk aortopathy	2
Coronary artery disease	2
No prior cardiac intervention	1
Late pregnancy assessment	1
Score	**Risk**
1	5%
2	10%
3	15%
4	22%
>4	41%

(CARPREG: cardiac disease in pregnancy; LVEF: left ventricular ejection fraction; NYHA: New York Heart Association; RVSP: right ventricular systolic pressure)

TABLE 4: ZAHARA risk score.

Predictor	Score
Prior arrhythmia	1.5
NYHA >II	0.75
Use of cardiovascular drugs before pregnancy	1.5
Severe LV obstruction (AV area <1 cm^2, AV gradient >50 mm Hg)	2.5
Moderate/severe systemic AV defect	0.75
Moderate/severe systemic subpulmonary AV defect	0.75
Mechanical valve prosthesis	4.5
Cyanotic heart disease (treated/untreated)	1
Score	**Risk**
0	2.9%
0–1.5	7.5%
1.51–2.5	17.5%
2.51–3.5	43.1%
>3.5	70%

(AV: aortic valve; LV: left ventricular; NYHA: New York Heart Association; ZAHARA: Zwangerschap bij Aangeboren Hartafwijking)

TABLE 5: Modified World Health Organization (mWHO) classification of maternal cardiovascular risk.

WHO pregnancy risk classification (risk of pregnancy by medical condition)	Cardiovascular conditions by WHO risk class
WHO risk class I: No detectable increased risk of maternal mortality and no or mild increase in morbidity	• *Uncomplicated, small, or mild:* 　– Pulmonary stenosis 　– Patient ductus arteriosus 　– Mitral valve prolapse • Successfully repaired simple lesions (atrial or ventricular septal defect, patent ductus arteriosus, anomalous pulmonary venous drainage) • Atrial or ventricular ectopic beats, isolated
WHO risk class II (If otherwise well and uncomplicated): Small increased risk of maternal mortality or moderate increase in morbidity	• Unoperated atrial or ventricular septal defect • Repaired tetralogy of Fallot • Most arrhythmias
WHO risk class II or III (depending on individual): Risk as indicated in class II (above) or class III (below)	• Mild left ventricular impairment • Hypertrophic cardiomyopathy • Native or tissue valvular heart disease not considered WHO I or IV • Marfan syndrome without aortic dilatation • Aorta <45 mm in bicuspid aortic valve • Repaired coarctation
WHO risk class III: Significantly increased risk of maternal mortality or severe morbidity. Expert counseling required. If pregnancy is decided upon, intensive specialist cardiac and obstetric monitoring needed throughout pregnancy, childbirth, and the puerperium	*Mechanical valve:* • Systemic right ventricle • Fontan circulation • Cyanotic heart disease (unrepaired) • Other complex congenital heart disease • Aortic dilatation 40–45 mm in Marfan syndrome • Aortic dilatation 45–50 mm in aortic disease associated with bicuspid aortic valve
WHO risk class IV (pregnancy contraindicated): Extremely high risk of maternal mortality or severe morbidity; pregnancy contraindicated. If pregnancy occurs termination should be discussed. If pregnancy continues, care as for class III	• Pulmonary arterial hypertension of any cause • Severe systemic ventricular dysfunction (LVEF <30% mm) • Previous peripartum cardiomyopathy with any residual impairment of left ventricular function • Severe symptomatic mitral or aortic stenosis • Marfan syndrome with aorta dilated >45 mm • Aortic dilation >50 mm in aortic disease associated with bicuspid aortic valve • Native severe coarctation

(LVEF: left ventricular ejection fraction)

■ STENOTIC LESIONS

The greatest challenge in stenotic lesions is that of coping with increased (up to 50%) cardiac output. Left-sided stenotic lesions pose the highest risk in pregnancy.[4]

Mitral Stenosis

Rheumatic MS is more common than congenital MS.

The symptoms in MS may range from asymptomatic individuals to those having dyspnea, orthopnea, paroxysmal nocturnal dyspnea, or productive cough with pink, frothy sputum. On examination, one may see mitral facies, tapping apex, loud S1 with opening snap and a low-pitched mid-diastolic murmur. Diagnosis and evaluation of severity is done by echocardiogram. Mild MS is generally well tolerated in pregnancy. Half of women with mitral valve area (MVA) <1.5 cm^2 and one-third of women with MVA <1 cm^2 have heart failure.[8,12] Owing to hemodynamic changes in pregnancy, an asymptomatic woman may deteriorate as second and third trimester approaches.

Management in pregnancy includes medical therapy to avoid tachycardia (risk of heart failure as diastolic filling time of LV is decreased in an already compromised LV filling due to stenosis) and fluid overload. Beta blockers must be initiated if the woman is symptomatic, belongs to NYHA >II, MVA is <1 cm^2 or right ventricular systolic pressure (RVSP) is >50 mm Hg. Physical activity must be restricted. Diuretics may be prescribed if symptoms persist.[4,7,8] Anticoagulation is recommended in cases of LA area >6 cm^2, paroxysmal or permanent atrial fibrillation (AF), LA thrombus or prior history of embolism.[4,7,8]

Surgical management includes balloon valvotomy or closed mitral commissurotomy. Both may be done after 20 weeks of gestation in cases of NYHA >II, RVSP >50 mm Hg or in women with recurrent episodes of pulmonary edema despite medical management.[4,7,8]

Obstetric management includes antenatal check-ups every month till 28 weeks and fortnightly thereafter. At each visit, one must enquire about cardiac symptoms, check vitals, look for any change in murmur, assign NYHA class, measure symphysio-fundal height and educate the woman about signs of heart failure. Fetal evaluation must be done by first trimester screening for aneuploidies by ultrasound and biochemical markers, second trimester targeted screening for structural anomalies and assessing fetal growth, and liquor third trimester onward.

Women with mild MS and no other complications may be allowed for vaginal delivery (cut short second stage to avoid maternal exhaustion). However, women with NYHA >II or those with complications of MS such as heart failure or AF must undergo a planned caesarean section. Tachycardia must be avoided by providing adequate hydration, pain relief, practicing asepsis, and active management of third stage of labor.

There is <10% risk of AF due to left atrial (LA) dilatation. This may trigger heart failure or thromboembolic event.[8,12] Mortality is 0–3% in western countries, but higher in lower- and middle-income countries.[8] Complications such as AF, cardiac failure or pulmonary edema must be managed as one would do in a non-pregnant state. Those with MVA <1 cm^2, NYHA >II, RVSP >30 mm Hg are poor predictive factors.[7,8,12]

Aortic Stenosis

Aortic stenosis due to bicuspid aortic valve is commoner than rheumatic AS.

Women with AS may be asymptomatic for a long time. Symptoms appear once there is LV hypertrophy due to outflow obstruction. They include dyspnea, exercise intolerance, angina, and syncope. Examination reveals sustained apical impulse and a harsh crescendo-decrescendo systolic murmur. Diagnosis is confirmed by echocardiography. Exercise tolerance must be evaluated prior to pregnancy. Pregnancy must be discouraged in those with poor exercise tolerance, symptomatic patients or impaired LV function.[4,7,8] These women must be offered valve replacement before embarking on pregnancy.

Pregnancy is usually well tolerated even in women with severe AS, provided their exercise tolerance is good. The risk of cardiac failure is <10% in those who were asymptomatic before pregnancy and in those with moderate AS, while it is 25% in symptomatic women. The risk of arrhythmias and mortality is low with optimal management. Women with bicuspid valve and those with AV area <50 mm^2 have low risk of aortic dissection.[8,12]

Medical management includes physical activity restriction, heart rate control (beta blockers, which also help in coronary circulation) and decongestive therapy (diuretics).[4,8] Surgical options include valvotomy and valve replacement. Both may be done in second trimester in symptomatic women despite drugs.[8]

Fetal risks include genetic transmission of LV outflow tract malformations (in women with bicuspid valve) miscarriage (<5%) preterm birth, and low birth weight (20-25%).[8] Antenatal and intrapartum care must be provided as described in MS. Vaginal birth must be considered in asymptomatic women with moderate AS. Others must undergo a planned cesarean section.[8]

Tricuspid Stenosis and Pulmonary Stenosis

Tricuspid stenosis is generally not seen in women of childbearing age. Pregnancy is well tolerated even in severe pulmonary stenosis.[4]

■ REGURGITANT LESIONS

Regurgitant lesions are generally well tolerated in pregnancy. This is because systemic vasodilatation leads to fall in peripheral vascular resistance, which helps to reduce regurgitation. In pre-pregnant state, evaluation with echocardiogram must be done to look for LV function and diameter. Pregnancy is well negotiated if there is no LV dysfunction.[7,8]

Mitral Regurgitation

It is seen due to rheumatic, congenital, or degenerative causes. Some women may be asymptomatic. Others may show symptoms due heart failure or pulmonary hypertension. On examination, one may find high pitched systolic murmur at apex, radiating to axilla. Echocardiogram confirms the diagnosis.

There is 20-25% risk of cardiac failure in women with moderate and severe MR. Fetal risks include 5-10% risk of growth restriction.[8,12]

Management involves management of fluid overload (diuretics). Acute severe regurgitation must be managed by medications for heart failure and treatment of cause when warranted (example—repair of chordae tendineae rupture).[8,12]

Antenatal and intrapartum periods must be managed as discussed in MS. Vaginal birth must be offered if there are no complications such as LA dilatation and pulmonary hypertension and NYHA class is <II. Others may undergo a planned cesarean.

Aortic Regurgitation

The cause of aortic regurgitation can be either rheumatic, congenital, or degenerative. AR may remain asymptomatic for a long time. Symptoms appear when LV dilatation takes place and there is congestive cardiac failure. Symptoms may be chest pain, palpitations, dyspnea or orthopnea. Examination reveals low-pitched diastolic murmur at the apex, wide pulse pressure, and a hyperdynamic apex. Peripheral signs of AR may be seen too. Echocardiogram confirms the diagnosis.

Maternal risk is that of cardiac failure if there is LV dilatation. Fetal risks are similar to risks with MR. Medical management is by decongestion therapy (diuretics) and heart rate control (beta blockers). Antepartum and intrapartum management must be done as is described in MS. Vaginal birth may be offered if NYHA class is <II and there are no complications.

Acute aortic regurgitation is a medical emergency. Management includes stabilization of the woman and surgical repair or replacement of the valve. It can be done in any trimester of pregnancy. But if fetus is of viable gestational age, then delivery should precede valve surgery.[8]

Tricuspid Regurgitation

Tricuspid regurgitation (TR) is usually due to Ebstein's anomaly or endocarditis. In symptomatic women with severe TR, valve repair must be done prior to pregnancy. Maternal risk in TR in pregnancy is determined by presence of pulmonary hypertension (poor prognosis). Even with severe TR, heart failure in pregnancy can be managed with standard protocols. Valve repair in pregnancy is done when there is annular dilatation (>40 mm).[4,8,12]

Prosthetic Valves

Women with tissue valves are at an advantage that they may escape anticoagulation. However, when there is valve dysfunction, the risk of complications (valve thrombosis, pulmonary edema due to non-functional valve) increases. Those with mechanical valves pose greatest risk to the mother and fetus and must be discussed prior to pregnancy.

The risks to mother are thrombosis (4.1-9%), thromboembolism (16%) and severe morbidity (41%) and mortality (20%) as quoted in various studies.[8,12] This risk of thrombosis was reduced to 1-4% with vitamin K antagonists (VKA). Anticoagulation with unfractionated heparin (UFH) poses a risk of valve thrombosis in first trimester (9-33%), osteoporosis and thrombocytopenia.[8,12,13] Amongst all anticoagulation drugs available, VKA throughout pregnancy poses least risk of thrombosis. Low molecular weight heparin (LMWH) seems better than UFH for prevention of thrombosis.[8,13]

Fetal risks are miscarriage (women on VKA in first trimester have higher risk as compared to those on LMWH and UFH -28.6 vs 9.2%), growth restriction, intracranial hemorrhage, and warfarin embryopathy.[12] Fetal loss is higher in VKA + LMWH regimen (22.7%) than that with LMWH alone (12.2%). The risk of warfarin embryopathy is 0.6-10% with VKA in first trimester and 0.7-2% fetopathy (ocular and central nervous system abnormalities, intracranial hemorrhage) with VKA in second trimester.[8,12,13] The risk of intracranial hemorrhage in vaginal delivery in fetus is high when the mother is on VKA, hence vaginal delivery is contraindicated.[8,13]

Taking these issues into account, one must balance maternal risks versus fetal risks. Avoiding VKA in first trimester and using LMWH and then switching over to VKA (aim INR of 2.5-3) from 14 to 34 weeks, and then again using LMWH seems a logical option. This will allow clearance of VKA from fetus at the time of delivery and lower the risk of intracranial hemorrhage.[4,7,8,13]

Low molecular weight heparin must be discontinued once the woman enters active phase of labor. Adequate hydration, pain relief (epidural may be sited if 24 hours have elapsed since last dose of LMWH), thromboembolic stockings, aseptic precautions, ambulation (in early labor) must be practiced. The time elapsed since last anticoagulant dose must be considered during labor because this is the most vulnerable time for thrombosis considering the factors that the woman is not ambulatory, oral hydration may be compromised and there is a risk of infection. Second stage of labor may be cut short. LMWH may be started after 8 hours of vaginal birth and 12 hours of cesarean section (depending on postpartum bleeding).[7,8,13] VKA must be started 5–7 days after delivery (overlap with LMWH considering 48 hours for action of VKA to initiate) and continue at least 6 weeks postpartum.[4,7,8,13]

In an event that delivery needs to be conducted in a fully anticoagulated woman, action of VKA may be reversed with vitamin K and that of LMWH with protamine sulfate. In both cases, fresh frozen plasma and factor VIII concentrates must be kept ready for use if needed.[7,8]

■ ANTIBIOTIC PROPHYLAXIS

Subacute bacterial endocarditis prophylaxis must be given as per standard guidelines (*see* **Table 3**).[8] Whenever recommended, amoxycillin 2 g intravenous and gentamycin 1.5 mg/kg intravenous must be given at the onset of active labor or at rupture of membranes or prior to cesarean. In women sensitive to penicillins, vancomycin 1 g intravenous over 1–2 hours can be given.

■ CONTRACEPTION

Contraception must be discussed in all women seeking prepregnancy and postpartum care. Each contraceptive method must be evaluated using medical eligibility criteria as given by WHO.[14] A team of health care professionals must guide the couple and help them make a right choice of method of contraception.

TAKE HOME MESSAGES

- Left-sided valvular lesions pose more risk to mother than right sided ones.
- Regurgitant lesions fare better than stenotic ones.
- The conditions where pregnancy is contraindicated and valve repair must be done are—MVA <1 cm^2, annular aortic valve >40 mm, critical aortic stenosis, and any symptomatic aortic or mitral valve disease. Pregnancy is discouraged in women with LV failure, pulmonary hypertension and in those with recurrent thrombosis.
- Women with mechanical valves are associated with significant risks to mother and fetus. Anticoagulation is a critical aspect of management of these women.
- Contraception must be discussed with these women so that pregnancy is planned in an optimal maternal condition.

■ REFERENCES

1. UNICEF. (2014). Maternal health. [online] Available from: https://www.unicef.org/india/what-we-do/maternal-health#:~:text=Maternal%20Mortality%20Ratio(MMR)%20of,live%20births%20in%202014%2D16 [Last accessed February, 2023].
2. Meh C, Sharma A, Ram U, Fadel S, Correa N, Snelgrove JW, et al. Trends in maternal mortality in India over two decades in nationally representative surveys. BJOG. 2022;129(4):550-61.
3. Moussa HN, Rajapreyar I. ACOG Practice Bulletin No. 212: pregnancy and heart disease. Obstet Gynecol. 2019;134(4):881-2.
4. Mehta LS, Warnes CA, Bradley E, Burton T, Economy K, Mehran R, et al. Cardiovascular considerations in caring for pregnant patients: a scientific statement from the American Heart Association. Circulation. 2020;141(23):e884-903.
5. Agrawal S, Agrawal A, Bhandari M, Siddiqui SS, Koonwar S. Critical analysis of all pregnancies with heart disease, misses and near misses over 1-year period along with expert group so as to optimize outcome and

improve patient care–Need-based analysis. Heart India. 2019;7(2):55.
6. Kumari A, Kumar K, Sinha AK. The pattern of valvular heart diseases in India during pregnancy and its outcomes. Cureus. 2021;13(7): e16394.
7. Nelson-Piercy C. Handbook of obstetric medicine. Boca Raton, Florida: CRC Press; 2020.
8. Regitz-Zagrosek V, Roos-Hesselink JW, Bauersachs J, Blomstrom-Lundqvist C, Cifkova R, De Bonis M, et al. 2018 ESC guidelines for the management of cardiovascular diseases during pregnancy. Kardiol Pol. 2019;77(3):245-326.
9. Siu SC, Sermer M, Colman JM, Alvarez AN, Mercier LA, Morton BC, et al. Prospective multicenter study of pregnancy outcomes in women with heart disease. Circulation. 2001;104(5):515-21.
10. Silversides CK, Grewal J, Mason J, Sermer M, Kiess M, Rychel V, et al. Pregnancy outcomes in women with heart disease: the CARPREG II study. J Am Col Cardiol. 2018;71(21): 2419-30.
11. Drenthen W, Boersma E, Balci A, Moons P, Roos-Hesselink JW, Mulder BJ, et al. Predictors of pregnancy complications in women with congenital heart disease. Euro Heart J. 2010;31(17):2124-32.
12. Roos-Hesselink J, Baris L, Johnson M, De Backer J, Otto C, Marelli A, et al. Pregnancy outcomes in women with cardiovascular disease: evolving trends over 10 years in the ESC Registry of Pregnancy and Cardiac disease (ROPAC). Euro Heart J. 2019;40(47):3848-55.
13. Xu Z, Fan J, Luo X, Zhang WB, Ma J, Lin YB, et al. Anticoagulation regimens during pregnancy in patients with mechanical heart valves: a systematic review and meta-analysis. Can J Cardiol. 2016; 32(10):1248-e1.
14. World Health Organization, (2010). Reproductive Health. Medical eligibility criteria for contraceptive use.

CHAPTER 13

Heart Failure in Pregnancy

Susruta Bandyopadhyay

■ INTRODUCTION

The American Heart Association defines heart failure as a complex clinical syndrome with symptoms and signs that result from any structural or functional impairment of ventricular filling or ejection of blood.[1] Physiologically pregnancy increases the burden on the heart by several ways. There is an increase in the blood volume, there is tachycardia, and decrease in systemic vascular resistance. All these add up to increase the cardiac output. The cardiac output measured in the left lateral decubitus increases almost by 45% in the second trimester in the singleton pregnancies. Increase in the cardiac output also increases myocardial oxygen demand.[2] A few salient changes in the physiology of the cardiovascular system during pregnancy are shown in the **Table 1**.

It is apparent that the increase in stroke volume, the heart handling a larger blood volume, increased sodium and water, increased heart rate, all makes any pregnant subject with a propensity to have a heart failure. During labor, increase in the sympathetic activity, puts further strain on the heart. There is an increase in the systemic vascular resistance, heart rate, and

TABLE 1: Physiology of the cardiovascular system during pregnancy.

Parameter	Change in pregnancy
Cardiac output	Increases (45% by the second trimester). Initially the increase is due to increased myocardial contraction, in later weeks, the increase is due to heart rate
Cardiac chamber sizes	Increase in left ventricular end-diastolic volume and mass. All four chamber dimensions are increased. Mitral, pulmonary, and tricuspid regurgitations may appear
Blood pressure	There is a decrease in systolic, diastolic, and mean arterial pressures. Overweight and obese subjects may show no drop or even increase in the blood pressures (observed from body mass index >25 upward)
Blood volume and red cell mass	The blood volume increases by 20–100% (average 45%). The red cell mass is increased by 40%
Sodium and water	Due to increased renin angiotensin system activity and mineralocorticoid action there is increase in both water and sodium in the body (water accumulation is proportionately more)

blood pressure during delivery. The pressure of the pregnant uterus on the inferior vena cava is removed after the delivery, which suddenly returns 300–500 mL of blood to the system. Hence, the preload is increased. Procedures like spinal anesthesia may also precipitate hemodynamic instability and heart failure in patients with compromised cardiac function.[3] Due to all these changes a pregnant woman is very liable to develop cardiac problems and particularly acute decompensated heart failure during and after the pregnancy, if she has an underlying heart disease.

THE EPIDEMIOLOGY OF HEART FAILURE IN PREGNANCY

In the developed countries, heart diseases are the major cause of death in pregnant women. As per the Centers for Disease Control and Prevention in the USA, 24% of the pregnancy-related deaths in the last decade have been due to cardiomyopathies and other heart diseases. This makes heart diseases the leading cause of death in the pregnant women. There has been also increase in the number of women with preexisting heart diseases becoming pregnant. The increase in high risk cardiac conditions such as heart failure and pulmonary arterial hypertension has increased by 18% from 2003 to 2012 in the USA. Both these conditions are high risk disease states in pregnancy as per the World Health Organization, increasing both morbidity and mortality substantially **(Table 2)**. Heart failure causes 9% death in all hospitalized pregnant women. Of the heart diseases, cardiomyopathies remain the largest group which faces cardiac complications, all most 50% of such patients have complications.[4]

Heart failure is mostly studied in elderly people. There has been a dearth of studies on the incidence of heart failure in pregnancy. A few studies done to look into the incidence of heart failure in pregnancy have come with some interesting findings. A large retrospective study specifically looked into heart failure in pregnant women in the USA. Nationwide Inpatient Sample (NIS) was used to look into >50 million pregnant women who were admitted to hospitals from 2001 to 2011. Women of 13–49 years of age were included in this study. The inpatients were categorized into antepartum, delivery, and postpartum groups. The incidence of heart failure was 112/100,000 pregnancies. Although postpartum admissions were 1.5% of the total admissions, 60% heart failures occurred in postpartum patients. Heart failure in antepartum patients was 13% and during delivery was 27%. The incidence of heart failure increased from 2001 to 2011 in both the postpartum and the antepartum group, but remained stable in the delivery group. Over 9% of the maternal deaths were attributed to heart failure, making it one of the major causes of maternal mortality in the developed world. There was an increase in maternal mortality related to heart failure in the study period.[5] An international registry: Registry on Pregnancy and Cardiac Disease (ROPAC) studied 1,321 pregnant women with preexisting heart disease. 13% of these patients developed heart failure. The most common group was with congenital heart disease followed by valvular heart disease, followed by cardiomyopathy.[6] A smaller Indian study looking into 281 Indian women with pregnancy and heart disease found that almost 70% of them had valvular heart disease and the most common complication was heart failure.[7] Risk factors for precipitating heart failure in pregnancy are given in **Table 3**.

TABLE 2: The World Health Organization (WHO) classification of cardiac risks in the pregnant women.

WHO classification of cardiovascular risk in pregnant women	Cardiovascular condition in this class
WHO risk class I: No detectable increased risk of maternal mortality and no or mild increase in morbidity	• *Uncomplicated, small or mild:* Pulmonary stenosis • Patient ductus arteriosus, mitral valve prolapse • Successfully repaired simple lesions (atrial or ventricular septal defect, patent ductus arteriosus, anomalous pulmonary venous drainage) • Atrial or ventricular ectopic beats, isolated
WHO risk class II (if otherwise well and uncomplicated): Small increased risk of maternal mortality or moderate increase in morbidity	• Unoperated atrial or ventricular septal defect • Repaired tetralogy of Fallot • Most arrhythmias
WHO risk class II or III (depending on individual): Risk as indicated in class II (above) or class III (below)	• Mild left ventricular impairment • Hypertrophic cardiomyopathy • Native or tissue valvular heart disease not considered WHO I or IV • Marfan syndrome without aortic dilatation • Aorta <45 mm in aortic disease associated with bicuspid aortic valve • Repaired coarctation
WHO risk class III: Significantly increased risk of maternal mortality or severe morbidity. Expert counseling required. If pregnancy is decided upon, intensive specialist cardiac and obstetric monitoring needed throughout pregnancy, childbirth, and the puerperium	• Mechanical valve • Systemic right ventricle • Fontan circulation • Cyanotic heart disease (unrepaired) • Other complex congenital heart disease • Aortic dilatation 40–45 mm in Marfan syndrome • Aortic dilatation 45–50 mm in aortic disease associated with bicuspid aortic valve
WHO risk class IV (pregnancy contraindicated): Extremely high risk of maternal mortality or severe morbidity; pregnancy contraindicated. If pregnancy occurs, termination should be discussed. If pregnancy continues, care as for class III	• Pulmonary arterial hypertension of any cause • Severe systemic ventricular dysfunction (left ventricular ejection fraction <30%, New York Heart Association class III–IV) • Previous peripartum cardiomyopathy with any residual impairment of left ventricular function • Severe symptomatic mitral or aortic stenosis • Marfan syndrome with aorta dilated >45 mm • Aortic dilation >50 mm in aortic disease associated with bicuspid aortic valve • Native severe coarctation

Heart failure prolongs hospital stay, increases mortality, causes adverse fetal outcome. The indicators for poor outcomes include advanced age, black race, multiple comorbidities, etc.[4]

DIAGNOSIS OF HEART FAILURE IN PREGNANCY

The diagnosis of heart failure may be tricky, especially early in its course. Normal clinical symptoms and signs of heart failure may

TABLE 3: Risk factors for precipitating heart failure in pregnancy.

Nonmodifiable risk factors	• Race • Advanced age
Modifiable risk factors	• Obesity • Dyslipidemia • Smoking • Alcohol or other substance abuse
Comorbidities	• Hypertension • Diabetes mellitus • Preexisting heart failure • Kidney disease • WHO cardiovascular risk 3 or 4
Obstetric conditions	• Preeclampsia/eclampsia • Gestational hypertension/diabetes • Amniotic fluid embolism • Conditions causing blood loss like placenta previa • Multiple pregnancies
Cardiac diseases	• Peripartum cardiomyopathy • Other cardiomyopathies • Valvular heart disease • Pulmonary hypertension • Ischemic heart disease • Congenital heart disease including Eisenmenger syndrome • Chronic hypertension (low risk for complications)

occur in pregnancy in absence of heart failure. Mild dyspnea tachypnea may occur in pregnancy due to several causes. Extra volume of blood in pregnancy may give rise to mild edema, raised jugular venous pressure and systolic murmurs due to high blood flow through the aortic and pulmonary valves. The heart rate may be high and there may be some benign arrhythmias and the patient may complain palpitations. However, severe shortness of breath, orthopnea, paroxysmal nocturnal dyspnea, presyncope, and chest pain may point toward pathological conditions and hence call for a work up. Murmurs found in places other than the left parasternal area and of higher grades, gallop sounds may also point toward a heart failure.[8] The various cardiac investigations, their safety in pregnancy, and their limitations in pregnancy are listed in the **Table 4**.

MATERNAL AND FETAL RISK WITH MATERNAL HEART FAILURE

The data on the outcome of the heart failure during the pregnancy may give an incomplete picture. Pregnancy is a continuum, and many patients may have increased mortality or morbidity related to heart failure during postpartum period or antepartum period. A heart failure occurring in a different admission than that during the delivery may not be recorded as pregnancy related complaint. The ROPAC (mentioned earlier) data showed that the pregnant women had a mortality of 4.8% vis-à-vis

TABLE 4: Tests done for the diagnosis of heart failure and ancillary conditions, their safety during pregnancy, and their limitations.[9,10]

Test	Safety of doing the test during pregnancy	Predictive value and limitations during pregnancy
ECG	Safe	• Nonspecific ST segment and T wave changes left axis deviation of the QRS • Small pathological q (all may be present without a cardiac disease)
Chest X-ray	Safe	• False mitralization of the pulmonary border and cardiomegaly may occur in pregnancy • It cannot differentiate between cardiogenic and noncardiogenic pulmonary edema
Echocardiogram (transthoracic)	Safe	Preferred method to assess cardiac structure and function
Echocardiogram (transesophageal)	Usually done only in case of absolute necessity	
CT scan (chest)	Safe (with precautions)	
Cardiac MRI	Safe (after the first trimester)	
Troponin I	Safe	Valid test for myocardial damage (not affected by pregnancy)
Coronary angiogram	Unsafe, to be done only when absolutely necessary and to be done with uterine shielding	
NT-proBNP	Safe	It may be valuable to pick up heart failure and also to predict heart failure in patients with preeclampsia

(CT: computed tomography; ECG: electrocardiogram; MRI: magnetic resonance imaging; NT-proBNP: N-terminal pro-brain natriuretic peptide)

0.5% in those without the heart failure. The pregnant patient with a diagnosis of heart failure has an increased risk of pulmonary edema, renal failure, cerebrovascular accidents, need for ventilation support, longer stay, and even death. They are more likely to undergo cesarean section. The risks increase with advancing age, black race, and multiple comorbidities. Several studies have looked into the fetal risks for the mothers who have heart failure during their pregnancy are low birth weight, premature delivery, low Apgar score, respiratory distress syndrome, and increased mortality. The predictors of poor outcome are the New York Heart Association (NYHA) class more than two symptoms or cyanosis, smoking during pregnancy, obstructive cardiac lesions (e.g., stenotic valves), and multiple pregnancies.[4]

TREATMENT OF HEART FAILURE IN PREGNANCY

In addition to the drugs mentioned in **Table 5**, acute decompensated heart failure in pregnancy may require treatments such as:
- Vasopressors and inotropes
- Ventilatory assist devices such as noninvasive and invasive ventilation
- Left ventricular assist devices
- Renal replacement therapy.

Treatment of specific disease entities such as percutaneous coronary intervention, treatment of arrhythmias, and treatment

TABLE 5: Drugs for the treatment of heart failure in pregnancy.[4,11]

Drug	Special consideration in pregnancy	Contraindication
Diuretics	• They may reduce intravascular volume and hence reduce the placental perfusion • They are not beneficial in patients with preeclampsia and eclampsia	Relative contraindication in preeclampsia and eclampsia
β blockers	• Only selective β_1 blockers are used. Labetalol and carvedilol are also safe • They are beneficial for the mother but may cause (rarely) fetal growth impairment, fetal hypoglycemia, and even increased fetal perinatal mortality	
Angiotensin-converting enzyme inhibitors (ACEI) and angiotensin receptor blockers (ARB)	They have been proven to be detrimental for both the mother and the fetus	Contraindicated during pregnancy but not during lactation
Spironolactone	It is teratogenic	Contraindicated during pregnancy but not during lactation
Bromocriptine	It is recommended in peripartum cardiomyopathy as a prolactin degradation product has been shown to be responsible for apoptosis of the cardiomyocytes	
Nitrates	They are beneficial in treating decompensated heart failure in the patients of eclampsia and preeclampsia	
Hydralazine	This can be a replacement for the ACEI and ARB drugs as a vasodilator	
Digoxin		Safe
Anticoagulation	• Heparin and low molecular heparin are safe • Vitamin K antagonists can be used only in low doses from the second trimester	
Ivabradine	Inadequate data	Contraindicated
Amiodarone	Should be used only to treat life-threatening arrhythmias	Relative contraindication

of some diseases which precipitate heart failure such as infection and anemia are part of the treatment spectrum. While doing an angiography or a related procedure, shield to protect the fetus should be used. A multidisciplinary approach is required.

DELIVERY

Cesarean section is not an absolute must in delivering the babies from the pregnant mother with heart failure. Rather individualized approach is needed. There are added risks for both during vaginal delivery (which may call for interventions like forceps delivery) as well as the cesarean section. Many of the fetuses may be small for the date or may need premature delivery. Preeclampsia precipitating heart failure is one of the conditions calling for an immediate delivery.[8]

TAKE HOME MESSAGES

- Heart failure remains one of the leading causes of morbidity and mortality in pregnant women.
- Some of the patients presenting with heart failure in pregnancy have preexisting heart diseases aggravated by pregnancy. Others have diseases associated with pregnancy. Of the latter group, preeclampsia and peripartum cardiomyopathy remain major causes.
- The diagnosis of heart failure in pregnancy may be difficult, more so in its early stages. This is because many early signs of heart failure may be confused with the physiological changes in pregnancy.
- The drug therapy for heart failure in pregnancy is similar to the standard care for heart failure, but with some specific contraindications to some drugs. In every situation, the risk benefit ratio should be carefully assessed before starting a drug.
- The patients should be followed well into the postpartum period because heart failure has been shown to have the maximum mortality during that period.

REFERENCES

1. Heidenreich PA, Bozkurt B, Aguilar D, Allen LA, Byun JJ, Colvin MM, et al. 2022 AHA/ACC/HFSA Guideline for the Management of Heart Failure: A Report of the American College of Cardiology/American Heart Association Joint Committee on Clinical Practice Guidelines. Circulation. 2022;145: e895-1032.
2. Mahilmaran A. Heart failure in pregnancy. Indian J Cardiovasc Dis Women WINCARS. 2018;3:161-6.
3. Sanghavi M, Rutherford JD. Cardiovascular physiology of pregnancy. Circulation. 2014;130(12):1003-8.
4. Bright RA, Lima FV, Avila C, Butler J, Stergiopoulos K. Maternal heart failure. J Am Heart Assoc. 2021;10(14):1-17.
5. Mogos MF, Piano MR, McFarlin BL, Salemi JL, Liese KL, Briller JE. Heart Failure in Pregnant Women: A Concern Across the Pregnancy Continuum. Circ Heart Fail. 2018;11(1):e004005.
6. Ruys TEP, Roos-Hesselink JW, Hall R, Subirana-Domènech MT, Grando-Ting J, Estensen M, et al. Heart failure in pregnant women with cardiac disease: data from the ROPAC. Heart. 2014;100(3):231-8.
7. Hiralal K, Snehamay C. Pregnancy complicated by maternal heart disease: a review of 281 women. J Obstet Gynecol India. 2012;62(3):301-6.
8. Sliwa K, Anthony J. Decompensated Heart Failure in Pregnancy. Card Fail Rev. 2016;2(1):20-6.
9. Nanda S, Nelson-Piercy C, Mackillop L. Cardiac disease in pregnancy. Clin Med (Lond). 2012;12(6):553-60.
10. Ker JA, Soma-Pillay P. NT-proBNP: When is it useful in Obstetric Medicine? Obstet Med. 2018;11(1):3-5.
11. Regitz-Zagrosek V, Roos-Hesselink JW, Bauersachs J, Blomström-Lundqvist C, Cífková R, De Bonis M, et al. 2018 ESC Guidelines for the management of cardiovascular diseases during pregnancy. Eur Heart J. 2018;39:3165-241.

CHAPTER 14

Renal Disorders and Drug Dosing

Acute Kidney Injury including Hemolytic Uremic Syndrome in Pregnancy

Ranajit Chatterjee, Priyanka H Chhabra

■ INTRODUCTION

Acute kidney injury (AKI) during pregnancy (PR-AKI) poses dual risks to both mother and fetus. PR-AKI in mother can be secondary to obstetric complications such as abruptio placentae, puerperal sepsis, hemolysis, elevated liver enzymes, and low platelets (HELLP) syndrome, etc. and may be associated with adverse fetal outcomes. Its association with diabetes, hypertension, and obesity poses an important public health problem in India. Pregnancy-associated thrombotic microangiopathies (P-TMAs) are an important cause of AKI during pregnancy, especially hemolytic uremic syndrome (HUS) and thrombotic thrombocytopenic purpura (TTP). Differentiating between the two distinct clinical entities requires a good clinical acumen. Apart from thrombotic microangiopathies (TMAs), urinary tract infections (UTIs) during pregnancy also constitute a major problem. Appropriate antibiotic therapy is also essential in proper management of patients with UTIs.

■ EPIDEMIOLOGY AND MAGNITUDE OF HEALTH PROBLEM

Although the incidence of PR-AKI is declining, it still continues to be a major public health problem in India. PR-AKI affects 20–40% obstetric patients in 1960s and now, it has declined to a mere 0–1% in the last decade.[1] Most of these cases (80%) were in the rural areas and were associated with poor perinatal care. However, the big difference in the incidence of PR-AKI amongst developing and developed nation is primarily due to its increased detection due to changed definitions of quantifying AKI or might be due to enhanced surveillance.[2,3] The incorporation of risk of renal failure, injury to the kidney, failure, loss of kidney function, and end-stage renal failure (RIFLE) and acute kidney injury network (AKIN) criteria in the updated definition of PR-AKI has raised its incidence from 1.66 to 2.68/10,000 pregnancies from 2003 to 2010 in Canada. Apart from bias in reporting, its incidence can also be increased due to increasing maternal age, diabetes, chronic kidney disease (CKD), and hypertension among pregnant women.

Pregnancy-related acute kidney injury usually has a bimodal distribution showing two peaks—one occurring in first trimester due to septic abortions, lupus nephritis, and hyperemesis gravidarum. The second peak is seen in third trimester because of preeclampsia, HUS, TTP, acute fatty liver of pregnancy (AFLP), and other obstetric complications.

PHYSIOLOGICAL CHANGES IN KIDNEYS DURING PREGNANCY

A number of physiological changes take place in the kidneys during pregnancy. There is renal vascular and interstitial vascular expansion leading to increase in anatomical size of kidney by about 1–1.5 cm. Pelvicalyceal system undergoes dilatation and hydronephrosis is normal in pregnancy. Several factors contribute to this dilatation of urinary system—compression on urinary system by the gravid uterus, hormonal effects of progesterone, and changes in ureteral wall. These changes promote stasis in the ureters often leading to urinary tract infection and renal stones. Glomerular filtration rate also increases by up to 50% owing to vasodilatory state. Also, renal plasma flow rate also increases by up to 85%. Hence, serum creatinine value of 0.4–0.5 is normal in pregnancy. Consequent to the hyperfiltration state, fall in serum sodium, and urine osmolality by 4–5 mEq/dL is normal in pregnancy. Glycosuria and proteinuria are also normal in pregnancy. **Table 1** depicts normal physiological changes occurring in urinary system. Pregnancy also affects the hepatic drug metabolism by affecting CYP450 enzymes. **Figure 1** depicts various anatomical and physiological changes occurring during pregnancy.

ACUTE KIDNEY INJURY DURING PREGNANCY—WHAT ARE THE CAUSES?

More than half of the cases of PR-AKI occur in the third trimester. As already discussed, there are two incidence peaks of PR-AKI—one in first trimester and another in third trimester. Preeclampsia is the most common cause for PR-AKI.[4] Other causes—septic abortion, hemorrhagic complications—antepartum hemorrhage (APH) or postpartum hemorrhage (PPH), TMAs. All causes of PR-AKI are listed in **Table 2**.

Preeclampsia

Preeclampsia is a serious disorder characterized by heterogeneity in presentation. Preeclampsia is defined as new onset hypertension (BP >140/90 mm Hg) and proteinuria (>300 mg/dL) after 20 weeks of gestation. It is

TABLE 1: Renal changes of normal pregnancy.

Anatomical changes	Physiological changes
Increase in kidney size	Renal blood flow increases by 50%, renal plasma flow increases by 80%
• Dilatation of collecting system, hydronephrosis • Kidney volume increases by 30%	• Serum creatinine falls to 0.3–0.5 mg/dL • Serum sodium falls by 4–5 mmol/L • Serum osmolality also falls around 270 mOsm/L

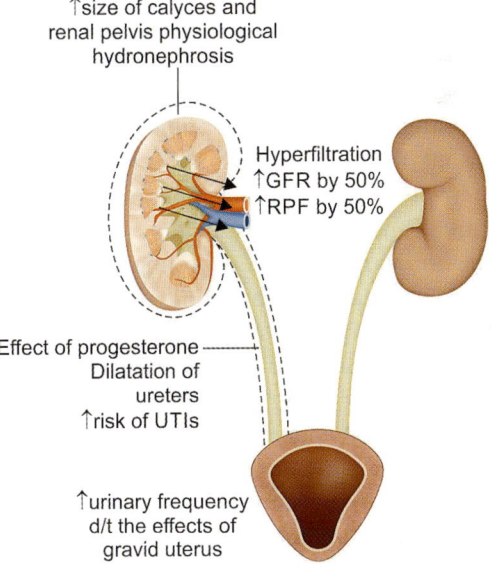

Fig. 1: Diagrammatic representation of anatomic and physiological changes of pregnancy. (GFR: glomerular filtration rate; RPF: renal plasma flow; UTIs: urinary tract infections)

TABLE 2: Causes of PR-AKI along with their timing in pregnancy.

Causes of AKI during pregnancy	Trimester	AKI
Obstetric complications		
Septic abortion (20–30% cases)	First trimester	Intrarenal
Antepartum hemorrhage—placenta previa, abruptio placentae	Third trimester	Prerenal
Postpartum hemorrhage—puerperal sepsis (25% cases)	Third trimester	Prerenal
Intrauterine fetal death	Third trimester	Intrarenal
Pregnancy specific diseases		
Preeclampsia/eclampsia (36%, most common cause)	Second/third trimester	Intrarenal
HELLP syndrome (3–15% cases)	Third trimester	Intrarenal
AFLP (20–100% cases)	Third trimester	Intrarenal
Atypical hemolytic uremic syndrome	Postpartum	Intrarenal
TTP	Any trimester	Intrarenal
Hyperemesis gravidarum	First trimester	Prerenal
Other causes		
Lupus nephritis	Any trimester	Intrarenal
Hydronephrosis	Third trimester	Postrenal

(AFLP: acute fatty liver of pregnancy; AKI: acute kidney injury; HELLP: hemolysis, elevated liver enzymes, and low platelets; TTP: thrombotic thrombocytopenic purpura)

primarily a clinical diagnosis. It complicates 3–10% of all pregnancies. Apart from hypertension, other features are upper epigastric pain (most common), thrombocytopenia, elevated liver enzymes, pulmonary edema, visual disturbances, and seizures. Basically, it involves defects in placentation and widespread endothelial dysfunction. There occurs an imbalance between proangiogenic factors [vascular endothelial growth factor (VEGF) and placental growth factor (PlGF)] and antiangiogenic factors (soluble endoglein 1 and soluble fms-like tyrosine kinase sflt-1). In preeclampsia, concentrations of seng-1 and sflt-1 are increased, which leads to widespread endothelial dysfunction. Dysfunction of endothelial cells in glomeruli leads to proteinuria.

Preeclampsia is one of the leading causes of PR-AKI. Approximately, 40–50% of patients with PR-AKI have preeclampsia.[4]

HELLP syndrome is a variant of preeclampsia which is characterized by HELLP. Decreased platelet count in pregnant women should raise a clinical suspicion of HELLP syndrome. Diagnostic criteria for HELLP syndrome are:
1. Microangiopathic hemolytic anemia—characterized by the presence of schistocytes on peripheral smear, serum bilirubin >1.2 mg/dL, lactate dehydrogenase (LDH) >600 U/L
2. Raised liver enzymes—AST >60 U/L
3. Platelet count <1,00,000 cells/mm^3.

However, HELLP syndrome is associated with a good overall prognosis. Almost all patients of HELLP syndrome experience complete renal recovery during lifetime.

Thrombotic Microangiopathies

Thrombotic microangiopathies during pregnancy are a group of rare disorders characterized by the presence of platelet fibrin thrombi in walls of arterioles and capillaries leading to platelet consumption and hemolytic anemia. As it frequently affects small vessels in glomeruli, it leads to PR-AKI. TMAs are characterized by a triad of clinical symptoms—thrombocytopenia, acute kidney injury, and microangiopathic hemolytic anemia (MAHA).[5] TMAs constitute two distinct entities namely—atypical HUS (aHUS) and TTP.

■ HEMOLYTIC UREMIC SYNDROME

Hemolytic uremic syndrome is a serious, life-threatening disease characterized by thrombocytopenia, AKI, and presence of schistocytes in blood. There are two variants of HUS—typical and atypical HUS.

Typical HUS is seen, usually in children, secondary to infection caused by Shiga-like toxin (verotoxin) producing *Escherichia coli* (*E. coli*) and by Shiga toxin producing *Shigella dysenteriae* (*S. dysenteriae*). Several other infections are also associated with HUS—*Clostridium difficile, Streptococcus pneumoniae, Haemophilus influenzae*, HIV, CMV, Epstein–Barr virus, hepatitis A, B, C, etc., to name a few.[6] It accounts for roughly 90% of the cases of HUS.[7]

Pregnancy-related HUS is usually atypical and occurs in postpartum period. It accounts for remaining 10% of the cases of HUS.[7] It can either be sporadic in 80% cases or familial due to generic defect in 10% cases. It is associated with a defect in complement factor H, which is responsible for activation of alternative complement pathway **(Fig. 2)**.[6]

Hemolytic uremic syndrome—alternative complement pathway is primarily affected.

Diagnosis of aHUS is purely clinical, renal involvement is usually severe and neurological manifestations are rare.[6] It occurs in the postpartum period. Often in these patients, antepartum and intrapartum period is uneventful. It is usually associated with poor prognosis, up to 60% patients' progress to end-stage renal dysfunction (ESRD) within a year of presentation. **Figure 3** depicts diagnosis of hemolytic uremic syndrome.

Treatment involves several rounds of plasma exchange and administration of monoclonal antibody eculizumab.

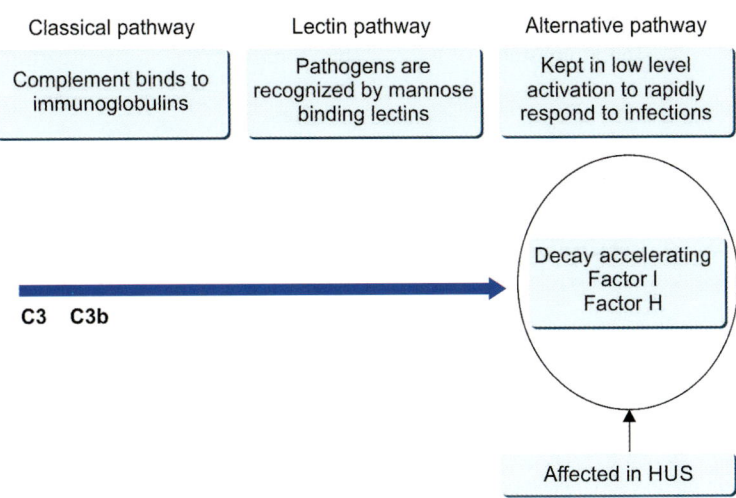

Fig. 2: Complement system activation. (HUS: hemolytic uremic syndrome)

Eculizumab is humanized form of anti-C5 antibody, which selectively inhibits a sub-portion of the complement cascade. Data concerning the use of eculizumab in pregnant women has confirmed its safety in pregnant women.[8] However, its safety and efficacy is proven only in few case reports.[9,10] Large scale studies are required in this direction to confirm its safety and efficacy. Patients with defects in complement gene should be counselled before pregnancy. There is 20–30% chance of acquiring the disease in offspring.[4]

THROMBOTIC THROMBOCYTOPENIC PURPURA

Thrombocytopenic purpura is a clinical syndrome characterized by fever, thrombocytopenia, hemolytic anemia, and predominant neurological symptoms (seizures, ataxia, and disorientation). The primary cause is deficiency of ADAMTS-13 (a disintegrin and metalloproteinase with a thrombospondin type 1 motif member-13). It can occur at any time during pregnancy usually in second and third trimesters.

The clinical features of TMAs (HUS, TTP, AFLP) are quite overlapping during pregnancy. **Table 3** shows various TMAs and their different clinical features. All the TMAs have MAHA, thrombocytopenia, and renal disease. **Figure 4** shows P-TMAs—aHUS and TTP.

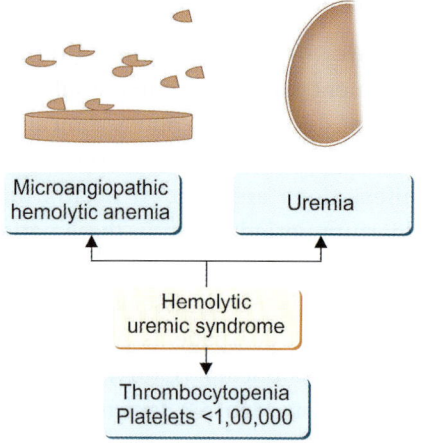

Fig. 3: Diagnosis of hemolytic uremic syndrome constitutes a triad of microangiopathic hemolytic anemia, uremia, and thrombocytopenia.

TABLE 3: Differences among various clinical syndromes (aHUS, TTP, AFLP).

Clinical feature	aHUS	TTP	AFLP
Onset	Third trimester	Third trimester, sometimes second trimester	Postpartum
Clinical features	Triad of hemolysis, renal failure and thrombocytopenia	Fever and neurological symptoms also in addition to triad	Deranged liver functions
Defect	Defect in a complement factor H	ADAMTS-13 deficiency	Deficiency of enzyme LCHAD (long-chain 3-hydroxyacyl-CoA dehydrogenase)
CNS manifestations	Absent	Present and dominant	Absent
Management	Plasma exchange, eculizumab	Plasma exchange	Supportive, delivery

(ADAMTS-13: a disintegrin and metalloproteinase with a thrombospondin type 1 motif member-13; AFLP: acute fatty liver of pregnancy; aHUS: atypical hemolytic uremic syndrome; TTP: thrombotic thrombocytopenic purpura)

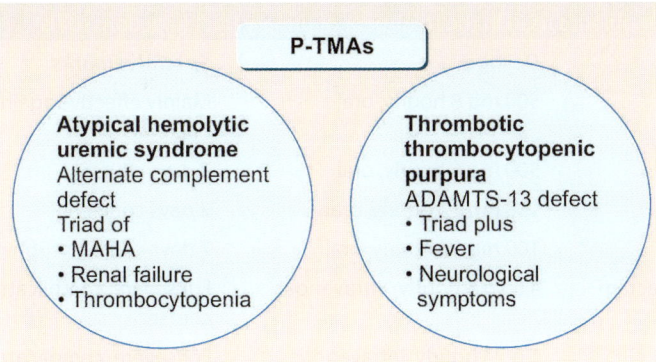

Fig. 4: Pregnancy thrombotic microangiopathies are of two types—atypical HUS and TTP. (ADAMTS-13: a disintegrin and metalloproteinase with a thrombospondin type 1 motif member-13; MAHA: microangiopathic hemolytic anemia; P-TMAs: pregnancy-associated thrombotic microangiopathies)

ACUTE FATTY LIVER OF PREGNANCY

Acute fatty liver of pregnancy is a rare cause of AKI in pregnant women. It occurs due to fetal deficiency of long-chain 3-hydroxyacyl-CoA dehydrogenase (LCHAD). Deficiency of this enzymes leads to accumulation of excess free fatty acids, which cross placenta and are toxic to the mother. Pregnant women usually presents in third trimester with vomiting, fatigue, raised liver enzymes, hypoglycemia, renal failure, and metabolic acidosis. Patients may have concomitant preeclampsia. Liver biopsy reveals ballooning of hepatocytes and microvesicular steatosis. Management includes supportive care, plasmapheresis, and liver transplantation.

Differences amongst aHUS, TTP, and AFLP are summed up in **Table 3** to avoid confusion.

HYPEREMESIS GRAVIDARUM

Hyperemesis gravidarum is the most common cause of AKI in early course of pregnancy primarily the first trimester. Excess vomiting leads to severe volume depletion and prerenal failure. Management is usually supportive and includes giving fluids.

PYELONEPHRITIS

Asymptomatic bacteriuria and pyelonephritis have a high incidence in pregnancy as compared to normal population. Symptomatic bacteriuria often progresses to cause urinary tract infection, pyelonephritis, and sepsis. Asymptomatic bacteriuria might be asymptomatic for the mother but in the fetus, it increases the incidence of preterm births and low-birth-weight babies. Thus, American College of Obstetrics and Gynecologists (ACOG) recommends screening of all pregnant women for asymptomatic bacteriuria. Causative organisms include *E. coli, Klebsiella, Proteus, Enterobacter* species and group B *Streptococcus*. Oral antibiotics are generally preferred for uncomplicated UTI and cystitis.

Nitrofurantoin, cephalexin, amoxycillin, and cefpodoxime are usually recommended. However, pyelonephritis requires treatment with parenteral antibiotics. Fluoraquinolones and aminoglycosides are not preferred due to the risk of fetal toxicity (arthropathy, ototoxicity). Aztreonam, imipenem/cilastatin, and meropenem can also be given. **Table 4** shows various antibiotics used to manage UTIs.

TABLE 4: Various antibiotics used in the treatment of urinary tract infections (UTIs).

Drug	Dosage	Special remarks
Amoxicillin	500 mg 8 hourly, oral	Mainly effective against gram-positive bacteria
Cephalexin	500 mg 6 hourly, oral	7 days course
Cefpodoxime	100 mg 12 hourly, oral	7 days course
Nitrofurantoin	100 mg 12 hourly, oral	7 days course, prophylaxis
Piperacillin–Tazobactam	4.65 g 6 hourly, intravenous	For severe, complicated UTI, 7–14 days course
Ceftriaxone	1 g 24 hourly, intravenous	For severe, complicated UTI, 7–14 days course
Meropenem	1 g 8 hourly, intravenous	For severe, complicated UTI, 7–14 days course
Imipenem/Cilastatin	500 mg 6 hourly	For severe, complicated UTI, 7–14 days course

Suppressive therapy with low dose nitrofurantoin is indicated in women developing frequent UTIs (>3 episodes of UTI per year). It reduces the rates of relapse by 90%.[11] However, it should be used in caution in women having G6PD deficiency due to the risk of hemolytic anemia in such women.

■ MANAGEMENT OF PR-AKI

The goals of management of PR-AKI are to ensure safety of both mother and the fetus. A team of multidisciplinary doctors—obstetricians, nephrologist, and intensivists—is generally required for optimal outcomes. Key to optimal management is patient stabilization and symptomatic management.
- *Stabilize the patient:* In case of ongoing bleeding in antepartum or postpartum hemorrhage, try to secure bleeding areas and treat the underlying cause.
- *Protect kidneys from further damage:* This is an essential part of management of a patient with PR-AKI. Adequate hemodynamic monitoring should be done and dynamic parameters should be assessed to decide on fluid responsiveness and resuscitation. Crystalloids are the fluids of choice. Colloids, though are needed in less amount and are better volume expanders than crystalloids, should be avoided as they increase the chances of AKI and renal replacement therapy (RRT). In acidotic patients with hyperchloremia, balanced salt solutions are preferred over normal saline. Volume overload should be avoided. The mean arterial pressure should be kept above 65 mm Hg. For hypertensive patients a higher target of 80–85 mm Hg should be set. Adequate glycemic control should be achieved and blood sugar should be kept below 180 mg/dL. If patients are on vasopressors, nor-adrenaline should be the vasopressor of choice. Also, nephrotoxic medications should be avoided. If at all used, monitoring of blood concentration of such drugs should be done. Dosing or interval of antibiotics should be modified

accordingly. Nutritional requirements in PR-AKI patients vary widely. However, patients should receive energy up to 25–30 kcal/kg/day equivalent to 100–130% of resting energy expenditure. Protein intake should be around 1.3 g/kg/day which may go up to 1.7 g/kg/day if patients are on continuous renal replacement therapy (CRRT).

- *Symptomatic management:*
  - *Hyperkalemia:* Hyperkalemia should be corrected with glucose insulin drip, salbutamol nebulization, potassium binding resins, and diuretics. In refractory cases hemodialysis should be performed.
  - *Metabolic acidosis:* Intravenous bicarbonate should preferably be avoided to correct metabolic acidosis unless the pH < 7.15 and HCO_3 < 15 mmol/L.
  - *Renal replacement therapy:* RRT should be done as and when required in cases of severe volume overload, refractory metabolic acidosis, severe, refractory hyperkalemia, uremic encephalopathy, pericarditis, etc. CRRT should be preferred in hemodynamically unstable patients with uncertain volume of distribution. It is also the preferred modality in patients of cerebral edema and acute liver failure. SCUF (slow continuous ultrafiltration) is effectively used in treating patients of hemodynamically unstable cardiogenic pulmonary edema. Intermittent hemodialysis may be preferred in hemodynamically stable patients. Obstetric patients often require alternate day dialysis schedule until improvement of urine output and recovery of renal function is achieved. Several trials[12] have evaluated the safety and efficacy of starting RRT early (with the onset of fluid overload) versus starting RRT late (for abovementioned indications). The recent consensus is in the favor of starting RRT late.[13] Early onset, high intensity dialysis only for minimal fluid overload should be avoided and specialist nephrologist opinion should always be sought in this regard.[13]
- *Disease specific management:*
  - *Preeclampsia/AFLP:* Delivery should be expedited whenever possible. Steroids should be given to expedite lung maturity, in case of delivery before 28 weeks.
  - *Obstetric hemorrhage:* Immediate intervention to stop bleeding. Blood and blood products should be replaced as and when necessary.
  - *Placenta previa:* It may require cesarean section to stop bleeding.
  - However, conservative approach can be done in case of mild bleeding.
  - *Ectopic pregnancy:* Immediate surgery and removal of gestational sac is required. In case of hemodynamically stable patient, methotrexate injection may be given.
  - *Placental abruption:* Immediate surgical intervention is required in case of severe placenta abruption. Expectant management may be required in less severe cases.
- *Antibiotics:* In cases of infection, appropriate antibiotics should be given, preferably, as per culture sensitivity report.
- *Follow up and monitoring:* Essential once the patient improves.
- *Renal transplant* may be considered after 6 months of delivery in case of requirement of long-term dialysis. It is not indicated during pregnancy.

TABLE 5: Maternal and fetal implications of PR-AKI.

Causes of PR-AKI	Maternal implications	Fetal implications
Preeclampsia	• Disseminated intravascular coagulation (DIC)) • Acute kidney injury (AKI) • End-stage renal dysfunction (ESRD) leading to requirement of renal replacement therapy • HELLP (hemolysis, elevated liver enzymes, and low platelets) syndrome • Pulmonary edema • Placental abruption • Increased maternal mortality	• Intrauterine fetal death • Intrauterine growth retardation • Prematurity • Birth defects
Thrombotic microangiopathies (TMAs)	• Hemolytic uremic syndrome—ESRD • Requirement of dialysis • Failure of renal transplantation • Neurological manifestations (seizures, ataxia, disorientation, headache, aphasia)	Chances of acquiring the microangiopathy
Acute fatty liver of pregnancy	• Headache, vomiting, hypoglycemic episodes, fatigue • Co-presentation with preeclampsia • Elevated liver enzymes, lactic acidosis, hemolytic abnormalities • ESRD • Requirement of dialysis	Chances of acquiring the microangiopathy
Pyelonephritis	• Urinary tract infection • Sepsis	Low birth weight babies and preterm births

MATERNAL AND FETAL IMPLICATIONS OF PR-AKI

PR-AKI has several maternal and fetal implications, which are summed up aptly in **Table 5**.

CONCLUSION

- Acute kidney injury is a common problem in critically ill patients.
- Antibiotics should be given in usual doses in patients with AKI for 48 hours.
- Appropriate antibiotic dosing is the key to management of sepsis in patients with AKI.
- Chronic kidney disease is another important problem requiring adjustment of antibiotic dosage.
- Several pharmacokinetic (P/K) and pharmacodynamics (P/D) factors affect drug concentrations in plasma in patients on RRT.
- Rule of thumb is loading dose does not require dosage modification in patients with AKI.
- Hence, drug dosing in patients with AKI and CKD depends on a complex interplay of factors.

TAKE HOME MESSAGES

- Overall incidence of AKI is decreasing throughout the world.
- Establishing a diagnosis is often challenging in clinical syndromes with overlapping features—HELLP syndrome, HUS, TTP, AFLP.
- Expertise and clinical acumen plays a crucial role in making correct diagnosis.
- Treatment of PR-AKI is generally supportive good quality intensive care.
- Plasma exchange may be useful modality in PR-TMAs. Eculizumab may be useful in patients with atypical HUS.

REFERENCES

1. Stratta P, Besso L, Canavese C, Grill A, Todros T, Benedetto C, et al. Is pregnancy-related acute renal failure a disappearing clinical entity?. Ren Fail. 1996;18:575-84.
2. Mehrabadi A, Liu S, Bartholomew S, Hutcheon JA, Magee LA, Kramer MS, et al. Hypertensive disorders of pregnancy and the recent increase in obstetric acute renal failure in Canada: population based retrospective cohort study. BMJ. 2014;349:g4731.
3. Mehrabadi A, Dahhou M, Joseph KS, Kramer MS. Investigation of a rise in obstetric acute renal failure in the United States, 1999–2011. Obstet Gynecol. 2016;127:899-906.
4. Prakash J, Ganiger VC. Acute kidney injury in pregnancy-specific disorders. Indian J Nephrol. 2017;27(4):258-70.
5. Noris M, Remuzzi G. Hemolytic uremic syndrome. J Am Soc Nephrol. 2005;16(4):1035-50.
6. Sheerin NS, Glover E. Haemolytic uremic syndrome: diagnosis and management. F1000Res. 2019;8:F1000 Faculty Rev-1690.
7. Jim B, Garovic VD. Acute kidney injury in pregnancy. Semin Nephrol. 2017;37(4):378-85.
8. Hallstensen RF, Bergseth G, Foss S, Jæger S, Gedde-Dahl T, Holt J, et al. Eculizumab treatment during pregnancy does not affect the complement system activity of the newborn. Immunobiology. 2015;220(4):452-9.
9. Ardissino G, Wally Ossola M, Baffero GM, Rigotti A, Cugno M. Eculizumab for atypical hemolytic uremic syndrome in pregnancy. Obstet Gynecol. 2013;122(2 Pt 2):487-9.
10. Canigral C, Moscardo F, Castro C, Pajares A, Lancharro A, Solves P, et al. Eculizumab for the treatment of pregnancy-related atypical hemolytic uremic syndrome. Ann Hematol. 2014;93(8):1421-2.
11. Fihn SD. Clinical practice. Acute uncomplicated urinary tract infection in women. N Engl J Med. 2003;349(3):259-66.
12. Zarbock A, Kellum JA, Schmidt C, Van Aken H, Wempe C, Pavenstädt H, et al. Effect of early vs delayed initiation of renal replacement therapy on mortality in critically ill patients with acute kidney injury: The ELAIN randomized clinical trial. JAMA. 2016;315(20):2190-9.
13. Jeong R, Wald R, Bagshaw SM. Timing of renal-replacement therapy in intensive care unit-related acute kidney injury. Curr Opin Crit Care. 2021;27(6):573-81.

CHAPTER 15

Chronic Kidney Disease and Pregnancy

Manisha Pradhan

■ INTRODUCTION

Chronic kidney disease (CKD) is defined as kidney damage with alteration in morphology, imaging, or function of the kidney, or, alternatively, an estimated glomerular filtration rate (eGFR) of <60 mL/min/1.73 m^2 for at least 3 months. The Kidney Disease Improving Global Outcomes (KDIGO) classifies CKD into five stages of increasing severity dependent on the eGFR as seen in **Table 1**.[1]

Due to dynamic nature of pregnancy and postpartum changes in renal function, creatinine-based equations for eGFR are not validated for pregnant women and may underestimate or overestimate eGFR in pregnancy. Calculation of creatinine clearance requires 24 hours urine collection, which is inconvenient and often incomplete thus limiting its use. Serum creatinine concentration should be used to assess renal function in pregnancy **(Table 2)**.[2] Relative changes in creatinine have greater clinical utility than absolute value. Currently there are no validated formulas in pregnancy to calculate eGFR.

Common etiologies in young women include glomerular diseases (focal segmental glomerulonephritis, immunoglobulin A nephropathy, minimal change disease), vascular diseases (thrombotic microangiopathies), tubulointerstitial diseases (nephrolithiasis and reflux nephropathy), and cystic diseases (polycystic kidney disease). Further, systemic diseases that often involve the kidneys are diabetes, systemic lupus erythematous, and vasculitis.[3]

Preconception CKD stage is an important determinant of obstetric and perinatal outcomes and impact of pregnancy on maternal

TABLE 1: Staging of chronic kidney disease outcomes quality initiative (KDOQI).[1]

Stage	Description	GFR (mL/min/1.73 m^2)
1	Abnormal renal morphology or function with normal or increased GFR	≥90
2	Abnormal renal morphology or function with mildly decreased GFR	60–89
3	Moderate decrease in GFR	30–59
4	Severe decrease in GFR	15–29
5	End-stage renal disease (ESRD)	<15 or dialysis dependent

(GFR: glomerular filtration rate)

TABLE 2: Degree of renal impairment in pregnancy.[3]			
Degree of CKD	Serum creatinine (mg/dL)	Creatinine clearance (mL/min)	Stage of CKD
Mild	<1.4	>70	1–2
Moderate	1.4–2.4	40–70	2–3
Severe	>2.4	<40	3–4

(CKD: chronic kidney disease)

renal health. In women with CKD, normal renal and hemodynamic adaptations to pregnancy may not occur, leading to adverse pregnancy outcomes. For some women hypertension, proteinuria, or hematuria detected at routine antenatal booking visit may uncover previously undiagnosed CKD.

Pregnancies in CKD patients should be considered "high risk" due to potential maternal and fetal complications and follow-up by a multidisciplinary team, with individually tailored plan is essential for successful fetomaternal outcome.

Epidemiology and Magnitude of the Problem

The global prevalence of CKD has been recently estimated to be approximately 13.4%, with men being affected more than women.[4] The prevalence of CKD in women of child-bearing age is relatively low, approximately 0.1–4%.[5] Pregnancy with CKD can have a turbulent course with grave complications. Stages 1 and 2 (normal or mild renal impairment with persistent albuminuria) affect up to 3% of women of child-bearing age group (20–39 years). Stages 3–5 (glomerular filtration rate <60 mL/min) affect around one in 150 women of child-bearing age group, but reduced fertility and early miscarriages make these cases infrequent in antenatal care.[6]

India does not have a renal registry, making availability of data in the Indian scenario difficult to interpret. Diabetes and hypertension account for over 2/3rd of the cases of CKD in western countries as well as in India. As per recent Indian Council of Medical Research data, prevalence of diabetes in Indian adult population has risen to 7.1–28%. Likewise, the reported prevalence of hypertension in the adult population today is 17%. With increasing prevalence of these diseases in India, we can extrapolate that the prevalence of CKD is expected to increase.[7]

IMPLICATIONS FOR MATERNAL AND FETAL HEALTH

As expected, the advanced stages of CKD are associated with adverse outcomes but even the earlier stages can have serious implications. It is not just the stage of the disease itself, but also associated hypertension, worsening serum creatinine (or a fall <10% from prepregnancy values) and proteinuria that are important predictors of pregnancy outcomes **(Table 3)**.[8]

EFFECT OF PREGNANCY ON CHRONIC KIDNEY DISEASE

Main risks for CKD mothers:
- *Worsening of renal function:* This may be irreversible. The degree and persistence of this decline is typically determined by the severity of the underlying renal disease.[10]
- *Worsening proteinuria:* It indicates superimposed preeclampsia or deteriorating renal disease. However, it can also be a physiological response to pregnancy or

TABLE 3: Pregnancy outcomes based on stage.[9]

Creatinine (mg/dL)	Adverse pregnancy outcomes (%)	Successful obstetric outcomes (%)	Permanent loss of GFR (%)
<1.5	26	96	10
1.5–2.5	47	89	20 10% progression to ESRD
>2.5	86	46	Very high chance of ESRD
Creatinine (mg/dL)	**Fetal growth restriction/ preterm birth (%)**	**Preeclampsia (%)**	**Live birth rate (%)**
<1.5	30	22	>90
1.5–2.5	60	40	About 85%
>2.5	>90	60	High fetal loss rates

(ESRD: end-stage renal disease; GFR: glomerular filtration rate)

a result of withdrawal of angiotensin-converting enzyme inhibitors/angiotensin receptor blockers.

a. *Mild renal impairment (stages 1-2):* Most women with CKD who become pregnant have mild renal dysfunction and pregnancy does not usually affect renal prognosis.[6]

b. *Moderate-to-severe renal impairment (stages 3-5):* The further deterioration of renal function in pregnancy depends on the baseline compromise, presence of uncontrolled hypertension, and proteinuria. Women with end-stage renal disease of any age group are at risk of increased morbidity and even mortality. Thus, women should be counseled accordingly and encouraged to plan pregnancies at earlier stages of the disease.[3] Pregnancy in women with CKD stages 3-5 advances the need for dialysis or renal transplantation by 2.5 years.[8]

EFFECT OF CHRONIC KIDNEY DISEASE ON PREGNANCY

While considering effect of CKD on pregnancy outcomes, the stage of CKD along with proteinuria, hypertension or preeclampsia have more impact as compared to the etiology of CKD. The only exception is SLE nephritis especially when associated with antiphospholipid antibodies and membranoproliferative glomerulonephritis, where poorer outcomes are noted.[10]

Risks to Mother

- Preeclampsia
- Potential flare of underlying disease
- Transient or persistent loss of renal function
- Requirement for dialysis/permanent loss of renal function
- Maternal mortality.

Compared to the general population, the risk of developing preeclampsia for women with CKD, increases with worsening renal function (20% for patients with mild renal impairment, and 60–80% with severe impairment, compared to approximately 5% in the general population).[11]

For patients on dialysis, additional risks include polyhydramnios related to uremia, preterm labor, and preterm premature rupture of membranes and placental abruption. Full heparinization requirements during hemodialysis further increase the risk of bleeding. The specific problems with peritoneal dialysis include peritonitis and limitation in the volume of exchanges in later pregnancy.[2]

Fetal Risks

- Spontaneous miscarriage
- Congenital malformations
- Growth restriction
- Prematurity
- Still birth
- Inheritance of maternal disease and side effects of maternal therapies.

Adverse fetal outcomes occur in approximately 20% of pregnancies in mothers with CKD, compared to 9% in those without CKD.[11] Studies have reported high live birth rates of 98% in pregnancies progressing beyond 20 weeks' gestation of women with CKD 3-5, but these pregnancies were complicated by preterm delivery (56%) and birthweight <10th centile (36%).[8]

Management Steps/Algorithm

The heightened risk for adverse maternal and neonatal outcomes in women with CKD, especially in those with advanced disease, necessitates multidisciplinary care that includes nephrologist, maternal medicine specialist, and neonatologist. Several management strategies exist to optimize outcomes, beginning with preconception care through delivery and postpartum period, and are applicable to all stages of CKD including those on dialysis and post-renal transplantation.

While managing CKD in pregnancy most important aspect is managing associated clinical features, rather than the type of kidney disease (except in lupus nephritis). **Tables 4 and 5** outline the management of CKD in pregnancy. **Table 6** summaries information on most commonly used antihypertensives and immunosuppressive drugs used in CKD.

Principles of Care

- *Hypertension:* Optimum control of blood pressure is imperative to preserve renal function and avoid adverse pregnancy outcomes. But there is a lack of randomized controlled trials to guide regarding what is the optimal blood pressures in pregnancy. As per CHIPS (Control of Hypertension in Pregnancy Study) trial, the target has been advocated to be 140/90 mm Hg and the same has been recommended.[3]
- *Proteinuria:* Progression of underlying renal disease during pregnancy and adverse pregnancy outcomes are associated with the degree of proteinuria.[3] Thus, formal quantification of proteinuria is essential. Dipstick testing of urine with reagent strips has high false positive and false negative results and 24-hour urine protein estimation is cumbersome and often incomplete. Urine protein—creatinine ratio is faster with better sensitivity and specificity.[2]
- *Preeclampsia in CKD:* High risk for development of superimposed preeclampsia. Criteria for diagnosis are:
  1. Blood pressure >160/110 mm Hg
  2. Blood control suddenly worsening after a period of good control
  3. Development of proteinuria >2,000 mg/day or abrupt worsening of proteinuria
  4. Serum creatinine increasing to >1.2 mg/dL

There are no separate trials or studies for preeclampsia prevention in CKD but use of aspirin in higher doses (150 mg) may be effective as per ASPRE trial. Cochrane also advocates use of calcium

TABLE 4: Algorithm for management of pregnancy with chronic kidney disease.[3]

Prepregnancy	• Timing of conception • Contraceptive advice • Fertility assessment • Determine disease activity. Repeat biopsy confirmation if necessary • Blood pressure optimization • Change to non-teratogenic medications • Provide reassurance about continuation of safe medications in pregnancy Explain risk of pregnancy complications and need for heightened surveillance

Antenatal	**Maternal management**
	• *Investigations:*
	  – Complete blood count—higher incidence of anemia with CKD
	  – Renal function test—baseline and serially depending on stage of disease. More frequently for disease stages 3–5 and in the second half of pregnancy
	• Urine examination—every 4–6 weeks check for:
	  – Infection—identification/management of urinary tract infection
	  – Proteinuria—need of thromboprophylaxis
	  – Hematuria—if present, perform microscopy for red cell casts, which suggest active renal parenchymal disease. Normal red cell morphology suggests urological pathology—seek urological advice
	• *Oral glucose tolerance test*—especially important in women taking steroids or calcineurin inhibitors
	• *Baseline renal ultrasound*—at booking (around 12 weeks' gestation) for pelvicalyceal dimensions. Repeat if symptoms suggest obstruction
	• Markers of disease activity, e.g., systemic lupus erythematosus
	• Monitoring drug levels, e.g., calcineurin
	• *Renal biopsy*—preferred preconception. In pregnancy <32 weeks of gestation (technically difficult >32 weeks) only if:
	  – New-onset nephrotic syndrome
	  – Significant glomerular disease needing confirmation of diagnosis for treatment choice
	  – Sudden deterioration in renal function (well-controlled hypertension, no coagulopathy)
	• *Disease specific management*
	• *Hypertension management:*
	  – Target BP <140/90 mm Hg
	  – Preferred medications—methyldopa (maximum 3 g/day), labetalol (maximum 1.2 g/day), nifedipine XL (maximum 90 mg/day), hydralazine (50 mg/day)
	  – Contraindication—angiotensin-converting enzyme inhibitors, angiotensin receptor blockers
	  – Preeclampsia prevention—start low-dose aspirin, consider vitamin D and calcium supplements
	• *Proteinuria management:*
	  – Immunological treatment vs. non-immunological treatment—depending on disease etiology
	  – Edema—extremity elevation, furosemide (judicious use), albumin infusions (severe cases)

Contd...

Contd...	
	– Anticoagulation with low molecular weight heparin (LMWH): - High-grade proteinuria with low serum albumin levels (<2.0–2.5 g/dL) - Lesser degrees of proteinuria with kidney diseases having higher risks of thrombosis (e.g., membranous nephropathy and vasculitis or additional risk factors, including prolonged periods of immobility, obesity) - In patients with impaired renal function dose adjustments for LMWH may be required and monitoring of factor Xa levels can sometimes be helpful • *Supportive measures:* – Avoid nephrotoxins, nonsteroidal anti-inflammatory drugs – Reduce doses of medications with renal clearance – Cautious use of magnesium sulfate – *Electrolyte imbalance:* Dietary counseling for a low-potassium diet. Binding resins can be used. Extreme cases may require to initiate dialysis. – *Bone mineral metabolism:* Treat associated hypocalcemia and hyperphosphatemia (due to secondary hyperparathyroidism) with oral calcium carbonate supplementations, calcium-based binders, and vitamin D analogs **Fetal management** • Genetic counseling should be offered to women with inheritable renal disease • First and second trimester screening • Serial growth scans after 28–32 weeks • Doppler studies (if indicated) • Cardiotocography • Cardiac monitoring in Ro+/La+ women
Delivery	• Deliver if presence of maternal or fetal decompensation • Corticosteroid administration for fetal lung maturation at least 24 hours and up to 7 days prior to anticipated delivery if <34 weeks gestation • Aim for vaginal delivery if possible. Cesarean for obstetric indication • Intrapartum stress dose of steroid (if on long-term steroid therapy) • Judicious fluid management • Antibiotic cover
Postpartum	• Encourage breastfeeding • Continue venous thromboembolism prophylaxis for at least 6 weeks • *Contraception:* Progesterone-only pill ("mini pill"), contraceptive implant, and Mirena coil are safe and effect

supplementation in high-risk populations with low baseline calcium intake.

- *Anemia:* It is commonly seen in pregnancy with CKD and needs early oral/parenteral iron supplementation to maintain target hemoglobin (Hb) of 10–11 g/dL. Erythropoietin might be needed if the Hb is low with normal or high serum ferritin. It is safe to use in pregnancy and breastfeeding. However, there is a theoretical risk of exacerbating preexisting or causing new-onset hypertension.[12]

- *Maternal acidosis:* It can lead to progressive fetal acidemia. Initiation of sodium bicarbonate therapy or in extreme cases dialysis should be considered to maintained maternal serum pH >7.2.[3]

TABLE 5: Management of specific kidney diseases during pregnancy.[6,15]

Specific renal disease	Associated complications	Summary of management
Lupus nephritis	*Lupus flare:* To be differentiated from preeclampsia (normal complement levels and dsDNA, no active urinary sediment, sFlt-1/PlGF ratio)	• Immunosuppressive therapy • Hydroxychloroquine • Prognosis favorable if disease in remission prior to pregnancy
Diabetic nephropathy	Worsening of renal function	• Good glycemic control • If significant proteinuria—only condition in which ACE inhibitors are to be continued till 8 weeks of pregnancy
Primary glomerulonephritis	Hypertension, proteinuria, recurrent infection	• Treatment of associated clinical features • Outcome relates to control of clinical features and severity of renal impairment
Autosomal dominant polycystic kidney disease	Impaired renal function, hypertension	Fetal work-up includes genetic counseling and prenatal diagnosis
Congenital urinary tract obstruction	Recurrence of obstruction despite initial correction	• Renal ultrasound • Serial assessment of renal function • Urine culture • Hypertension management
Vesico-ureteric reflux nephropathy	Recurrent urinary tract infection, ureteral obstruction, hypertension	• Prophylactic antibiotics • Drainage of obstruction
Nephrolithiasis	Renal colic, ureteric obstruction	Magnetic resonance urography can be used in diagnosis to avoid exposure to radiation

- *Prenatal screening for aneuploidies:* Women with abnormal renal function have potentially increased false positive rate in first trimester combined screening as the multiple of the median may be increased for beta-human chorionic gonadotrophin. Noninvasive prenatal testing (NIPT) can be offered as an alternative.[13]

  The cell-free fetal fraction of deoxyribonucleic acid (DNA) in NIPT and placental growth factor (PlGF) is also affected in dialysis patients. In these cases, first trimester prenatal screening becomes less reliable, and other options may need to be explored, including chorionic villus sampling or amniocentesis, with its inherent risks and limitations.[14]

- *Dialysis in pregnancy:* Dialysis is indicated in cases with severe metabolic acidosis (pH <7.2) and hyperkalemia (Sr Potassium >6 mmol/L) that is not amenable to treatment, along with congestive heart failure due to volume overload, uremic symptoms, and persistent blood urea nitrogen (BUN) >50 mg/dL.[2]

  Hemodialysis is preferred in pregnancy. The duration and the frequency of dialysis must be increased to >20 hours/week, (ideally 36 hours week) and 5–6 days/week.

TABLE 6: Pharmacological considerations.

Drugs	Maternal factors	Fetal factors	Lactation
Labetalol	Avoid if asthmatic	No anomalies, reduced birth weight, neonatal bradycardia (2%), and hypoglycemia (5%)	Safe
Nifedipine	None	No anomalies	Safe
Methyldopa	Avoid in depression or risk of depression	No association with anomalies	Risk of postnatal depression
Hydralazine	Risk of hypotension, tachycardia	No anomalies	Safe
Beta-blockers	• Avoid in asthmatics • Used in maternal indication	• No anomalies • Reduced birth weight, neonatal bradycardia (1%), and hypoglycemia (3%)	Safe
ACE inhibitors	None	Fetotoxic in 2nd and 3rd trimester leads to fetal and neonatal renal failure, bone and aortic arch malformations, oligohydramnios, and pulmonary hypoplasia	Safety data for captopril and enalapril
Angiotensin receptor blockers (ARBs)	None	Fetotoxic in 2nd and 3rd trimester like ACE inhibitors	No data
Thiazide diuretics	Reduce plasma volume expansion in pregnancy	No jaundice, thrombocytopenia	Suppress lactation
Corticosteroids	Potential risk—diabetes mellitus (DM), hypertension, preeclampsia (PE), preterm premature rupture of membranes (PPROM). Aim for minimum maintenance dose	Fetus exposed to <10% maternal dose due to placental deactivation. Increase in oral cleft	• Small amount in breast milk • Feed 4 hours post administration
Azathioprine	None	No anomalies	Safe
Cyclosporin/tacrolimus	May need higher dose in pregnancy. Increased risk of gestational diabetes mellitus (GDM)	No anomalies	Safe
Hydroxychloroquine	Withdrawal may precipitate lupus flare. Continued throughout pregnancy in lupus nephritis	No anomalies. May reduce risk of congenital heart block (CHB) if maternal Ro/La antibodies	Safe

Contd...

Contd...

Drugs	Maternal factors	Fetal factors	Lactation
Mycophenolate mofetil (MMF)	None	Effective contraception for 6 weeks after treatment. Teratogenic causing ear, heart, eye, lips/palate, kidney and bone abnormalities, tracheo-esophageal fistula (TEF)	Avoid in lactation
Cyclophosphamide	None	Teratogenic causing abnormalities of skull, ear, face, limb, and visceral organs	• Excreted in milk • Discontinue breastfeeding for 36 hours after treatment
Rituximab	Indicated for severe disease. Aim to give before and in early pregnancy to avoid neonatal B cell depletion	Active transfer in 2nd and 3rd trimester. Neonatal B cell depletion	Unclear. Neonatal abnormalities unlikely
Sirolimus/Everolimus	Impaired wound healing and proteinuria	Likely placental transfer, toxicity in animal studies	Limited data. Avoid during lactation

Women on peritoneal dialysis will also need increased exchange frequency and lower exchange volumes.[2]

Nutrition and supplementation requirements include increased protein (1.5–1.8 g/kg/day), increased folate (5 mg/day), increased dose of erythropoietin, double doses of multivitamins, liberal dosages of dietary phosphate, and vitamin D.

Heparin-free dialysis is to be instituted prior to delivery so as to be able to offer regional anesthesia and reduce risk of postpartum hemorrhage.

Serial ultrasound scan for cervical length assessment and supplementation with progesterone should be done for preterm prevention in such cases.

Neonates born to women on dialysis have a higher BUN and creatinine resulting in osmotic diuresis needing close monitoring and correction of fluid and electrolyte imbalance.

TAKE HOME MESSAGES

- Pregnancy in CKD is studded with risks to both mother and the fetus necessitating multidisciplinary team care.
- Management starts in the prepregnancy period with counseling, medication review, and health optimization.
- Strict maternal and fetal surveillance to be done during the antenatal period and pregnancy plan to be decided on individual basis.
- Delivery should be at a tertiary care center with neonatal intensive care unit (NICU) facilities.
- Pregnant women on dialysis and post-renal transplant pregnancies need specialist care.

■ REFERENCES

1. Kidney Disease: Improving Global Outcomes (KDIGO) CKD Work Group. KDIGO 2012 Clinical Practice Guideline for the Evaluation and Management of Chronic Kidney Disease. Kidney Int Suppl. 2013;3:1-150.
2. Wiles K, Chappell L, Clark K, Elman L, Hall M, Lightstone L, Mohamed G, et al. Clinical

practice guideline on pregnancy and renal disease. BMC Nephrol. 2019;20(1):401.
3. Hui D, Hladunewich MA. Chronic kidney disease and pregnancy. Obstet Gynecol. 2019;133(6):1182-94.
4. Hill NR, Fatoba ST, Oke JL, Hirst JA, O'Callaghan CA, Lasserson DS, et al. Global prevalence of chronic kidney disease: a systematic review and meta-analysis. PLoS One. 2016;11:e0158765.
5. Piccoli GB, Alrukhaimi M, Liu ZH, Zakharova E, Levin A, World Kidney Day Steering Committee. What we do and do not know about women and kidney diseases; Questions unanswered and answers unquestioned: Reflection on World Kidney Day and International Woman's Day. Physiol Int. 2018;105(1):1-18.
6. Williams D, Davison J. Chronic kidney disease in pregnancy. BMJ. 2008;336(7637):211-5.
7. Varma PP. Prevalence of chronic kidney disease in India: Where are we heading? Indian J Nephrol. 2015;25(3):133-5.
8. Wiles K, Webster P, Seed PT, Bennett-Richards K, Bramham K, Brunskill N, et al. The impact of chronic kidney disease Stages 3-5 on pregnancy outcomes. Nephrol Dial Transplant. 2021;36(11):2008-17.
9. Brown MA, Mangos GJ, Peek MJ, Plaat F. Chapter 7. Renal Disease in Pregnancy. In: Powrie RO, Greene MF (Eds). de Swiet's Medical Disorders in Obstetric Practice, 5th edition. Oxford, UK: Wiley-Blackwell, 2010. pp. 182-208.
10. Piccoli GB, Cabiddu G2, Attini R3, Vigotti FN4, Maxia S2, Lepori N, et al. Risk of adverse pregnancy outcomes in women with CKD. J Am Soc Nephrol. 2015;26:2011-22.
11. Brunskill NJ. Renal disease in pregnancy. Obstet Gynaecol Reprod Med. 2019;29: 15-20.
12. Sanchez-Gonzalez LR, Castro-Melendez SE, Angeles-Torres AC, Castro-Cortina N, Escobar-Valencia A, Quiroga-Garza A. Efficacy and safety of adjuvant recombinant human erythropoietin and ferrous sulfate as treatment for iron deficiency anemia during the third trimester of pregnancy. Eur J Obstet Gynecol Reprod Biol. 2016;205:32-6.
13. Valentin M, Muller F, Beaujard MP, Dreux S, Czerkiewicz I, Meyer V, et al. First-trimester combined screening for trisomy 21 in women with renal disease. Prenat Diagn. 2015;35:244-8.
14. Wehmann RE, Amr S, Rosa C, Nisula BC. Metabolism, distribution and excretion of purified human chorionic gonadotropin and its subunits in man. Ann Endocrinol (Paris). 1984;45:291-5.
15. Giorgina B, Cabiddu G, Attini R, Vigotti F, Fassio F, Rolfo A, et al. Pregnancy in chronic kidney disease: questions and answers in a changing panorama. Best Pract Res Clin Obstet Gynaecol. 2015;29(5):625-42.

CHAPTER 16

Urinary Tract Infections in Pregnancy

Kallur Sailaja Devi

■ INTRODUCTION

Urinary tract infections (UTIs) are one of the most frequent complications during pregnancy. Incidence is around 8%.[1] Bacteriuria rates in pregnant and nonpregnant are similar; however, bacteriuria during pregnancy has a greater tendency to progress to ascending infection than in nonpregnant women. Physiological and anatomical changes associated with pregnancy increase the risk of urinary stasis which can alter the course of infection leading to an increased risk of recurrent UTI and progression to acute pyelonephritis.

Urinary tract infection in pregnancy is associated with maternal and fetal complications, increases the risk of preterm birth, low birth weight fetus, maternal anemia, and acute pyelonephritis leading to sepsis.[2,3]

Risk factors for UTI in pregnancy include diabetes, history of infection, steroids or immunosuppressive drugs, and anatomical urinary tract abnormality.

Historically UTI is classified as lower urinary tract acute cystitis or upper urinary tract pyelonephritis (acute pyelonephritis) with bacteriuria as a predisposing factor.

■ ASYMPTOMATIC BACTERIURIA

Incidence: It affects 5–10% of pregnant women.[4] In pregnant women, treat at the time of first positive urine culture while in nonpregnant women, treat when two consecutive voided cultures with >10^5 colony-forming units of the same bacteria are present.

Screening methods: Screening test is by clean catch specimen, which involves the collection of mid-stream specimen of urine after cleaning of the perineum to minimize contamination of skin flora.

Screening by complete urine examination in the first trimester for bacteriuria (leukocyte esterase and nitrite positive), protein, and blood may help to exclude UTIs. World Health Organization (WHO) recommends routine screening by midstream specimen of urine (MSU) for culture to diagnose asymptomatic bacteriuria. Between 14 and 16 weeks of pregnancy, do urine culture and sensitivity test.[5] Repeat complete urine examination in the third trimester, especially for cases that are at risk of infection.

Criteria for asymptomatic bacteriuria are considered as 10^5 colony forming units/mL of urine, the chance of contamination at this level is <1%. There is a 50% chance of contamination when the colony count is 10^3–10^4 colony forming units/mL of urine.

Bacteriology

Escherichia coli (*E. coli*) accounts for 80–90% of infection, other gram-negative bacilli include *Proteus, Klebsiella pneumoniae,* and *Pseudomonas*.[6] Gram-positive beta-hemolytic *Streptococci* and *Staphylococcus saprophyticus* account for 10% of infections. Group B streptococci have implications in pregnancy; need to consider antibiotics in the intrapartum period. Less common organisms include *Gardnerella vaginalis* and ureaplasma urealyticum.

Treatment

Treatment is based on antibiotic sensitivity patterns in the culture report. If untreated there is a 20-40% risk of pyelonephritis. Cochrane review in 2000 showed that antimicrobial treatment was compared with placebo or no treatment, and treatment was effective in clearing asymptomatic bacteriuria (RR: 0.25, 95% CI: 0.14-0.48), reducing the risk of pyelonephritis (RR: 0.23, 95% CI: 0.13-0.41), and reducing the incidence of low birth weight babies (RR: 0.66, 95% CI: 0.49-0.89).[7]

Antibiotics should cover the most common infecting organism such as gram-negative gastrointestinal organisms and should be safe for the mother and fetus. Earlier ampicillin was the drug of choice, but resistance was found in 20-30% of *E. coli* cultured from urine in an outpatient setting.[8] Antibiotics that are safe in pregnancy include penicillin (ampicillin, amoxicillin), and cephalosporins (cephalexin, cefuroxime, cefotaxime) clindamycin, and macrolides (azithromycin, erythromycin). For asymptomatic bacteriuria consider antibiotic for 5-7 days based on culture sensitivity report.[9,10] Nitrofurantoin is a good choice because of urinary antiseptic with higher urinary concentration and acts mainly on gram-negative bacteria such as *E. coli*. **Table 1** shows common drug dosages in pregnancy. Repeat test to ensure eradication of organism as 15% of women have a recurrence. Recurrence of infection needs evaluation, consider scan to rule out anatomical abnormalities and low dose antibiotic till delivery. **Table 2** shows drugs that are contraindicated in pregnancy.

■ CYSTITIS

Incidence: It occurs in 1-3% of pregnant women.[11]

Clinical features: It usually presents with pain, dysuria, urinary frequency, and urgency.

Diagnosis: Cystitis is diagnosed by midstream urine sample culture to find out the organism and sensitivity pattern to an antibiotic.

Treatment: Empirical antibiotic to be started based on symptoms and change antibiotic based on sensitivity pattern of the organism, consider antibiotic for 7 days. National Institute for Clinical Excellence guidance quotes that no evidence was found on cranberry products or urine alkalinizing agents to treat UTIs.[12] **Box 1** shows the preventive measures to reduce recurrence of UTIs.

■ ACUTE PYELONEPHRITIS

Incidence: It occurs in around 1-2% of pregnant women, common in the second

TABLE 1: Antibiotics recommended in pregnancy.

Antibiotic	Dose	Duration	Safety
Co-amoxiclav	625 mg thrice daily	5 or 7 days	Safe in 1, 2, 3 trimester, and lactation period
Cefuroxime axetil	500 mg twice daily	5 days	Safe in 1, 2, 3 trimester, and lactation period
Nitrofurantoin	100 mg twice daily	7 days	Avoid near term and lactation period

TABLE 2: Antibiotics to be avoided in pregnancy.[16]

Antibiotic	Trimester	Risk
Tetracyclines	1, 2, 3	Effect on skeletal development and teeth discoloration
Quinolones	1, 2, 3	Arthropathy
Chloramphenicol	1, 2, 3	Neonatal Gray syndrome
Trimethoprim	1	Teratogenicity risk
Aminoglycosides	2, 3	Vestibular damage
Sulphonamides	3	Neonatal hemolysis, methemoglobinemia
Nitrofurantoin	Term	Neonatal hemolysis

BOX 1: Measures to prevent recurrent urinary tract infections.

- Increasing fluid intake leads to frequent voiding and a high volume of dilute urine.
- Empty bladder after intercourse—helps to wash out microorganisms that have migrated to the urethra from the perineum into the bladder.
- Double voiding so that no residual urine is left in the bladder after micturition.
- Clean perineum from front to back—to minimize the risk of bowel organisms colonizing the urethra.

and third trimesters.[13,14] Most are due to undiagnosed or inadequately treated lower UTIs.

Points to Check in History Taking

- Current urinary symptoms such as dysuria, hematuria, frequency, urgency, and suprapubic pain. Frequency can be a physiologic change of pregnancy, difficult to differentiate in the absence of testing.
- History of previous UTI—the risk of recurrence is more in pregnancy.
- Coexisting vaginal discharge and sexual history should be taken.
- Systemic symptoms—such as shivering, fever, vomiting, loin pain.
- Relevant medical history—diabetes, on any drugs such as steroids and immunosuppressants, neuropathic bladder (spina bifida, multiple sclerosis).

Steps in an Examination

1. Record respiratory rate and pulse, look for any hypotension, temperature, and oxygen saturation.
2. Check for any loin, groin, or suprapubic tenderness, which may give clues for urinary tract calculi or infection.
3. Check for fetal heart rate, fetal growth, and amniotic fluid. Based on gestational age do the nonstress test.

Differential diagnosis includes pneumonia, viral infections, cholecystitis, biliary colic, preeclampsia, acute appendicitis, gastroenteritis, placental abruption, and degenerating uterine fibroid.

Management of Acute Pyelonephritis

- Admission to the hospital until clinical symptoms improved.
- Investigations include complete blood picture, serum creatinine, urine examination, and urine culture and renal scan.
- Renal ultrasonography is useful to show kidney size and collecting system obstruction. In most causes no significant findings are seen on scan.

- Consider intravenous fluids if dehydrated due to fever, pain, and vomiting.
- Consider antipyretics and analgesics for pain. Nonsteroidal anti-inflammatory agents may cause oligohydramnios and premature closure of patent ductus arteriosus, hence avoid in pregnancy.
- Based on clinical symptoms start intravenous antibiotics after obtaining urine culture samples. The first choice is intravenous penicillin or cephalosporin for 24–48 hours, based on clinical improvement change to an oral antibiotic. Antibiotics should be continued for a period of at least 2 weeks.
- If sepsis is suspected consider third-generation cephalosporins and aminoglycoside antibiotics and monitor with renal function test.
- At the risk of deep vein thrombosis (DVT) because of reduced mobility, identify any other risk factors for DVT and consider thromboprophylaxis with stockings and low molecular weight heparin.
- Women are at risk of preterm delivery, anemia, and preeclampsia.[15]
- Avoid steroid prophylaxis for lung maturity during an episode of acute infection.

PROPHYLAXIS

Pregnant women who had confirmed and documented two or more UT in pregnancy need renal scans and antibiotic prophylaxis throughout pregnancy. Antibiotics include low-dose amoxicillin or low dose cephalosporin (cephalexin 250 mg) or nitrofurantoin 50 mg once daily dose.

Group B streptococcal infection in pregnancy is associated with chorioamnionitis and neonatal disease. When diagnosed with Group B streptococcal bacteriuria, give a 7-day course of antibiotic and intrapartum antibiotic prophylaxis with a loading dose of benzylpenicillin followed by a 4-hourly dose till birth.

TAKE HOME MESSAGES

- Asymptomatic bacteriuria in pregnancy is common and is associated with maternal and fetal complications.
- Pregnant women should be screened for asymptomatic bacteriuria by urine culture and treated with appropriate antibiotics.
- Pregnancy women with recurrent infection needs long-term low dose antibiotic cover till delivery.

REFERENCES

1. Hooton TM, Stamm WE. Diagnosis and treatment of uncomplicated urinary tract infection. Infect Dis Clin. 1997;11(3): 551-81.
2. McDermott S, Daguise V, Mann H, Szwejbka L, Callaghan W. Perinatal risk for mortality and mental retardation associated with maternal urinary-tract infections. J Fam Pract. 2001; 50:433-7.
3. Romero R, Oyarzun E, Mazor M, Sirtori M, Hobbins JC, Bracken M. Meta-analysis of the relationship between asymptomatic bacteriuria and preterm delivery/low birth weight. Obstet Gynecol. 1989;73:576-82.
4. Kass EH. Maternal urinary tract infection. N Y State J Med. 1962;2822-6.
5. U.S. Preventive Services Task Force. Guide to clinical preventive services: report of the U.S. Preventive Services Task Force. 2nd edition. Baltimore: Williams & Wilkins, 1996.
6. Polk BF. Urinary tract infection in pregnancy. Clin Obstet Gynecol. 1979;22(2):285-92.
7. Smaill FM, Vazquez JC. Antibiotics for asymptomatic bacteriuria in pregnancy. Cochrane Database Syst Rev. 2019(11):CD000490.
8. Sanders CC, Sanders WE. Beta-lactam resistance in gram-negative bacteria: global trends and clinical impact. Clin Infect Dis. 1992;15:824-39.
9. Widmer M, Gulmezoglu AM, Mignini L, Roganti A. Duration of treatment for

asymptomatic bacteriuria during pregnancy. Cochrane Database Syst Rev. 2015(11): CD000491.
10. WHO recommendation on antibiotic prophylaxis to prevent recurrent urinary tract infections 09 March 2018.
11. Harris RE, Gilstrap LC 3rd. Cystitis during pregnancy: a distinct clinical entity. Obstet Gynecol. 1981;57:578-80.
12. NICE Guideline [NG109]. (2018). Urinary tract infection (lower): antimicrobial prescribing. [online] Available form: https://www.nice.org.uk/guidance/ng109 [Last accessed February, 2023].
13. Gilstrap LC 3rd, Cunningham FG, Whalley PJ. Acute pyelonephritis in pregnancy: an anterospective study. Obstet Gynecol. 1981;57:409-13.
14. Hill JB, Sheffield JS, McIntire DD, Wendel Jr GD. Acute pyelonephritis in pregnancy. Obstet Gynecol. 2005;105(1):18-23.
15. Mazor-Dray E, Levy A, Schlaeffer F, Sheiner E. Maternal urinary tract infection: is it independently associated with adverse pregnancy outcome?. J Matern Fetal Neonatal Med. 2009;22(2):124-8.
16. Safety advice from the British National Formulary.

CHAPTER 17

Drug Dosing in Renal Failure

Shrikant Sahasrabudhe, Beena Daniel

■ INTRODUCTION

It is a well-known fact that pregnant women are usually healthy. By and large they do not need any medications. It is not very easy to find drug dosing guidelines and clearance predictions pertaining to pregnant women as only occasionally are drug kinetics in pregnancy investigated. Due to the above mentioned fact, pregnancy is an exclusion criterion for most of the drug pharmacokinetic studies. Pregnant women can have renal disease (acute/chronic/or acute on chronic) or may require renal replacement therapy. They may be on immunosuppressants, antimicrobials, antihypertensives, anticonvulsants, and anticoagulants. It would be a good practice to avoid drugs other than those needed to treat underlying disease in pregnancy. In this particular chapter, we will try to embark on the drug dosing in renal failure in pregnancy.

■ EPIDEMIOLOGY AND MAGNITUDE OF THE PROBLEM

It has been found that about 75-99% of pregnant women consume some or the other medicine during pregnancy.[1]

We will first look at how and what are the physiological changes occurring in pregnancy pertaining to drug dosing.

In normal pregnancy, there is approximately 25% increase in glomerular filtration rate (GFR).[2] Due to this factor, they might need higher than normal dose of common antibiotics such as cefazolin, cefuroxime, and ampicillin in absence of any kidney disease in pregnant women.[1] There are few factors which get affected and other factors counter them. On one hand, it is assumed that there is decrease in protein binding and decrease in metabolic capacity of liver which is due to decrease in hepatic albumin synthesis by about 20% in the mid pregnancy.[3] On the other hand, there is about 50% increase in plasma volume and in turn total body water increases by about 8 liters.[4]

As against this, a pregnant woman with any kidney disease will influence the drug elimination and distribution and will pose a challenge for drug dose adjustment. For an example, higher doses of cyclosporine and methadone are required in pregnant women with kidney ailment due to increased hepatic clearance.

■ IMPLICATIONS FOR MATERNAL HEALTH

Anemia is very common in pregnancy. Iron therapy is very commonly prescribed in this setting, but supplementation is to be given in women only with documented deficiency.[5]

Folic acid is more effective in the first 4 weeks of pregnancy but most often women are not yet aware of their pregnancy status.[6] Pregnancy in women with renal impairment poses three problems:
1. Progress in renal disease
2. Teratogenicity and embryo toxicity
3. Inadequate information on dose adjustment.

IMPLICATIONS FOR FETAL WELL-BEING

It is imperative on a part of treating doctor to prescribe folic acid supplement to all pregnant women who are on folate antagonists such as aminopterin sodium, methotrexate, sulfasalazine, pyrimethamine, triamterene, trimethoprim, carbamazepine, phenytoin, and phenobarbitone which will reduce the risk of cardiovascular defects, oral clefts, and urinary tract defects in the fetus.

Drug-induced risk for fetus should be weighed against the disease related risk for the mother with kidney disease. Nonsteroidal anti-inflammatory drugs (NSAIDs) and COX-2 inhibitors are better avoided in the third trimester due to risk of fetal nephrotoxicity.[7] Angiotensin-converting enzyme (ACE) inhibitors are to be avoided in third trimester. Misoprostol and methotrexate can induce Moebius syndrome and other malformations during first trimester. Similarly, idarubicin given during the second trimester for pregnant women with acute lymphoblastic leukemia can cause cardiotoxicity in infants.[8] Risk of fetal malformation increases almost six to seven times with antineoplastic drugs mainly during first week after conception.[4] Irradiation to mother also poses risk of fetal abnormalities. Tetracyclines can cause tooth and bone dysplasias in infants. Quinolones causes cartilaginous defects whereas gentamicin can induce oligonephronia in the fetus. Fetal growth retardation is increased when maternal blood pressure comes down below 160/100 mm Hg. ACE inhibitors and losartan use in mother can cause ACE inhibitor-related fetopathy with vascular malformations, pulmonary hypoplasia, and neonatal anuria. Warfarin or dicoumarol can potentially cause fetal bleeding, stillbirth, teratogenicity, special warfarin syndrome, and warfarin embryopathy. Carbamazepine and valproic acid use can cause malformations. Lithium use can cause lithium-induced teratogenicity in first trimester with perinatal death and cardiovascular abnormalities.

MANAGEMENT STEPS AND ALGORITHM

For the sake of simplicity and understanding, let us divide renal ailment in pregnancy in to three broad categories and discuss various drugs being used and their dose adjustments in the mentioned three board categories:
1. Pregnancy with acute kidney injury (AKI)/insufficiency
2. Pregnancy in a case of chronic kidney disease (CKD) on or not on dialysis
3. Pregnancy after kidney transplantation.

Let us discuss each clinical scenario with emphasis on drug dosing in that particular scenario.

Pregnancy with Acute Kidney Insufficiency and Drug Dosing

Practically any kidney disease can occur in pregnancy. It can be AKI due to any reasons responsible for it as seen with nonpregnant state. Other diseases which are encountered in this scenario are hemolytic uremic syndrome (HUS), lupus nephritis, antiphospholipid syndrome, diabetes mellitus, immunoglobulin A (IgA) nephritis and hydronephrosis and obstructive nephropathy caused due to physiological reflux seen due to pregnancy. For patients with lupus nephritis—steroids, azathioprine, calcineurin inhibitors, intravenous immunoglobulin, and plasma exchange can be used.[9] Important to note here is pregnancy loss was more seen in women with preexisting kidney disease compared to those without kidney disease. Let us start with various drug categories and strategies for their dosing.

- *Antimicrobials:* Antibiotics is the category which is most frequently prescribed in pregnancy (12-29%).[1] As a dictum even asymptomatic bacteriuria (>104 bacteria/mL) should be treated with antibiotics like penicillins or other beta lactams.[10] Itraconazole is an antifungal of choice for vaginal yeast infections as compared to fluconazole. Aminoglycosides (gentamicin and netilmicin), cotrimoxazole, quinolones, rifampicin, tetracyclines, thallium, and trimethoprim are not recommended.
- *Antiviral agents:* Antiretroviral drugs are rated as nontoxic in animal studies. They are mainly didanosine, saquinavir, ritonavir, and nelfinavir.[11] Proven toxic agents are efavirenz, delavirdine mesylate, zalcitabine, and zidovudine. Lamivudine, aciclovir, and ganciclovir needs dose adjustment.
- *Antihypertensives:* ACE inhibitors and angiotensin II AT1 receptor blockers are contraindicated.[12] ACE inhibitors should be discontinued in second or third trimester. Also furosemide and triamterene use is not recommended. Use of beta blockers, diuretics, and calcium channel blockers is controversial.
- *Immunosuppressants:* Recommendations for immunosuppressant medications in pregnancy are given in **Table 1**.[13]
- *Anticoagulants:* Patients with nephrotic syndrome and antiphospholipid syndrome have high propensity to develop thromboembolic complications. As overall risk of thromboembolism in pregnancy is six times more than in a nonpregnant state. Warfarin or dicoumarol use is discouraged. Agents preferred are low dose aspirin, parenteral heparin, or subcutaneous low molecular weight heparin.
- *Erythropoietin:* No risk is associated with its use. High dose has to be used due to its low drug potency.[14]
- *Anticonvulsants:* Interaction with folic acid and metabolism of vitamin K with the risk of neural tube defects and early neonatal bleeding. Anticonvulsant drug level monitoring along with that of vitamin K is advisable.
- *Antidepressants:* Dose adjustment to renal function is required for lithium. Dose of lithium needs to be lowered in a pregnant patient with renal insufficiency. Valproic acid is teratogenic.
- *Tocolytics:* Nifedipine is the first choice. Ritodrine and terbutaline can cause hypokalemia which can be exacerbated in patients with salt losing interstitial renal syndromes.
- *Lipid lowering drugs/antidiabetics:* Atorvastatin and pravastatin should not be used. Also antidiabetic agent metformin is not recommended.

Pregnancy with CKD and the Choice of Drugs Used with the Dose Dosing[9]

It can be divided as:
- *Prepregnancy care:*
  - Contraception—progesterone only pill is recommended
  - Angiotensin receptor antagonists to be discontinued in advance of pregnancy

TABLE 1: Recommendations for immunosuppressant medications in pregnancy.

Drug	Pregnancy effects	Recommendation in pregnancy
Prednisolone	• Maternal hypertension and GDM • Risk of thymic hyperplasia and adrenal suppression in neonate with high doses	• May be continued • Avoid prolonged high doses
Azathioprine	• No teratogenicity • Unable to be activated by fetal liver	May be continued
Tacrolimus	• Potential increased risk of GDM • Risk of transient neonate renal dysfunction and hyperkalemia	• Monitor and adjust levels • Early OGTT in pregnancy, especially if combined with prednisolone • Check neonatal biochemistry
Cyclosporine A	• No teratogenicity • Associated with maternal hypertension • Reversible effect on fetal lymphocytes	• May be continued • Monitor and adjust levels
Mycophenolate mofetil	• Teratogenic and embryopathic • Multiple congenital defects of ears, digits, and oral cavity • Increased pregnancy loss	Cease 12 weeks prior to conception
Cyclophosphamide	• Teratogenic in first trimester • Affects ovarian function and fertility	• Cease 12 weeks preconception • Use in later pregnancy if critical to maternal life
Sirolimus and everolimus (mTOR inhibitors)	Animal studies suggest teratogenicity, effects on bone and fetal growth. Data remain very limited	Cease 12 weeks preconception due to lack of data to support safe use

(GDM: gestational diabetes mellitus; mTOR: mammalian target of rapamycin; OGTT: oral glucose tolerance test)

- *Preeclampsia prophylaxis:*
  - Low dose aspirin (75–150 mg)
  - Same dose of aspirin to kidney donors as well
- *Blood pressure management:*
  - Labetalol, nifedipine and methyldopa are preferred
  - ACE inhibitors, angiotensin receptor blocker (ARBs), and diuretics are not to be used
- *Thromboembolic prophylaxis:* Low molecular weight heparin
- *Anemia:*
  - Parenteral iron only if indicated
  - Erythropoietin if indicated
- *Bone health:* Vitamin D supplements for deficient pregnant women
- *Postnatal care:*
  - NSAIDs should not be given
  - Medicines given which are compatible with breastfeeding
- *Diabetic nephropathy:* ACE inhibitors to be continued until conception.

Pregnancy after Kidney Transplant and Drug Dosing

Use of low dose prednisolone with 7.5 mg/day rather than 10 mg/day dose has more favorable outcome. Breastfeeding is discouraged in patient taking cyclosporine. Other best practice guidelines as regards use of drugs include use of azathioprine of 2 mg/kg or less and cyclosporine <5 mg/kg per day.

Experience with the use of tacrolimus is increasing and it is suggested that it is reasonably safe with similar side effect profile as that of cyclosporine.

As far as the treatment for graft rejection is concerned, use of steroids and intravenous immunoglobulin are found to be safe but the safety profile of antilymphocyte globulins and rituximab are unknown.

PHARMACOLOGICAL CONSIDERATIONS

For all practical purposes, creatinine clearance (ClCr) is the most reliable noninvasive means to adjust drug dose in patients with renal impairment. When it comes to pregnant women, Cockcroft and Gault formula is well certified as it takes in to account the actual pregnancy body weight. Relation between the drug clearance and estimated ClCr is almost linear.

At this juncture, it is imperative for us to understand significance of half-life of a drug as it gives us the best estimate of effect of renal impairment on pharmacokinetics. The half-life is a direct determinant for the duration time of drug effect. Half-life and drug clearance are inversely proportional to each other.

There are two dose adjustment rules:
1. Luzius Dettli rule = Proportional dose reduction rule

    (D/I) individual = (D/I) norm CL individual/CL norm

    Where D = Dose
    I = Administration interval
    Individual = Individual half-life
    CL = Drug clearance
2. Calvin Kunin rule = Half dosage rule

    D individual = 1/2 D start/$t_{1/2}$ individual

There is a third method to calculate dose adjustment which is called as Nicholas Holford method and needs computer-based system. Experience tells us that Luzius Dettli rule leads to calculate insufficiently low doses of a particular drug.

As far as the drug dosing of a particular drug when the patient is undergoing hemodialysis there is a formula as follows:

$$D\ HD = D\ anur + D\ suppl$$

D HD is dose post hemodialysis
D anur is dose off dialysis
D suppl is dose supplementing the dialysis effect.

It is a well-known fact that under dosing of a drug would be more deleterious than overdosing. This is especially applicable to antimicrobials and more importantly in critical area like intensive care unit patients who are on renal replacement therapy. Higher doses are justified in pregnant patients as the volume of distribution increases for water-soluble drugs. These are the same drugs whose elimination depends upon renal function. Usually drug dose proposals are given for extremes of normal and functional anuric renal function. Individual dose is then calculated by interpolating between the two extreme values.

TAKE HOME MESSAGES

- Women with underlying kidney disease can be pregnant in the safest possible way and disease ailments can now be effectively treated due to good understanding of pharmacokinetics.
- One cap does not fit all. We need to have individualized approach for drug dosing for pregnant women with kidney disease.
- It is easy to remember which drugs are contraindicated in pregnancy and avoid them for mother and fetal safety.
- Overdosing and not underdosing is preferred in pregnancy with kidney ailment due to increase in volume of distribution.

- Most effective antihypertensive drugs and immunosuppressive drugs are available now and sound knowledge about them should guide us towards timely and optimum treatment for both mother and child safety.

■ REFERENCES

1. Berkovitch M, Elbirt D, Addis A, Schuler-Faccini L, Ornoy A. Fetal effects of metaclopramide therapy for nausea and vomiting of pregnancy. N Eng J Med. 2000;343:445-6.
2. Loebstein R, Lalkin A, Addis A, Costa A, Lalkin I, Bonati M, et al. Pregnancy outcome after gestational exposure to terfenadine: a multicenter, prospective controlled study. J Allerg Clin Immunol. 1999;104:953-6.
3. Roubenoff R, Hoyt J, Petri M, Hochberg MC, Hellmann DB. Effects of anti-inflammatory and immunosuppressive drugs on pregnancy and fertility. Semin Arthritis Rheum. 1988;18:88-110.
4. Doll DC, Ringenberg OS, Yarbro JW. Antineoplastic agents and pregnancy. Semin Oncol. 1989;16:337-46.
5. Donati S, Baglio G, Spinelli A, Grandolfo ME. Drug use in pregnancy among Italian women. Eur J Clin Pharmacy. 2000;56:323-8.
6. Nulman I, Laslo D, Koren G. Treatment of epilepsy in pregnancy. Drugs. 1999;57(4):535-44.
7. Komhoff M, Wang JL, Cheng HF, Langenbach R, McKanna JA, Harris RC, et al. Cyclooxygenase-2-selective inhibitors impair glomerulogenesis and renal cortical development. Kidney Int. 2000;57(2):414-22.
8. Achtari C, Hohlfeld P. Cardiotoxic transplacental effect of idarubicin administered during the second trimester of pregnancy. Am J Obstet Gynacol. 2000;183:511-2.
9. Wiles K, Chappell LC, Clark K, Elman L, Hall M, Lightstone L, et al. Clinical practice guideline on pregnancy and renal disease. BMC Nephrol. 2019;20:401.
10. Robinson AJ, Ridgway GL. Concurrent gonococcal and chlamydial infection. Drugs. 2000;59:801-13.
11. Carr A, Cooper DA. Adverse effects of antiretroviral therapy. Lancet. 2000;356:1423-30.
12. Hou S. Pregnancy in chronic renal insufficiency and end stage renal disease. Am J Kidney Dis. 1999;33(2):235-52.
13. KDIGO, clinical practice guideline for the care of kidney transplant recipients. Am J Transplant. 2009;9(Suppl 3):S1-S155.
14. Thorp M, Pulliam J. Use of recombinant erythropoietin in a pregnant renal transplant recipient. Am J Nephrol. 1998;18(5):448-51.

Metabolic Conditions

CHAPTER 18

Hyperosmolar State in Pregnancy: Diabetic Ketoacidosis and Hyperosmolar Hyperglycemic Syndrome

Ritesh Shah, Anuj Clerk

INTRODUCTION

Diabetic ketoacidosis (DKA) and hyperosmolar hyperglycemic syndrome (HHS) are the medical and obstetric emergencies requiring multidisciplinary approach and aggressive intensive care unit (ICU) management. Hyperglycemic emergencies in pregnancy can occur in patients with Type 1 or Type 2 or gestational diabetes. Incidence of DKA in pregnancy is approximately 0.5–3%[1] in diabetes patients. Pregnancy predisposes poor glycemic control in diabetics. The exact incidence of HHS in pregnancy is not well defined. Lack of early recognition and aggressive management leads to poor perfusion status, multiorgan failure, and even death. The maternal mortality rate of DKA is <1% but the perinatal mortality rate and morbidity are quite high (9–35%). As onset of both of the conditions can be insidious and can become life-threatening to mother and/or fetus, it requires prompt diagnosis and treatment. It is often diagnosed late because of relative euglycemic state. A multidisciplinary team approach (team including obstetrician, intensivist, and fetal physician) is required to prevent the complications. Prevention is the key.

PRECIPITATING FACTORS[2-4]

- Accelerated starvation because of intractable vomiting
- Inadequate insulin management
- Resistance to insulin
- Steroid use for fetal lung maturation
- Intercurrent infection
- Counter-regulatory actions of hormones—prolactin, human placental lactogen, progesterone, and cortisol
- Compensatory respiratory alkalosis, which decreases buffer capacity
- Unrecognized new onset diabetes
- Insulin pump failure
- Stress of labor
- Gastroparesis
- Thyrotoxicosis
- Myocardia infarction
- Abdominal crisis
- Trauma
- Drug related, e.g., atypical antipsychotics, lithium, diuretics, phenytoin, calcium channel blockers, beta blockers, etc.

PATHOPHYSIOLOGY OF DIABETIC KETOACIDOSIS (FIG. 1)[3-6]

Because of lack of endogenous insulin (absolute insulin deficiency), hyperglycemia develops. This induces polyuria, dehydration and catabolic state which result into breakdown of proteins and fats. This leads to high levels of ketone bodies and free fatty acids. Eventually metabolic acidosis develops and it's adverse consequences develop.

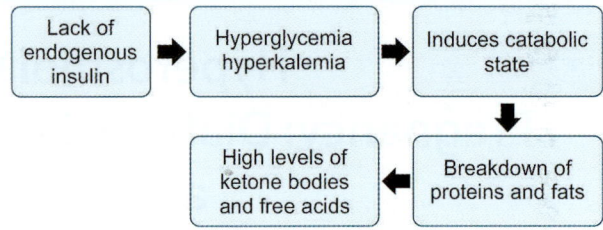

Fig. 1: Pathophysiology of diabetic ketoacidosis.

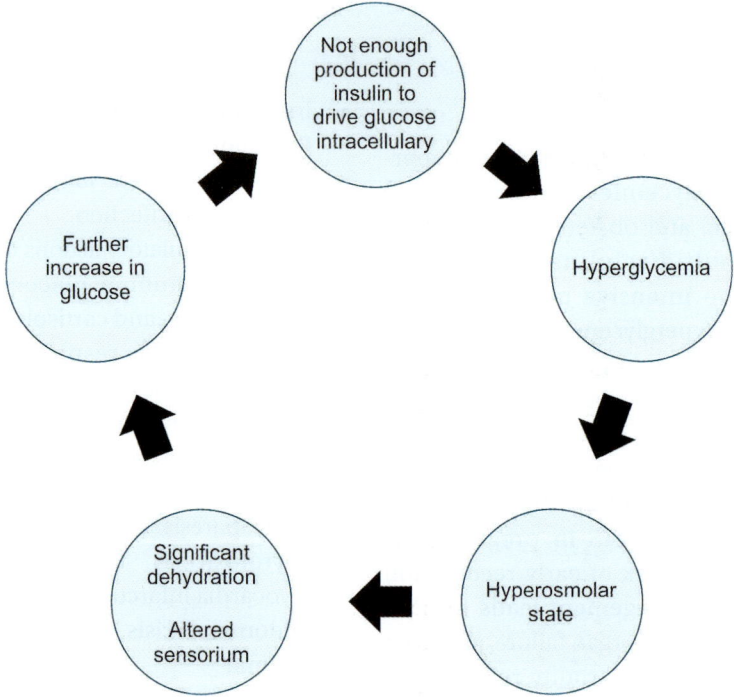

Fig. 2: Pathophysiology of hyperosmolar hyperglycemic syndrome.

PATHOPHYSIOLOGY OF HYPEROSMOLAR HYPERGLYCEMIC SYNDROME (FIG. 2)[3-6]

Usually patients produce sufficient amount of insulin to drive potassium intracellularly and to inhibit the breakdown of proteins and fats but not enough insulin to drive glucose intracellularly. There is enough insulin to block a catabolic state so ketoacidosis and hyperkalemia are not seen frequently in HHS.

MECHANISM OF MATERNAL AND FETAL DISTRESS (FIG. 3)[2]

- Hyperglycemia causes diuresis which ultimately caused uncontrolled water loss which may hamper maternal and fetal hydration.
- There is reduction in glucose utilization in peripheral tissues which increases gluconeogenesis, glycogenolysis and lipolysis. This ultimately initiates a cascade of events including hypovolemia,

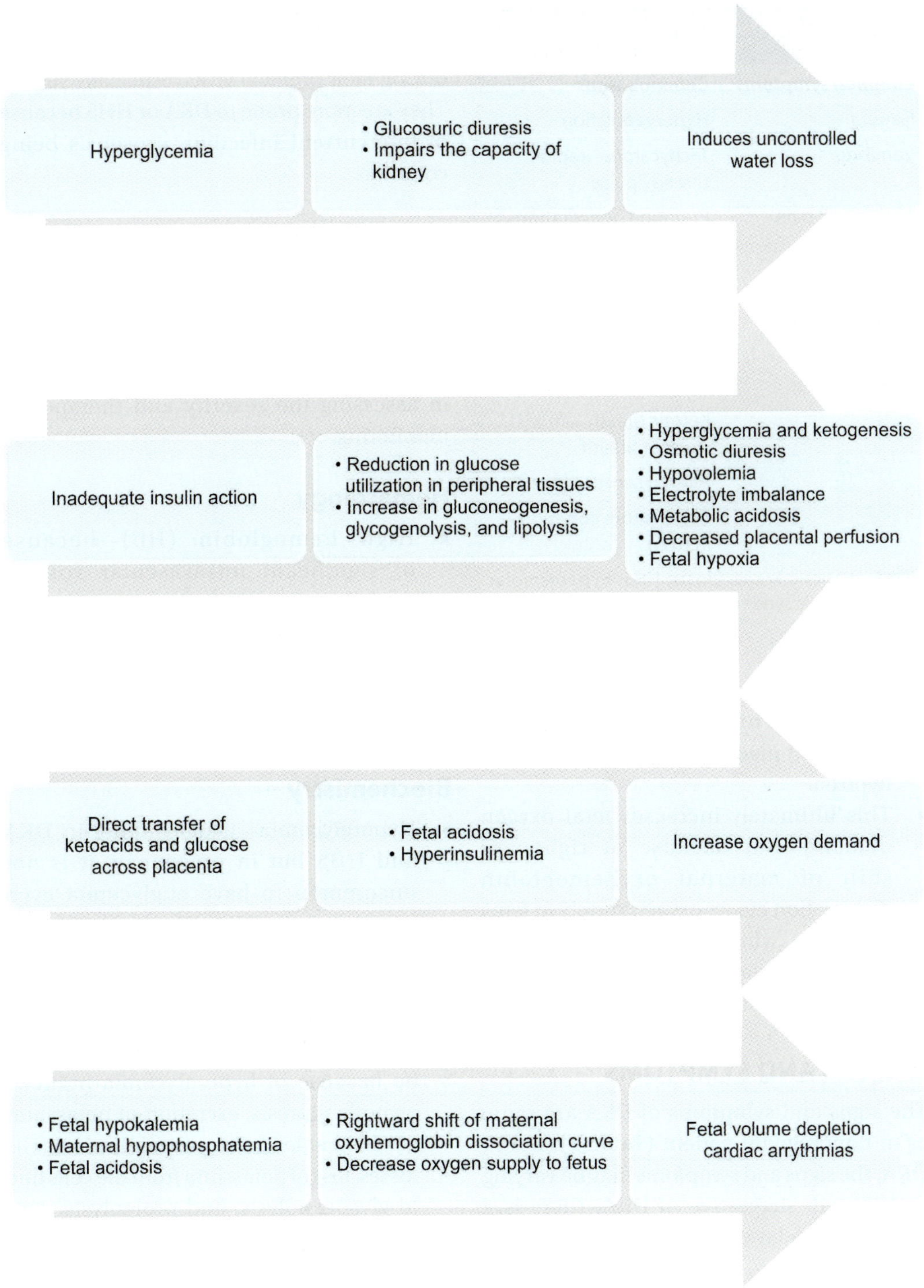

| Hyperglycemia | • Glucosuric diuresis
• Impairs the capacity of kidney | Induces uncontrolled water loss |

| Inadequate insulin action | • Reduction in glucose utilization in peripheral tissues
• Increase in gluconeogenesis, glycogenolysis, and lipolysis | • Hyperglycemia and ketogenesis
• Osmotic diuresis
• Hypovolemia
• Electrolyte imbalance
• Metabolic acidosis
• Decreased placental perfusion
• Fetal hypoxia |

| Direct transfer of ketoacids and glucose across placenta | • Fetal acidosis
• Hyperinsulinemia | Increase oxygen demand |

| • Fetal hypokalemia
• Maternal hypophosphatemia
• Fetal acidosis | • Rightward shift of maternal oxyhemoglobin dissociation curve
• Decrease oxygen supply to fetus | Fetal volume depletion cardiac arrythmias |

Fig. 3: Mechanisms of maternal and fetal distress.

TABLE 1: Common symptoms and signs of DKA and HHS.

Common symptoms	Common signs
Nausea	Hyperventilation
Vomiting	Tachycardia—rapid thready pulse
Abdominal pain	Profound dehydration
Polyuria	Poor skin turgor
Polydipsia	Sunken eyeballs
Feeling sleepy or drowsiness	Cool extremities
Breathlessness	Hypotension
	Ketotic breath—fruity smell of breath
	Altered sensorium
	Coma (more common in HHS)

(DKA: diabetic ketoacidosis; HHS: hyperosmolar hyperglycemic syndrome)

electrolyte imbalance and metabolic acidosis. This ultimately leads to decreased placental perfusion and fetal hypoxia.
- This ultimately increases fetal oxygen demand. But because of rightward shift of maternal oxyhemoglobin dissociation curve, oxygen supply to fetus decreases which causes fetal hypoxia and it's consequences including cardiac arrythmias and fetal death.

SIGNS AND SYMPTOMS[3-5]

The signs and symptoms of DKA are same as in nonpregnant patient **(Table 1)**. But in DKA, the signs and symptoms may be varying and though suggestive of DKA, there is a tendency to delay medical help as many signs such as vomiting, nausea, abdominal pain, malaise, and hyperventilation are common in pregnancy, so taken for granted.

Pregnant diabetic patients need to be monitored thoroughly and aggressively during their prenatal visits, especially sugars. They are more prone to DKA or HHS because of intercurrent infection, urosepsis being common.

LABORATORY INVESTIGATIONS[6-10]

Prompt laboratory diagnosis is one of the most important diagnoses as it helps not only in diagnosis of DKA or HHS but also helps in assessing the severity and therapeutic monitoring.

Hematology
- High hemoglobin (Hb)—because of significant intravascular volume depletion
- High white blood cell (WBC) with shift to left—may be because of infection
- Platelets may be low because of pregnancy and/or infection.

Biochemistry
- Hyperglycemia—usual finding in DKA and HHS but in pregnancy, it is not uncommon to have euglycemia even if patient is in DKA. The level of blood glucose is different in DKA and HHS (discussed later) **(Table 2)**.
- Hypokalemia—common finding but normal K level is not unlikely. It may be because of hyperglycemia-induced osmotic diuresis, excretion of potassium ketoacid anion salts, gastrointestinal (GI) losses, loss of potassium from the cells due to glycogenolysis, and proteolysis. And during treatment due to insulin therapy which shifts potassium intracellular.
- Hyperkalemia—if acute kidney injury is associated

TABLE 2: The difference between DKA and HHS.[3,4,6,7,11,12]

	DKA	HHS
Onset	Acute	Subacute or chronic
Age	Any age group	Elderly
Comorbidities	Less common	More common
Nausea, vomiting	More common	Less common
Abdominal pain	More common	Less common
Gastric stasis and ileus	More common	Less common
Glucose	Usually 250–600 mg/dL	Usually >600 mg/dL
Ketoacidosis	Profound	Minimal
Urine ketones	Positive	Negative or small
Metabolic acidosis	Moderate to severe	Mild
Serum bicarbonate	5–15 mEq/L	20–24 mEq/L
Anionic gap	>12	Variable
Osmolality	Variable but usually 300–325 mOsm/kg	>350 mOsm/kg
Endogenous insulin level	Very low	May be normal
Seizures	Less common	More common
Coma	Only in very severe cases	Common
Mortality	Very low <1%	10–20%

(DKA: diabetic ketoacidosis; HHS: hyperosmolar hyperglycemic syndrome)

- Hypernatremia—secondary to intravascular volume depletion
- Hypomagnesemia
- Low serum bicarbonate—due to metabolic acidosis
- Arterial blood gas:
  - Metabolic acidosis with respiratory alkalosis
  - Elevated anion gap
  - Mixed disorder—metabolic acidosis with respiratory alkalosis with metabolic alkalosis (contraction alkalosis) may coexist
- High serum osmolality
- Altered blood urea nitrogen and creatinine—due to acute kidney injury secondary to dehydration
- *Positive or elevated serum ketones:* Three ketone bodies are produced—acetoacetic acid, beta-hydroxybutyric acid, and acetone. Detected with nitroprusside test or by direct assay of beta-hydroxybutyrate levels.
- Positive urine ketone (by dipstick test-nitroprusside test)
- Elevated serum lactate—if patient is in septic shock
- Altered liver function tests (LFTs)—due to uncontrolled diabetes.

DIAGNOSIS[3,4,6,7,9,11,12]

Pregnant patient presenting with breathlessness, hyperglycemia, high anionic gap metabolic acidosis, and positive urine ketones suffice for diagnosis of DKA.

Pregnant patient presenting with significant hyperglycemia (>600 mg/dL), mental obtundation, negative urine ketone, high serum osmolality, and no or mild metabolic acidosis suffice for diagnosis of HHS.

PREVENTION[9,12]

Preconception Care

Educate diabetic women regarding the probable adverse consequences of uncontrolled diabetes including teratogenic effects of persistent hyperglycemia. Strict diet control, reduction of obesity, exercise, etc. help to prevent complications during pregnancy.

During Pregnancy

More frequent monitoring and strict control of diabetes play a key role. There are some data stating sodium-glucose cotransporter-2 (SGLT2) inhibitors lowering threshold of DKA.

Assessment and Prevention of Complications

Hypertension

Diabetic women are more prone to develop hypertension during pregnancy as compared to nondiabetic women. The incidence is higher in nulliparous women. This may complicate pregnancy in terms of development of preeclampsia and eclampsia. So hypertension needs to be diagnosed and treated early during antenatal visits.

Cardiovascular Disease and Kidney Disease

Diabetic women are more prone to develop cardiovascular and kidney disease. These diseases need to be screened and treated during antenatal visits. These diseases worsen the prognosis if patient develops DKA or HHS during pregnancy.

■ MANAGEMENT[4,7-9,11-16]

All patients should be admitted in either ICU or high dependency unit (HDU) **(Box 1)**.

Airway-Breathing-Circulation

Whenever unstable patient presents to ER, airway-breathing-circulation (ABC) is the key to save a life. We need to anticipate difficult

> **BOX 1:** Goals of treatment.
> - Airway-breathing-circulation
> - Correction of intravascular volume deficit and restoration of perfusion
> - Control of blood sugar
> - Acid–base and electrolyte(s) correction
> - Treatment of the primary or precipitating cause
> - Prevention or treatment of complications

airway in pregnant patients. Even vascular access might be difficult especially when patient is severely dehydrated.

Correction of Intravascular Volume Deficit and Restoration of Perfusion

Patients with DKA suffer from huge volume deficit. The goal of fluid therapy is to expand extracellular volume and stabilization of cardiovascular status. Correction of intravascular volume deficit lowers plasma osmolality, increases insulin responsiveness, reduces vasoconstriction, reduces stress hormone levels, and improves tissue perfusion.

The initial choice of fluids is 0.9% saline. The usual deficit is approximately 100 mL/kg of body weight in DKA and 100–200 mL/kg in HHS.[4] Typically in mild to moderate cases of DKA, the fluid deficit is 3–5 liters whereas in severe cases 5–6 liters. In HHS, the usual fluid deficit is approximately 9–10 liters.

Many fluid regimens are studied and available but the principles remain the same. Start with 10–20 mL/kg fluid bolus (in absence of cardiac compromise), assess and reassess, monitor hemodynamics, urine output, and tissue perfusion. Repeat fluid bolus if required. Once hemodynamics are optimized, switch over to per hour base regimen like 250–500 mL/h under strict monitoring of hemodynamics, perfusion status, serum sodium level, and evidence of volume overload.

Once the intravascular volume is corrected, switch over to 0.45% saline if the Sodium (Na) level is normal or elevated and continue with 0.9% saline if hyponatremia. Once blood sugar drops to 200 mg/dL in DKA and 250–300 mg/dL in HHS, switch fluid to dextrose in saline.

Few studies compared 0.9% saline versus RL versus balanced salt solutions which suggested balanced salt solution raises bicarbonate level faster than 0.9% saline but at the same time takes longer time to reduce blood glucose level. Use of balanced salt solutions also prevents hyperchloremic metabolic acidosis secondary to large volume resuscitation with 0.9% saline.

Invasive hemodynamic monitoring for intravascular volume status and fluid responsiveness might be helpful.

Control of Blood Sugar

Patients with DKA and HHS require insulin therapy till adequate control of sugar and resolution of ketoacidosis. At the same time, prevention of hypoglycemia is most important as it may increase maternal and fetal morbidity and mortality.

Before starting insulin, it is imperative to start correction of hypokalemia if it exists. Insulin drives potassium intracellularly which may lead to dangerous hypokalemia and life-threatening arrhythmias including ventricular tachycardia, fibrillation, and torsades de pointes.

Insulin Strategy

Various recommendations are available for insulin therapy in DKA and HHS but the most common is to start with intravenous insulin bolus of 0.1 unit/kg followed by 0.1 unit/kg/h and titrate as per sugar level. Usually short-acting insulin is used to manage. The rationale behind insulin bolus is to saturate insulin receptors. Few studies suggested no difference in outcome, sugar control, length of stay between bolus versus no bolus insulin.

The target sugar is 150–200 mg/dL for DKA and 200–300 mg/dL for HHS. It is absolutely necessary to monitor sugar frequently to prevent hypoglycemia.

Acid–Base and Electrolyte Correction

Sodium and Potassium

Diabetic ketoacidosis and HHS-induced osmotic diuresis causes significant hypokalemia. The usual potassium deficit in both DKA and HHS is approximately 3–5 mEq/kg. Many patients present with hyperkalemia, which develops because of transmembrane shift of potassium secondary to acidosis, insulin deficiency, and hypertonicity.

The rate of potassium supplementation should be as per patient's initial potassium level, degree of metabolic acidosis or any other reason. If K level is >5 mEq/kg, potassium should not be administered. If K level is 4–5 mEq, the rate of potassium supplementation should be approximately 10 mEq/h. If initial K is 3–4 mEq/L, then supplement 20 mEq/h. If <3 mEq/L, stop insulin and supplement at the rate of 20–30 mEq/h. Potassium should be monitored 4–6 hourly initially.

Bicarbonate for Correction of Metabolic Acidosis

Bicarbonate therapy is controversial because of lack of benefit. There are many harmful effects also:
- Paradoxical intracellular acidosis

- Can reduce hyperventilatory drive which leads to fall in cerebral pH
- May slow the rate of recovery of ketosis.

Few studies suggested its use in pH ≤6.9 on presentation with severe hemodynamic instability till pH raises to >7.0.

Magnesium and Phosphate

Magnesium should be corrected if moderate-to-severe hypomagnesemia or refractory hypokalemia.

Phosphate correction should be done only if symptomatic hypophosphatemia (serum phosphate is <1) causing muscle weakness, respiratory depression, hemolytic anemia, cardiac dysfunction, etc.

Treat the Precipitating Cause

Most essential step in management of DKA/HHS is treating the precipitating cause as delay in identifying and treating can worsen the prognosis.

Correction and Treatment of Complications

Organ dysfunction and failure may set in because of DKA/HHS. Organ support in terms of respiratory support, renal support, cardiac support, etc., is required till DKA/HHS resolves.

■ MONITORING[17,18]

Maternal Monitoring

Hemodynamic status, neuromonitoring, respiratory monitoring, and urine output monitoring are crucial as it warrants therapeutic modification at frequent intervals.
- Sugar—1 hourly initially, once start getting under control—2–4 hourly
- K—4–6 hourly
- Na—4–6 hourly
- ABG—2 hourly, later 4-6 hourly and then as required.

Urine ketones: Four hourly initially only. But it should not be used to monitor resolution of ketoacidosis. It is measured by nitroprusside test, which reacts mainly with acetoacetate, acetone (though weak reaction) and not with beta-hydroxybutyrate. Treating ketoacidosis shifts the reaction toward acetoacetate which may give positive urine ketone test even after resolution of ketoacidosis. It also detects acetone which actually is not an acid and it is slowly eliminated via lungs.

Organ functions: Liver function test, Renal Function Tests (RFT) daily for first 2–3 days.

Decision to go for delivery should be individualized based on maternal condition, fetal complications, and fetal maturity. Usually DKA/HHS does not warrant early delivery as prompt diagnosis and treatment prevent or reverse the complications.

Once DKA/HHS resolve, insulin therapy should be modified as per clinical status and switched over to subcutaneous regimen. Electrolytes and fluid supplementation should be de-escalated as soon as possible to prevent therapy related complications such as volume overload.

Fetal Monitoring

Fetal heart rate should be monitored frequently. Fetal biophysical profile and Doppler study monitoring are usually not required unless persistent DKA/HHS.

■ COMPLICATIONS

Diabetic ketoacidosis/HHS can cause cerebral edema, vascular occlusion (secondary to hyperosmolar state) such as mesenteric ischemia, myocardial infarction, DIC, cardiac arrhythmias, coma, or any other organ failure.

Euglycemic Diabetic Ketoacidosis in Pregnancy[10,11]

It is a situation where the blood sugar is normal or low with ketoacidosis.

Mechanisms

- Increase in pregnancy hormones such as estrogen and progesterone, which increase maternal usage of blood glucose
- Higher plasma volume of pregnancy dilutes effect on blood glucose
- Decrease maternal glycogenolysis
- Use of glucose by fetoplacental unit
- High Glomerular Filtration Rate (GFR) increases renal loss of glucose
- Excessive vomiting leads to starvation ketosis without increase in blood glucose.

Clinical Importance

It may lead to delayed recognition and increase chances of complications of DKA.

Management

Same principles as hyperglycemic DKA except addition of dextrose in saline while administering fluids. High index of suspicion and screening helps in early diagnosis.

■ CONCLUSION

Diabetic ketoacidosis and HHS are not uncommon in pregnancy. These are obstetrics emergencies, which impact maternal and perinatal mortality. Pregnancy can precipitate diabetes or worsen existing diabetes. If unrecognized and unmonitored, it can lead to adverse complications. One must ensure adequate sugar control during pregnancy and postpartem period.

TAKE HOME MESSAGES

- Early recognition (including euglycemic DKA) and prompt treatment usually control DKA/HHS and prevent complications.
- ABC remains the basic principle.
- Aggressive Insulin therapy to control sugar and prevention of hypoglycemia should be done.
- Rapid correction of fluid deficit and electrolytes under close monitoring are life saving for mother and fetus.
- Treatment of the precipitating cause should never be forgotten.

■ REFERENCES

1. Sibai BM, Viteri OA. Diabetic ketoacidosis in pregnancy. Obstet Gynecol. 2014; 123(1):167-78.
2. Mohan M, Baagar KAM, Lindow S. Management of diabetic ketoacidosis in pregnancy. Obstet Gynaecolt. 2017;19(1):55-62.
3. Dingle HE, Slovis C. Diabetic Ketoacidosis and Hyperosmolar Hyperglycemic Syndrome Management. Emerg Med. 2018; 50(8):161-71.
4. Malz R. Management of the hyperosmolar hyperglycemic syndrome. Am Fam Physician. 1999;60(5):1468-76.
5. Diguisto C, Strachan MWJ, Churchill D, Ayman G, Knight M. A study of diabetic ketoacidosis in pregnant population in the United Kingdom: Investigating the incidence, aetiology, management and outcomes. Diabet Med. 2022;39(4):e14743.
6. Coutada RS, Cunha SS, Goncalves ES, Gama AP, Silva JP, Pinheiro PM. Diabetic ketoacidosis in pregnancy. Int J Reprod Contracept Obstet Gynecol. 2018;7:2945-7.
7. Kamalakannan D, Baskar V, Barton DM, Abdu TA. Diabetic ketoacidosis in pregnancy, Postgrad Med J. 2003;79(934):454-7.
8. Sharma S, Tembhare A, Inamdar S, Agarwal HD. Impact of diabetic ketoacidosis in pregnancy. J South Asian Feder Obst Gynae. 2020;12(2):113-5.

9. Carroll MA, Yeomans ER. Diabetic ketoacidosis in pregnancy. Crit Care Med. 2005;33(10 Suppl):S347-53.
10. de Veciana M. Diabetes ketoacidosis in pregnancy. Semin Perinatal. 2013;37(4):267-73.
11. Dalfra MG, Burlina S, Sartore G, Lapolla A. Ketoacidosis in diabetic pregnancy. J Matern Fetal Neonat Med. 2019;29(2016):2889-95.
12. Alghamdi MA, Alzahrani AM, Alshams, HA, Maqdad H, Al-Saif MH, Ahlam M, et al. Hyperosmolar hyperglycemic state management in the emergency department. Arch Phar Pract. 2021:12(1):37-40.
13. Diabetes Canada Clinical Practice Guidelines Expert Committee; Goguen J, Gilbert J. Hyperglycemic emergencies in adults. Can J Diabetes. 2018;42 Suppl 1:S109-14.
14. Nyenwe EA, Kitabchi AE. The evolution of diabetic ketoacidosis: an update of its etiology, pathogenesis and management. Metabolism. 2016;65(4):507-21.
15. Fayfman M, Pasquel FJ, Umpierrez GE. Management of hyperglycemic crises: diabetic ketoacidosis and hyperglycemic Hyperosmolar state. Med Clin North Am. 2017;101(3):587-606.
16. Van Zyl DG, Rheeder P, Delport E. Fluid management in diabetic acidosis-Ringer's lactate versus normal saline: a randomized controlled trial. QJM. 2012;105(4):337-43.
17. Dargel S, Schleußner E, Kloos C, Groten T, Weschenfelder F. Awareness of euglycaemic diabetic ketoacidosis during pregnancy prevents recurrence of devastating outcomes: a case report of two pregnancies in one patient. BMC Pregnancy Childbirth. 2021;21(1):552.
18. Kitabchi AE, Fisher JN, Murphy MB, Rumbak MJ. Diabetic ketoacidosis and the hyperglycemic hyperosmolar nonketotic state. In: Kahn CR, Weir GC (Eds). Joslin's Diabetes Mellitus, 13th edition. Philadelphia: Lea and Febiger; 1994. p. 738.

CHAPTER 19

Thyroid Disorders in Critically Ill Pregnant Lady

Bhagyesh Shah

INTRODUCTION

Thyroid hormone is important for normal functioning of multiple organs and has complex but significant effect on the human body. Pregnancy is all together a unique condition in a woman's life where there is a little life inside the womb growing and fully dependent on the mother for full term of 36 weeks. To allow this unique phenomenon to take place in the best way a mother's body undergoes multiple changes in all organs where hormones play a significant part. Thyroid hormones weather in access or in scarcity too can cause noteworthy contributions to maternal and fetal health. Prevalence of hypothyroidism in Indian women is around 11%.[1]

Hyperthyroidism is not as common as hypothyroidism in pregnancy but cannot be ignored as it also has grave consequences if left untreated.

Thyroid dysfunction has been found to increase morbidity and mortality in critically ill patient.[2] Add to this a critically ill pregnant patient with thyroid disorder. It literally calls for war horns. For a critical care specialist, it is important to keep cautious approach while dealing with a pregnant patient with thyroid disorder in intensive care unit (ICU).

PHYSIOLOGY

A normal fetal development warrants adequate supply of thyroid hormone from maternal glands from early conception period. So the reference range for thyroid hormone levels needs to be known and followed to guide for selection of patient and dose for supplementation. Commonly used serum thyroid-stimulating hormone (TSH) range for different trimesters is from 0.1 to 2.5, 0.2 to 3.0, and 0.3 to 3.0, respectively for first, second, and third trimester.[3]

Serum TSH levels in mother's blood starts declining from first trimester and gradually come to prepregnancy levels near full term. Free T4 levels usually decline over the term of pregnancy.

Placental human chorionic gonadotropin (hCG) with help of estrogen can increase release of thyroid-binding globulin (TBG) and in turn can have thyrotrophic effect. Although, fetal thyroid hormone production starts by 18th week in pregnancy, exposure to maternal hormone and their effects starts from 5th week and continue till full term.[4]

All of these may be affected by placental development and protein levels in mother making it a multifactorial management of thyroid hormones in the pregnant female.

EPIDEMIOLOGY AND MAGNITUDE OF THE PROBLEM

In a meta-analysis of 61 studies and >60,000 study subjects from India done in 2021, prevalence of hypothyroidism in pregnant patients was found to be around 11%.[1]

After iodine deficiency, the second most frequent cause for hypothyroidism is autoimmune or Hashimoto's thyroiditis. Thyroid autoantibodies are seen positive in almost 30–60% pregnant women.[5]

Thyroid disorders in pregnancy can be divided into broadly two ends of the spectrum:
1. Hypothyroid
2. Hyperthyroid

Hypothyroid can be subdivided into following subtypes:
- *Overt hypothyroidism*: It is defined as high TSH and below normal fT4 levels.
- *Subclinical hypothyroidism*: It is defined as high TSH and normal fT4 levels.

Hyperthyroid condition in pregnancy has been defined as hyperfunction of thyroid gland causing symptoms due to hypermetabolism and hyperactivity. Common cause is Graves' disease. Less common causes are toxic multinodular goiter and toxic adenoma. Thyroid receptor antibody [thyrotropin receptor antibody (TRAb)] levels and ultrasonography (USG) of neck are primary investigations along with thyroid function tests.

Isolated Hypothyroxinemia

It is defined as normal serum TSH associated with low fT4 levels.

A specific mention is required for thyroid peroxidase (TPO) antibodies is required as they are quite commonly seen positive in women of childbearing age and associated with maternal and fetal complications in many studies requiring aggressive treatment plans. This has been proven by certain populations' studies showing prevalence of TPO antibody in women of around 5.4–20% and in women who had miscarriages and infertility showed 14–33% prevalence.[6]

IMPLICATIONS FOR MATERNAL HEALTH

Overt hypothyroidism if not treated properly can result in spontaneous pregnancy loss, pregnancy-induced hypertension (PIH), preeclampsia, and even postpartum hemorrhage.[7]

Subclinical hypothyroidism is also associated with miscarriages, preeclampsia, breech presentation, preterm delivery, etc.[8]

Isolated hypothyroxinemia has also increased risk of placental abruption, breech delivery, and preterm delivery.[9]

IMPLICATIONS FOR FETAL WELL-BEING

As pregnancy itself is a very dynamic process the role of thyroid hormone in placental and fetal development is significant. Both overt and subclinical hypothyroidism has been shown to cause neurodevelopmental deficits and neurocognitive issues in offspring. Although there are different studies suggesting contradictory results there is an established belief how crucial role maternal thyroid hormones play in overall fetal and neonatal growth.

MANAGEMENT AND PHARMACOTHERAPY

Management of thyroid disorders in pregnant patient starts with preconception screening and counseling.

Routine screening of all pregnant females for thyroid disorder has not been recommended except for few high-risk cases.

A high-risk case group will be as follows:
- Resident of iodine deficiency area
- Morbidly obese
- History of hypo- or hyperthyroidism
- History of thyroid surgery
- History of infertility-related treatment

- History of previous complicated pregnancy
- History of drug use such as amiodarone and lithium
- History of neck surgery or radiation
- History of autoimmune diseases or endocrine diseases
- Older age (>30 years)

Such a high-risk case group will require ideally preconception counseling for pregnancy-related issues and then a frequent monitoring during the term of pregnancy.

In a diagnosed case of hypothyroid disorder, the pregnant woman will require monthly check of serum TSH and/or fT4 levels till 20th weeks and then at a lesser frequency.

Chances of conception are less with hyperthyroid status but if conception happens then they also require regular blood levels of TSH, fT4 checked as we do for diagnosed hypothyroid cases. Check of TSH should be done every 2 weeks and then may be every 4th week once the levels are looking under control.

All women hyperthyroid patient in child-bearing age should be properly counseled for chances of pregnancy and related complications. Along with that if they are planning pregnancy they should be euthyroid before attempting for pregnancy and even medical management should be planned according to risk benefits to the future offspring.

The common high-risk group of pregnant patient with Graves' disease which requires to check for TRAb levels are:
- History of thyroidectomy for hyperthyroidism in pregnancy
- History of delivery of hyperthyroid infant
- Mothers with untreated or medically treated hyperthyroidism with pregnancy
- History of Graves' disease treated with radioactive iodine or thyroidectomy.

The management of hypothyroid cases is done with levothyroxine (LT4) being given orally with the reference range target of TSH kept in mind.

Mind well that the start of thyroxin supplement happens early from first diagnosis and may continue in postpartum or lactational period.

It is usually seen that increase of around 20–30% of dose is needed from prepregnancy level in a prior diagnosed hypothyroid case.[2]

A regular fetal and maternal sonography and Doppler studies are required to identify and correct fetomaternal issues during pregnancy.

Cordocentesis as a routine is not recommended in all cases of autoimmune thyroid disorders.

For hyperthyroid cases, propylthiouracil (PTU) is given in first 16 weeks and later changed to carbimazol for remaining period to avoid chances of fetal anomalies. Other drugs such as beta-blockers and calcium channel blockers are used for crisis and emergency to avoid complications.

PHARMACOLOGICAL CONSIDERATIONS

Iodine Supplementation

Although the use of iodized salt has covered >70% of world population iodine deficiency remains one of the major reason for hypothyroidism. The iodine supplementation as an iodized salt is cost effective option but the target of 250 μg per day of daily allowance is preferred for pregnant and lactating women as per the World Health Organization (WHO). If not achieved, one dose of 400 mg iodized oil postdelivery can supplement neonates well.

Iron Supplementation

As TPO is a heme-containing enzyme, iron deficiency can worsen hypothyroidism and in pregnancy iron deficiency is common specifically in Indian women. Iron supplementation is must for hypothyroid pregnant patients.

Nutritionally, there has not been any clear advantage of selenium supplements.

Thyroid Supplements for Hypothyroid Patients

LT4 is indicated for all hypothyroid females who are being treated or evaluated for infertility or undergoing controlled ovarian hyperstimulation.

LT4 is started in all pregnant patients with TSH above 2.5 and/or TPO antibodies positive status.

LT4 is given to all pregnant females with TSH >10.

For hypothyroid females who are on LT4 supplementation before pregnancy must be increasing their doses by at least 20–30% of their prepregnancy doses.

Post-delivery a titration back to prepregnancy dose is done by frequently checking serum TSH levels **(Fig. 1)**.

With proper public and private obstetric safety programs, it is very rare to find untreated hypothyroid pregnant patient who are prone for myxedema coma. The treatment for the same requires intravenous (IV) thyroxin and steroids along with supportive care protecting airway, breathing, and circulation.

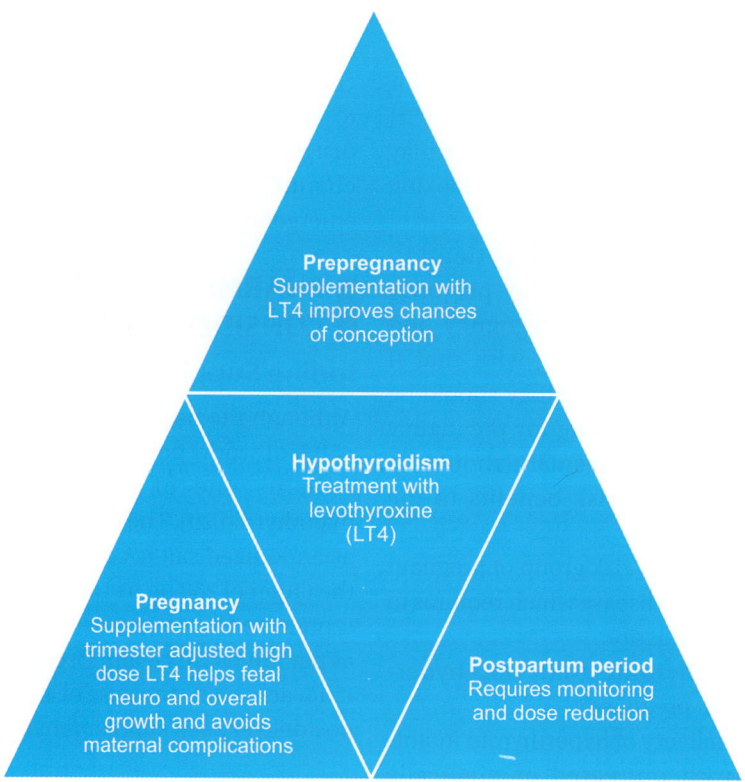

Fig. 1: Routine management of hypothyroid patient.

Medical Management of Hyperthyroid Patients

For pregnant patient with active thyrotoxic symptoms surgery after second trimester can be an option but the ideal way would be avoid antithyroid drugs unless necessary. If at all needed, PTU can be given till 16–18 months and then carbimazole can be added. Beta-blockers for tachycardia and blood pressure control is preferred choice before trying calcium-channel blockers as a second option.

For TRAb positive patients treated with radioactive iodine it is advised to avoid pregnancy at least for 6 months. They need regular monitoring of their thyroid hormone levels till they normalize or up to 6 weeks postpartum.

There are few specific conditions which require special mention as they mimic thyroid disorders or influence the plan of management when presented with thyroid disorders.

■ POSTPARTUM THYROIDITIS

Postpartum thyroiditis (PPT) is an autoimmune condition mostly an inflammatory reaction presenting with transient phase of hyperthyroidism followed by period of hypothyroidism. It happens in first year of postpartum period and resolves by end of the year to euthyroid levels and happens mostly in females who were euthyroid before pregnancy.

The Graves' thyrotoxicosis may mimic the PPT. The easy identifier will be late onset after 6 months postpartum is usually Graves' if no clinical signs like nodule or ophthalmopathy is absent.

The symptoms of PPT are mild and rather less in hyperthyroid phase than in hypothyroid phase. In hyperthyroid phase, the symptoms can be palpitation, irritability, and early fatigue. Beta-blockers are sufficient for these symptoms.

While in hypothyroid phase we may see complaints of depression, cold intolerance, dry skin, paresthesia, and impaired concentration. You may need to supplement with LT4 till the symptoms resolve and follow TSH levels till 1–2 months. If planning pregnancy again, then do not decrease or taper doses till at least 1 year.

■ GESTATIONAL THYROTOXICOSIS

Gestational thyrotoxicosis may present along with hyperemesis gravidarum and it is thought to be caused by higher levels of beta-hCG. It is limited to first half of pregnancy only and may have severe nausea, vomiting, dehydration along with palpitation, anxiety, irritability, tremors, and heat intolerance. It requires maintaining hydration and supportive treatment in acute phase.

■ PERIOPERATIVE AND CRITICAL PATIENT MANAGEMENT

In hypothyroid cases, it is advisable to allow planned surgeries once TSH target levels are achieved. For emergency surgeries, we can use IV thyroxin, if available.

Hypothyroid pregnant patients are more sensitive to sedatives and anesthetic drugs and may add challenge by adding hypoventilation and kidney dysfunction due to the thyroid status. Worst can be myxedema coma which may precipitate due to surgical stress or infections characterized by altered sensorium, heart failure, etc. The management needs IV thyroxin and ventilator support along with stress dose steroids. Continue oral thyroxin in perioperative period.

Hypothyroid	Hyperthyroid
☐ IV thyroxine and/or thyronine	☐ Propyl thiouracil/carbimazole
☐ Hydration	☐ Beta-blockers/calcium-channel blockers
☐ Steroids	☐ Circulatory support and steroids

Fig. 2: Management of thyroid disorder in pregnant critical patient.

In hyperthyroid cases, it is best to avoid planned surgeries till postpartum period. If at all needed ICU stay with perioperative beta-blockade and symptomatic support needs to be discussed with family and patient beforehand.

Hyperthyroid patients may show hypermetabolic signs such as arrhythmia, confusion, cardiovascular dysfunction ultimately leading to shock and needs invasive hemodynamic monitoring to support circulatory status. Beta-blockers are main drugs in acute scenario to support cardiovascular system. Calcium-channel blockers can be used when beta-blockers does not help. Steroids in acute conditions are having supportive role by decreasing the conversion to active hormones. Iodine, lithium and cholestyramine have not been recommended routinely for pregnant patients. Antithyroid drugs like PTU or carbimazole must be continued in perioperative period **(Fig. 2)**.

Overall for thyroid disorder in critically ill pregnant patient, the aim should be to get to euthyroid status as soon as possible while managing active symptoms with specific medications.

The role of intensivist is started from first visit till postpartum in high-risk pregnant patient with thyroid disease and with a primary target to prevent complications both in mother and the fetus due to thyroid disease.

TAKE HOME MESSAGES

- Thyroid disorders are common and requires monitoring and counseling along with medical management.
- As far as possible, maintaining euthyroid status is the key to prevent complications in mother as well as the fetus.
- Availability of high-risk obstetrics critical care units is must to manage pregnant patients with complications due to thyroid disorders.
- Thyrotoxicosis and pregnancy is strict No-No when avoidable. If facing them together, prepare for the worst with the best you have.
- Hypothyroid needs to be corrected in view of future development of fetus and to avoid maternal complications remaining within local reference range of target serum TSH values which are trimester specific.

■ REFERENCES

1. Yadav V, Dabar D, Goel AD, Bairwa M, Sood A, Prasad P, et al. Prevalence of hypothyroidism in pregnant women in India: a meta-analysis of observational studies. J Thyroid Res. 2021;2021:5515831.
2. Slag MF, Morley JE, Elson MK, Crowson TW, Nuttall FQ, Shafer RB. Hypothyroxinemia in critically ill patients as a predictor of high mortality. JAMA. 1981;245:43-5.
3. Stagnaro-Green A, Abalovich M, Alexender E, Azizi F, Mestman J, Negro R, et al. Guidelines of the American Thyroid Association for the Diagnosis and Management of the Thyroid Disease during Pregnancy and Postpartum. Thyroid. 2011;21:1081-25.
4. Calvo RM, Jauniaux E, Gulbis B, Asunción M, Gervy C, Contempré B, et al. Fetal tissues

are exposed to biologically relevant free thyroxin concentrations during early phases of development. J Clin Endocrinol Metab. 2002;87:1768-77.
5. Korevaar TI, Schalekamp-Timmermans S, de Rijke YB, Visser WE, Visser W, de Muinck Keiser-Schrama SM, et al. Hypothyroxinemia and TPO antibody positivity are risk factors for premature delivery: the generation R study. J Clin Endocrinol Metab. 2013;98: 4382-90.
6. Poppe K, Velkinier B, Glinoer D. The role of thyroid autoimmunity in fertility and pregnancy. Nat Clin Pract Endocrinol Metab. 2008;4:394-405.
7. LaFranchi SH, Haddow JE, Hollowell JG. Is thyroid inadequacy during gestation a risk factor for adverse pregnancy and developmental outcomes? Thyroid. 2005; 15:60-71.
8. Chan S, Boelaert K. Optimal management of hypothyroidism, hypothyroxinaemia and euthyroid TPO antibody positivity preconception and in pregnancy. Clin Endocrinol (Oxf). 2015;82(3):313-26.
9. Pop VJ, Brouwers EP, Wijnen H, Oei G, Essed GG, Vader HL. Low concentrations of maternal thyroxin during early gestation: a risk factor of breech presentation. BJOG. 2004;111:925-30.

Electrolyte Disorders

CHAPTER 20

Disorders of Sodium Homeostasis and Fluid Balance in Pregnancy

Santanu Bagchi, Saurabh Debnath

■ INTRODUCTION

The fluid compartment inside an adult's body is wide and segmented. During pregnancy there are additional physiologic changes which make the fluid homeostasis altered and more complicated. Fluid homeostasis is altered during normal pregnancy due to changes in hormonal levels, particularly increased levels of antidiuretic hormone (ADH) and aldosterone. These hormones play a crucial role in regulating fluid balance by increasing the reabsorption of water and salt in the kidneys. As a result, there is an increase in total body water and blood volume, which is essential for the growth and development of the fetus. This altered fluid homeostasis can lead to an increase in blood pressure and an increased risk of edema, particularly in the legs and ankles.[1] The fluid compartments contain different electrolytes and among these, sodium is the predominant electrolyte of the extracellular fluid compartment. The disorder of sodium homeostasis, as it is in normal adults, is primarily a function of altered water balance during pregnancy as well.[2] A thorough understanding of the fluid distribution and dynamics along with renal function during pregnancy is required for the optimization of both resuscitative and maintenance fluid management.

■ PHYSIOLOGICAL ALTERATION IN PREGNANCY

Sodium and Volume Homeostasis

In a normal human adult, the total body water proportion varies from 55 to 65% of body weight and it is divided into two compartments, extracellular and intracellular, with the former being smaller (one-third) and the latter being the larger (two-thirds) component. The extracellular compartment, further, comprises intravascular (25%) and interstitial (75%) spaces. In a pregnant woman, the individual fluid compartment volumes get altered, most notably involving the extracellular compartment and invariably the total body water gets increased by approximately 6-8 liters, leading to physiological hypervolemia during pregnancy.[2] There is approximately a 4-6 liters increase in extracellular fluid volume and both intravascular (plasma) and interstitial spaces also get swelled up with additional fluids. The rise in plasma volume is usually higher during the second trimester reaching as high as about 50% above baseline. The interstitial fluid volume, on the other hand, reaches its peak during late pregnancy. The plasma volume ratio with total extracellular fluid volume also gets increased. During the postpartum period, the plasma volume starts decreasing within the initial 24 hours and reaches prepregnancy level usually by 6–9 weeks postpartum.[3-5]

Renal functioning and sodium handling have a dominant role in volume homeostasis. There is an increase in both renal plasma flow and the glomerular filtration rate during pregnancy, particularly during the early second trimester. The possible mechanism can be multifactorial including, but not limited to, the increased plasma and extracellular fluid volume, hypoalbuminemia leading to decreased intrarenal oncotic pressure and hormonal interference like that by relaxin and prolactin.[6-8]

The filtered sodium load, during pregnancy, increases from nonpregnant levels of about 20,000–30,000 mmol per day. Several aspects of tubular function are affected by pregnancy. There is renal retention of approximately 950 mEq of sodium during pregnancy. Several factors contribute to enhanced renal sodium reabsorption in pregnancy.[2,8]

The different determining factors responsible for sodium excretion in pregnancy have been enumerated in **Table 1**.

Osmoregulation

In a normal adult human, the renin-angiotensin-aldosterone system (RAAS) regulates renal sodium handling, whereas renal water handling is managed primarily by the posterior pituitary originated hormone arginine vasopressin (AVP).[9]

Pregnant state results in a fall in plasma osmolarity, particularly during early gestation. On an average, it has been found that the plasma osmolarity falls by 10 mOsm/L and sodium by 4–5 mEq/L from their prepregnancy level. The basic underlying mechanism of this fall in osmolarity has been pointed out to be resetting of osmotic threshold (decrement), which in turn results from pregnancy-induced vasodilation with arterial underfilling, stimulating AVP release and thirst.

The central hormone, AVP, does its osmoregulatory action through R1 receptors, located on basolateral membrane of collecting duct cells. On positive activation, these receptors cause insertion of water absorbing aquaporin-2 channels on the basolateral membrane. During pregnancy, the action of AVP gets altered by both osmotic and nonosmotic stimuli. The resetting of osmoreceptor at a lower value at hypothalamus comes under osmotic stimulus. There has been a role of the hormone human chorionic gonadotropin (hCG) in osmotic stimulus, by causing increased stimulation of thirst center.

TABLE 1: Factors affecting sodium excretion in pregnancy.[1]

Increased excretion	*Decreased excretion*
Increased progesterone	Increased plasma aldosterone
Marked increase in glomerular filtration rate	Increased plasma angiotensin II
Increased neurophysins	Increased deoxycortisone
Increased prostaglandins	Increased placental lactogen
Increased melanocyte-stimulating hormone	Increased plasma estrogen
Decreased plasma albumin	Increased plasma prolactin
Decreased postglomerular oncotic pressure	Increased postglomerular oncotic pressure
Decreased vascular resistance	Increased ureteral pressure
	Maternal posture (supine or upright)

In a nonpregnant state, hCG levels are close to zero or undetectable. However, as pregnancy progresses, hCG levels increase dramatically, typically doubling every 2–3 days in the first weeks of pregnancy. By the end of the first trimester, hCG levels have usually decreased to about 100,000 mIU/mL or lower.[10] The resultant arterial vasodilation results in neurohumoral and sympathetic stimulation which act as nonosmotic stimuli for increased AVP secretion. Additional alteration in pregnancy happens due to release of the enzyme vasopressinase by placental trophoblast. This enzyme is a cystine aminopeptidase and it rapidly cleaves AVP. Therefore, these opposing mechanisms of increased production and increased degradation of AVP during human pregnancy ultimately help in keeping serum sodium level slightly lower than normal level, during normal pregnancy. However, any further derangements in sodium value should be considered pathological and accordingly managed.[11,12]

Figures 1 and 2 depict the sodium homeostasis mechanism in nonpregnant and pregnant state respectively.

DISORDERS OF SODIUM HOMEOSTASIS

Hyponatremia

In pregnancy, pathological hyponatremia is considered when serum sodium goes below 130 mEq/L, which in turn has been postulated to be caused by various reasons peculiar to pregnancy itself.[13] Oxytocin, a polypeptide secreted from posterior pituitary and having structural similarity with AVP, has been found to have action on collecting duct like AVP, acting on R2 receptors. Iatrogenic hyponatremia risk rises significantly when infused rapidly a hypotonic solution (e.g., 5% dextrose) due to maximal antidiuretic effect mimicking AVP like action. Hyperemesis gravidarum is another risk factor and in severe cases can cause hypovolemic

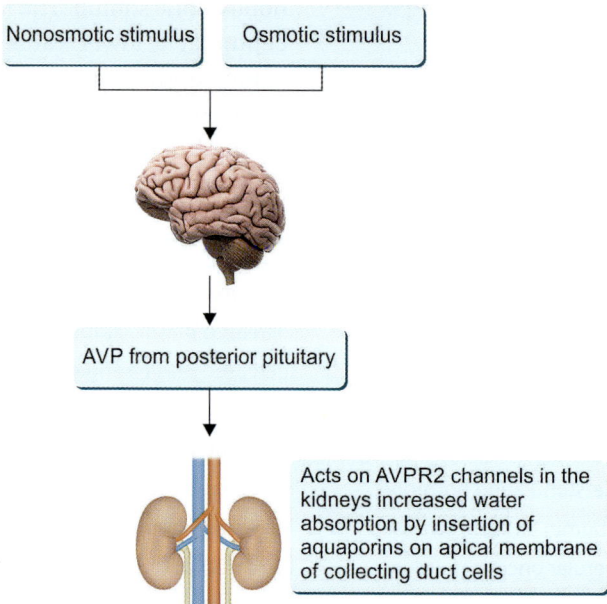

Fig. 1: Sodium homeostasis in nonpregnant states. (AVP: arginine vasopressin)

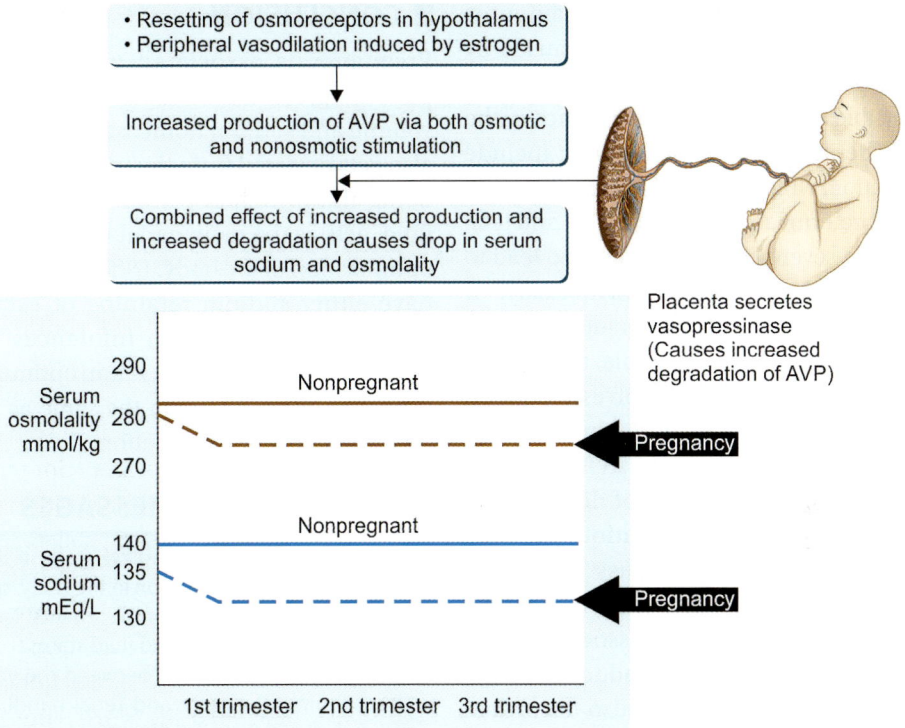

Fig. 2: Sodium homeostasis during pregnancy. (AVP: arginine vasopressin)

hyponatremia. Again, in rare situations, preeclampsia had been found to cause euvolemic or hypervolemic hyponatremia. Additionally, uncommon situations such as Sheehan's syndrome and hypothyroidism can also cause hyponatremia. In Sheehan's syndrome, the underlying mechanism has been postulated to be adrenocorticotropin deficiency and inappropriate ADH secretion.

The clinical features, grading and management usually do not differ from that of nonpregnant state, in most of the situations. However, for hyponatremia caused by syndrome of inappropriate antidiuretic hormone secretion (SIADH), the conventional approach of fluid restriction, as in nonpregnant state, can be harmful in pregnancy, as it can increase the risk of oligohydramnios and dehydration.

Therefore, management of this condition during pregnancy necessitates optimum water intake restriction (approximately 1.5 L/day) and monitoring amniotic fluid index (ultrasound guided) in order to further titrate fluid intake.[14]

Hypernatremia

Hypernatremia in pregnancy is termed when the serum sodium value exceeds 145 mEq/L, the same as in a nonpregnant state. It is a hyperosmolar state. Among pregnancy-specific causes, gestational diabetes insipidus (GDI) is a leading cause, alongside unmasking of preexisting central or nephrogenic diabetes insipidus or any iatrogenic causes (e.g., use of hypertonic saline and sodium bicarbonate infusion). GDI is a condition that occurs during pregnancy and is characterized by excessive thirst and the production of large amounts of dilute urine. This condition is caused by a decrease in the levels of ADH, which is responsible for regulating fluid balance in the body. The implications of GDI can include dehydration, which can lead to complications such as preterm labor, preeclampsia, and fetal distress. In severe cases, GDI can also lead to maternal and fetal morbidity and mortality.[15] It can lead to serious implications such as severe oligohydramnios, hypernatremia, and altered sensorium. Pathogenesis involves increased secretion of placental vasopressinase, which causes rapid degradation of AVP hormone and subsequent production of dilute urine, hypernatremia, and dehydration. Patients with increased placental mass (e.g., twin pregnancy) and pregnancies conceived via in vitro fertilization can be associated with increased vasopressinase production. High levels of vasopressinase can also occur due to abnormalities of liver function, as seen in preeclampsia, hemolysis, elevated liver enzymes, low platelets, or chronic liver disease due to hampered vasopressinase degradation in the liver. Patients with placental abruption can develop diabetes insipidus due to the sudden release of a large amount of vasopressinase. GDI typically resolves in 4–6 weeks after delivery with a gradual degradation of circulating vasopressinase.[12]

Treatment consists of a synthetic analog of AVP hormone named desmopressin (DDAVP). Desmopressin is resistant to placental vasopressinase and can be safely used in pregnancy as it has not been found to have a vasopressor activity or increased incidence of preeclampsia. There is a theoretical risk of desmopressin causing increased uterine contractility due to its similarity to oxytocin, but its intranasal use has 75 times less oxytocic action as compared to oxytocin.

■ CONCLUSION

Pregnancy is associated with significant physiological alterations. Consequently, volume and sodium homeostasis of the body also gets deviated from the baseline. Sodium, being the principal cation of extracellular fluid, acts as the main variable in fluid status optimization of the body. Different hormones have either sodium retaining or excreting action and this in turn influences water balance in the body. The sodium optimization principles grossly remain the same as in the nonpregnant adult population.

TAKE HOME MESSAGES

- Pregnancy is a physiological state in which there is water accumulation in the body, spread over different volume compartments, leading to alteration in sodium and fluid status.
- Generally, it is a balance between the various neurohumoral effects and renal handling of excess plasma flow and filtered solute load. It is usually manageable and after delivery the body quickly returns to its prepregnant state.
- Sodium level below 130 mEq/L or above 145 mEq/L is considered hypo- and hypernatremia, respectively, during pregnancy.
- Usual corrective actions for nonpregnant state with similar disorders should be undertaken.
- In SIADH with pregnancy, because of the risk of oligohydramnios and dehydration, the conventional approach of fluid restriction is tempered.

■ REFERENCES

1. Department of Obstetrics and Gynecology, University of Alabama at Birmingham. (2021). Fluid and Electrolyte Balance During Pregnancy. [online] Available from: https://www.uab.edu/medicine/obgyn/patient-care/obstetrical-care/pregnancy-information/fluid-and-electrolyte-balance-during-pregnancy. [Last accessed February, 2023].
2. Lindheimer MD, Katz AI. Normal and abnormal pregnancy. In: Arieff AI, DeFronzo R (Eds).

Fluid, Electrolyte and Acid-Base Disorders. New York: Churchill Livingstone; 1985. pp. 1041-65.
3. Davison JM, Lindheimer MD. Volume homeostasis and osmoregulation in human pregnancy. Baillieres Clin Endocrinol Metab. 1989;3(2):451-72.
4. Gallery ED, Brown MA. Volume homeostasis in normal and hypertensive human pregnancy. Baillieres Clin Obstet Gynaecol. 1987;1:835-51.
5. Brown MA, Zammit VC, Mitar DM. Extracellular fluid volumes in pregnancy-induced hypertension. J Hypertens. 1992;10:61-8.
6. Ueland K. Maternal cardiovascular dynamics. VII. Intrapartum blood volume changes. Am J Obstet Gynecol. 1976;126:671-7.
7. Lund CJ, Donovan JC. Blood volume during pregnancy. Significance of plasma and red cell volumes. Am J Obstet Gynecol. 1967;98:394-403.
8. Davison JM, Dunlop W. Renal hemodynamics and tubular function normal human pregnancy. Kidney Int. 1980;18:152-61.
9. Dafnis E, Sabatini S. The effect of pregnancy on renal function: Physiology and pathophysiology. Am J Med Sci. 1992;303:184-205.
10. American Pregnancy Association. (2021). Human Chorionic Gonadotropin (hCG) Levels. [online] Available from: https://americanpregnancy.org/pregnancy-complications/hcg-levels/. [Last accessed February, 2023].
11. Lindheimer MD, Davison JM. Osmoregulation, the secretion of arginine vasopressin and its metabolism during pregnancy. Eur J Endocrinol. 1995; 132:133-43.
12. Rosenbloom AA, Sack J, Fisher DA. The circulating vasopressinase of pregnancy: species comparison with radioimmunoassay. Am J Obstet Gynecol. 1975;121:316-20.
13. Baker PN. Hyponatremia in pregnancy: causes, consequences, and management. Br J Anaesth. 2017;118(3):285-92.
14. Moen V, Brudin L, Rundgren M, Irestedt L. Hyponatremia complicating labour: Rare or unrecognised? A prospective observational study. BJOG. 2009;116:552-61.
15. Molitch ME. Gestational Diabetes Insipidus. Endocr Rev. 2017;38(4):401-11.

CHAPTER 21

Disorders of Potassium Homeostasis

Soumya Sharma, Sai Saran

■ INTRODUCTION

There exists a high prevalence of electrolyte disturbances in pregnant patients, the most common being hyponatremia due to fluid retention and edema. Disturbances in serum potassium (K) levels are the second most common electrolyte abnormalities seen in pregnant patients.[1] There are very few large nationwide population studies to analyze the prevalence and risk factors associated with K disturbances in pregnancy. In the critically ill patients, hypokalemia, hyperkalemia, and K variability are independently related to increased mortality, as shown by the bell-shaped curve in a large retrospective study performed in more than 10,000 patients and 200,000 serum K measurements between 2002 and 2011 in the intensive care unit (ICU) of a teaching university hospital.[2] However, little is known about the importance of serum K levels in pregnant critically ill patients.

PHYSIOLOGICAL CHANGES LEADING TO POTASSIUM DISTURBANCES

Serum K levels are maintained by a balance between reabsorption (cellular and proximal tubular uptake) and secretion (collecting duct). The secretion is increased by elevation in glomerular filtration rate (GFR) by almost 50%, with a concomitant decrease in serum creatinine, urea, and uric acid. Activation of the renin-angiotensin-aldosterone system (RAAS) leads to increased aldosterone levels leading to net gain of sodium approximately 900–1,000 mEq, along with enhanced tubular K excretion. However, increased levels of progesterone having aldosterone antagonistic action, and systemic vasodilation act to maintain normal (or slightly lower) serum K levels during pregnancy. Total body K stores in non-pregnant females is approximately 3,500 mEq (50 mEq/kg), out of which 2% is extracellular. In pregnant females, an additional 300–350 mEq are retained, out of which 200 mEq is within the product of conception. Overall, there is a net gain of sodium and K, and retention of water up to 1–1.6 L. Raised GFR also leads to a net loss of magnesium from urine causing mild hypomagnesemia which coexists with mild hypokalemia. Among acid-base changes, respiratory alkalosis is normal in pregnancy, however, there is no significant change in K level despite the reduction in serum osmolality and rising circulating volume.

■ HYPOKALEMIA

Defined as serum K level <3.5 mEq/L (3.5 mmol/L) and classified as mild:

3–3.4 mmol/L; moderate: 2.5–3 mmol/L, and severe: <2.5 mmol/L, respectively.

Epidemiology and Magnitude of the Problem

Although, a US based study performed from 2012 to 2014 National Inpatient Sample (NIS) showed that hypokalemia is a rare condition seen in pregnancy related hospitalization with a prevalence of <1%, the prevalence in low-middle income and low-income countries would have been higher (other studies citing the prevalence between 6.7 and 21%). The result from the study also showed a strong association between hypokalemia and hyperemesis gravidarum (20%), overexpression of certain angiotensin genes leading to alteration in the RAAS system, with other risk factors for hypokalemia being younger age (<18 years), low socioeconomic status, and diseases such as preeclampsia, eclampsia, congestive heart failure, cirrhosis, and sickle cell disease.[3] Pregnant women with hyperemesis gravidarum are also at increased risk of development of refeeding syndrome which is characterized by hypokalemia, hypomagnesemia, hypophosphatemia, and hypocalcemia, especially in those who are fed after a prolonged phase of starvation and poor nutritional intake.

Special Conditions Leading to Hypokalemia in Pregnancy

- One of the most important concerns in obstetrics patients is the use of intravenous (IV) β_2 adrenergic agonist (e.g., ritodrine) in the management of preterm labor. Stimulation of β_2 receptor results in metabolic effects such as glycogenolysis and gluconeogenesis, subsequently causing a rise in glucose and later on insulin secretion from pancreatic islet cells. The $Na^+K^+ATPase$ pump transports K intracellularly without changing total body K^+ via direct stimulation of β_2 receptor and insulin.[4] A significant decrease in serum K occurs within a minute after IV β_2 agonist administration. This fall in K level is more pronounced if pretreatment serum K is already low. Serum K <2.5 mEq/L requires replacement, before treatment with β_2 agonist.
- Hyperemesis gravidarum typically presents in the first trimester as refractory vomiting leading to severe volume depletion and electrolyte abnormalities. Severe hypokalemia causing rhabdomyolysis is seen in the setting of hyperemesis gravidarum. This patient should be hospitalized and should receive volume replacement with isotonic fluid, thiamine, and K chloride which correct both hypokalemia and metabolic alkalosis.
- Bartter and Gitelman syndromes are rare autosomal recessive disorders seen in pregnancy requiring an increase in K supplementation. Over one-third of patients suffering from Bartter syndrome have low serum magnesium levels and need magnesium supplementation too. These cases can present as persistent hypokalemia and hypomagnesemia. Presence of hypertension along with hypokalemia points toward primary hyperaldosteronism (second most common cause of hypertension in pregnancy).[5] Geller syndrome (rare) due to functional mutation of mineralocorticoid receptor causing inappropriate activation of mineralocorticoid receptor by progesterone, unlike Bartter and Gitelman syndrome, this condition is associated with low aldosterone level and renin

levels. Hypokalemia and hypertension seen in this disorder respond to amiloride and improve postdelivery.
- Pica in pregnancy (clay eating) can also result in hypokalemia, resulting from impaired intestinal K absorption due to clay binding to K.[6]

Causes of hypokalemia in pregnancy are mentioned in **Flowchart 1**.

Clinical Features

The severity of clinical manifestations is proportional to the degree and duration of K reduction. Symptoms generally do not manifest until serum K level is below 3 mEq/L. Symptoms usually resolve with the correction of hypokalemia. Symptoms can be categorized according to the affected system.

- *Neurological symptoms*: Leg cramps, muscle weakness which can progress to symmetric ascending paralysis, hypotonia, altered mentation
- *Cardiovascular symptoms:* Palpitations, fatigue, and arrhythmia
- *Respiratory symptoms*: Can lead to respiratory failure due to muscle weakness
- *Gastrointestinal symptoms*: Gastrointestinal hypomotility manifesting as nausea, vomiting or ileus/constipation.

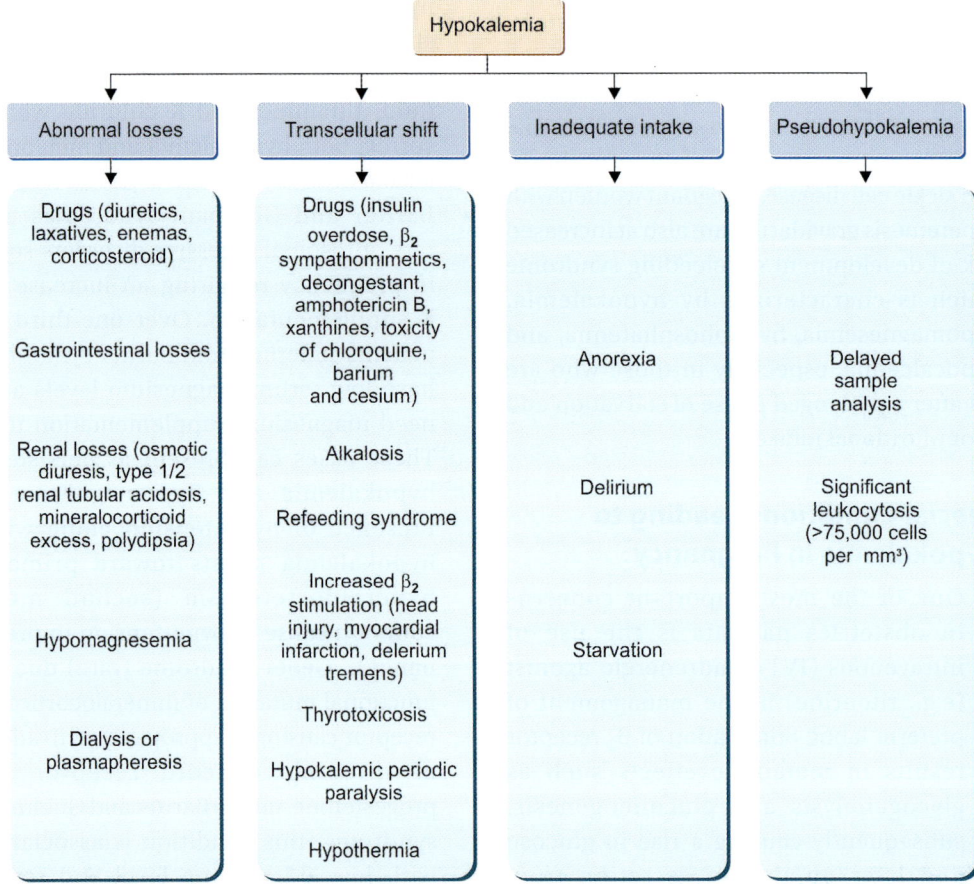

Flowchart 1: Causes of hypokalemia.

Diagnosis

The first step in the diagnosis is history and physical examination to identify the precipitating cause and treat it accordingly such as vomiting, diarrhea, or diuretic use. Identify conditions causing transcellular shift like drugs (insulin, β_2 agonists, catecholamines, etc.), hypothermia, and alkalosis (respiratory and metabolic). Simultaneously, a repeat serum K measurement should be done, along with serum magnesium, glucose, urine K, and creatinine levels. Urinary K excretion is best assessed by "24 urine collection". Normal kidney excretes up to 15-30 mEq per L of K per day.[7] Urine K of <30 mEq/day (spot K/C ratio: urine K: creatinine ratio: <13 mEq per g) suggests extrarenal losses or redistribution within the body and greater values are suggestive of renal loss. In patients with renal K losses, concomitant metabolic acidosis (HCO_3 <24 mEq/L) can suggest renal tubular acidosis. In cases of hypokalemia associated with metabolic alkalosis, urine chloride is measured, which when <10 mEq/L suggests gastrointestinal losses with conditions such as vomiting and nasogastric suctioning and when >10 mEq/L is seen with diuretic, steroid therapy and mineralocorticoid excess **(Flowcharts 2 and 3)**.[8]

Electrocardiogram Changes

Electrocardiogram (ECG) changes occur in 50% of patients with hypokalemia and

Flowchart 2: Approach to hypokalemia.

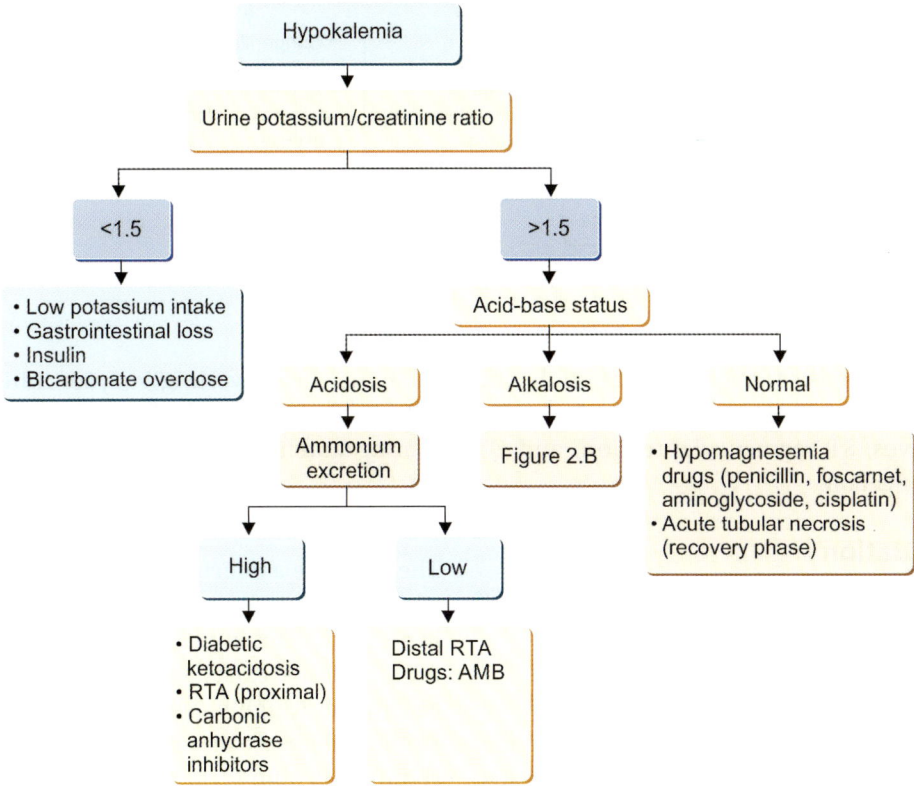

(AMB: amphotericin B; RTA: renal tubular acidosis)

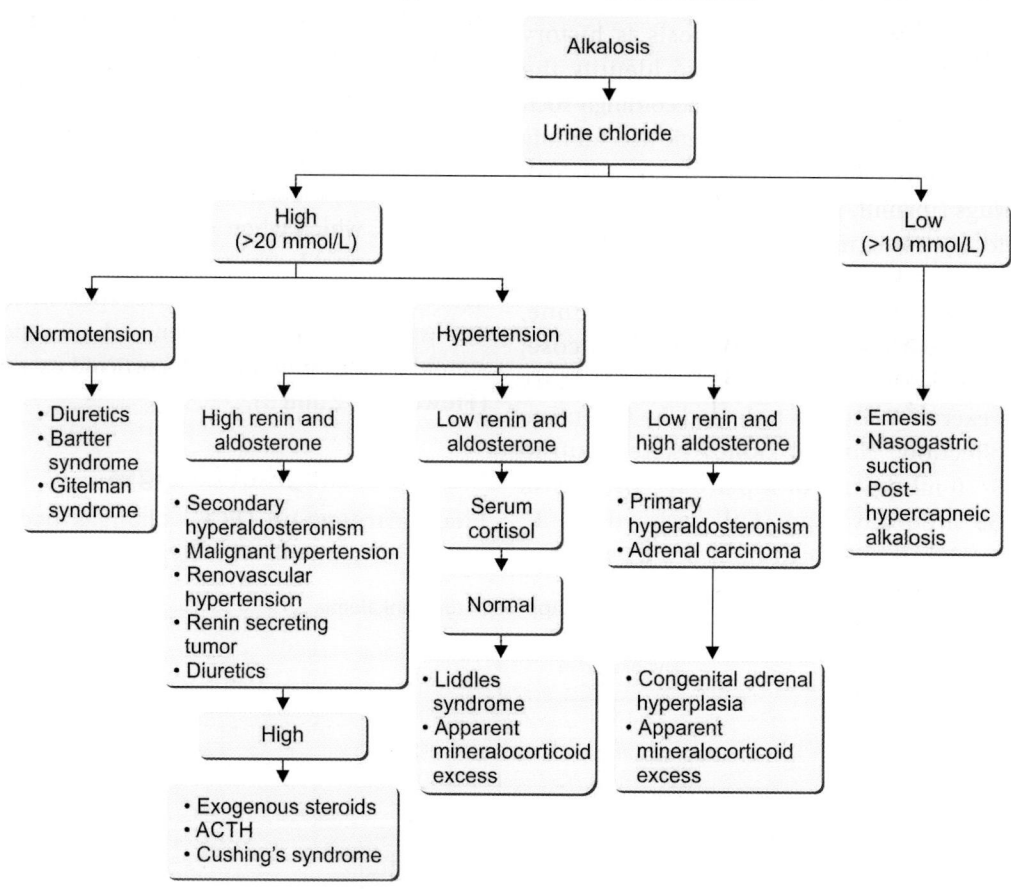

Flowchart 3: Hypokalemia with metabolic alkalosis.

(ACTH: adrenocorticotropic hormone)

involve decrease in T wave amplitude and appearance of U waves. ECG shows flat T waves, ST segment depression, and QT prolongation.

Evaluation

Evaluation of hypokalemia in pregnancy is illustrated in **Flowcharts 2 and 3**.

Management Steps/Algorithm

Identify the precipitating factor and treat it: Stop or decrease dose of drugs causing hypokalemia or use K-sparing drugs (angiotensin-converting enzyme inhibitor, aldosterone receptor blocker, and potassium-sparing diuretics).

Deficit Estimation

There will be a deficit of approximately 10% of total body K for every 1 mEq/L decrease in serum K^+. But in pregnancy as additional requirements exists the deficit could be estimated roughly as 12–14% for every 1 mEq/L decrease in serum K^+.[4] For example serum K fall from 3.5 to 2.5 means 12% deficit accounting for 300 mEq in 50 kg pregnant patient (total K store of 2,500). Based on the severity of symptoms the replacement can be oral or IV.

Treatment

Dietary supplementation in mild asymptomatic cases (serum K 3–3.5 mEq/L) with K-rich foods such as banana, dry fruit, spinach, milk, and coconut water can be initiated. The effectiveness of such supplementation is low as most of the dietary supplements are coupled with phosphates. Usually, serum chloride levels are low (hypochloremia) in patients with hypokalemia, which gets corrected with potassium chloride (KCl) supplementation. Oral KCl salts are good source as they contain around 13.6 mEq/g. Oral syrups like KCl (20% solutions, 2.6 mEq K and chloride per mL) achieve faster correction than K citrate [each mL contains 2 mEq K ion and is equivalent to 2 mEq bicarbonate (HCO_3)] albeit with complications like hyperchloremia.[4,5] Citrate formulations can be preferred in patients with concomitant metabolic acidosis, such as renal tubular acidosis. IV potassium chloride (2 mEq/mL K^+ and Cl^-) is used in symptomatic hypokalemia and serum K < 3 mEq/L, as this is a hyperosmolar solution (4,000 mOsm/kg H_2O), which can cause pain and phlebitis in the injected vein. So, these are reserved in conditions of hypokalemia associated with ECG changes, physical signs or symptoms, and unable to tolerate oral supplementation. The best and fastest results can be achieved with a combination of IV and oral routes. Replacement through peripheral IV route rate should not exceed 20 mEq/L and standard administration is 20–40 mmol per 1 liter of normal saline (avoid in dextrose-containing solutions as they can stimulate insulin release and aggravate hypokalemia). Through central venous catheters, the replacement can be up to 40 mEq/hour based on the severity of symptoms and the intensity of monitoring available, especially for any arrhythmias. The other solution which is available for IV replacement is potassium phosphate (4.4 mEq/mL of K and 3 mmol/mL of phosphorus), which has a role in cases of coexisting hypophosphatemia. Correction of coexisting hypomagnesemia also should be done, especially in cases of alkalosis, as hypokalemia can be refractory if hypomagnesemia is not corrected.

■ HYPERKALEMIA

Defined as serum K >5.5 mEq/L. It can be classified as mild (5.5–6.5 mEq/L), moderate (6.5–7.5 mEq/L), and severe (>7.5 mEq/L) hyperkalemia. During sample collection, it is important to know which laboratory specimen is taken for analysis, as during the clotting process, platelets release K. Pseudohyperkalemia occurs when serum K^+ exceeds the plasma K^+ by 0.5 mEq/L. Pseudohyperkalemia can occur due to the movement of K out of the cell during or after blood sample collection. Hemolysis during vein puncture, thrombocytosis (>1 million/mm^3), leukocytosis (>1.2 lakh/mm^3), and delayed processing time can cause pseudohyperkalemia. True hyperkalemia occurs as a result of redistribution within the body, increased K intake, or reduced renal excretion.[3,6] Normally kidneys account for 90% of K^+ excretion and serum K^+ rise can occur only when renal function falls by <25%.

Epidemiology and Magnitude

A study performed in 26,960 pregnant women between 2000 and 2012 at Soroka University medical Centre showed that a level of serum K >5 mEq/L showed a significant association with severe atherosclerotic morbidity in the future, as it might be an indication for occult metabolic and renal dysfunction. Another study conducted in the labor ward of general hospital in Nigeria between 2008 and 2011 showed an association between prolonged labor and hyperkalemia.

Etiology

Impaired Potassium Excretion

Reduced renal K$^+$ excretion occurs due to renal failure (GFR <10 mL/min or reduce urine output to <1 L/day), reduced aldosterone secretion or responsiveness, reduced distal sodium and water delivery, as seen in congestive heart failure, cirrhosis, acute kidney injury (AKI), and advanced chronic kidney disease (CKD). Obstetric AKI, especially in the last trimester and immediate postpartum, with ongoing hemolysis still remains a leading cause of hyperkalemia in obstetric critically ill patients. However, with improved care and survival, pregnancies in women with advanced CKD are on the rise, and obstetric complications are much higher in this special population.[2,7] Relatively rarer causes include aldosterone deficiency due to Addison's disease and hyperreninemic hypoaldosteronism, seen in diabetic nephropathy and tubulointerstitial diseases and Gordon syndrome due to defect in WNT1 or WNT4 channel (with reduced activity of thiazide sensitive sodium chloride cotransporter in the distal tubule causing hypertension, hyperkalemia, hyperchloremic acidosis, and chronic hypertension).

Transcellular Shifts

Mechanisms that promote the exit of K from the cells or impede its entrance can lead to redistributive hyperkalemia. As 98% of total body K is intracellular, any pathophysiology with increased cell turnover like rhabdomyolysis, tumor lysis syndrome, and conditions associated with a high plasma osmolality (uremia and diabetes mellitus) and metabolic acidosis, result in movement of K into extracellular space due to exchange of extracellular H$^+$ with intracellular K$^+$.

Medication-induced Hyperkalemia

Angiotensin-converting enzyme inhibitor, angiotensin receptor antagonist, K sparing diuretics, and nonsteroidal anti-inflammatory drugs cause reduce aldosterone level and hyperkalemia. Hyperkalemia is also reported in pregnancy with use of magnesium sulfate causing hypermagnesemia. Other drugs that can lead to hyperkalemia are mentioned in **Box 1**.

Special Causes Leading to Hyperkalemia in Pregnancy

Pregnancy-associated complications such as hemolysis, elevated liver enzymes, and low platelet count (HELLP syndrome), severe preeclampsia, and conditions characterized by hemolysis are associated with hyperkalemia. Life-threatening arrhythmia and cardiac arrest due to hyperkalemia have been reported in pregnancies due to the use of succinylcholine for anesthesia prior to cesarean section, especially in women with prolonged bed rest and immobilization. This is attributed to upregulation of extrajunctional acetylcholine

---

BOX 1: The causes of hyperkalemia in pregnancy.

- Impaired excretion (Angiotensin-converting enzymes inhibitors, angiotensin receptor blockers, nonsteroidal anti-inflammatory drugs, potassium sparing diuretics, trimethoprim, heparin, lithium, calcineurin inhibitors)
- Transcellular shift (Mannitol, beta-blockers, digoxin toxicity, somatostatin, succinylcholine)
- Increased intake (Penicillin G potassium)

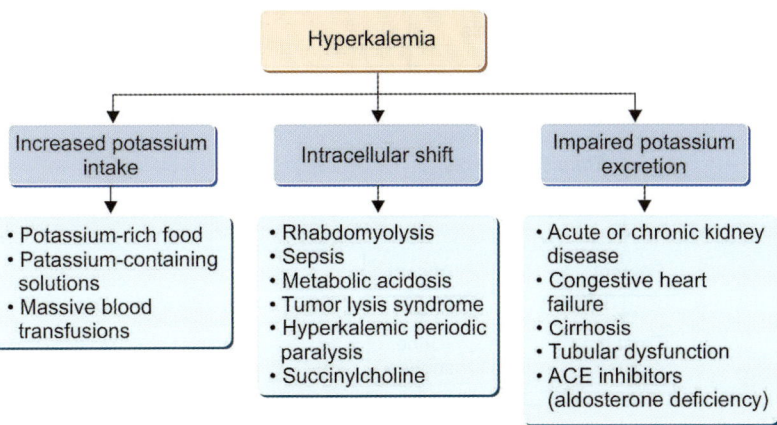

Flowchart 4: Causes of hyperkalemia.

(ACE: angiotensin-converting enzyme)

receptors causing the release of K from the whole muscle instead of the neuromuscular junction. Hyperkalemia is also seen in patients with hypermagnesemia due to magnesium sulfate administration. Causes of hyperkalemia are mentioned in **Flowchart 4**.

Clinical Features

Absence of symptoms does not exclude severe hyperkalemia, as it is often asymptomatic. The most dominant features of hyperkalemia are skeletal muscle and cardiac conduction abnormalities. Neuromuscular weakness, including flaccid paralysis, is seen. Other nonspecific symptoms such as fatigue, paresthesia, and motor paralysis are usually seen in severe cases. The most important consequence of hyperkalemia is a reduction in myocardial resting membrane potential.

Electrocardiogram Changes

Electrocardiographic changes begin when the K reaches 6 mEq/L and are universal when serum level of 8.0 mEq/L is reached. But there exists no correlation of serum K with ECG changes. These changes may be milder or blunted in patients with preexisting CKD. The earliest changes are tall, peaked, narrow base T wave in precordial leads V_{2-4} followed by P-wave flattening, P-R interval prolongation, widening of QRS complex followed by sine waves, ultimately progressing to ventricular arrhythmias (ventricular tachycardia and ventricular fibrillation), and asystole.

Workup Required

Repeat measurements should be performed to definitively exclude pseudohyperkalemia. Etiology of hyperkalemia can be determined primarily by history taking, physical examination (blood pressure and intravascular volume status to identify the cause of renal hypoperfusion), and laboratory tests (such as blood urea nitrogen, urine electrolyte, creatinine, acid base status, serum glucose, serum renin, aldosterone, and cortisol).[6,7] The clinician should review medications and any salt containing K if ongoing should be stopped. ECG should be done if K reaches 6 mEq/L, or with suspicion of rapid onset hyperkalemia or with any new onset of hyperkalemia with underlying kidney disease, heart disease, or cirrhosis.

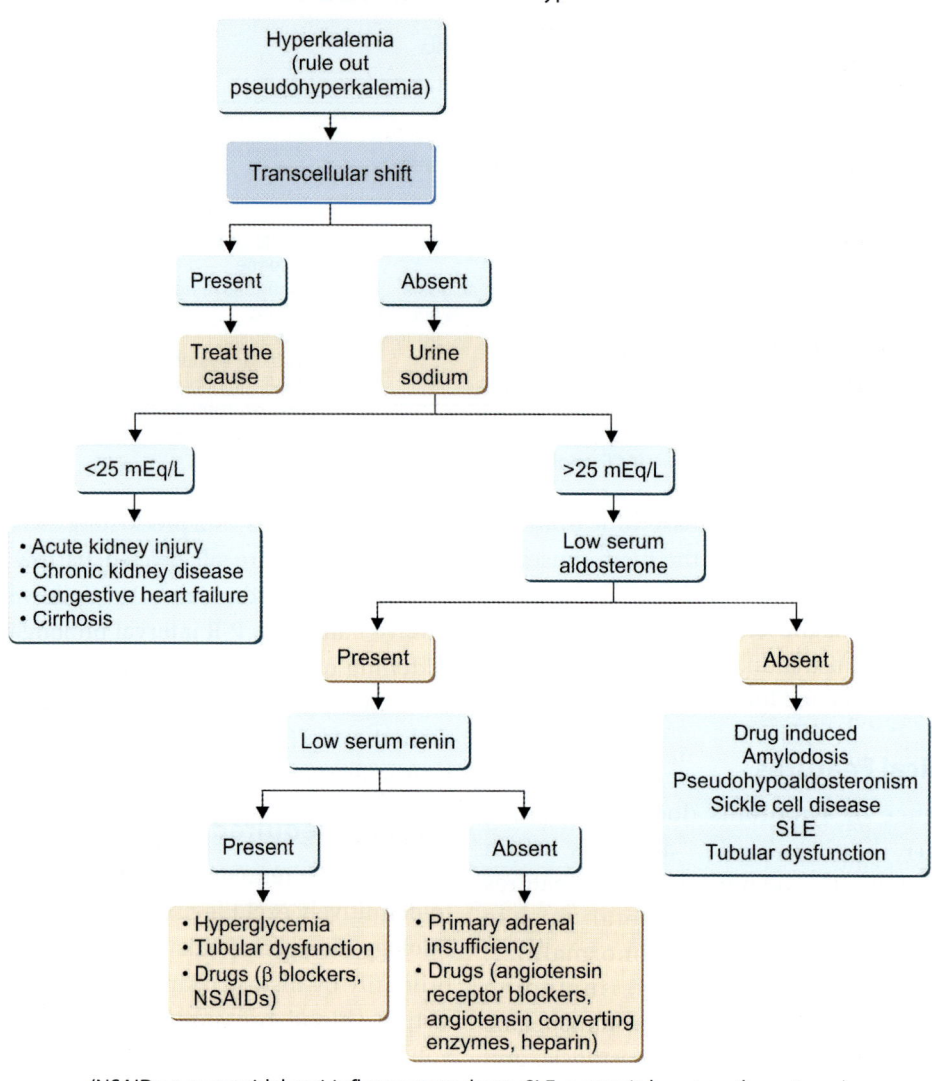

Flowchart 5: Evaluation of hyperkalemia.

(NSAIDs: nonsteroidal anti-inflammatory drugs; SLE: systemic lupus erythematosus)

Evaluation

Evaluation of hyperkalemia in pregnancy is mentioned in **Flowchart 5**.

Management Steps/Algorithm

Prompt treatment should be initiated when ECG changes are evident; the serum K levels are >6 mEq/L, and rapid onset, especially associated with underlying heart disease cirrhosis or kidney disease.

Urgent Treatment

Intravenous calcium: Calcium (Ca) salts (Ca gluconate and Ca chloride) are used to achieve a membrane-stabilizing effect due to hyperkalemia in order to prevent further arrhythmias, although they have no effect on serum K levels. Usual dose of Ca gluconate is 1,000 mg (10 mL of a 10% solution) and calcium chloride is 500–1,000 mg (5–10 mL of a 10% solution) infused over 2–3 minutes, with cardiac monitoring through ECG. Ca gluconate is most commonly used as it is less irritant to veins, even though, calcium chloride contains three times the concentration of elemental calcium compared with calcium gluconate. While the onset of action is immediate, the duration of effect ranges from 30 to 60 minutes.

Insulin and glucose: Insulin administration lowers the serum K concentration by driving K into the cells, primarily by enhancing the activity of the Na-K-ATPase pump in skeletal muscle. The usual dose is 10 units followed by 25 g of glucose (50 mL of 50% glucose). In patients with blood glucose levels of >250 mg/dL, glucose administration could be deferred. The onset of action ranges from 10 to 15 minutes, with a duration of around 2 hours. As the fetus cannot depend on gluconeogenesis for glucose production and is completely dependent on maternal glucose diffusion, it is always preferable to use insulin and dextrose together in pregnancy.

Inhaled β_2 agonists: Usual doses needed are four to eight times the respiratory nebulization dose at approximately 10–20 mg of salbutamol, the dose can further be increased in patients on mechanical ventilatory support, in order to enhance the delivery apart from using vibrating mesh nebulizers or ultrasonic nebulizers. The onset of action ranges from 15 to 30 minutes, with a duration of around 2 hours. Fetal heart rate should be monitored as rarely it may cause fetal tachycardia (defined as a sustained fetal heart rate >210 beats/min) or tachyarrhythmia (supraventricular tachycardia).

Sodium bicarbonate (NaHCO$_3$): As adjuvant therapy in conditions associated with metabolic acidosis. Raising the systemic pH with NaHCO$_3$ results in hydrogen ion release from the cells as part of the buffering reaction. This change is accompanied by K movement into the cells to maintain electroneutrality.

Subacute treatment: These play a pivotal role in removing K from the body.

Loop diuretics: Can increase renal K losses and cause mild metabolic alkalosis (synergistic in reducing serum K levels), and should preferably be used in hypervolemic states, even with mild to moderate renal impairment (though higher doses required).

Resins: Gastrointestinal cation exchangers such as sodium polystyrene sulfonate (SPS), and sodium zirconium cyclosilicate (SZC), bind K in exchange for Na and thereby lower total body K. Adverse effects such as gastrointestinal tract injury (intestinal necrosis) and constipation apart from delayed onset of action preclude their usage in acute and emergent treatments. These resins are preferably avoidable in pregnant patients with AKI.

Dialysis: When quick serum K reduction is required, especially in life-threatening situations, intermittent hemodialysis and sustained low-efficiency dialysis (when hemodynamically unstable) should be utilized. Using K-free baths in hemodialysis should be limited to the first hour of hemodialysis, as prolonged use may precipitate cardiac arrhythmias. Slower modalities such as continuous renal replacement therapy and rarely, peritoneal dialysis can also be utilized effectively in patients with renal failure and hyperkalemia. Internal jugular veins are preferable as inferior vena cava compression by gravid uterus can further aggravate aortocaval compression syndrome which can lead to fetal compromise. Peritoneal dialysis catheter placement can be done from supraumbilical approach to avoid trauma to the gravid uterus.[6,7]

CONCLUSION

Disorder of K homeostasis is rare in obstretic population. They are mostly due to imbalance between secretion and reabsorption of K. Hypokalemic symptoms mostly occur at K <3 mEq/L whereas in hyperkalemia symptoms are seen when K >5.5 mEq/L. Diagnosis is based on history (use of any drugs causing hypo- or hyperkalemia is important) and physical examination, laboratory and ECG findings. Treatment is done on symptomatic patient and underlying cause should be treated accordingly. Under and overcorrection should be avoided for maternal and fetal benefit.

TAKE HOME MESSAGES

- Potassium disturbances are the most common electrolyte abnormalities seen after sodium disturbances worldwide; however, their prevalence in pregnancy is low.
- Potassium homeostasis in pregnant females is governed by aldosterone and progesterone and there is an additional 300–350 mEq requirement per day.
- Evaluation of potassium disorders should primarily focus on proper history taking and biochemical evaluation to ascertain cause, and the clinician should actively look for the presence of any warning signs.
- Treatment should continue in symptomatic patients and underlying causes should be treated accordingly.
- Under and overcorrection in treatment should be strictly avoided, to prevent maternal and fetal harm.

REFERENCES

1. Yang C-W, Li S, Dong Y. The Prevalence and Risk Factors of Hypokalemia in Pregnancy-Related Hospitalizations: A Nationwide Population Study. Int J Nephrol. 2021;2021:9922245.
2. Tanacan A, Erol SA, Anuk AT, Yetiskin FDY, Tokalioglu EO, Sahin S, et al. The Association of Serum Electrolytes with Disease Severity and Obstetric Complications in Pregnant Women with COVID-19: a Prospective Cohort Study from a Tertiary Reference Center. Geburtshilfe Frauenheilkd. 2022;82:326-32.
3. Wolak T, Shoham-Vardi I, Sergienko R, Sheiner E. High potassium level during pregnancy is associated with future cardiovascular morbidity. J Matern Neonatal Med. 2016;29:1021-4.
4. Barta V, Koncicki H. Electrolyte disorders in pregnancy. In: Sachdeva M, Miller I (Eds). Obstetric Gynecologic Nephrology. Cham: Springer International Publishing; 2020. pp. 113-27.
5. Kardalas E, Paschou SA, Anagnostis P, Muscogiuri G, Siasos G, Vryonidou A. Hypokalemia: a clinical update. Endocr Connect. 2018;7:R135-46.
6. Viera AJ, Wouk N. Potassium disorders: Hypokalemia and hyperkalemia. Am Fam Physician. 2015;92:487-95.
7. Cheung KL, Lafayette RA. Renal Physiology of Pregnancy. Adv Chronic Kidney Dis. 2013;20(3):209-14.
8. Moustakakis MN, Bockorny M. Gitelman syndrome and pregnancy. Clin Kidney J. 2012;5(6):552-5.

CHAPTER 22

Disorders of Calcium, Magnesium, and Phosphorus Homeostasis

Prashant Kumar, Mukta Seth

INTRODUCTION

Calcium, magnesium, and phosphorus are the chemical elements required for enzymatic functions or structural elements in human health. Disorders of mineral metabolism involving abnormalities of calcium, phosphorus, and magnesium homeostasis are common.[1] Human body maintains a physiologic range of these minerals and their abnormalities can range from minor symptoms to fatal consequences depending on many other factors. An understanding of normal physiology is necessary to accurately diagnose and treat disorders of mineral metabolism during pregnancy.

EPIDEMIOLOGY AND MAGNITUDE OF THE PROBLEM

Mineral disorders are common in pregnancy **(Table 1)**. The prevalence of hypocalcemia was 29.20% among the pregnant women and 14.20% among the nonpregnant women whereas hypercalcemia in pregnancy is uncommon, occurring in approximately 0.03% of women of reproductive age. Prevalence of hypomagnesemia (magnesium serum level cut-off <0.66 mmol/L/<0.8 mmol/L) was 34.0%/78.9% in pregnant women and 21.4%/54.8% in women with hormone-related conditions (HRC).[1] The highest prevalence of magnesium deficiency was observed for osteoporosis and climacteric syndrome. Hypermagnesemia is an uncommon laboratory finding and symptomatic hypermagnesemia is even less common in normal renal function. This disorder has a low incidence of occurrence because the kidney can eliminate excess magnesium by rapidly reducing its tubular reabsorption to almost negligible amounts.

IMPLICATIONS FOR MATERNAL HEALTH

The pregnant females require minerals for their own health and that for the fetal health. Fetal accumulation of calcium occurs mainly during the third trimester. By the end of normal pregnancy, the fetus acquires approximately 28 g of calcium and 16 g of phosphorus. The additional calcium required during pregnancy is needed mainly for the fetal skeleton. Magnesium during pregnancy is important for almost every system in the mother and the baby. Depending on the age, 350–400 mg of magnesium is needed every day during the pregnancy. Phosphorus is a mineral that helps build bones of the mother and the baby during pregnancy. Getting adequate magnesium during pregnancy

TABLE 1: Mineral disorders during pregnancy.

Disorder	Proposed pathophysiology/features	Treatment options
Osteoporosis in pregnancy[6]	Genetic predisposition, excessive resorption of skeleton during pregnancy, usually seen in first pregnancy, ankle and other lower limb fractures are common	Optimization of calcium and vitamin D intake, correction of nutritional deficiencies, appropriate weight bearing
Primary hyperparathyroidism[7]	Diagnosis may be obscured by physiological hypocalcemia in pregnancy	Surgical option, calcitonin, bisphosphonates, high dose magnesium, dialysis, hydration, and correction of electrolyte abnormalities
Familial hypercalciuric hypercalcemia[8]	Genetic, hypercalcemia in the mother, fetal and neonatal parathyroid suppression leading to tetany in the newborn	Treatment of hypercalcemia in the mother if symptomatic, watch/treat baby for hypocalcemia
Hypoparathyroidism[9]	Preexisting condition may aggravate during pregnancy	Albumin-corrected calcium should be maintained in the mid normal range
Pseudohypoparathyroidism[10]	Genetic disorder casing resistance to parathyroid hormone (PTH) leading to hypocalcemia, hypophosphatemia and high PTH	Maintain albumin-corrected calcium in the mid normal range
Vitamin D deficiency and insufficiency[11]	Nutritional deficiency	Vitamin D supplementation
Genetic vitamin D resistance syndrome[12]	Genetic disorder of vitamin D physiology	Maintain albumin-corrected calcium in the mid normal range with oral calcium
24-hydroxylase deficiency[13]	Causes high calcitriol and mild hypercalcemia	Increased hydration moderately restricted calcium diets
Hypercalcemia of malignancy[14]	Generally, a terminal condition for the mother	Monitor cord blood for calcium, risk of neonatal hypoparathyroidism

can help prevent preterm labor and other complications during pregnancy.[2]

IMPLICATIONS FOR FETAL WELL-BEING

Calcium and phosphorus help strengthen fetal rapidly developing bones and teeth, and boost muscle, heart, and nerve development. Magnesium is an essential mineral required to regulate body temperature, nucleic acid, and protein synthesis with an important role in maintaining nerve and electrical potentials of the muscle cells. It may reduce fetal growth restriction and preeclampsia as well as increase birth weight.

MANAGEMENT STEPS/ALGORITHM

Both excess and deficiency of the mineral can present with symptoms. Since the symptoms of mineral deficiency can be variable, it is not possible to diagnose them clinically. A general nutritional assessment and laboratory test can contribute to the assessment.

Plasma Calcium

The calcium in plasma is present in three forms, ionized calcium (nearly half of the total), which is active and complexed (with albumin, protein, and sulfates), which is inactive. It is better to order for the ionized calcium separately since the total calcium depends on some other factors (such as hypoalbuminemia). Intestinal calcium and phosphate absorption doubles during the pregnancy driven by 1,25-dihydroxyvitamin D and other factors. The serum (total) calcium is decreased during pregnancy, while the ionized calcium remains normal. Serum phosphate and magnesium concentrations remain normal during pregnancy. Hypercalcemia and hypocalcemia cannot be diagnosed based on the total calcium level. Parathyroid hormone is reduced, and serum calcitonin level is raised in pregnancy.[3]

Blood collection for measuring ionized calcium should not contain air bubbles (which can lower carbon dioxide) and anticoagulants (which can bind the ionized calcium).

Laboratory Values

Normal laboratory values of calcium, magnesium, and phosphorus are listed in **Table 2**.

Predisposing Conditions for Hypocalcemia

- Magnesium depletion
- Sepsis
- Blood transfusion
- Drugs (such as aminoglycosides and heparin)
- Renal failure
- Pancreatitis
- Vitamin D deficiency.

Clinical Manifestations

Hypocalcemia leads to enhanced cardiac and neuromuscular excitability and reduced contractile force in the cardiac and vascular muscles. It may lead to tetany, hyperreflexia, paresthesia, and seizures. Chvostek's sign and Trousseau's sign can be positive in some but are unreliable for diagnosis. In extreme ionized hypocalcemia cardiovascular manifestation may be present (hypotension, decreased cardiac output, ventricular ectopic, etc.).

Calcium Replacement Regimen (Table 3)

Intravenous (IV): Generally, for the symptomatic hypocalcemia 200 mg of elemental calcium is given intravenously over 10 minutes followed by continuous infusion in dose range of 1–2 mg/kg/h for 6–12 hours. Calcium gluconate has lower osmolarity (680 mOsm/L) than calcium chloride (2,000 mOsm/L).

TABLE 2: Normal laboratory values of calcium, magnesium and phosphorus.

Parameter	Normal value
Serum calcium	8.6–10.3 mg/dL (2–2.5 mmol/L)
Serum magnesium	1.7–2.2 mg/dL (0.85–1.10 mmol/L)
Serum phosphorus	2.8–4.5 mg/dL (1.12–1.45 mmol/L)

TABLE 3: Elemental calcium content in calcium chloride and calcium gluconate.

	Calcium preparation solution	
Solution	Elemental calcium	Unit volume
Calcium chloride	27 mg/mL	10 mL ampules
Calcium gluconate	9 mg/mL	10 mL ampules

Monitoring ionized calcium during therapy is recommended.

Adverse Effects of Intravenous Calcium

Sudden correction leads to vasoconstriction, ischemia in vital organs, and cellular injury particularly in patients with circulatory shock. Therefore, IV calcium should be reserved for the patients in whom hypocalcemia correction is likely to benefit.

Oral maintenance therapy of 2–4 g/day in the adults is given in the form of calcium carbonate or calcium gluconate tablets.

Hypercalcemia

In the intensive care unit (ICU) up to 23% patient may have an episode of hypercalcemia. Hypercalcemia in pregnancy is uncommon, with associated adverse obstetric and perinatal outcomes for both the mother and the fetus.

Clinical Manifestation

Nonspecific symptoms have been noticed in hypercalcemia such as gastrointestinal (nausea, vomiting, constipation, ileus, pancreatitis, etc.), cardiovascular (hypovolemia, hypotension, shortened QT interval), renal (polyurea), neurologic (confusion, altered sensorium, coma), etc. Clinical features are common in rapid rise in the serum calcium such as in malignancy.

Treatment

One or more of the following based on severity and response:
- Active treatment is recommended for symptomatic hypercalcemia.
- Hydration—isotonic saline 200–500 mL/h maintaining urine output 100–150 mL/h.
- Loop diuretic—furosemide 40–80 mg IV stat with infusion 10 mg/h.
- Calcitonin—4 units/kg SC/IM 12 hourly.
- Steroids—injection hydrocortisone 200–400 mg/day.
- Bisphosphonates—zoledronate 4–8 mg IV over 15 minutes.
- Dialysis is recommended for renal patients with low urine output.

Hypophosphatemia

Phosphate is predominantly intracellular anion where it participated in glycolysis and adenosine triphosphate (ATP) production. Serum phosphate <2.5 mg/dL (0.8 mmol/L) is reported in 17–29% in critically ill patients. Intestinal phosphate absorption is doubled during normal pregnancy.

Causes

- Glucose loading—phosphate moves into cell with glucose
- Hyperglycemia—osmotic diuresis leads to loss of phosphate in urine
- Respiratory alkalosis
- Beta agonists promote the movement of phosphate into the cells
- Sepsis and systemic inflammation
- Phosphate biding agents such as sucralfate.

Clinical Manifestations

Hypophosphatemia causes symptoms of impaired energy metabolism such as low cardiac output, hemolytic anemia, poor oxygen unloading at tissues, muscle weakness, respiratory failure, etc.

Phosphate Correction

- Phosphate dosing is calculated based on the body weight and initial serum phosphate level.
- Oral replacement (phosphate level 1.0–1.9 mg/dL)—250–500 mg 3–4 times/day.

- IV replacement (phosphate <1.0 mg/dL)—dose (0.08–0.20 mmol/kg)—switch to oral when phosphate level reaches >1.5 mg/dL.

Hyperphosphatemia

Hyperphosphatemia results from either reduced excretion (e.g., renal failure) or excess loading from the disrupted cells (e.g., tumor lysis syndrome, rhabdomyolysis, etc.).

Hyperphosphatemia can manifest as symptoms of hypocalcemia such as tetany or as deposition of calcium phosphate complexes in the soft tissues on the long run.

Management

Sucralfate and aluminum containing antacids bind the phosphate in the intestinal lumen and make a loss thereby ultimately reducing to total systemic load [gastrointestinal (GI) dialysis]. Hemodialysis is another option in the renal patients.

Magnesium

Approximately 24 g of magnesium is distributed in the body mainly in the bone (53%), muscle (27%), soft tissues (19%), red blood cell (RBC) (0.7%) with <1% in the plasma **(Table 4)**.

TABLE 4: Serum magnesium and clinical condition/toxicity.

mEq/L	Effects
1.3–2	Normal serum level
4–7	Therapeutic level
5–7	Depression of deep tendon reflexes
5–10	Prolongation of p-q interval
7–10	Loss of deep tendon reflexes
10–12	Respiratory paralysis
>15	Sinoatrial and atrioventricular block
>25	Cardiac arrest

Total serum magnesium is 1.7–2.4 mg/dL and ionized is 0.8–1.1 mEq/L whereas urinary magnesium excretion is 5–15 mEq/24 h. Serum magnesium does not reflect total magnesium stores in the body. Urinary magnesium loss is more important to assess the magnesium deficiency. In condition of magnesium deficiency, the urinary loss is conserved.

Magnesium Deficiency

Magnesium deficiency is one of the common underdiagnosed conditions. Significant decrease of magnesium levels in serum is observed in pregnancy.[4] Magnesium supplementation during pregnancy improves maternal health and fetal outcome. Magnesium supplementation reduces the incidence of preterm labor and vaginal hemorrhage. Premature delivery is significantly reduced from 8.2 to 2.8%. In preeclampsia and eclampsia IV magnesium in pharmacological doses is the standard of care.

Predisposing conditions for hypomagnesemia:
- Nutritional deficiency
- Drug therapy (furosemide, aminoglycosides, amphotericin, digitalis, cisplatin, etc.)
- Diarrhea
- Alcohol use
- Diabetes mellitus
- Acute myocardial infarction (MI).

Clinical significance of magnesium in obstetric critical care: There are no specific symptoms related to magnesium deficiency. Other electrolytes deficiency may indicate toward magnesium deficiency.

Intrauterine growth retardation: Magnesium deficiency in the mother has been linked to the low birth weight and premature labor.

Preterm labor: Magnesium deficiency is a risk for preterm labor, which can be prevented and cured with magnesium supplementation, which is a tocolytic.

Preeclampsia and eclampsia: It has been claimed that magnesium supplementation can prevent at least half of the cases of preeclampsia. In addition, magnesium supplementation prevents the progress of preeclampsia to eclampsia and the maternal death.[5]

Sudden infant death syndrome: An association of infant death in the first year and magnesium deficiency has been proposed and needs further research.

Fetal neuroprotection: Magnesium should be considered for fetal neuroprotection in antenatal patients presenting <30 weeks in preterm gestation.

Nocturnal leg cramps: Several mechanisms of leg cramps such as disorder of oxygen uptake, energy production, and electrolyte balance have been discussed and magnesium supplementation has been proposed in pregnant ladies for this symptom.

Postoperative analgesia: Studies on magnesium role in postoperative analgesia have given mixed results. Several studies have shown reduced opioid requirement for pain in postoperative patients. Intrathecal $MgSO_4$ (100 mg) has also been used to enhance the pain relief.

Diagnosis

Serum magnesium should be done. But this is unlikely to reveal the total deficiency.

Magnesium retention test: If <50% of the infused magnesium is recovered in the urine in 24 hours, magnesium deficiency is likely. This is both diagnostic and partially therapeutic. A total of 6 g of $MgSO_4$ is given slow IV over 2 hours and magnesium level is tested in urine collected in 24 hours to calculate the total loss in urine.

Magnesium Replacement

Oral magnesium can be used in the dose of 5 mg/kg in the normal subjects. IV magnesium in the form of magnesium sulfate is available (1 g = 8 mEq). In mild hypomagnesemia, the dose is 1–2 mEq/kg. Assuming 50% loss in urine, twice the dose calculated is given. For example, a 50-kg-person's total dose is 100 mEq (100/8 = 12.5 g), 50% of the total dose is given in first 24 hours and the remaining in the next 3–4 days.

Hypermagnesemia

Hypermagnesemia is less commonly observed (5%) in the hospitalized patients.

Predisposing Factors

- Renal insufficiency
- Homolysis
- Other conditions such as diabetes ketoacidosis, adrenal insufficiency, hyperparathyroidism, lithium intoxication.

Clinical Features

The manifestations depend on the level of serum magnesium such as hyperreflexia 1st degree atrioventricular (AV) block.

Management

- Hemodialysis is the treatment of choice for severe hypermagnesemia.
- IV calcium gluconate (1 g slow IV over 2–3 minutes) is given, which antagonizes the effects of magnesium in the heart.

- Crystalloid infusion with loop diuretic—in nonoliguric patients, crystalloid administration with a loop diuretic can increase the urinary loss of magnesium.

TAKE HOME MESSAGES

- Mineral disorders not related to pregnancy can effect during pregnancy and it should be evaluated and treated keeping in consideration of the altered physiology during pregnancy.
- During normal pregnancy total calcium is low, parathyroid hormone is high, calcitriol level is high and calcitonin level is high. Ionized calcium should be used to assess the calcium status, which is in the normal range and should be used for concluding a "true" case of hypocalcemia.
- Phosphorus falls during pregnancy until the 11th–13th week before delivery, followed by an equal rise until term. Phosphorus deficiencies are very rare and usually seen only in cases of starvation. By the end of a full-term gestation about 30 g calcium, 20 g phosphorus, and 0.8 g magnesium are required to mineralize the fetal bones. Phosphorus disorders during other critical illness during pregnancy should be treated in the same manner as nonpregnant state.
- Magnesium status is relevant in fetal development during gestation and for growth of the newborn during the perinatal period. Moreover, magnesium can influence fetal programming and disease presentation in childhood or even adulthood. Magnesium has been used to treat preeclampsia and eclampsia for the last several decades.
- Magnesium is used to blunt stress response during induction of anesthesia, reduce analgesic requirement during intraoperative and postoperative period, fetal neuroprotection and maternal leg cramps etc. Very small amount of magnesium reaches the brain after systemic administration.

■ REFERENCES

1. Sharon MM. Disorders involving calcium, phosphorus, and magnesium. Prim Care. 2008;35(2):215-37, v-vi.
2. Farias PM, Marcelino G, Santana LF, de Almeida EB, Guimarães RCA, Pott A, et al. Minerals in pregnancy and their impact on child growth and development. Molecules. 2020;25(23):5630.
3. Kovacs CS. Calcium and Phosphate Metabolism and Related Disorders During Pregnancy and Lactation. In: Feingold KR, Anawalt B, Boyce A, Chrousos G, de Herder WW, Dhatariya K, et al. (Eds). Endotext. South Dartmouth (MA): MDText.com, Inc.; 2000.
4. Spätling L. Magnesium in obstetrics and gynecology. Gynakol Geburtshilfliche Rundsch. 1993;33(2):85-91.
5. Smith JM, Lowe RF, Fullerton J, Currie SM, Harris L, Felker-Kantor E, et al. An integrative review of the side effects related to the use of magnesium sulfate for pre-eclampsia and eclampsia management. BMC Pregnancy Childbirth. 2013;13:34.
6. Herath M, Wong P, Trinh A, Allan CA, Wallace EM, Ebeling PR, et al. Minimal-trauma ankle fractures predominate during pregnancy: a 17-year retrospective study. Arch Osteoporos. 2017;12(1):86.
7. Schnatz PF, Curry SL. Primary hyperparathyroidism in pregnancy: evidence-based management. Obstet Gynecol Surv. 2002;57:365-76.
8. Jones AR, Hare MJ, Brown J, Yang J, Meyer C, Milat F, et al. Familial Hypocalciuric hypercalcemia in pregnancy: diagnostic pitfalls. JBMR Plus. 2020;4:e10362.
9. Khan AA, Clarke B, Rejnmark L, Brandi ML. Management of endocrine disease: hypoparathyroidism in pregnancy: review and evidence-based recommendations for management. Eur J Endocrinol. 2019; 180(2):R37-44.
10. Vidailhet M, Monin P, André M, Suty Y, Marchal C, Vert P. Neonatal hyperparathyroidism secondary to maternal hypoparathyroidism. Arch Fr Pediatr. 1980;37(5):305-12.
11. Kovacs CS, Ward LE. Disorders of calcium, phosphorus, and bone metabolism during fetal and neonatal development. In:

Kovacs CS, Deal CL (Eds). Maternal-Fetal and Neonatal Endocrinology: Physiology, Pathophysiology, and Clinical Management. San Diego: Academic Press; 2019. pp. 755-82.
12. Rosen CJ, Adams JS, Bikle DD, Black DM, Demay MB, Manson JE, et al. The nonskeletal effects of vitamin D: an Endocrine Society scientific statement. Endocr Rev. 2012;33:456-92.
13. Carpenter TO. CYP24A1 loss of function: clinical phenotype of monoallelic and biallelic mutations. J Steroid Biochem Mol Biol. 2017;173:337-40.
14. Rey E, Jacob CE, Koolian M, Morin F. Hypercalcemia in pregnancy – a multifaceted challenge: case reports and literature review. Clin Case Rep. 2016;4(10):1001-8.

Neurological Disorders

CHAPTER 23

Severe Preeclampsia and Eclampsia

Pallavi Chandra Ravula, Tarakeswari Surapaneni

INTRODUCTION

Maternal mortality and severe maternal morbidity continue to be a major challenge worldwide. Hypertensive disorders in pregnancy are one of the three leading causes of maternal morbidity and mortality globally.[1] In one study in India, the maternal mortality rate due to preeclampsia/eclampsia was 24.4% of all maternal deaths.[2]

DEFINITIONS AND DIAGNOSTIC CRITERIA OF HYPERTENSIVE DISORDERS IN PREGNANCY[3,4]

1. *Chronic hypertension:* Systolic blood pressure of 140 mm Hg or more or diastolic blood pressure of 90 mm Hg or more before pregnancy or before 20 weeks of gestation.
2. *Gestational hypertension:* Systolic blood pressure of 140 mm Hg or more or diastolic blood pressure of 90 mm Hg or more, or both, on two occasions at least 4 hours apart after 20 weeks of gestation in a woman with a previously normal blood pressure. Gestational hypertension is considered to be severe when systolic blood pressure reaches 160 mm Hg or diastolic blood pressure reaches 110 mm Hg or both. About 50% of women with gestational hypertension progress to preeclampsia.
3. *Preeclampsia:* It is a multisystem disorder, and the definition has been recently broadened. According to the International Society for the Study of Hypertension in Pregnancy (ISSHP) preeclampsia is defined as systolic blood pressure at ≥140 mm Hg and/or diastolic blood pressure at ≥90 mm Hg on at least two occasions measured 4 hours apart in previously normotensive women and is accompanied by ≥1 of the following new-onset conditions at or after 20 weeks of gestation. This definition has been endorsed by FIGO.[3,4]

Preeclampsia de novo: Gestational hypertension accompanied by ≥1 of the following new-onset conditions at or after 20 weeks of gestation:
1. *Proteinuria:* 24-hour urine protein ≥300 mg/day; spot urine protein/creatinine ratio ≥30 mg/mmoL or ≥0.30 mg/dL, or urine dipstick testing ≥2+.
2. *Other maternal organ dysfunction:* Acute kidney injury (creatinine ≥90 µmol/L; >1.1 mg/dL); liver involvement [such as elevated alanine aminotransferase (ALT) or aspartate transaminase (AST) >40 IU/L with or without right upper quadrant or epigastric pain]; neurological complications (including eclampsia, altered mental status, blindness, stroke,

or more commonly hyperreflexia when accompanied by clonus, severe headaches, and persistent visual scotomata); hematological complications (thrombocytopenia—platelet count <150,000/mcL, disseminated intravascular coagulation, hemolysis)
3. Uteroplacental dysfunction (such as fetal growth restriction, abnormal umbilical artery Doppler waveform or stillbirth).
Preeclampsia can be further classified into:
- *Early-onset preeclampsia:* Delivery before 34 weeks of gestation
- *Preterm preeclampsia:* Delivery before 37 weeks of gestation
- *Late-onset preeclampsia:* Delivery at or after 34 weeks of gestation
- *Term preeclampsia:* Delivery at or after 37 weeks of gestation

Early-onset preeclampsia is associated with adverse maternal and perinatal outcomes when compared to late-onset preeclampsia.
4. *Superimposed preeclampsia on chronic hypertension:* Women with chronic essential hypertension develop any of the above maternal organ dysfunctions consistent with preeclampsia. In the absence of pre-existing proteinuria, new-onset proteinuria in the setting of a rise in blood pressure is sufficient to diagnose superimposed preeclampsia.
5. *Hemolysis, elevated liver enzymes, and low platelets (HELLP):* It is one of the severe forms of preeclampsia. It comprises of hemolysis (LDH >600 IU/L), elevated liver enzymes (ALT and AST elevated more than twice the upper limit) and low platelet count (<1,00,000/L).
6. *Eclampsia:* A convulsive manifestation of hypertension defined by new-onset tonic-clonic, focal, or multifocal seizures in the absence of other causative conditions such as epilepsy, cerebral arterial ischemia and infarction, intracranial hemorrhage, or drug use.

EPIDEMIOLOGY AND MAGNITUDE OF THE PROBLEM

Hypertensive disorders are one of the leading causes of maternal and perinatal morbidity and mortality worldwide. Globally, 2–5% of pregnancies are complicated by preeclampsia.[5,6] The women in low-income countries are affected the most. Eclampsia is one of the leading causes of severe maternal morbidity and mortality and is a life-threatening emergency with a mortality rate as high as 22%.[7]

IMPLICATIONS FOR MATERNAL HEALTH

Serious complications of preeclampsia are eclampsia, abruption, HELLP syndrome, acute pulmonary edema, respiratory distress syndrome, and intracranial hemorrhage. Long-term complications include chronic hypertension, cardiovascular diseases, cardiovascular accident, atherosclerosis, metabolic syndrome, and end-stage renal disease.

IMPLICATIONS FOR FETAL WELL-BEING

Preeclampsia is associated with perinatal morbidity and mortality; it is mostly associated with placental lesions. The short-term complications include fetal growth restriction, oligohydramnios, intrauterine fetal demise, preterm birth, low APGAR scores, nonreassuring fetal heart rate in labor and the need for neonatal intensive care unit (NICU) admissions. Long-term complications include cerebral palsy, low IQ, hearing loss, visual impairment, insulin-resistant diabetes mellitus, coronary artery disease, and hypertension.

MANAGEMENT OF PREECLAMPSIA

In the past decade, major efforts have been made to identify strategies for risk categorization and prediction of preeclampsia. Management of preeclampsia depends on screening, prevention strategies and medication.

Universal screening for preeclampsia in the first trimester: All pregnant women should be screened for preeclampsia in the first trimester. Screening identifies women at high risk of developing preeclampsia at a very early stage and this helps to use strategies to prevent preeclampsia. The best-combined test is maternal risk factors, measurement of mean arterial blood pressure (MAP), maternal serum pregnancy-associated plasma protein A (PAPP-A), serum placental growth factor (PLGF), and uterine artery pulsatility index (UTPI). A woman is considered high risk when the risk is 1 in 100 or more based on the first-trimester combined test with maternal risk factors (MAP, PLGF, and UTPI).[8]

Risk factors for preeclampsia are mentioned in **Table 1**.[9]

Uterine artery pulsatility index (PI): An ultrasound examination at 11–13^{+6} weeks gestational age by doing a uterine artery PI is an integral part of screening for preeclampsia.

Bioscreening: Biochemical markers increase the sensitivity screening for preeclampsia. In a recent study, the preferred biochemical marker was PLGF rather than PAPP-A. However, if PAPP-A was to be used rather than PLGF, the same detection rate can be achieved but at a higher screen-positive rate.[10] The PELICAN study showed that the Triage PLGF test had a negative predictive value of 98% when used to rule out preeclampsia that needed delivery within the next 14 days. These tests were valid in women presenting with suspected preeclampsia, which includes women with hypertension, proteinuria, fetal growth restriction, or symptoms suggestive of preeclampsia such as headaches or epigastric pain.[11] In screening for risk of development of preterm preeclampsia by a combination of maternal factors, MAP, UTPI, and PLGF, the detection rate was 82%.[12]

Prophylactic measures: The ASPRE trial has shown that in pregnancies at high risk for preeclampsia, administration of aspirin 150 mg/day from 11 to 14^{+6} to 36 weeks

TABLE 1: Risk factors for preeclampsia.[9]

High risk factors	Moderate risk factors	Others
• Previous pregnancy with preeclampsia • Multifetal gestation • Chronic kidney disease • Systemic lupus erythematosus • Antiphospholipid antibody syndrome • Thrombophilias • Type 1 or Type 2 diabetes mellitus • Chronic hypertension	• Nulliparity • Maternal age 35 or more • BMI of >30 kg/m^2 • Family history of preeclampsia • Low socioeconomic status • Previous stillbirth • Previous history of abruption • In vitro fertilization • Previous SGA adverse outcomes • Pregnancy with >10 years interval	• Assisted reproductive techniques • Gestational diabetes • Gestational HTN • Migraine • Hydatidiform mole • Hyperthyroidism

(BMI: body mass index; HTN: hypertension; SGA: small for gestational age)

gestation reduces the rate of early preeclampsia with delivery at <34 weeks gestation by about 80% and that of preterm preeclampsia with delivery at <37 weeks by 60%. But there is little evidence of a reduction in the incidence of preeclampsia with delivery at ≥37 weeks.[13,14] The updated guidelines by the American College of Obstetricians and Gynecologists (ACOG), the Society for Maternal-Fetal Medicine (SMFM), US Preventive Services Task Force (USPSTF) and the American Diabetes Association have been for low-dose aspirin (81 mg/day) prophylaxis between 12 and 28 weeks of gestation, preferably before 16 weeks in pregnant individuals at high risk of preeclampsia.[13] The detection rates in screening with use of the USPSTF recommendations were 90% and 89%, at 64.3% false-positive rates.

MATERNAL AND FETAL SURVEILLANCE[15]

The PIERS models (pre-eclampsia integrated estimate of risk scores) include a maternal assessment by components such as maternal laboratory testing, fetal ultrasonographic assessment of growth, umbilical artery Doppler, and fetal cardiotocography.

Maternal surveillance: Initial maternal evaluation involves end organ evaluation with tests such as complete blood picture with platelet count, liver function tests, renal function tests, lactate dehydrogenase, complete urine examination with urine protein, spot protein creatinine ratio, coagulation profile with prothrombin time and activated partial thromboplastin time.

Fetal evaluation: Fetuses are at increased risk of fetal growth restriction and stillbirths. Ultrasound can be performed once every 2 weeks to assess fetal growth and liquor volume. Umbilical artery Doppler and other vessel Dopplers must be done as per obstetric indications. Fetal cardiotocography (CTG) to monitor the fetal condition should be a part of the fetal surveillance once a viable gestational age is achieved.

Antihypertensive medication: The threshold for treatment of hypertension in pregnancy is a systolic blood pressure ≥140 mm Hg and/or a diastolic blood pressure ≥90 mm Hg. Treatment reduces the likelihood of developing severe maternal hypertension and other associated complications with it.[16]

Target blood pressure: Different guidelines suggest varied target blood pressure levels as shown in **Table 2**. The target blood pressure for antihypertensive treatment should be a diastolic blood pressure of 85 mm Hg.

Goal of antihypertensive medications: Control of blood pressure to minimize end-organ damage, avoid acute hypotension, avoid maternal side-effects and long-term control of blood pressure and delivery when indicated. Oral labetalol, nifedipine, and methyldopa must be considered as first-line antihypertensive agents for nonsevere hypertension. The antihypertensive medication, mechanism of action, dosage, and important considerations are mentioned in **Table 2**. Oral nifedipine, oral labetalol, intravenous labetalol, and intravenous hydralazine are considered as first-line antihypertensive agents for severe hypertension as mentioned in **Tables 3 and 4**.

ECLAMPSIA

The development of convulsion or unexplained coma in pregnancy or postpartum period in a woman with preeclampsia is called eclampsia. The spectrum of signs such as severe hypertension, severe proteinuria, and generalized

TABLE 2: Guidelines showing treatment thresholds and target blood pressure.

Guideline	Treatment threshold (mm Hg)	Treatment target (mm Hg)
ACOG, 2020	≥160/105 with a diagnosis of chronic HTN ≥160/110 if acute/chronic HTN	120–159/80–105 120–159/80–109 if chronic
WHO, 2020	Not specified	Above lower limits of normal
NICE, 2019	≥140/90	≤135/85
SOGC Canada, 2020	≥140/90	DBP- 85 <140/90 with comorbidities
International Society for Study of Hypertension in Pregnancy, 2018	≥140/90 in office ≥135/85 at home	110–140/85
European Society of Cardiology, 2018	≥150/95 ≥140/90 with end-organ damage/Gest HTN	Not specified
Society of Obstetric Medicine of Australia and New Zealand, 2014	≥160/100 ≥140/90, optional	Based on clinical assessment

(ACOG: American College of Obstetricians and Gynecologists; HTN: hypertension; NICE: National Institute for Health and Clinical Excellence; SOGC: Society of Obstetricians and Gynaecologists; WHO: World Health Organization)

TABLE 3: Oral antihypertensives in pregnancy.

Drug	Mechanism of action	Dose	Precautions	Adverse effects
Nifedipine category C	• Calcium channel blocker • Reduces peripheral vascular resistance • Uterine relaxant	30–120 mg/day of a slow-release preparation	Avoid sublingual	Headache
Labetalol category C	• Selective α1 and non-selective β receptor antagonist • Reduces afterload, reduces cardiac contractility and heart rate but maintains cardiac output	200–2,400 mg/day in two or three divided doses	Bronchial asthma	May cause fetal growth restriction if used early in pregnancy
Hydralazine category C	• Direct smooth muscle relaxant • Decreased peripheral vascular resistance • Increased cerebral and renal blood flow	50–300 mg/day in 2–4 divided doses	Use in combination with a sympatholytic agent to prevent reflex tachycardia	
Methyldopa category B	Binding to alpha (α)-2 adrenergic receptors as an agonist, leading to the inhibition of adrenergic neuronal outflow and reduction of vasoconstrictor adrenergic signals	0.5–3.0 g/day in two or three divided doses		

TABLE 4: Antihypertensive agents for urgent control of blood pressure in pregnancy.

Drug	Dosage	Onset of action	Note
Labetalol	10–20 mg IV, then 20–80 mg every 10–30 minutes to a maximum cumulative dosage of 300 mg; or constant infusion 1–2 mg/min IV	1–2 minutes	• Tachycardia is less common with fewer adverse effects. 1–2 minutes • Avoid in women with asthma, preexisting myocardial disease, decompensated cardiac function, and heart block and bradycardia
Hydralazine	5 mg IV or IM, then 5–10 mg IV every 20–40 minutes to a maximum cumulative dosage of 20 mg; or constant infusion of 0.5–10 mg/h	10–20 minutes	Higher or frequent dosages associated with maternal hypotension, headaches, and abnormal fetal heart rate tracings; may be more common than other agents
Nifedipine (immediate release)	10–20 mg orally, repeat in 20 minutes if needed; then 10–20 mg every 2–6 hours; maximum daily dose is 180 mg	5–10 minutes	May observe reflex tachycardia and headaches

edema may be present. Eclampsia can occur in the absence of hypertension, proteinuria, or edema.

Differential diagnosis: Hypertensive encephalopathy, seizure disorder, hypoglycemia, hyponatremia, thrombotic thrombocytopenic purpura, vasculitis, amniotic fluid embolism, cerebrovascular accident, hemorrhage, or thrombosis.

Maternal complications of eclampsia are: Abruption: 7–10%, Pulmonary edema: 3–5%, acute renal failure: 5–9%, aspiration pneumonia: 2–3%, and cardiopulmonary arrest: 2–5%.

Magnesium Sulfate for Prevention of Eclampsia

One important reason for the grave complications of eclampsia is delayed magnesium sulfate prophylaxis used for its prevention. The Maternal Early Warning Trigger tool has a pathway to address the four major causes of maternal morbidity and mortality—hemorrhage, sepsis, hypertension in pregnancy, and cardiovascular dysfunction.[17] The original article showed a significant reduction in eclampsia and maternal morbidity rates. The current practice as per guidelines had magnesium sulfate prophylaxis when they had imminent symptoms of eclampsia (headache, vomiting, blurring of vision, epigastric pain) or severe features which were many times subjected to the doctor's decision. One of the landmark trials, the Magpie trial has proven beyond doubt that $MgSO_4$ should be given in women with preeclampsia. Magnesium sulfate not only halves the risk of eclampsia, but it also reduces the risk of maternal death. There does not appear to be substantive harmful effects to the mother or baby in the short term.[17] The dosage for magnesium sulfate is mentioned in **Figure 1**.

The toxicity levels at different values are mentioned in **Table 5**.[18]

Timing of delivery in hypertensive disorders[4]: The timing of delivery in hypertensive disorders is based on the type of the disease and organ involvement and gestational age of

Availability: 2 mL ampules, 50% solution, 1 g MgSO$_4$

Dosage
IV loading dose
4 g, 20% solution
(Two 10 cc syringes, each with 2 ampules of MgSO$_4$, diluted to 10 cc with distilled water)
Given slowly not to exceed 1 g/min or 5 cc/min
Maintenance dose
Continuous infusion at 1 g/hour
(20 ampules of MgSO$_4$, added in 500 mL RL, 25 mL = 1 g)

Indications to stop MgSO$_4$ infusion
(Decision to be taken by the Doctor)
- Urine output <100 mL in 4 hours or <25 mL/hr for 2 consecutive hours
- Absent deep tendon reflexes
- Respiratory rate of <15/min
- 24 hours postdelivery

Magnesium levels
- Normal: <2 mEq/L
- Therapeutic levels aimed: 4–7 mEq/L
- Patellar reflexes disappear at 10 mEq/L
- Respiratory paralysis and arrest occurs at 12–15 mEq/L

Renal impairment
(S. creatinine >1.3 mg/dL)
Loading dose: Remains the same
Maintenance dose: Halved

Antidote: Calcium gluconate (1 g slow intravenously)

Fig. 1: Magnesium sulfate regime for eclampsia.

TABLE 5: Serum magnesium concentration and toxicities.[18]

	mmol/L	mEq/L	mg/dL
Therapeutic range	2–3.5	4–7	5–9
Loss of patellar reflexes	>3.5	>7	>9
Respiratory paralysis	>5	>10	>12
Cardiac arrest	>12.5	>25	>30

the fetus. Cesarean section should be limited for obstetric indications. The mode of delivery depends on gestational age, fetal condition, and other obstetric conditions.

Chronic hypertension: For women with chronic hypertension and no other comorbidities, expectant management up to 37 weeks of gestation is recommended with maternal and fetal monitoring.

Gestational hypertension and preeclampsia without severe features: For women with gestational hypertension and preeclampsia without severe features expectant management up to 37 weeks of gestation is recommended. Fetus is monitored with an ultrasound scan every 2 weeks for fetal weight and liquor. The nonstress test (NST) must be done every week. Maternal monitoring must include initial inpatient management for 48–72 hours. If the mother and fetus are stable, then outpatient basis management may be planned. The woman should be educated about premonitory symptoms of preeclampsia and asked to check her blood pressure at home once a day. Laboratory parameters must be done every week. Antenatal checkups must be scheduled every week.

Preeclampsia with severe features: For women diagnosed with preeclampsia with severe features at or beyond 34 weeks of gestation, delivery should be planned after maternal stabilization and administration of corticosteroids for fetal lung maturity.

For women diagnosed with preeclampsia with severe features before 34 weeks of gestation, expectant management is based on strict criteria and is based on resources available for maternal and neonatal care. Expectant management should not be advised when neonatal survival is not anticipated. An expectant woman must be monitored inpatient. In the hospital, blood pressure must be checked 4 hourly, premonitory symptoms should be enquired about, and laboratory parameters be repeated twice a week. Fetal monitoring must be done by NST every day and ultrasound for fetal growth and liquor every 2 weeks, while waiting with expectant management delivery is recommended at any time in case of maternal or fetal deterioration.

For women with eclampsia delivery should be expedited (irrespective of gestational age) after maternal stabilization and maternal and fetal evaluation.

The HYPITAT trial has proven that women with gestational hypertension and preeclampsia without severe features after 36 weeks of gestation induction of labor was associated with a significant reduction in a composite of adverse maternal outcome including new-onset severe preeclampsia, HELLP syndrome, eclampsia, pulmonary edema, or placental abruption.[19] The PHOENIX trial suggests delivery will reduce maternal morbidity.[20]

CONDITIONS PRECLUDING EXPECTANT MANAGEMENT (IRRESPECTIVE OF GESTATIONAL AGE)

Maternal

- Uncontrolled severe-range blood pressures (persistent systolic blood pressure 160 mm Hg or more or diastolic blood pressure 110 mm Hg or more) not responsive to antihypertensive medication.
- Persistent headaches, refractory to treatment
- Epigastric pain or right upper quadrant pain unresponsive to repeat analgesics
- Visual disturbances, motor deficit, or altered sensorium
- Stroke
- Myocardial infarction
- HELLP syndrome
- New or worsening renal dysfunction (serum creatinine >1.1 mg/dL or twice baseline)
- Pulmonary edema
- Eclampsia
- Suspected acute placental abruption or vaginal bleeding in the absence of placenta previa.

Fetal

- Abnormal fetal testing
- Fetal death
- Fetus with no expectation for survival at the time of maternal diagnosis.
- Persistent reversed end-diastolic flow in the umbilical artery.

Postpartum care: Women with preeclampsia need monitoring postdelivery because the blood pressure will start peaking 3–6 days postpartum. Antihypertensive medication that was given during the antenatal period should be continued postdelivery as long as required to maintain blood pressure and to avoid long-term cardiovascular complications. The choice of antihypertensive drugs in the postpartum period is wide. Most antihypertensive agents, including ACE inhibitors, are acceptable in breastfeeding.

Contraception: Most women, with or without hypertension, will not have an adverse effect on blood pressure from any form of contraception. Progestin-only methods, including the pill, injection, subdermal implant, and intrauterine device, are safe in women with hypertension, even if blood pressure is poorly controlled. Estrogen-containing methods, including the pill, patch, and ring, have all been shown to increase blood pressure, although the degree of increase has not been well established in the literature.

TAKE HOME MESSAGES

- All pregnant women should be screened for preeclampsia in the first trimester. The best strategy is to combine maternal risk factors, and measurement of MAP, PAPP-A, PLGF, and UTPI.
- Goal of antihypertensive therapy is to control blood pressure to minimize end-organ damage, avoid acute hypotension, avoid maternal side effects and long-term control of blood pressure, and delivery when indicated.
- Timing of delivery in hypertensive disorders is based on the type of the disease and organ involvement and gestational age of the fetus.
- Hypertension that proves increasingly difficult to control is an indication to terminate the pregnancy.
- Antihypertensive agents acceptable for use in breastfeeding are nifedipine, labetalol, methyldopa, captopril and enalapril.
- Progestin-only methods, including the pill, injection, subdermal implant, and intrauterine device, are safe in women with hypertension for contraception, even if blood pressure is poorly controlled.

■ REFERENCES

1. Steegers EA, von Dadelszen P, Duvekot JJ, Pijnenborg R. Pre-eclampsia. Lancet. 2010; 376(9741):631-44.
2. Singla A, Rajaram S, Mehta S, Radhakrishnan G. A ten year audit of maternal mortality: millennium development still a distant goal. Indian J Community Med. 2017;42(2):102-6.
3. Gestational Hypertension and Preeclampsia: ACOG Practice Bulletin, Number 222. Obstet Gynecol. 2020;135(6):e237-60.
4. Brown MA, Magee LA, Kenny LC, Karumanchi SA, McCarthy FP, Saito S, et al. The hypertensive disorders of pregnancy: ISSHP classification, diagnosis and management recommendations for international practice. Pregnancy Hypertens. 2018;13:291-310.
5. Ronsmans C, Graham WJ. Maternal mortality: who, when, where, and why. Lancet. 2006;368:1189-1200.
6. Villar K, Say L, Gulmezoglu A, Meraldi M, Lindheimer MD, Betran AP, et al. Eclampsia and pre-eclampsia: a health problem for 2000 years. In: Critchly H, MacLean A, Poston L, Walker J (Eds). Pre-eclampsia. London: RCOG Press, 2003. pp. 189-207.
7. Nobis PN, Hajong A. Eclampsia in India Through the Decades. J Obstet Gynaecol India. 2016;66(Suppl 1):172-6.
8. Poon LC, Magee LA, Verlohren S, Shennan A, von Dadelszen P, Sheiner E, et al. A literature review and best practice advice for second and third trimester risk stratification, monitoring, and management of pre-eclampsia: Compiled by the Pregnancy and Non-Communicable Diseases Committee of FIGO (the International Federation of Gynecology and Obstetrics). Int J Gynaecol Obstet. 2021;154(Suppl 1):3-31.
9. Garovic VD, Dechend R, Easterling T, Karumanchi SA, McMurtry Baird S, Magee LA, et al. Hypertension in pregnancy: diagnosis, blood pressure goals, and pharmacotherapy: a scientific statement from the American Heart Association. Hypertension. 2022;79(2):e21-41. Erratum in: Hypertension. 2022;79(3):e70.

10. Mazer Zumaeta A, Wright A, Syngelaki A, Maritsa VA, Da Silva AB, Nicolaides KH. Screening for pre-eclampsia at 11–13 weeks' gestation: use of pregnancy-associated plasma protein-A, placental growth factor or both. Ultrasound Obstet Gynecol. 2020;56(3):400-7.
11. Chappell LC, Duckworth S, Seed PT, Griffin M, Myers J, Mackillop L, et al. Diagnostic accuracy of placental growth factor in women with suspected preeclampsia: a prospective multicenter study. Circulation. 2013;128:2121-31.
12. Tan MY, Wright D, Syngelaki A, Akolekar R, Cicero S, Janga D, et al. Comparison of diagnostic accuracy of early screening for pre-eclampsia by NICE guidelines and a method combining maternal factors and biomarkers: Results of SPREE. Ultrasound Obstet Gynecol. 2018;51:743-50.
13. Rolnik DL, Wright D, Poon LCY, Syngelaki A, O'Gorman N, de Paco Matallana C, et al. ASPRE trial: performance of screening for preterm pre-eclampsia. Ultrasound Obstet Gynecol. 2017;50(4):492-5. Erratum in: Ultrasound Obstet Gynecol. 2017;50(6):807.
14. Rolnik DL, Wright D, Poon LC, O'Gorman N, Syngelaki A, de Paco Matallana C, et al. Aspirin versus placebo in pregnancies at high risk for preterm preeclampsia. N Engl J Med. 2017;377(7):613-22.
15. Magee LA, von Dadelszen P, Singer J, Lee T, Rey E, Ross S, Asztalos E, et al. The CHIPS Randomized Controlled Trial (Control of Hypertension in Pregnancy Study): Is severe hypertension just an elevated blood pressure? Hypertension. 2016;68(5):1153-9.
16. Shields LE, Wiesner S, Klein C, Pelletreau B, Hedriana HL. Use of maternal early warning trigger tool reduces maternal morbidity. Am J Obstet Gynecol. 2016;214(4):527: e1-527.e6.
17. Altman D, Carroli G, Duley L, Farrell B, Moodley J, Neilson J, et al. Do women with pre-eclampsia, and their babies, benefit from magnesium sulphate? The Magpie Trial: a randomised placebo-controlled trial. 2002;359(9321):1877-90.
18. Lu JF, Nightingale CH. Magnesium sulfate in eclampsia and pre-eclampsia: pharmacokinetic principles. Clin Pharmacokinet. 2000;38(4):305-14.
19. Koopmans CM, Bijlenga D, Groen H, Vijgen SM, Aarnoudse JG, Bekedam DJ, et al. Induction of labour versus expectant monitoring for gestational hypertension or mild pre-eclampsia after 36 weeks' gestation (HYPITAT): a multicentre, open-label randomised controlled trial. HY- PITAT study group. Lancet. 2009;374:979-88.
20. Chappell LC, Brocklehurst P, Green ME, Hunter R, Hardy P, Juszczak E, et al. Planned early delivery or expectant management for late preterm pre-eclampsia (PHOENIX): a randomised controlled trial. Lancet. 2019;394(10204):1181-90.

CHAPTER 24

Central Venous Sinus Thrombosis

Sulagna Bhattacharjee, Gaurav Mittal, Souvik Maitra

■ INTRODUCTION

Cerebral venous sinus thrombosis (CVST) is an unusual form of stroke that commonly occurs during pregnancy and puerperium. With a wide variety of clinical presentations and outcomes, the challenge lies in early diagnosis to initiate appropriate therapy and reduce mortality and long-term sequel.

■ EPIDEMIOLOGY AND MAGNITUDE OF THE PROBLEM

Overall, 75% of all CVSTs occur in women. The incidence in developed world is 11.6/100,000 deliveries per year, accounting for 6–64% of pregnancy-related strokes. In developing countries like India, the estimated incidence from hospital-based studies was higher (4.5/1,000 obstetric admissions), although the exact figure is unknown due to lack of population-based studies. It results in 9–15% overall mortality and dependency rate in pregnant patients. More than three-fourths of all cases occur during the 1–4 weeks puerperium.[1,2]

■ RISK FACTORS

The systemic and local factors that increase the risk of CVST in general population include:[3]
- *Transient like*:
  - Infection (meningitis, otitis media, head, and neck)
  - Head injury, trauma, surgery, and lumbar puncture (LP)
  - Pregnancy and puerperium
  - Dehydration
  - Drugs like oral contraceptive pills
- *Permanent like*:
  - Inflammatory disease [systemic lupus erythematosus (SLE), Behçet's, and vasculitis]
  - Malignancy
  - Hematologic conditions with pro-thrombotic states like protein C and S deficiency
  - Nephrotic syndrome
  - Congenital heart disease
  - Thyroid disorders.

The possible risk factors for CVST in pregnancy include cesarean section, anemia, traumatic delivery, dehydration, elevated homocysteine levels, and low cerebrospinal fluid (CSF) pressure due to dural puncture. However, their specific role in the disease outcome remains yet to be determined.[2]

Cerebral venous sinus thrombosis has also been reported with coronavirus disease-2019 (COVID-19) without the presence of any other risk factor.[4] It has also been found in association with vaccine-induced thrombotic thrombocytopenia among patients immunized with the adenovirus-vector ChAdOx1 nCov-19 (AstraZeneca COVID-19) and Ad26.COV2.S (Janssen COVID-19) vaccines.[5]

IMPLICATIONS FOR MATERNAL AND FETAL HEALTH

In pregnant women with a past history of CVST, the incidence of recurrent CVST and noncerebral venous thromboembolism (VTE) is higher than the general population; the incidence of spontaneous abortion was similar. History of CVST is not a contraindication for future pregnancy.[6]

PATHOGENESIS

Although the pathogenesis of CVST is incompletely understood, two principal mechanisms contribute to its development,[7] which are elucidated in **Flowchart 1**.
- Thrombosis of cortical veins leading to parenchymal lesion (stroke)
- Thrombosis of dural sinuses leading to reduced CSF absorption causing raised intracranial pressure.

CLINICAL FEATURES

Clinically, the presentation of CVST is highly variable, ranging from acute, subacute, or chronic. The most common presentation is a new onset headache or of isolated intracranial hypertension. Others include seizures, focal neurological deficits, and encephalopathy. The signs and symptoms of CVST can be broadly grouped as three syndromes:[7]
1. Isolated intracranial hypertension syndrome in about 25% of patients (headache with or without vomiting, papilledema, and visual problems).
2. Focal syndrome (focal deficits, seizures, or both).
3. Encephalopathy (multifocal signs, mental status changes, stupor, or coma).

The severity of presentation depends on age, sex, number of veins or sinuses involved, extent of parenchymal lesions, and onset of CVT to presentation.

Headache is the most common presentation occurring in up to 89% patients.[8] It occurs more commonly in females, is usually the first symptom to appear, can be localized or diffuse and is usually gradual, increasing in intensity over days.

Seizures can be generalized or focal and can present as status epilepticus. It occurs in about 39% patients[8] being a common feature in CVST among all cerebrovascular diseases.

Clinical features of other sinuses or veins involved are depicted in **Figure 1**.

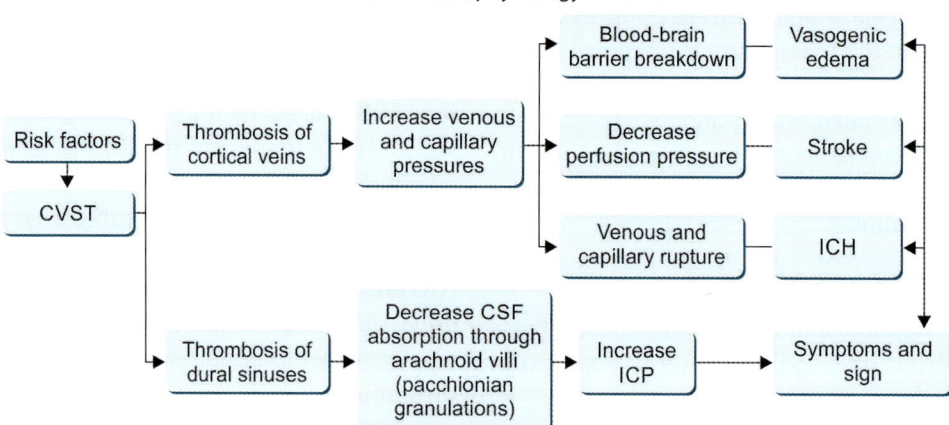

Flowchart 1: Pathophysiology of CVST.

(CSF: cerebrospinal fluid; CVST: cerebral venous sinus thrombosis; ICH: intracerebral hemorrhage; ICP: intracranial pressure)

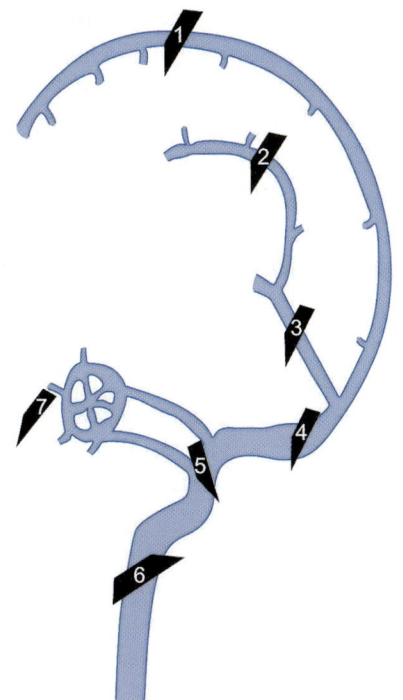

Fig. 1: Clinical features of other sinuses or veins involved.
1. Superior sagittal sinus thrombosis—motor deficits and seizures
2. Inferior sagittal sinus thrombosis—motor deficits and seizures
3. Straight sinus thrombosis—motor deficits and mental status changes
4. Transverse sinus thrombosis—raised intracranial pressure (ICP), tinnitus, aphasia, and cranial nerve palsy
5. Sigmoid sinus
6. Internal jugular vein thrombosis—neck pain, tinnitus, and cranial nerve palsy
7. Cavernous sinus thrombosis—orbital pain, chemosis, proptosis, and cranial nerve palsy

Source: Adapted from Piazza G. Cerebral venous thrombosis. Circulation. 2012;125(13):1704-9.

Cerebral venous sinus thrombosis should be suspected in the presence of:
- New-onset headache
- Headache with features that differ from the usual pattern (e.g., progression or change in attack frequency, severity, or clinical features) in patients with a previous primary headache
- Symptoms or signs of intracranial hypertension
- Encephalopathy.

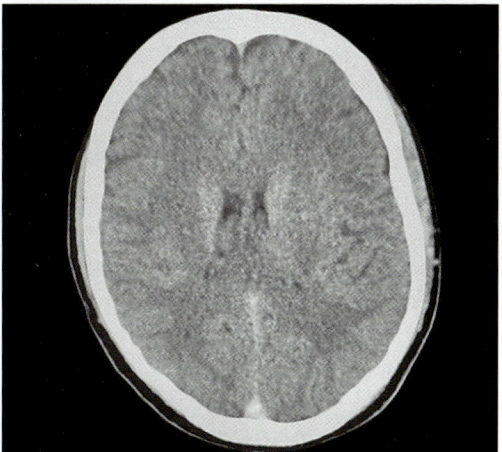

Fig. 2: Plain computed tomography brain showing hyperdensity in superior sagittal sinus suggesting thrombosis.

■ INVESTIGATIONS

Clinical suspicion of CVST warrants urgent neuroimaging. The principal modalities are discussed here.

Magnetic Resonance Imaging

Brain magnetic resonance imaging (MRI) with gradient echo T2-weighted sequences with MR venography is the most sensitive modality to detect thrombus in the occluded veins or sinuses. Depending on the age of the thrombus, the characteristic findings include:[9]
- 0 to day 5, the thrombosed sinuses isointense on T1-weighted images and hypointense on T2-weighted images (Fig. 2)
- >5 days hyperintense on both T1- and T2-weighted images
- >30 days variable pattern of signal, may appear isointense.

Parenchymal brain lesions secondary to venous occlusion, such as brain swelling, vasogenic edema, and venous infarction, are hypointense or isointense on T1-weighted and hyperintense on T2-weighted.

Magnetic Resonance Venography

It is performed using the time-of-flight (TOF) technique, can demonstrate absence of flow in the cerebral venous sinuses (**Fig. 3**). Its interpretation is confounded by normal anatomic variants such as sinus hypoplasia and asymmetric flow.

Computed Tomography Brain

Computed tomography (CT) brain can be normal in about one-third of the cases. In another third, direct signs of CVST can be appreciated (*see* **Fig. 2**).
- Cord sign—linear or curvilinear hyperdensity from a thrombosed cortical vein
- Dense triangle sign—for a thrombosed sinus on cross sectional view
- Empty delta sign—a triangular pattern of contrast enhancement surrounding a nonenhanced central region.

Indirect signs such as intense contrast enhancement of falx and tentorium, dilated transcerebral veins, small ventricles and parenchymal abnormalities like hemorrhagic (intracerebral bleed, hemorrhagic infarcts, or subarachnoid bleed) or nonhemorrhagic (infarcts and edema). These can be present in 60–70% of the patients.[9]

Computed Tomography Venography

It is useful in situations where MRI is contraindicated or unavailable. Head CT plus computed tomography venography (CTV) has an overall accuracy of 90–100% and has a sensitivity and specificity of 95% and 91%, respectively as compared to digital substraction angiography. The findings include filling defects, sinus wall enhancement, and increased collateral venous drainage. Although helpful in subacute or chronic situations, it can miss thrombosis of the deep veins.[9]

Conventional Angiography

It is reserved for situations where MRI or CT with venography is inconclusive. Sudden termination of a cortical vein followed by dilated tortuous collaterals "cork screw" veins is pathognomonic. However, the accuracy of angiography can also be limited by anatomical abnormalities.

Lumbar Puncture

Lumbar puncture can help to distinguish meningitis from isolated intracranial hypertension and to measure and decrease CSF pressure in case of threatened vision. CSF picture in CVST shows nonspecific changes such as lymphocytic pleocytosis, increased red blood cells, and protein. However, LP is not helpful in the absence of clinical suspicion of meningitis or focal neurological findings. It is contraindicated in large lesions due to the risk of herniation.[7,8]

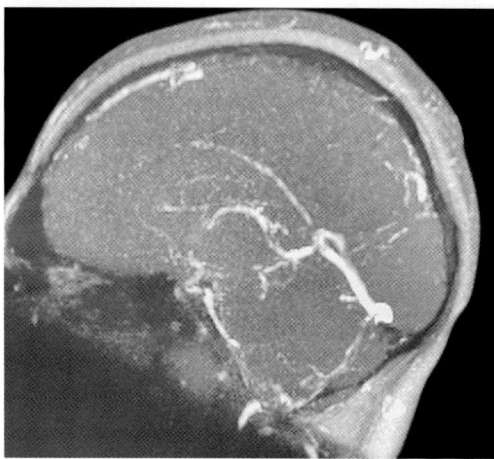

Fig. 3: Magnetic resonance venography showing absence of flow-related enhancement in superior sagittal sinus and torcula.

Laboratory Tests

Complete hemogram, serum chemistry, prothrombin time, and activated partial thromboplastin time should be done as recommended by the American Heart Association, Stroke Association guidelines.[9] In addition:

- *D-dimer*: An elevated level of D-dimer supports the diagnosis of CVST, but a normal level does not exclude it. From a meta-analysis of 14 studies, the sensitivity and specificity of D-dimer in diagnosing CVST were 89% and 83%, respectively.[10]
- Tests for thrombophilias.

Differential diagnoses are discussed in **Table 1**:[11]

- Posterior reversible encephalopathy syndrome
- Preeclampsia/eclampsia
- Reversible cerebral vasoconstriction syndrome (RCVS)
- Hypercoagulable states.

TABLE 1: Differential diagnoses

Clinical features	PRES	RCVS	CVST	Eclampsia
Mode of onset	Rapid, postpartum	Abrupt, postpartum	Third trimester or later, usually gradual	Antepartum, intrapartum, or postpartum
Key findings	Seizures may be associated with stupor, visual loss, or hallucination. The headache is usually dull and throbbing	Thunderclap headache. Seizures are less common, and transient focal deficits	Headache is universal, progressive, and diffuse. 40% cases of seizures	Seizures, frequent visual symptoms, abdominal pain, hyperreflexia, hypertension, and proteinuria
Evolution over time	If BP is controlled, it resolves within the short period	Changes over time, second week—ICH, third week—ischemic complications	Evolve over several days, nonarterial territorial infarcts and hemorrhages might develop	Can evolve (from preeclampsia) gradually or abruptly
CSF findings	Usually, normal	Often normal, 50% of cases have pleocytosis and raised proteins	Pressure raised in 80%, 30–50% have increased proteins and cell counts	Usually normal unless complicated by hemorrhage
Imaging	CT positive 50%, MRI shows prominent T2-weighted and FLAIR abnormalities nearly always in parieto-occipital lobes but can involve other brain regions; ICH in 15%	CT usually normal (if no SAH); 20% show localized convexal SAH on MRI, CT angiogram, and MR angiogram show typical string of beads arteries, DSA cervical artery dissection	CT is often negative, and MRI might show nonarterial. Territorial infarcts; hemorrhages common; MRV shows intraluminal clot flow voids. Although MRV is preferred, CT venogram is also sensitive	Same as PRES, some patients have a coincident acute ischemic stroke or ICH

(BP: blood pressure; CSF: cerebrospinal fluid; CT: computed tomography; CVST: cerebral venous sinus thrombosis; DSA: digital subtraction angiography; FLAIR: fluid-attenuated inversion recovery; ICH: intracerebral hemorrhage; MRV: magnetic resonance venography; PRES: posterior reversible encephalopathy syndrome; RCVS: reversible cerebral vasoconstriction syndrome; SAH: subarachnoid hemorrhage)

MANAGEMENT

The goals of management include:
- To promote recanalization of the occluded veins and to prevent progression of the thrombus
- To treat associated complications
- To treat underlying prothrombotic states to prevent thrombosis of other sites
- To prevent future recurrence.

Initial Anticoagulation

Low-molecular-weight heparin (LMWH) or intravenous unfractionated heparin (UFH) should be used at therapeutic doses for initial anticoagulation, even in patients with hemorrhagic complications, in the absence of any contraindications. LMWH does not cross the placenta and has a good safety profile. The advantages of UFH include a short half-life, therapeutic monitoring with activated partial thromboplastin time (aPTT), and presence of antagonist agent protamine. However, UFH can cross placenta, and can be associated with increased risk of fetal bleeding and teratogenicity. Limited evidence suggests that LMWH is superior to UFH in terms of efficacy. The 2017 European Stroke Organization guidelines recommend LMWH over UFH.[9,12]

Endovascular Treatment

It is indicated in progressive neurological worsening despite adequate anticoagulation, in centers experienced with these mechanisms. A meta-analysis involving 185 patients from 42 studies with CVST receiving mechanical thrombectomy (using AngioJet, balloon angioplasty, rheolytic catheter, stents and microsnare) has shown a good outcome in 84% patients, with mortality of 12%.[7,13]

Supportive Therapies[9]

- Increased intracranial pressure should be treated urgently. In patients with increased intracranial pressure, progressive visual loss should be monitored. In case of severe mass effect due to intracranial hypertension or hemorrhage, decompressive craniectomy may be considered.
- Antiseizure medication should be considered in patients with seizure and supratentorial parenchymal lesions, to prevent the development of early seizures. Valproate or levetiracetam is preferred to phenytoin so as to avoid pharmacological interactions with warfarin.
- In case of CVST with suspected bacterial infection, appropriate antibiotics should be started. Surgical intervention required for any source of infection should be done.
- Steroids should not be used even in the presence of parenchymal lesions.
- Admission to a stroke unit is reasonable for optimum management of such cases.

Management Postacute Phase

Long-term Anticoagulation[9,14]

For pregnancy-related CVST, anticoagulation with LMWH should be continued throughout pregnancy and till 6 weeks postpartum with LMWH or vitamin K antagonist like warfarin. Although, results from trials regarding newer oral anticoagulants (dabigatran and rivaroxaban) are promising, equally efficacious, and safe, their safety profile has not been studied in pregnancy. The current consensus is not to use novel oral anticoagulants (NOACs) in the acute phase of CVST and pregnancy.

Duration of anticoagulation therapy should be stratified according to prothrombotic risk. Anticoagulation should be continued for a minimum total duration of 6 months in case of transient risk factors. In case of unprovoked CVST, anticoagulation for 6–12 months is recommended. In the presence of severe thrombophilias, anticoagulation may be continued indefinitely. Future pregnancies in CVST are not contraindicated. It is reasonable to advise prophylactic anticoagulation during pregnancy with a history of CVST.

Other clinical features like headache may be persistent with recurrent CVST or sinus stenosis due to occlusion. Visual impairment is a rare event. Approximately, 50% of the patients suffer from cognitive and psychiatric problems such as depression, anxiety, and language deficits.

Algorithm for the management of CVST is summarized in **Flowchart 2**.

■ PROGNOSIS

From the International Study on Cerebral Vein and Dural Sinus Thrombosis (ISCVT) study, the predictors of mortality at 30 days include:[8]

- Depressed consciousness
- Altered mental status
- Thrombosis of the deep venous system
- Right hemisphere hemorrhage
- Posterior fossa lesions.

Flowchart 2: Algorithm for management of CVST.

```
Clinical suspicion of CVST
            ↓
MRI T2WI + MRV
CT brain/CTV if MRI unavailable  →  Consider other differentials
            ↓
    CVST confirmed
            ↓
Anticoagulation (LMWH/UFH)
       ↓              ↓
Neurological     Neurological deterioration
improvement/     despite anticoagulation
stable              ↓          ↓
   ↓          Severe mass    No/mild
Continue      effect/ICH     mass effect
anticoagulation    ↓             ↓
according to   May consider   May consider
etiology       decompressive  endovascular
               craniectomy    therapy
```

(CTV: computed tomography venography; CVST: cerebral venous sinus thrombosis; ICH: intracerebral hemorrhage; LMWH: low-molecular-weight heparin; MRV: magnetic resonance venography; UFH: unfractionated heparin)

Source: Adapted from Saposnik G, Barinagarrementeria F, Brown RD Jr, Bushnell CD, Cucchiara B, Cushman M, et al. Diagnosis and management of cerebral venous thrombosis: a statement for healthcare professionals from the American Heart Association/American Stroke Association. Stroke. 2011;42(4):1158-92.

The most common cause of death was due to transtentorial herniation due to a unilateral focal mass effect or diffuse brain edema and multiple parenchymal lesions.[8]

Predictors of poor long-term prognosis in CVST are as follows:[8]
- Central nervous system infection
- Any malignancy
- Thrombosis of the deep venous system
- Hemorrhage on head CT or MRI
- Glasgow Coma Scale score <9 on admission
- Mental status abnormality
- Age >37 years
- Male sex.

A cerebral venous thrombosis risk score was devised from the ISCVT cohort to assess the functional outcome of patients with CVST at 6 months:[15]
- Presence of malignancy—2 points
- Coma on admission—2 points
- Thrombosis involving the deep venous system—2 points
- Mental status disturbance on admission—1 point
- Male sex—1 point
- Intracranial hemorrhage on admission—1 point.

A CVST risk score ≥3 was associated with a poor outcome, defined as a modified Rankin Scale score of >2 (dependency or death), with a high sensitivity but poor specificity (96 and 14%, respectively). Complete recovery was significantly more in females.

RECURRENCE

The risk of recurrent CVST is about 2–4%, while the risk of recurrent VTE in other locations after CVST ranges from 4 to 7%.[7]

RECANALIZATION

Recanalization happens during the first few months after anticoagulation, and can take up to 1 year. Recanalization is achieved in up to 85% patients on follow-up imaging, with about 49% patients achieving complete recanalization,[16] and is associated with good functional recovery. Follow-up imaging is recommended to assess recanalization at 3–6 months.[14]

CONCLUSION

Central venous sinus thrombosis is a life-threatening neurological complication in pregnant and parturient women. Early diagnosis by MRI, and prompt management with therapeutic anticoagulation, along with supportive therapy, in an intensive care unit, with multidisciplinary collaboration, usually leads to an excellent outcome.

REFERENCES

1. Roeder HJ, Lopez JR, Miller EC. Ischemic stroke and cerebral venous sinus thrombosis in pregnancy. Handb Clin Neurol. 2020; 172:3-31.
2. Liang ZW, Gao WL, Feng LM. Clinical characteristics and prognosis of cerebral venous thrombosis in Chinese women during pregnancy and puerperium. Sci Rep. 2017;7:43866.
3. Dash D, Prasad K, Joseph L. Cerebral venous thrombosis: An Indian perspective. Neurol India. 2015;63(3):318-28.
4. Baldini T, Asioli GM, Romoli M, Dias MC, Schulte EC, Hauer L, et al. Cerebral venous thrombosis and severe acute respiratory syndrome coronavirus-2 infection: A systematic review and meta-analysis. Eur J Neurol. 2021;28:3478-90.
5. Perry RJ, Tamborska A, Singh B, Craven B, Marigold R, Arthur-Farraj P, et al. Cerebral venous thrombosis after vaccination against COVID-19 in the UK: a multicentre cohort study. Lancet. 2021;398:1147-56.
6. Aguiar de Sousa D, Canhão P, Crassard I, Coutinho J, Arauz A, Conforto A, et al. Safety of Pregnancy after Cerebral

Venous Thrombosis: Results of the ISCVT (International Study on Cerebral Vein and Dural Sinus Thrombosis)-2 PREGNANCY Study. Stroke. 2017;48(11):3130-3.
7. Ferro JM. (2022). Cerebral Venous Thrombosis: Etiology, Clinical Features and Diagnosis. [online] Available from: https://www.uptodate.com/contents/cerebral-venous-thrombosis-etiology-clinical-features-and-diagnosis#H3. [Last accessed February, 2023].
8. Ferro JM, Canhão P, Stam J, Bousser MG, Barinagarrementeria F; ISCVT Investigators. Prognosis of cerebral vein and dural sinus thrombosis: results of the International Study on Cerebral Vein and Dural Sinus Thrombosis (ISCVT). Stroke. 2004;35(3):664-70.
9. Saposnik G, Barinagarrementeria F, Brown RD Jr, Bushnell CD, Cucchiara B, Cushman M, et al. Diagnosis and management of cerebral venous thrombosis: a statement for healthcare professionals from the American Heart Association/American Stroke Association. Stroke. 2011;42(4):1158-92.
10. Dentali F, Squizzato A, Marchesi C, Bonzini M, Ferro JM, Ageno W. D-dimer testing in the diagnosis of cerebral vein thrombosis: a systematic review and a meta-analysis of the literature. J Thromb Haemost. 2012; 10(4):582-9.
11. Edlow JA, Caplan LR, O'Brien K, Tibbles CD. Diagnosis of acute neurological emergencies in pregnant and post-partum women. Lancet Neurol. 2013;12(2):175-85.
12. Ferro JM, Bousser MG, Canhão P, Coutinho JM, Crassard I, Dentali F, et al. European Stroke Organization guideline for the diagnosis and treatment of cerebral venous thrombosis—Endorsed by the European Academy of Neurology. Eur Stroke J. 2017;2(3):195-221.
13. Siddiqui FM, Dandapat S, Banerjee C, Zuurbier SM, Johnson M, Stam J, et al. Mechanical thrombectomy in cerebral venous thrombosis: systematic review of 185 cases. Stroke. 2015;46(5):1263-8.
14. Piazza G. Cerebral venous thrombosis. Circulation. 2012;125(13):1704-9.
15. Ferro JM, Bacelar-Nicolau H, Rodrigues T, Bacelar-Nicolau L, Canhão P, Crassard I, et al. Risk score to predict the outcome of patients with cerebral vein and dural sinus thrombosis. Cerebrovasc Dis. 2009;28(1):39-44.
16. Aguiar de Sousa D, Lucas Neto L, Canhão P, Ferro JM. Recanalization in Cerebral Venous Thrombosis. Stroke. 2018;49(8):1828-35.

Rheumatological Disorders

CHAPTER 25

Systemic Lupus Erythematosus Flare during Pregnancy

Ritu Singh, Suruchi Ambasta, Sanjeev Kumar

■ INTRODUCTION

Systemic lupus erythematosus (SLE) is a chronic and autoimmune disease that involves multiple organs and is characterized by inflammation affecting the skin, joints, kidneys, serous membranes, and central nervous system (CNS). It predominantly affects women of reproductive age and may have serious manifestations due to hormonal fluctuations during pregnancy. Its clinical course comprises disease flares followed by variable periods of remission.[1] Advances in medical care have led to an increased number of obstetric SLE patients with improved outcomes in pregnancy. Nonetheless, SLE pregnancy is still considered a high-risk pregnancy requiring a multidisciplinary approach, with close monitoring for an uneventful outcome.[2,3]

Adverse maternal and fetal outcomes associated with pregnancy in a woman with SLE prompted physicians to advise patients with SLE not to plan conception. However, with the present understanding of the disease course, better prevention and management of the existing complications have been achieved. The frequency of pregnancy loss in SLE has dropped over the last 40 years from levels as high as 43% in 1960–1965 to 17% in 2000–2003.[4]

Though the majority of SLE patients have favorable outcomes during pregnancy; however, there is an increased incidence and established risks of flares, and complications such as preeclampsia, fetal loss, intrauterine growth retardation, and preterm birth. Active lupus nephritis, if present during conception, is the leading factor for disease flares and adverse obstetric outcomes.

A quiescent disease state of at least 6 months prior to the pregnancy leads to the best prognosis in both mother and child. Disease flares during SLE pregnancy pose challenges with respect to distinguishing physiologic changes of pregnancy from disease-related manifestations. Thus, a multidisciplinary approach with close medical, obstetric, and neonatal monitoring is necessary to optimize both maternal and fetal outcomes.

▌ EPIDEMIOLOGY AND MAGNITUDE OF THE PROBLEM

Epidemiologically, SLE prevalence in India is approximately 3.2 per 100,000 of the population.[5] 80% of patients comprise females. The mean age of disease onset in women is approximately 30, whereas in men it is 40 years of age.

Problem Statement

Pregnancy in an SLE patient is considered high risk. A recent US study of 16.7 million pregnancies, comprising 13,555 lupus patients showed a 20-fold increase in maternal mortality and increased risks for maternal morbidity, including cesarean sections [odds ratio (OR): 1.7], preterm labor (OR: 2.4), and preeclampsia (OR: 3.0).

Disease flares are common during lupus pregnancies ranging from 13.5 to 65%. SLE patients have a very high risk of relapse with almost double incidences during pregnancy. These flares frequently involve the renal, musculoskeletal, and hematological systems. Rates of occurrence of a moderate-to-severe flare are between 15 and 30%.[6]

Lupus flares during pregnancy and most commonly affect the skin, joints, renal, and hematological systems. Joint flares are less common as compared to nonpregnant counterparts while renal and hematological flares have an increased frequency. About 15–30% of patients with flare have severe manifestations, with renal and many other internal organs involved.[3,6]

Signs and symptoms of lupus flare are very similar to normal pregnancy thus differentiation becomes difficult **(Table 1)**.

Pregnancy in SLE can have an unfavorable course due to immunological, neuroendocrinological, and clinical factors.

Immunological

Preterm birth and fetal demise may occur in SLE patients with low complement or positive anti-double-stranded deoxyribonucleic acid (dsDNA) in the second trimester. Immunological factors leading to complications include autoantibodies, antiphospholipid (aPL) antibodies, such as lupus anticoagulant (LAC), Th1, and Th2 cytokines, chemokines, soluble cytokine receptors, and soluble glycoproteins.[3]

Neuroendocrine

Hormones such as estrogen and prolactin mainly interact with the immune system to multiply the inflammatory effect leading to relapses. Estrogens, progesterone, testosterone, and dehydroepiandrosterone (DHEA) serum levels are high during the second

TABLE 1: Differences between lupus flare and mimics of normal pregnancy.

	Flares of lupus	*Normal pregnancy*
Clinical		
Joints/synovium	Inflammatory arthritis	Arthralgia
Pleura	Pleuritis	Edema of hands, legs, and face
Pericardium	Pericarditis	Mild dyspnea
Laboratory		
Erythrocyte sedimentation rate (ESR)	Increased	Increased
Anemia	Present	Present and dilutional
Thrombocytopenia	Present <1 lakh	Mild
Urine analysis	Hematuria or casts	Rare due to vaginal contamination
Proteinuria	>300 mg/dL	<300 mg/dL
dsDNA antibodies	Rising	Negative
Complement levels	Decrease	Normally increased

(dsDNA: double-stranded deoxyribonucleic acid)

trimester increasing the incidences of SLE flares.

Clinical

Though the clinical risk factors have not been completely elucidated, the following may contribute to relapses such as any disease activity within 6 months prior to conception, frequent disease exacerbations before conception, irregular treatment and follow-up during pregnancy, and associated comorbidities.

IMPLICATIONS FOR MATERNAL HEALTH

Preterm Birth

One-third of lupus patients may have preterm birth which constitutes a major problem and the most common complication.[4,7] Increased disease activity (marked by increasing dsDNA titers and low complements), high prednisone use (may lead to premature rupture of membranes), and comorbidities such as hypertension and thyroid may all contribute to preterm delivery. Preterm birth may also be associated with elevated serum uric acid as per a recent study.[6]

Preeclampsia

Higher rates of obstetric and fetal complications such as preeclampsia, pregnancy losses, and intrauterine growth retardation are seen in lupus as compared to the general population. Preeclampsia incidence increases two to three times in these patients as compared to the normal maternal population. Preeclampsia may be due to lupus nephritis-specific disease markers, the presence of aPL antibodies, thrombocytopenia, and reduced complement levels. Advanced maternal age, preexisting hypertension, diabetes, and obesity may also contribute as predisposing factors.[8,9]

The most challenging clinical conundrum is to differentiate SLE flare from the common maternal complication, i.e., preeclampsia. 20% of lupus pregnancies are may have preeclampsia. Treatment for preeclampsia is immediate delivery whereas immunosuppression is the key to management in a lupus flare. Hypertension, proteinuria, and thrombocytopenia are common in both conditions but urinalysis in preeclampsia rarely reveals active sediment than in SLE flare. Elevated liver function tests (LFTs) are more suggestive of preeclampsia. In lupus flares, leukopenia, lower complement levels, and uric acid are seen as compared to preeclampsia.[10] Preeclampsia and active lupus nephritis may be difficult to differentiate as similar symptoms such as proteinuria, hypertension, pedal edema, compromised renal status, and thrombocytopenia may be present. Both conditions may even coexist together. The American College of Obstetricians and Gynecologists has established guidelines for the diagnosis of superimposed preeclampsia. It includes new-onset proteinuria in a hypertensive woman before 20 weeks of gestation, a sudden increase in existing proteinuria, a sudden increase in hypertension, or the development of HELLP syndrome.

PREGNANCY LOSS AND ANTIPHOSPHOLIPID ANTIBODIES

Almost 25–50% of SLE patients may have aPL antibodies. It increases the risk of adverse pregnancy outcomes such as intrauterine growth retardation and preterm births.[11] The probable pathophysiology is thrombosis in uterine vasculature and binding of antibodies to trophoblasts, endothelial, and neuronal cells.[11,12]

IMPLICATIONS FOR FETAL WELL-BEING

Fetal Loss

Previously, fetal loss in SLE pregnancies was as high as 43% which has come down to 17% as per a study in 2002.[4] SLE pregnancies end in fetal death almost double the time as compared to non-SLE pregnancies. Risk factors include the presence of aPL antibodies, lupus nephritis, renal insufficiency, and increased lupus activity before 6 months or during conception.

Fetal Complications

Systemic lupus erythematosus pregnancies are prone to preterm delivery, particularly in patients with lupus nephritis and hypertension. Intrauterine growth restriction is seen in patients with hypertension, Raynaud's, and disease flares. A study conducted in Taiwan reported higher rates of intrauterine growth restriction, preterm birth, and stillbirth.[13] Similarly, an Italian group reported a higher risk of preterm delivery and a small for gestational-aged infants in their SLE cohort.[14]

Neonatal Lupus

Neonatal lupus (NL) can occur in 10% of babies delivered to SLE patients with anti-Ro/SSA and anti-La/SSB antibodies. It may present with cutaneous or cardiac manifestations. Cutaneous NL presents with photosensitive rash and elevated liver function tests which normalizes within 6 months of life. In 1–2% of fetuses of mothers with anti-Ro and anti-La antibodies, congenital complete heart block (CCHB) can occur. If there is a history of a previous child with CCHB then the incidence increases to 17%. Complete heart block is the most dangerous and fatal complication of NL leading to fetal mortality in 20% of the cases.

70% of the survivors require pacemaker insertion.[15]

MANAGEMENT

A well-planned approach is the key to minimizing the effects of SLE flares during pregnancy. The American College of Rheumatology (ACR) laid the road map in 2020 to improve maternal and fetal outcomes.[16] A multidisciplinary approach is desirable to execute this road map.

Prepregnancy Planning

For a better disease control, pregnancy needs to be planned and optimized for better outcomes. Pregnancy is absolutely contraindicated in SLE when it is associated with end-organ damages such as cardiomyopathy, severe pulmonary hypertension, renal insufficiency, and catastrophic aPL syndrome.

For others a proper preconceptual counseling has to be done before proceeding for pregnancy. A holistic counseling before conception reduces risk of unnecessary disease worsening, exposure to teratogenic disease modifying drugs and adverse pregnancy outcomes. For those who not wanting pregnancy proper contraceptive advice should be taken with respect to its diseases status.

Preconceptual Risk Assessment

In patients planning for pregnancy a complete remission or low lupus disease activity state (LLDAS) is the goal before pregnancy is attempted.[17] A minimum of 6 months of low activity or remission is required before pregnancy is planned. Women with SLE should be tested for the presence of anti-Ro/SSA, anti-La/SSB, and aPL antibodies and LAC. The risk to the fetus is higher in women who have moderate and high titers of aPL antibodies in combination with the LAC.[18,19]

TREATMENT APPROACH AND MEDICATION

Pregnancy with lupus flare-ups is a high-risk pregnancy and a multidisciplinary team consisting of a rheumatologist, obstetrician, nephrologists, and pediatric cardiologist should be there. Early recognition by regular assessment and differentiating physiological changes from SLE flare-ups is an important key. **Table 2** summarizes the important monitoring parameters and its necessary management plan.

Apart from these, medication management for lupus also poses certain maternal

TABLE 2: Pregnancy management.

Time frame	Monitoring parameters	Management
Preconception	• SLE clinical assessments scoring • Routine laboratory tests in plus disease specific anti-Ro/SSA, anti-La/SSB, antiphospholipid antibodies, and lupus anticoagulant	• Switch to pregnancy compatible medications • At least 6 months of remission should be ensured before conception • Start on or continue with HCQ as per dosing in SLE
First trimester	• Regular clinical checkups with early pick up of hypertension and SLE flares • Ultrasound to review fetal anomalies and establish gestational age • *Laboratory parameters:* Complete blood count (CBC), comprehensive metabolic profile (CMP), urinalysis and morning urine protein to creatinine ratio (UPCR), anti-double-stranded DNA (dsDNA) antibodies, complement levels (CH50, or C3 and C4), and serum uric acid	• To start aspirin (81 mg/day) early • Early consultation with obstetrician start prophylactic heparin • Patients with evidence of thrombosis should start full dose heparin • For SLE flare-ups early medications like HCQ should be started • Compliance of medication should be monitored
Second trimester	• Regular clinical assessment • Laboratory investigation for early pick up of gestational diabetes • Genetic screening • Fetal ECHO/USG to assess to evaluate fetal anatomy and to assess fetal growth and placental insufficiency	• Compliance of medication should be monitored • In fetuses with evidence for first- or second-degree heart block, oral dexamethasone 4 mg daily can be started and adjusted according to response • Avoid NSAIDs at 20 weeks and later
Third trimester	• Regular clinical assessment • *Laboratory parameters:* CBC, CMP, urinalysis and morning UPCR, anti-dsDNA antibodies, complement levels (CH50, or C3 and C4), and serum uric acid • Ultrasound examination regularly to evaluate fetal growth, adequacy of amniotic fluid and placental insufficiency	• Compliance of medication should be monitored • Preparation for delivery

Contd...

Contd...

Time frame	Monitoring parameters	Management
Postpartum and lactation	• Regular clinical checkups with early pick up of hypertension and SLE flares • Regular laboratory follow-ups	• Switch to lactation-compatible medications if breastfeeding is desired • Those patients who are on prednisone ≥20 mg/day should avoid breastfeeding at least 4 hours after dosing

(ECHO: echocardiogram; dsDNA: double-stranded deoxyribonucleic acid; HCQ: hydroxychloroquine; NSAIDs: nonsteroidal anti-inflammatory drugs; SLE: systemic lupus erythematosus; USG: ultrasonography)

and fetal risks. All patients with SLE should continue hydroxychloroquine during pregnancy, as fewer side effects are associated with its use.[19-22] During first trimester, it is recommended to use aspirin therapy (81 mg/day) in primigravida patients with hypertension, prior renal disease, presence of aPL antibodies, and older patients who are at risk of developing preeclampsia.[23] Immunosuppressive drugs such as sulfasalazine, cyclosporine, azathioprine, and tacrolimus are compatible with pregnancy.[23,24] Biologic drugs such as rituximab and belimumab can continue through conception but less supported with evidence.[23,24] Steroids are also a good option for managing flare but should be used cautiously, especially due to dysglycemia.[24]

Most of the drugs are safe during pregnancy; however, certain drugs should be avoided during lactation. Leflunomide, methotrexate, mycophenolate mofetil, and voclosporin should be stopped prior to pregnancy and avoided in lactating women.[25]

■ CONCLUSION

Pregnancy in women with SLE is a high-risk condition, which carries significantly high maternal and fetal morbidity and mortality. Disease should be well controlled for at least 6 months in patients planning pregnancy as disease activity usually worsens during pregnancy. Early recognition of clinical features suggestive of disease flare-ups is challenging as it is fraught with difficulties such as overlapping features, lack of specific diagnostic markers, and drug toxicities. Increased fetal loss, preterm births, and intrauterine growth restrictions are major concerns of fetal outcome. The key to management lies in multidisciplinary care with close monitoring. Early detection of threats to maternal and fetal well-being, with judicious use of appropriate medications, helps to achieve a positive outcome.

■ REFERENCES

1. Stojan G, Baer AN. Flares of systemic lupus erythematosus during pregnancy and the puerperium: prevention, diagnosis and management. Expert Rev Clin Immunol. 2012;8(5):439-53.
2. Lateef A, Petri M. Managing lupus patients during pregnancy. Best Pract Res Clin Rheumatol. 2013;27:435-47.
3. Jara LJ, Medina G, Navarro C, Saavedra MA, Blanco-Favela F, Espinoza LR. Pregnancy, hormones, and autoimmune rheumatic diseases. In: Walker S, Jara LJ (Eds). Endocrine Manifestations of Systemic Autoimmune Diseases. Amsterdam: Elsevier; 2008. pp. 185-98.
4. Clark CA, Spitzer KA, Laskin CA. Decrease in pregnancy loss rates in patients with systemic lupus erythematosus over a 40-year period. J Rheumatol. 2005;32(9):1709-12.

5. Malaviya AN, Singh RR, Singh YN, Kapoor SK, Kumar A. Prevalence of systemic lupus erythematosus in India. Lupus. 1993;2(2):115-8.
6. Clowse ME, Wallace DJ, Weisman M, James A, Criscione-Schreiber LG, Pisetsky DS. Predictors of preterm birth in patients with mild systemic lupus erythematosus. Ann Rheum Dis. 2013;72(9):1536-9.
7. Yan Yuen S, Krizova A, Ouimet JM, Pope JE. Pregnancy outcome in systemic lupus erythematosus (SLE) is improving: results from a case control study and literature review. Open Rheumatol J. 2008;2:89-98.
8. Hutcheon JA, Lisonkova S, Joseph KS. Epidemiology of preeclampsia and the other hypertensive disorders of pregnancy. Best Pract Res Clin Obstet Gynaecol. 2011;25(4):391-403.
9. Chakravarty EF, Colon I, Langen ES, Nix DA, El-Sayed YY, Genovese MC, et al. Factors that predict prematurity and preeclampsia in pregnancies that are complicated by systemic lupus erythematosus. Am J Obstet Gynecol. 2005;192(6):1897-904.
10. Bellos I, Pergialiotis V, Loutradis D, Daskalakis G. The prognostic role of serum uric acid levels in preeclampsia: a meta-analysis. J Clin Hypertens. 2020;22(5):826-34.
11. Gomez-Puerta JA, Cervera R. Diagnosis and classification of the antiphospholipid syndrome. J Autoimmun. 2014;48-49:20-5.
12. Levy RA, Dos Santos FC, de Jesus GR, de Jesús NR. Antiphospholipid antibodies and antiphospholipid syndrome during pregnancy: diagnostic concepts. Front Immunol. 2015;7(6):205.
13. Chen YJ, Chang JC, Lai EL, Liao TL, Chen HH, Hung WT, et al. Maternal and perinatal outcomes of pregnancies in systemic lupus erythematosus: a nationwide population-based study. Semin Arthritis Rheum. 2020;50(3):451-7.
14. Moroni G, Doria A, Giglio E, Tani C, Zen M, Strigini F, et al. Fetal outcome and recommendations of pregnancies in lupus nephritis in the 21st century. A prospective multicenter study. J Autoimmun. 2016;74:6-12.
15. Brito-Zerón P, Izmirly PM, Ramos-Casals M, Buyon JP, Khamashta MA. The clinical spectrum of autoimmune congenital heart block. Nat Rev Rheumatol. 2015;11(5):301-12.
16. Sammaritano LR, Bermas BL, Chakravarty EE, Chambers C, Clowse MEB, Lockshin MD, et al. 2020 American College of Rheumatology Guideline for the management of reproductive health in rheumatic and musculoskeletal diseases. Arthritis Rheumatol. 2020;72(4):529-56.
17. Dao KH, Bermas BL. Systemic Lupus Erythematosus Management in Pregnancy. Int J Womens Health. 2022;14:199-211.
18. Yelnik CM, Porter TF, Branch DW, Laskin CA, Merrill JT, Guerra MM, et al. Brief report: changes in antiphospholipid antibody titers during pregnancy: effects on pregnancy outcomes. Arthritis Rheumatol. 2016;68(8):1964-9.
19. Allen D, Hunter MS, Wood S, Beeson T. One key question®: first things first in reproductive health. Matern Child Health J. 2017;21(3):387-92.
20. Motta M, Tincani A, Faden D, Zinzini E, Lojacono A, Marchesi A, et al. Follow-up of infants exposed to hydroxychloroquine given to mothers during pregnancy and lactation. J Perinatol. 2005;25(2):86-9.
21. Friedman DM, Kim M, Costedoat-Chalumeau N, Clancy R, Copel J, Phoon CK, et al. Electrocardiographic QT intervals in infants exposed to hydroxychloroquine throughout gestation. Circ Arrhythmia Electrophysiol. 2020;13(10):e008686.
22. Huybrechts KF, Bateman BT, Zhu Y, Straub L, Mogun H, Kim SC, et al. Hydroxychloroquine early in pregnancy and risk of birth defects. Am J Obstet Gynecol. 2021;224(3):290.e1-290.e22.
23. Davidov D, Sheiner E, Wainstock T, Miodownik S, Pariente G. Maternal systemic lupus erythematosus (SLE) high risk for preterm delivery and not for long-term neurological morbidity of the offspring. J Clin Med. 2021;10(13):2952.
24. Butte NF. Carbohydrate and lipid metabolism in pregnancy: normal compared with gestational diabetes mellitus. Am J Clin Nutr. 2000;71(5 Suppl):1256S-61S.
25. Kim M, Rostas S, Gabardi S. Mycophenolate fetal toxicity and risk evaluation and mitigation strategies. Am J Transplant. 2013;13(6):1383-9.

CHAPTER 26

Catastrophic Antiphospholipid Antibodies Syndrome

Hetal Patolia, Shweta Bhatt Dave

INTRODUCTION

Catastrophic antiphospholipid syndrome (CAPS) is a life-threatening disease caused by the onset of rapidly progressive and widespread small vessel thrombosis in the presence of the antiphospholipid syndrome resulting in multi-organ failure. This accelerated form of antiphospholipid syndrome (APS) is rare but life-threatening with detrimental outcome for mother and fetus. Pregnancy and puerperium with its hypercoagulable stat can trigger CAPS in APS positive patients.

It is also called Asherson's syndrome after Robert Asherson who first described it in 1992. Diagnostic criteria for CAPS were proposed at 10th International Congress on APL in Sicily, Italy in 2002, which were validated and accepted in 2005.[1]

Criteria for CAPS include multiple small vessel thrombosis within 1 week time period involving at least three organs or tissue or system which is confirmed by histopathology and presence of antiphospholipid (APL) antibodies in blood test in at least one occasion. Patient having all four criteria termed as definite CAPL and patient having few but not all four criteria termed as probable CAPS showed here.

PRELIMINARY CRITERIA FOR CLASSIFICATION OF CATASTROPHIC ANTIPHOSPHOLIPID SYNDROME[2]

1. Evidence of involvement of three or more organs, systems and/or tissues.
2. Development of manifestations simultaneously or in less than a week.
3. Confirmation by histopathology of small vessel occlusion in at least one organ or tissue.
4. Laboratory confirmation of the presence of antiphospholipid antibodies (lupus anticoagulant and/or anticardiolipin antibodies).

Definite CAPS[2]

Abovementioned all four criteria.

Probable CAPS[2]

- All four criteria except for only two organs, systems, or tissue involvement.
- All four criteria except for the absence of laboratory confirmation at least 6 weeks apart due to death of patient in previously never tested for APL.
- Criteria 1, 2, and 4.
- Criteria 1, 3, and 4 and development of third event in >1 week but <1 month, despite anticoagulation.

This criterion has sensitivity of 90.3% and specificity of 99.4% in the diagnosis of CAPS. However, these criteria should be used for classification purpose and not as guideline for diagnosis.

The CAPS task force was developed at 13th International Congress at Texas, USA in 2010 to address the challenges in diagnosis and management of CAPS. As CAPS is a very rare disorder international registry was created by European forum on diagnosis of CAPS. The data from all over the world is pooled for evaluation. It can be freely assessed through the internet.

EPIDEMIOLOGY AND MAGNITUDE OF PROBLEM

Catastrophic antiphospholipid syndrome is rare and occurs in <1% patients with APS. It mostly occurs in third trimester and puerperium.[3]

Among the patients who develop CAPS in pregnancy, more than half have a primary APS or a history of APS manifestations such as previous abortions or fetal loses, previous DVT or arterial thrombosis. About 30% of CAPS are encountered in patients of SLE and the rest other autoimmune disorders such as rheumatoid arthritis, Sjögren syndrome, ulcerative colitis, systemic sclerosis, or relapsing polytonicities.

The mortality rate of CAPS over the years has decreased from 53% in patient diagnosed in 2000 to 33.3% in patients diagnosed between 2001 and 2005.[4] The decrease in mortality rate attributed to early diagnosis and use of triple therapy including glucocorticoids, anticoagulant, and plasmapheresis/intravascular immunoglobulins.

PATHOPHYSIOLOGY

It involves widespread rapid thrombosis in different organs in presence of APS.

The presence of APL represents the first hit, which increases the risk of thrombosis.

Certain environmental factors trigger the complement and immune activation leading to CAPS as a second hit leading to activation; of prothrombic and proinflammatory mediators and hence thrombosis of large and small vessels in multiple organs.

This in turn causes tissue necrosis and further complement activation causes a cytokine storm with multiorgan failure.

It is not clear why certain patients with APS go into the vicious cycle of complement activation. However certain triggers have been identified which predispose to CAPS.

Pregnancy with hypercoagulable state with increase in level of factor 2-5-7-9-10-12 and von Willebrand factor (vWF) and decrease in levels of protein S and activated protein C contributes to increase risk of CAPS.[5,6]

Pregnant women are at the high risk of CAPS during the postpartum period. First 3-4 weeks of delivery can be highest risk of thrombosis and hence CAPS.[1,7]

Preexisting risk factors associated with increase in thrombosis of pregnancy are age (>35 years), multiple pregnancy, personal and family history of deep venous thrombosis.[5-7]

Acquired transient risk factor simply due to pregnancy includes bed rest, immobility for 4 days or longer, pregnancy-induced hypertension (PIH), assisted reproductive technology (ART), weight gain of >21 kg, trauma to pelvis during delivery, all predispose toward hypercoagulations and CAPS.

A trigger for CAPS is identified in 65.4% of patients with the most common being infection endometritis, cesarean section (CS) wound or episiotomy infection or mastitis. Other precipitating factors

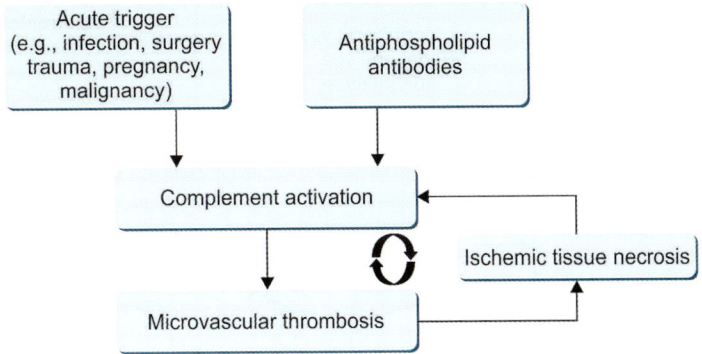

Fig. 1: Series of events in development of catastrophic antiphospholipid syndrome.

include neoplasm, surgical procedures, anticoagulant withdrawal or changeover with low level of INR and lupus flares. Hence it is very important to prevent infection and maintain an adequate anticoagulation in these patients with previous thrombosis and APL. Also pregnancy complication such as hemolysis, elevated liver enzymes, and low platelets (HELLP) syndrome, placental infection and pelvic thrombosis can lead to CAPS **(Fig. 1)**.

The exact mechanism of CAPS is not fully worked out but, this might capture some key elements. Dysregulation of the complement system leads to widespread microvascular thrombosis, causing tissue damage. A vicious spiral ensues, causing rapid clinical deterioration.

■ SIGNS AND SYMPTOMS

The clinical manifestations of CAPS depend on the organ involved and the extent of thrombosis. Most commonly affected organs are the kidneys, liver, lungs, brain, heart, and skin. Hepatic infarcts in pregnancy should raise a suspicion of APL and CAPS as well. The placental infarcts can affect fetus causing oligohydramnios, growth restriction, and intrauterine death **(Fig. 2)**.

Laboratory findings may reflect the dysfunction of the organ involved.

Thrombosis is seen in 67% of cases. Schistocytes thrombotic microangiopathy, disseminated intravascular coagulation (DIC) may also be present. Among the antiphospholipid antibodies, lupus anticoagulant, and immunoglobulin G (IgG) are most frequently positive.[2,8] Patients are often triple positive for [lupus anticoagulant (LA), anticardiolipin (aCL) beta-2-glycoprotein (anti-b2-GP)].[9] Anti-nuclear and anti-deoxyribonucleic acid (DNA) antibodies are also frequently present.

A false positive APL test can occur transiently during infection.

Also, anticoagulation with heparin or warfarin can result in both false positive and false negative result. False negative APL can also occur during acute APS events because of its consumption in process of coagulation.[10]

■ DIFFERENTIAL DIAGNOSIS

The differential diagnosis includes other thrombotic microangiopathies encountered with pregnancy. These include preeclampsia, HELLP syndrome, hemolytic uremic syndrome, thrombotic thrombocytopenic

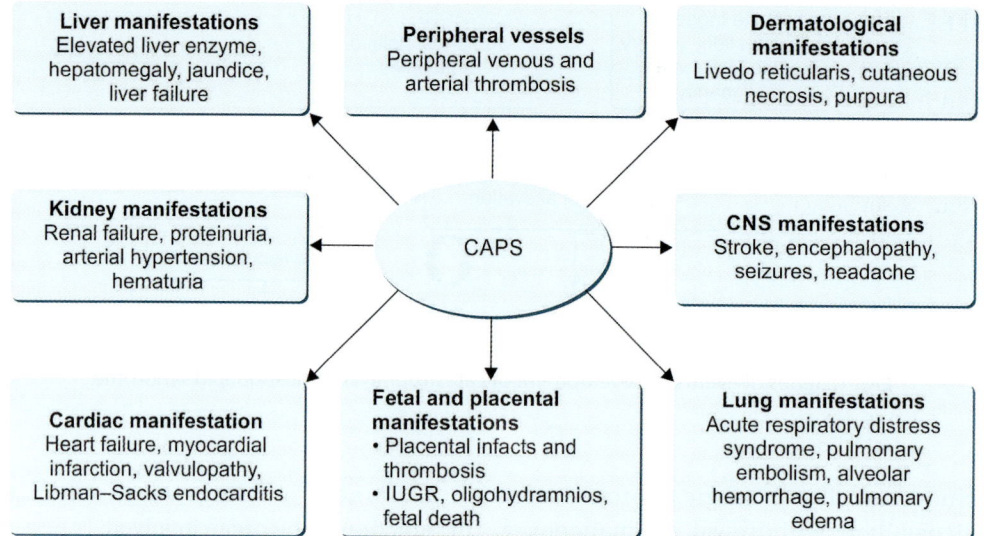

Fig. 2: Multisystem involvement in CAPS. (CAPS: catastrophic antiphospholipid syndrome; CNS: central nervous system; IUGR: intrauterine growth restriction)

purpura, lupus flare, DIC, and acute fatty liver of pregnancy.

All these differential diagnoses are characterized by microangiopathic anemia and thrombocytopenia.

Catastrophic antiphospholipid syndrome is rapidly progressive in nature with high morbidity and mortality so it is important to keep a high level of suspicion for probable CAPS diagnosis in certain cases. Timely assessment of different symptoms and comparisons of laboratory investigations is crucial in diagnosis of CAPS and the gold standard for diagnosis of CAPS is the APL positivity.

Specificity of CAPS diagnosis increases with higher antibody levels. However, multiple organ thrombosis with positive antibodies is not always CAPS so other differential diagnosis should be considered. Many infections can cause increase in APL levels giving a false positive value while during the period of thrombosis, due to consumption of APL, there is low level of antibodies leading to false negative APL. Hence, there is need of doing a retest for APL after 6 weeks of acute event for the confirmation.

MANAGEMENT

Following laboratory tests should be done. Complete blood count (CBC) with platelets mainly shows thrombocytopenia and presence of schistocytes in peripheral smear. Most common organ damage occurs in kidney and liver so both kidney and liver functions may be deranged. DIC may leads to deranged coagulation profile. Antiphospholipid antibody and antinuclear and anti-DNA antibodies may be positive. However thrombosis there may be consumption of antiphospholipid antibodies, which can lead to a negative test, hence repetition of test is required after 6 weeks in case of negative results.

TREATMENT

Following general measures have to be taken into consideration. For prevention of development of CAPS, identify the underlying cause which acted as a precipitating factor (example sepsis, any surgery, anticoagulants withdrawal) and first correct the factor. Aggressive management of infection is must in pregnant patient with APS. All infections should be treated with specific antibiotics and in case of unpredictable infections broad-spectrum antibiotics should be started. Necrosed tissue should be removed. Start aggressive management of hypertension if present, as intravascular hemolysis can worsen the condition and in patient of probable CAPS avoid intravascular punctures (mainly arterial line).

Patients with severe symptoms should be given intensive care. The patient should be managed by a multi-specialty team and should be monitored in intensive care unit. Critically ill patients may require ventilatory support and hemodialysis. According to clinical condition patients may require antihypertensives or vasopressors. Thrombolysis should be started and surgery should be postponed to allow anticoagulant therapy to work. Blood sugars should be strictly monitored and maintained. Patients may develop stress ulcers, for which prophylactic therapy should be given.

It is uncertain whether delivery of fetus will improve the condition. However, delivery is advised when fetals is mature. Trial of labor can be given but cesarean delivery is preferred depending upon the medical condition of patient, anticoagulant status, and willingness for labor.

Mainstay of treatment is identification and removal of precipitating factor and combination therapy with anticoagulants, glucocorticoids, and plasmapheresis or intravenous immunoglobulins.

Therapeutic anticoagulation should be initiated with intravenous unfractionated heparin for 7–10 days. This will allow rapid reversal of events, after which, patient can be put on oral anticoagulant or Low Molecular Weight heparin (LMWH). Other treatment focuses on immunosuppression. First line is usually corticosteroids, they are more effective when given in combination with anticoagulants. In addition to this intravenous immune globulin or plasma exchange is used for additional immunosuppression and treatment. In cases of refractory CAPS where there is no improvement with triple therapy other immunosuppressive therapies such as rituximab and eculizumab should be considered.

Anticoagulants: Heparin is the main anticoagulant used with very good results, and its anti-inflammatory property. Heparin infusion is used and it should be titrated against anti-Xa level. It is important to do this because many patients with lupus anticoagulant artificially increase the partial thromboplastin time (PTT). Heparin should be replaced with warfarin as oral anticoagulant.

Glucocorticoids: Steroids are very important part of treatment because they inhibit nuclear factor NF-κb, a mediator in both systemic inflammatory response and APL mediated thrombosis. CAPS involves a proinflammatory factors and steroids can be helpful in patients with underlying rheumatoid disorders and to lower the level of antiphospholipid antibodies. Methyl prednisolone 1,000 mg daily for 3–5 days can be used with anticoagulants.[1]

Plasmapheresis or intravenous immunoglobulins: These two techniques help to reduce the activity of antiphospholipid antibodies; plasmapheresis directly removes antibodies while intravenous immune globulin (IVIG) helps to lower their levels. Plasmapheresis is mainly selected for patients with microangiopathic hemolytic anemia or renal dysfunction, IVIG is selected mainly in patients with immune thrombocytopenia. The dose of IVIG is 0.4 mg/kg/day for 3–5 days. For plasmapheresis most commonly used protocol is to remove 2–3 liters of plasma daily for 3–5 days.

Monoclonal Antibodies Like Eculizumab and Rituximab

Eculizumab: The monoclonal antibody inhibits the breakdown of C5 and C5b by which inhibits terminal complement system. Given at initial dose of 900 mg weekly, it has shown its efficacy in inducing remission and preventing the recurrence of CAPS.

Rituximab: It is a monoclonal antibody against CD20 on B cells and may play a role in treatment for resistant CAPS; B cell suppression may be a good strategy with a target to reduce antiphospholipid antibody with this drug use.

LONG-TERM SEQUELAE OF CATASTROPHIC ANTIPHOSPHOLIPID SYNDROME

Microvascular thrombosis can lead to organ damage in long term. Few cases of CAPS with long-term maternal sequelae have been identified like permanent adrenal insufficiency, chronic liver insufficiency, hepatic infarction, diffuse alveolar hemorrhage, stroke, venous thrombosis, and sudden death. Fetal complications of CAPS are prematurity and fetal death.

Adverse obstetric outcome rate is very high in subsequent even after optimum management of CAPS pregnancy so women with first episode of pregnancy-related CAPS should be advised not to go for further pregnancy. If the women still want to become pregnant, they should be monitored very closely and provided multidisciplinary antenatal assistance.

TAKE HOME MESSAGES

- Catastrophic antiphospholipid syndrome is rare but life-threatening condition.
- High mortality rate of 33.3%.
- Early diagnosis and aggressive management is required to save the patient.
- Pregnancy may be a trigger for CAPS in patients with APS.
- HELLP syndrome in patients with APS indicates high risk for development of CAPS.
- APS patient going under surgical treatment prophylactic anticoagulation therapy should be started and maintained well to prevent flares. Heparin is the first line of management in CAPS.

REFERENCES

1. Cervera R, Rodríguez-Pintó I, Colafrancesco S, Conti F, Valesini G, Rosário C, et al. 14th International Congress on Antiphospholipid antibodies Task Force Report On catastrophic Antiphospholipis Syndrome. Autoimmun Rev. 2014;13(7):699-707.
2. Silver RM. Catastrophic antiphospholipid syndrome and pregnancy. Semin Perinatol. 2017;42(1):26-32.
3. Stojanovich L, Marisavljevic D, Rovensky J, Djokovich A, Kozáková D, Milinic N. Clinical and laboratory features of the catastrophic antiphospholipid syndrome. Clin Rev Allergy Immunol. 2009;36(2-3):74-9.
4. Bucciarelli S, Cervera R, Espinosa G, Gómez-Puerta JA, Ramos-Casals M, et al. Mortality in the catastrophic antiphospholipid syndrome: causes of death and prognostic factors. Autoimmun Rev. 2006;6(2):72-5.

5. Gómez-Puerta JA, Espinosa G, Cervera R. Catastrophic antiphospholipid syndrome: diagnosis and management in pregnancy. Clin Lab Med. 2013;33:391-400.
6. Gómez-Puerta Ja, Cervera R, Espinosa G, Bucciarelli S, Font J. Pregnancy and puerperium are high susceptibility periods for the development of catastrophic antiphospholipid syndrome. Autoimmun Rev. 2006;6:85-8.
7. Gómez-Puerta JA, Sanin-Blair J, Galarza-Maldonado C. Pregnancy and catastrophic antiphospholipid syndrome. Clin Rev Allergy Immunol. 2009;36:85-90.
8. Espinosa G, Bucciarelli S, Cervera R, Gómez-Puerta JA, Font J. Laboratory studies on pathophysiology of the catastrophic antiphospholipid syndrome. Autoimmun Rev. 2006;6(2):68-71.
9. Hanouna G, Morel N, Le Thi Huong D, Josselin L, Vauthier-Brouzes D, Saadoun D, et al. Catastrophic anti-phospholipid syndrome and pregnancy: an experience of 13 cases. Rheumatology. 2013;52:1635-41.
10. Avcin T, Toplak N. Antiphospholipid antibodies in response to infection. Curr Rheumatol Rep. 2007;9(3):212-8.

CHAPTER 27

Trauma

Polytrauma in a Pregnant Lady

Amrita Shah, Pradeep Rangappa, Ipe Jacob

INTRODUCTION

Trauma in pregnancy possesses unique challenges to the clinicians. There are significant anatomical and physiological changes normal to pregnancy which are adapted not only to aid the mother but also her baby.[1] These changes may pose a challenge during trauma management as they may lead to an altered response to treatment necessitating modification of treatment.

Any female presenting with minor or major trauma and is of child-bearing age should be considered pregnant until proven otherwise. Trauma may complicate 6–7% of pregnancies[2] and can cause severe maternal and fetal morbidity and mortality. Even minor injuries in the mother can cause significant fetal complications in 60–70% of cases, especially in late trimester.[3,4]

EPIDEMIOLOGY AND MAGNITUDE

The most common mechanisms of injury include motor vehicle collision resulting from poor compliance to passenger seat belts. Others include slip and fall, domestic violence, gunfire, burn, and toxins **(Figs. 1A and B)**.[2] Among abdominal injury, blunt trauma have been found to be more common

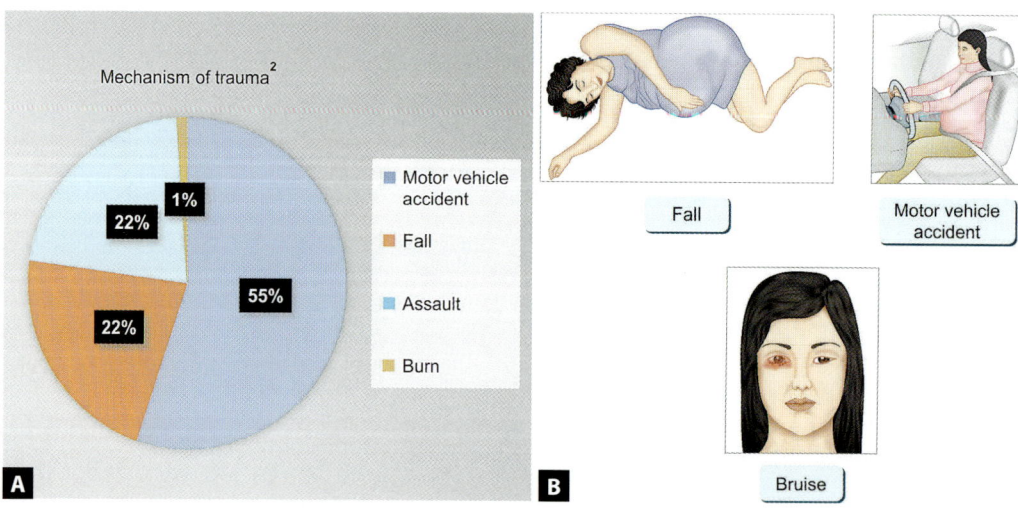

Figs. 1A and B: Common mechanisms of trauma in pregnancy.

than penetrating injuries. Gunshot injuries are more lethal than knife injury.[5]

The risk factors for maternal trauma include young age, alcohol use, drug use, and domestic violence. Pregnancy by itself may be a risk factor for trauma.[6] The risk factors for poor fetal as well as severe adverse maternal outcome include age of the gravid mother, month of gestation, hyperlactatemia, and injury severity score (ISS).[7-9] In a retrospective study on maternal trauma, an ISS >9 was found to have sensitivity and specificity of 100% and 98%, respectively, with area under the curve (AUC) of 0.998 for predicting poor perinatal outcome.[8] Though an ISS >9 predicts increased chances of fetal complications, a lower ISS score and hemodynamic stability of mother does not rule out fetal demise.

IMPLICATIONS FOR MATERNAL HEALTH

An understanding of the normal changes in anatomy and physiology during pregnancy is important.

Anatomical Differences

Postural changes resulting from weight gain and breast enlargement can pose challenges during intubation. An increased estrogen level and blood volume may lead to mucosal edema. Capillary engorgement of respiratory tract mucosa brings about naso-oropharyngeal and laryngeal swelling which further contributes to difficult intubation. Eight times higher incidence of failed intubation have been noted compared to other surgical patients.

Preeclamptic patients are more prone to regurgitation than other pregnant patients as they have narrower upper airway, increased tissue edema, and more soft tissue deposition around their neck.[5,10]

Pulmonary Changes (Table 1)

Implications

With increasing gestational age, the gravid uterus pushes the diaphragm upward causing premature closure of smaller airways

TABLE 1: Respiratory changes during pregnancy.

Respiratory parameters	Changes from normal
Tidal volume (TV) (mL)	Increased by 40%
Respiratory rate (breaths/min)	Increased by 15%
Minute ventilation (mL/min)	Increased by 40%
Functional residual capacity (FRC) (mL)	Decreased by 25%
Residual volume (RV) (mL)	Decreased by 20%
Oxygen consumption (mL/min)	Increased by 20%
Vital capacity (VC) (mL)	Unchanged
Inspiratory capacity (IC)	Increased by 15%
pH	7.41–7.46
Partial pressure of arterial oxygen (PaO_2)	↑105
Partial pressure of arterial carbon dioxide ($PaCO_2$)	↓27–32
HCO_3	↓19–24
Total lung capacity	Decreases by 5%
Colloid oncotic pressure	Decreases by 20%

and decrease in functional residual capacity (FRC). This decrease causes respiratory distress which is aggravated by reduced chest wall compliance due to increasing abdominal content. As term approaches, because of increased progesterone levels, oxygen demand increases. All these factors together decrease oxygen reserve in mother. Hence, close monitoring of oxygenation is mandatory in such patients.

In view of upward displacement of diaphragm, the chest tube insertion in pregnant trauma cases should be one or two spaces above the 5th intercostal space to prevent injury to abdominal organs.

An increased tidal volume and mild increase in respiratory rate results in increased minute ventilation. This causes an increase in arterial oxygen and decrease in carbon dioxide tension. pH is mildly increased reflecting respiratory alkalosis.[2,3] Diphosphoglycerate levels are increased but because of respiratory alkalosis, p50 levels remain unchanged.

There is decrease in colloid oncotic pressure with increased hydrostatic pressure favoring pulmonary edema.[5,11]

Cardiovascular Changes (Table 2)

Implications

Physiologic hypotension: With increase in cardiac output, systemic vascular resistance and blood pressure start decreasing. The vasodilation caused by progesterone, nitric oxide, and prostaglandin along with decreased resistance result in hypotension around the second trimester. Leftward shift of uterus to release the compression is necessary to relieve hypotension.

The enlarged uterus can cause aortocaval compression decreasing the blood flow distribution by 25%. There is pooling of blood in lower extremity veins which can precipitate hemorrhage and shock during lower limb injuries.

Electrocardiogram (ECG) may simulate myocardial contusion.[1,5,12]

Hematological Changes (Table 3)

Implications

- *Physiological anemia:* An increase in plasma volume much more than red blood cell (RBC) volume during pregnancy can result in a state of physiological anemia. In a gravid trauma scenario, because of such high blood volume, shock and tachycardia may be a late sign of hypovolemia whilst fetal compromise has already set in.
- The prothrombotic state of pregnancy along with blood stasis can predispose to increased thrombotic complications.[1]
- Fibrinogen levels may rise to as high as 500 mg/dL. A review article on critical obstetric hemorrhage suggested a massive transfusion target of at least 200 mg/dL for fibrinogen or 10 mm of A5 on rotational thromboelastometry (*ROTEM®*).[13]

TABLE 2: Cardiovascular changes during pregnancy.

Cardiac parameters	Changes from normal
Cardiac output (L/min)	Increases by 30–50%
Heart rate (beats/min)	Increases by 15–20 beats/min
Systemic vascular resistance (dynes.s.cm^{-5})	Decreases by 1,000–4,000
Electrocardiogram (ECG)	• Left axis deviation—15° • Flattened or inverted T waves in leads III and aVF

TABLE 3: Hematological changes during pregnancy.

Hematology parameters	Changes from normal
Blood volume (mL)	Increases by 30–50%
Plasma volume (mL)	Increases by 30–50%; maximum up to 34 weeks
Red blood cell (RBC) volume (mL)	Increases by 20–30% at term
Hematocrit (%)	32–42
Total count (mm)	Increases to 5,000–14,000
Coagulation factors	• *Increase:* Factors II, VII, VIII, X, XII, and von Willebrand factor • *Decrease:* Protein S, factor XIII, decreased fibrinolysis due to increased plasminogen activator inhibitor-1
Fibrinogen (mg/dL)	400–500

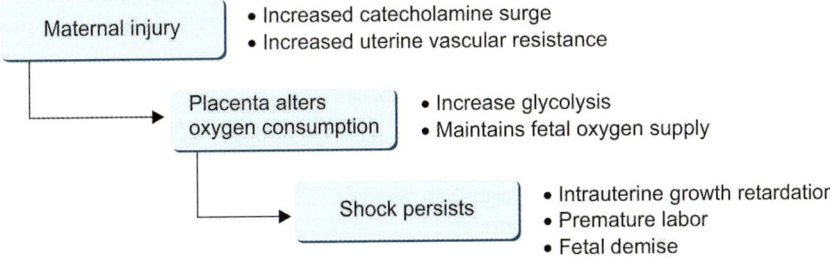

Flowchart 1: Pathophysiological changes during trauma in pregnancy.

Gastrointestinal Changes

Progesterone-mediated smooth muscle relaxation with cephalad displacement of stomach by the gravid uterus and decrease in lower esophageal sphincter tone escalates chances of gastric aspiration.

Renal Changes

Pregnancy results in increase in renal blood flow, decrease in glomerular filtration rate, and reduction in serum creatinine levels. Even a mild increase in creatinine level might reflect marked acute kidney injury.

Musculoskeletal Changes

There is increase in spinal lordosis with laxity of ligaments after 32 weeks resulting in increased incidence of fall.[5]

Vascular Changes

In case of pelvic fracture, engorged pelvic vessels (uteroovarian and infundibulopelvic vessels) can contribute to retroperitoneal bleed in an event of blunt abdominal obstetric trauma.[12]

Implications on Fetal Health (Flowchart 1)

Placental perfusion and oxygenation are valuable to baby's health. What happens to the fetus during maternal injury?

The severity of fetal injury also depends on the mechanism of trauma. Because of cushioning effect of amniotic fluid, abdomen and uterine musculature, direct fetal trauma is less in blunt injury compared to penetrating injuries. Penetrating trauma has a good maternal outcome (with 7% mortality) but very high fetal mortality (70%).[12,14]

■ MANAGEMENT STEPS

Assessment of an obstetric trauma case is similar to any other case presenting to the emergency department with injury. Trauma call is initiated; co-coordinating with surgeons, obstetricians, neonatologist, and emergency physician to optimize the patient and maximize outcome.

Primary Survey

Table 4 shows the steps of the primary survey on initial presentation.

Transfusion Practices

- In case of massive hemorrhage, massive transfusion protocol strategy should be activated.

TABLE 4: Steps of the primary survey in trauma.

Airway and cervical spine stabilization	• Early intubation is advocated in cases having airway compromise. Eight times higher incidence of failed intubation was noted compared to other surgical patients[5,14] • Manual-in-line stabilization for suspected cervical spine injury • Difficult airway cart with adjuncts to be ready • Fiberoptic intubation—cervical spine or facial injury and morbid obesity
Breathing and ventilation	• Oxygen saturation (SpO_2) levels are targeted at >95% • Chest tubes placed one or two spaces above the 5th intercostal[14]
Circulation and hemorrhage control	• Two large intravenous (IV) bore 14–16 G cannula secured • Send the necessary investigations including type-specific blood grouping and crossmatching and acid–base analysis • Crystalloids are the preferred choice of fluids. Colloids did not confer any mortality benefit over normal saline (SAFE trial)[5] • Vasopressors may be used only in cases of refractory hypotension as a last measure as they compromise fetoplacental perfusion • Supine hypotension syndrome → Manually displace the uterus to the left or log roll the patient or the spine board by 4–6 inches to the left using bolstering device or wedge for support[5]
Disability (neurologic examination)	• Differentiate headache and seizures in head injury from obstetric conditions like preeclampsia • Any drug or alcohol intake can also result in altered sensorium • Rule out neurogenic shock
Exposure/ environment	• Expose the patient to look of external injuries—bruises, gunshot entry-exit wound • Prevent hypothermia
Adjuncts for primary survey	• Extended Focused Assessment with Sonography in Trauma (E-FAST), pelvic or chest X-ray, urinary and feeding catheters, and capnography • Use pelvic binders in pelvic trauma
Recognize injury: Consider emergency surgery/thoracotomy/laparotomy	
If mother stable	Move to secondary survey
If mother dead/ unsalvageable	• Check fetus for viability • *Perimortem cesarean section*: In the event of maternal cardiac arrest and viable fetus, cesarean section is to be performed within 4 or 5 minutes of cardiac arrest

- Transfusion goals include hemoglobin >7 g/dL (in severe hemorrhage) but <10 g/dL[5], platelet count >75 × 10^9/L, prothrombin time (PT) <1.5 × mean control, activated PT <1.5 × mean control and fibrinogen >1.0 g/L.[15]
- Point of care testing—Thromboelastography (TEG) and rotational thromboelastometry® (ROTEM) can be used for clot analysis in suspicion of disseminated intravascular coagulation.
- In case a female of childbearing potential receives RhD positive red cells, anti-D immunoglobulin should be considered.
- In women of unknown blood group, it is recommended to use of O RhD negative transfusion as last retort.
- Tranexamic acid (1 g) should be initiated promptly within 3 hours of injury.[16]

Secondary Survey

Secondary survey begins as soon as primary survey ends. It is done to identify any condition which might later cause hemodynamic instability. History of the patient is taken including obstetric history, last menstrual period, pregnancy complications, expected date of delivery, fetal movements, and current events. **Table 5** describes common complications that may be seen.

Head-to-toe Examination

- Physical examination includes assessment of the fundal height.
- Extended Focused Assessment with Sonography in Trauma (E-FAST) should be reassessed.
- At 12 weeks, the uterus is a pelvic organ, by 20 weeks it lies at the level of umbilicus, at 32–36 weeks it lies at subcostal/below xiphoid process.
- Gestational age (weeks) can also be found by fundal height which is measured from pubic symphysis to top of fundus (in cm).
- A femur length of ≥4 cm is suggestive of fetal age of 22–24 weeks.[17]
- Abdominal examination includes presence or absence of uterine tenderness and contractions.
- Pelvic examination using a sterile speculum should be used to evaluate the presence of blood or amniotic fluid, cervical effacement, dilation, and fetal station.
- Vaginal examination to look for either leak of amniotic fluid and/or vaginal bleeding is vital. Amniotic fluid can be identified using nitrazine paper to detect pH. A pH of 7–7.5 suggests the presence of amniotic fluid.

Fetal Assessment

The fetus is assessed for movements and heart sounds by auscultation or Doppler probe. Doppler ultrasound can detect fetal heart tones by 10 weeks of gestation. Signs of fetal decompensation include abnormal fetal heart rate–saltatory pattern, frequent uterine activity, repetitive decelerations, absence of accelerations. or beat-to-beat variability.[5]

According to the Advanced Trauma Life Support (ATLS) 2018 guidelines, risk factors for fetal compromise include maternal tachycardia >110/min, ISS >9, evidence of placental abruption, fetal tachycardia >160/min or bradycardia <120/min, and dangerous mechanism of injury like ejection from motor vehicle crash. Patients with risk factors for fetal loss are advised observation with tocodynamometer for over 24 hours.[18]

Diagnostic peritoneal lavage, if performed, should be through an open surgical incision above the fundus.[5]

Imaging studies involving radiation are not a contraindication in pregnant trauma cases where benefit outweighs the risk. Risk to fetus depends on the dose of radiation and gestational age. Dose-related side effects are rare below 5 rad and beyond 17 weeks

TABLE 5: Complications unique to pregnancy and definite care.[5]

Placental abruption	• Suggested by vaginal bleeding (70% of cases), uterine tenderness, frequent uterine contractions, tetany, and irritability. In 30% of abruptions following trauma, vaginal bleeding may not occur • Its incidence is 6–35% for major injuries • Maternal mortality <1%, fetal mortality is between 20 and 30% • Laparotomy is indicated for the mother's stabilization
Uterine rupture	• Rare complication (0.06%); fetal mortality approaches 100%; mainly in third trimester • Associated with pelvic fractures and bladder injuries • Presentation—abdominal pain, distention, palpable fetal parts, and shock. However, due to peritoneum's insensitivity in the third trimester, there may be no pain • Treatment is exploratory laparotomy, delivery of fetus, and supportive care
Premature labor	• Presents as frequent uterine contraction, associated with cervical effacement and dilation • Suppression of labor is contraindicated: Maternal/fetal compromise, stable mother >36 weeks or <20 weeks • It is indicated if steroids course is ongoing for fetal lung maturity or transfer to another trauma care
Premature rupture of membranes	• If signs of viable fetus +/mother stable → induction and vaginal delivery • If fetal distress+/stable mother → cesarean section
Fetomaternal hemorrhage	• *Incidence:* 8–30% • *Increased risk:* Rhesus D (Rh D)-negative women; even <0.1 mL of transplacental hemorrhage can sensitize such patients • All unsensitized Rh-negative women who suffer trauma should be offered Rh D immunoglobulin (300 µg protects against 30 mL) of fetal blood • *Detection:* Flow cytometry > Kleihauer–Betke test

TABLE 6: Drugs requiring dose modification in pregnancy.

Drugs which easily cross placental barrier	Inhalational, induction agents, local anesthetics, antihypertensives, benzodiazepines and opioids, atropine, and ephedrine
Drugs which do not easily cross placental barrier	Depolarizing and nondepolarizing agents, glycopyrrolate, sugammadex, heparin, and phenylephrine

gestation. Lead apron can always be used to shield the uterus. Contrast CT has better sensitivity (almost 100%) than ultrasound in detection of placental abruption or fetomaternal hemorrhage. It, however, has a low specificity.[5]

Pharmacological Considerations

Drugs that show an increased transfer across the placenta include smaller sized molecules (<1,000 dalton), lipophilic, uncharged, albumin bound drugs (digoxin, midazolam, and phenytoin)[1] and drugs with high free and nonionized drug fraction in plasma **(Table 6)**. Hydrophilic drugs on the other hand may require a higher initial and maintenance dose, as pregnancy is a high volume of distribution state.

■ PREVENTION

It has been noted that an improper placement of seat belt can also cause uterine rupture and

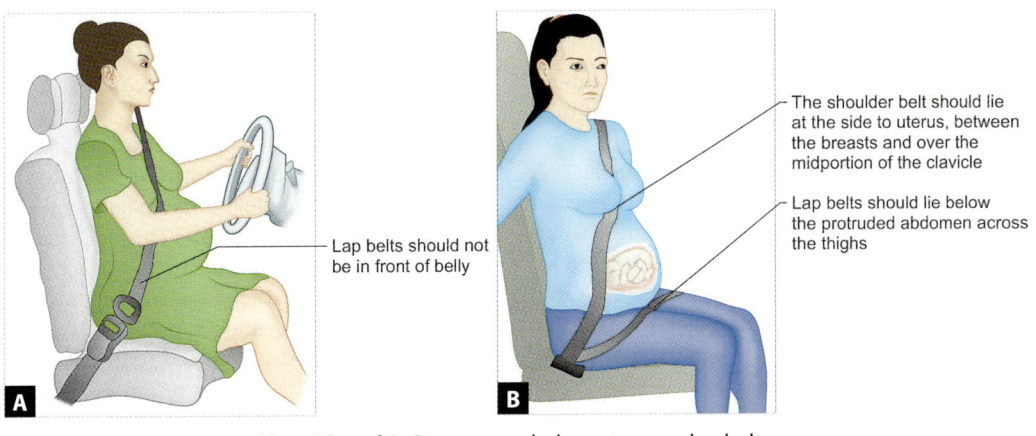

Figs. 2A and B: Recommended way to wear lap belts.

fetal death. The recommended way to wear lap belts is shown in **Figures 2A and B**.[12]

Outpatient department screening for domestic abuse and intimate partner violence when patients come with history of depression, and/or suicide attempts, injuries inconsistent with history, symptoms of substance abuse, and multiple outpatient visits is vital.[12,18]

■ CONCLUSION

Trauma in pregnancy poses unique challenges. While the initial examination of a pregnant trauma patient does not differ from the standard primary survey, further examination requires a clear understanding of the normal physiological changes that occur in pregnancy as well as complications that are unique to pregnancy.

TAKE HOME MESSAGES

- Obstetric trauma is dealt in a similar fashion as other trauma patients, however, clinicians must remember that two lives are involved; assessment and resuscitation of the mother always takes priority over fetus.
- The anatomical and physiological changes in a parturient can delay and complicate diagnosis and treatment particularly in a case of fetal decompensation.
- Activation of trauma call and coordination with various specialties can ensure optimal maternal and fetal care and survival.
- Complications specific to pregnancy and pharmacological consideration is important in recognizing a fetal demise/compromise even in the event of minor trauma or maternal stability.

■ REFERENCES

1. Costantine MM. Physiologic and Pharmacokinetic Changes in Pregnancy. Front Pharmacol. 2014;5:65.
2. Connolly AM, Katz VL, Bash KL, McMahon MJ, Hansen WF. Trauma and pregnancy. Am J Perinatol. 1997;14:331-6.
3. Taha E, Nasralla K, Khalid A, Ali AA. Blunt abdominal trauma to a pregnant woman resulting in a child with hemiplegic spastic cerebral palsy and permanent eye damage. BMC Res Notes. 2013;6:517.
4. Murphy NJ, Quinlan JD. Trauma in pregnancy: assessment, management, and prevention. Am Fam Physician. 2014;90(10):717-24.
5. Weinberg L, Steele RG, Pugh R, Higgins S, Herbert M, Story D. The Pregnant Trauma Patient. Anaesth Intensive Care. 2005;33(2):167-80.
6. Chames MC, Pearlman MD. Trauma during pregnancy: outcomes and clinical management. Clin Obstet Gynecol. 2008;51(2):398-408.

7. Aboutanos SZ, Aboutanos MB, Dompkowski D, Duane TM, Malhotra AK, Ivatury RR. Predictors of fetal outcome in pregnant trauma patients: a five-year institutional review. Am Surg. 2007;73(8):824-7.
8. Dalton S, McPherson J, Charles A, Stamilio DM. 717: Major trauma in pregnancy: Prediction of maternal and perinatal severe adverse outcomes. Am J Obstet Gynecol. 2020;222(1):S453-4.
9. Theodorou DA, Velmahos GC, Souter I, Chan LS, Vassiliu P, Tatevossian R, et al. Fetal death after trauma in pregnancy. Am Surg. 2000;66(9):809-12.
10. Munnur U, Boisblanc B, Suresh M. Airway problems in pregnancy. Crit Care Med. 2005;33(10 Suppl):S259-68.
11. LoMauro A, Aliverti A. Respiratory physiology of pregnancy: Physiology masterclass. Breathe (Sheff). 2015;11(4):297-301.
12. Hill CC, Pickinpaugh J. Trauma and surgical emergencies in the obstetric patient. Surg Clin North Am. 2008;88(2):421-40.
13. Matsunaga S, Takai Y, Seki H. Fibrinogen for the management of critical obstetric hemorrhage. J Obstet Gynaecol Res. 2019;45(1):13-21.
14. Jain V, Chari R, Maslovitz S, Farine D; Maternal Fetal Medicine Committee, Bujold E, et al. Guidelines for the Management of a Pregnant Trauma Patient. J Obstet Gynaecol Can. 2015;37(6):553-74.
15. Jadon A, Bagai R. Blood transfusion practices in obstetric anaesthesia. Indian J Anaesth. 2014;58(5):629-36.
16. Rudloff U. Trauma in pregnancy. Arch Gynecol Obstet. 2007;276(2):101-17.
17. Hadlock FP, Deter RL, Harrist RB, Park SK. Estimating fetal age: computer-assisted analysis of multiple fetal growth parameters. Radiology. 1984;152(2):497-501.
18. American College of Surgeons. Advanced Trauma Life Support. Chicago, IL: American College of Surgeons, Committee on Trauma; 2012.

Hematological Disorders

CHAPTER 28

Sickle Cell Crisis

Maimoona Ahmed, Tarakeswari Surapaneni

INTRODUCTION

Sickle cell disease (SCD) is a hemoglobinopathy with autosomal recessive inheritance. It encompasses different genotypes such as homozygous HbS sickle cell anemia (SS) as well as the double heterozygous sickle hemoglobin C disease (SC), sickle beta plus thalassemia (Sβ + thal), sickle alpha thalassemia (SS α thal) and sickle cell anemia with high fetal hemoglobin (SS + F).[1] SCD is characterized by a tumultuous course affecting all systems. Pregnancy, with its physiological changes such as increased metabolic demand, stress, increased blood viscosity, aggravates the disease. One such serious complication is sickle cell crisis with implications to both maternal and fetal well-being.[2]

Sickle cell crisis includes vaso-occlusive crisis, acute chest syndrome, acute stroke, and aplastic crisis. Vaso-occlusive crisis is most common and involves recurrent, acute onset, and severe episodes of pain. The pathophysiology of the pain is blockage of the micro-vasculature by the abnormal sickle-shaped red cells resulting in infarction and release of inflammatory mediators. The pain is unpredictable, can occur spontaneously but may be precipitated by dehydration, infections, or even stress.[3]

EPIDEMIOLOGY AND MAGNITUDE OF THE PROBLEM

Sickle cell disease ranks as the most common inherited disease worldwide with over 3 lakh affected newborns each year. Higher prevalence is reported in Africa, parts of Mediterranean, Middle East, and India.[4]

In India, SCD was first described among the tribals living in Nilgiri Hills in South India.[5] Since then, screening has revealed the prevalence of this condition among the scheduled castes, scheduled tribes, and other backward classes in India with prevalence of sickle cell carriers ranging from 1 to 40%. Being an autosomal recessive condition, consanguineous marriages (a part of Indian culture) also explain the higher prevalence rate. Altogether, India ranks second in the number of SCD births with an estimated 42,016 newborns with SCD in 2010.[5]

Improvement in neonatal screening methods and treatment modalities has increased the life expectancy of those born with SCD, with more affected women reaching reproductive age group and conceiving.[6] With migration and intermixing of populations, genetic conditions are no longer restricted to a particular ethnic group or confined to a geographical location.[7] Thus, management of this condition in pregnancy has now become an integral part of high risk obstetrics and critical care.

Vaso-occlusive (painful) crisis is the most frequent complication in SCD in pregnancy with a reported incidence of 27–50% in the antenatal period.[8] Intrapartum events, vaginal delivery or cesarean section, are a profound physiological challenge and can precipitate crisis. Even in postpartum period, it occurs in 7–25% of pregnancies.[9] Fetal complications are also more common, with a 21% risk of stillbirth, 32% risk of premature delivery, and 42% risk of intrauterine growth restriction.[10]

IMPLICATIONS FOR MATERNAL HEALTH

Women suffer from more frequent incidences of sickle cell crisis in pregnancy. Even those women who have a mild disease prior to conceiving are at risk during pregnancy and postpartum period.[11]

Painful crisis being the most common maternal complication in-turn starts the domino effect of increased hospital admission, need for ICU stay and critical care and in more complicated cases even need for respiratory support, and blood transfusion. Each transfusion carries the risk of blood-borne infections, volume overload, iron overload, lung injury, hyper-viscosity syndrome and alloimmunization.[12]

Release of prostaglandin during the crisis, can precipitate preterm labor. There is also an increase in the caesarean section rates.[13]

IMPLICATIONS FOR FETAL WELL-BEING

Sickle cell disease increases the risk of miscarriages and the crisis episodes further add to it with some studies reporting rates as high as 36%.[14]

Maternal hypoxia and acidosis during the crisis can be reflected by abnormal fetal heart changes on nonstress testing. These are usually transient and revert to normal as maternal condition improves. Vaso-occlusive crisis in the uteroplacental circulation can result in intrauterine fetal growth restriction or even fetal demise. Preterm labor and growth restriction lead to premature and low birth weight babies needing neonatal intensive care unit (NICU) admission.[13]

Women needing multiple blood transfusions are at risk of red cell alloimmunization and this can cause hemolytic disease of the newborn. Further, newborns of women needing chronic opioid therapy for pain episodes are at risk of neonatal withdrawal syndrome.[14] Thus, strict fetal surveillance goes hand-in-hand with the maternal management in view of associated morbidities.

MANAGEMENT

Sickle cell crisis in pregnancy needs a multidisciplinary team approach with inputs from the obstetrician, physician, anesthesiologist, and hematologist. As painful crisis is a hallmark of SCD, a pain management plan must be put in place beforehand, and both the patient and the treating team should be familiar with the same. The patient should be managed in high dependency unit or in the intensive care unit.

Vaso-occlusive Crisis/Painful Crisis

Initial Assessment

There should be a rapid evaluation to rule out other complications of SCD such as acute chest syndrome, severe anemia, splenic enlargement, and neurological complications such as stroke. Localized, painful swellings will need differentiation from acute osteomyelitis. Precipitating factors such as dehydration and infection must be looked for.[3] **Box 1** lists the investigations to be done in sickle cell crisis.

> **BOX 1:** Investigations during sickle cell crisis.[3]
>
> *Baseline investigations:*
> - Complete blood count
> - Serum creatinine
> - Serum urea and electrolytes
> - Urine routine
>
> *Directed evaluation:*
> - X-ray chest: Fever, dyspnea, cough, tachypnea, reduced O_2 saturation, chest signs
> - Arterial blood gas: O_2 saturation <95%, neurological symptoms
> - Liver function test (LFT), serum amylase: Jaundice, abdominal pain
> - Blood and urine cultures: Fever with chills and rigors, hypotension
> - Reticulocyte count: Severe anemia
> - Parvovirus B19 serology in case of reduced reticulocyte count
> - Imaging modalities: Ultrasound abdomen if splenomegaly, abnormal LFTs, abdominal pain. Magnetic resonance imaging in cases of stroke or to rule out osteomyelitis

Maternal monitoring should be documented on a Modified Obstetric Early Warning Chart.

Pain Management

The treatment is directed toward providing rapid pain relief. Analgesia should be started within 30 minutes of admission after the initial assessment and the pain should be adequately controlled within an hour of starting the medications.[15] The choice of drug should be as per the patient's analgesic history, pain tolerance, and previous side-effects.

There are no trials that have examined the management of painful crisis in pregnancy with SCD and so the treatment should be as per the recommendations for nonpregnant women.[6] However, the profile of medications should take into account fetal safety. The RCOG recommends use of the World Health Organization analgesic ladder as a guide for prescribing the medications.[15] The ladder mainly consists of three steps:

- First step—mild pain. Paracetamol can be used in such cases.
- Second step—moderate pain. Weak opioids (hydrocodone, codeine, tramadol, and co-dydramol) can be used. Non-steroidal anti-inflammatory drugs (NSAIDs) can be used between 12 and 28 weeks of gestation.
- Third step—severe pain. Strong opioids such as morphine or diamorphine are to be used.

Parenteral opioids can be given as bolus doses or as patient-controlled administration. Pethidine is not to be used due to risk of toxicity and seizures in SCD.[15]

Maternal monitoring should include assessment of pain relief and to rule out opioid related side-effects. Once the pain is sufficiently controlled, a detailed evaluation is to be done for underlying cause. **Box 2** outlines the algorithm for pain management in painful crisis.

Hydration

Fluid management is a simultaneous step in the treatment. Strict input-output chart should be maintained. The recommended fluid intake should be 60 mL/kg/24 hours either oral, nasogastric, or intravenous. Hydration should proceed with caution in case with associated comorbidities such as renal dysfunction and preeclampsia. Cannulation of veins in the lower limbs should be avoided due to risk of thrombosis and ulceration. Also central lines and urinary catheterization should be used with caution because of higher rate of infection.[3]

Antibiotics

Infection is a common precipitating cause of a crisis so appropriate assessment with cultures

> **BOX 2:** Algorithm for pain management in vaso-occlusive crisis.[3]
> - Initial rapid assessment to rule out complication and precipitating event
> - *Early initiation of analgesics as per the WHO stepwise ladder:* Paracetamol for mild pain, weak opioids/NSAIDs for moderate pain, strong opioids for severe pain
> - *Adjuvant medications:* Laxatives, antiemetic, anti-histaminic to combat opioid side effects
> - *Monitoring:* Pain, sedation, MEOWs chart. Every 30 minutes until pain controlled, then every 2 hours
> - Rescue doses of analgesia in case of break-through pain
> - *Fetal monitoring:* If viable gestational age. Fetal heart monitoring and/or biophysical profile
> - Reduce analgesia after 2–3 days and switch to oral medications
> - Discharge once pain is controlled with analgesics or needing acceptable oral doses
> - Advice regarding home care and follow-up
>
> (MEOWs: Modified Early Obstetric Warning Score; NSAIDs: non-steroidal anti-inflammatory drugs; WHO: World Health Organization)

and chest X-ray should be done. In cases of fever or a high clinical suspicion of infection, antibiotics should be started after collecting the culture specimens. Antibiotic choice depends on the local policy and likely pathogen. These patients are more susceptible to encapsulated organisms such as *Streptococcus pneumoniae*, *Haemophilus influenzae B*, *Meningococcus*, and *Salmonella* species due to hyposplenism.[3] Initial empiric antibiotic of choice is ceftriaxone. In case of cephalosporin allergy, clindamycin can be used. As the white cell count is commonly increased in SCD, isolated elevated counts are not indicative of infection. It needs further clinical correlation.[12]

Oxygen Therapy

Oxygen saturation should be monitored and oxygen should be provided by facial mask if the saturation falls below the patient's baseline or <95%.[15] The critical care team should be involved in the care if there are severe features with persistent hypoxia or in a deteriorating patient to consider ventilator support.[12]

Blood Transfusion

Current evidence does not support prophylactic blood transfusion over therapeutic transfusion. Studies have shown no significant difference in the complication rates or the frequency of the crisis with prophylactic blood transfusion.[6] Blood transfusion is indicated in cases of severe complications such as acute chest syndrome, stroke, acute anemia, intractable pain or in multiple pregnancy. Women who are already on long-term transfusion therapy should continue the same frequency during their pregnancy. By limiting the number, patients are less exposed to the inherent risk associated with blood transfusions as described before. The goal of transfusion is to lower the percentage of HbS to <40% and increase the hemoglobin to 10 g/dL.[12] The blood should be ABO blood group compatible, cytomegalovirus negative, HbS negative, and phenotypically matched with C, D, E, and Kell blood groups.[6]

Severe cases such as acute chest syndrome, suspected cerebrovascular disease and multiorgan dysfunction warrant need for exchange transfusion.[3]

Adjuvant Treatments

Sickle cell disease and pregnancy both are independent prothrombotic states and painful crisis further adds to the immobility. Prophylactic thromboprophylaxis with low molecular weight heparin should be prescribed for all the cases unless contraindicated. To counteract the side effects of opiates, antiemetics, laxatives, and antihistamines should also be added.[15]

Physiotherapy such as incentive spirometry can benefit patients with chest or back pain, chest infection, hypoxia, and reduces the risk of atelectasis and acute chest syndrome.[3]

Nonpharmacological avenues for pain management such as cognitive behavioral therapy can teach patients coping strategies during the pain episode. A small number of studies have shown beneficial effects of patient education, cognitive strategies, and biofeedback techniques but there is no exact guidance regarding their application. Local heat pads must be used with caution especially in cases of opioid sedation due to risk of inadvertent burn injury. There is no evidence to support use of other modalities such as transcutaneous electric nerve stimulation, acupressure, or acupuncture.[3]

Fetal Surveillance

Fetal monitoring is an integral part of the management if the fetus is of a viable gestational age. In such cases corticosteroid administration for fetal lung maturity should be considered in view of the increased risk of preterm labor, preterm premature rupture of membranes, and preeclampsia. The fetal well-being assessment can, however, be confounded by the use of opiates for pain relief as they can affect the nonstress testing and the biophysical profile scores. This effect is mostly transient and does not warrant delivery unless there are severe changes such as fetal bradycardia not responsive to intrauterine resuscitative measures.[12] There is no recorded evidence of teratogenicity with therapeutic opioid use in pregnancy but long-term exposure can result in neonatal abstinence syndrome immediately after birth.[15]

■ OTHER ACUTE SYNDROMES

Acute Chest Syndrome

The incidence of acute chest syndrome in pregnancy is 6%.[14] Diagnosis is suspected in case of fever with respiratory symptoms and signs and reduced oxygen saturation. Chest X-ray shows evidence of infiltrate similar to the findings of pneumonia. Management is by the critical care team with antibiotics, respiratory support, and blood transfusion. In cases of severe hypoxia where the hemoglobin levels are in range, exchange transfusion will be required. Another differential diagnosis is pulmonary embolism and thromboprophylaxis should be added.[8]

Acute Stroke

Both types of stroke—hemorrhagic and infarction—are increased in pregnancy with SCD. There should be a low threshold for suspicion if any woman presents with neurological symptoms and urgent MRI brain should be performed. Timely intervention can reduce long-term neurological sequelae in such cases.[14] Management should be guided by neurologists and hematologists as exchange transfusion is needed. Current evidence does not support thrombolysis in cases of infarction due to SCD.[15]

Acute Anemia

Sudden drop in hemoglobin associated with reticulocytopenia is a hallmark of this complication. Parvovirus serology should be sent to determine the cause.[8] The treatment is blood transfusion and isolation measures. Fetal medicine specialist should be a part of the management due to risk of vertical transmission and fetal anemia.[15]

TABLE 1: Medications for pain management in sickle cells crisis.[12]

Drug	Route and dose	Maternal side effect	Fetal effect
Acetaminophen	Oral: 300–1,000 mg every 4–6 h	Nausea, headache, rash, liver dysfunction	Inconsistent reports of childhood asthma and cryptorchidism
Ibuprofen	Oral: 600–800 mg every 6–8 h	Nausea, gastritis, gastrointestinal (GI) bleed, tinnitus	Premature ductal closure
Ketorolac	• Oral: 10 mg every 4–6 h • Parenteral: 30 mg every 6–8 h	Nausea, gastritis, GI bleed, headache	Premature ductal closure
Codeine	Oral: 15–60 mg every 3–6 h	Pruritus, constipation, sedation, respiratory depression	Neonatal abstinence syndrome (NAS)
Morphine	• Oral: 10–30 mg every 3–4 h • Parenteral: 5–10 mg every 2–4 h	Pruritus, constipation, sedation, respiratory depression	NAS
Hydromorphone	• Oral: 7.5 mg every 3–4 h • Parenteral: 1.5 mg every 3–4 h	Pruritus, constipation, sedation, respiratory depression	NAS

PHARMACOLOGICAL CONSIDERATIONS

Table 1 gives a brief summary of the medications used in sickle cell crisis along with their maternal and fetal side effects.

TAKE HOME MESSAGES

- Pregnant women are at risk for complications of SCD such as sickle cell crisis with adverse maternal and fetal implications.
- Sickle cell crisis management should be done by a multidisciplinary team with experience of high risk pregnancies.
- A clear management plan to deal with the painful crisis should be made prospectively and shared with the patient and treating staff.
- Timely assessment for complications, rapid initiation of analgesia, treatment of underlying cause, and supportive measures are the four pillars of management.
- Pregnant women with SCD should be educated regarding the complications along with the preventive measures and coping strategies.

REFERENCES

1. Koshy M. Sickle cell disease and pregnancy. Blood Rev. 1995;9(3):157-64.
2. Jain D, Atmapoojya P, Colah R, Lodha P. Sickle cell disease and pregnancy. Mediterr J Hematol Infect Dis. 2019;11(1):e2019040.
3. Rees DC, Olujohungbe AD, Parker NE, Stephens AD, Telfer P, Wright J, et al. Guidelines for the management of the acute painful crisis in sickle cell disease. Br J Haematol. 2003;120:744-52.
4. Serjeant GR. Sickle cell disease. Lancet. 1997;350(9079):725-30.
5. Colah RB, Mukherjee MB, Martin S, Ghosh K. Sickle cell disease in tribal populations in India. Indian J Med Res. 2015;141(5):509-15.
6. Oteng-Ntim E, Pavord S, Howard R, Robinson S, Oakley L, Mackillop L, et al. Management of sickle cell disease in pregnancy. A British Society for Haematology Guideline. Br J Haematol. 2021;194:980-95.
7. Weatherall DJ, Clegg JB. Inherited haemoglobin disorders: an increasing global

health problem. Bull World Health Organ. 2001;79:704-12.
8. Howard J, Oteng-Ntim E. The obstetric management of sickle cell disease. Best Pract Res. 2012;26(1):25-36.
9. Camous J, N'da A, Etienne-Julan M, Stéphan F. Anesthetic management of pregnant women with sickle cell disease – effect on postnatal sickling complications. Can J Anesth. 2008;55(5):276-83.
10. Oteng-Ntim E, Chase AR, Howard J, Khazaezadeh N, Anionwu EN. Sickle cell disease in pregnancy. Obstet Gynaecol Reproduct Med. 2008;18(10):272-8.
11. Al Jama FE, Gasem T, Burshaid S, Rahman J, Al Suleiman SA, Rahman MS. Pregnancy outcome in patients with homozygous sickle cell disease in a university hospital, Eastern Saudi Arabia. Arch Gynecol Obstet. 2009;280(5):793-7.
12. Marc P, Morrison JC. Sickle cell crisis and pregnancy. Semin Perinatol. 2013;37(4):274-9.
13. Sun PM, Wilburn W, Raynor BD, Jamieson D. Sickle cell disease in pregnancy: twenty years of experience at Grady Memorial Hospital, Atlanta, Georgia. Am J Obstet Gynecol. 2001;184(6):1127-39.
14. Kanda Rogers, Molokie R. Sickle cell disease in pregnancy. Obstet Gynecol Clin North Am. 2010;37(2):223-37.
15. Royal College of Obstetricians and Gynaecologists. Management of Sickle cell disease in pregnancy. RCOG Green Top Guideline No. 61; 2011.

CHAPTER 29

Thalassemia in Pregnancy

Y Subhashini

■ INTRODUCTION

Thalassemias are a group of abnormal hemoglobins (Hb) where there is quantitative defect in the production of alpha and beta chains leading to imbalance and unpaired chains. This leads to hemoglobinopathies, which are autosomal recessive in inheritance.

Alpha thalassemia is caused by reduced production of alpha chains and accumulation of excess beta-like chains. The severity of phenotype increases with loss of one (alpha thalassemia minima), two (alpha thalassemia minor), three (Hb H disease), or four functioning alpha globin alleles (Barts Hb).

Beta thalassemia is currently classified as transfusion dependent beta thalassemia (TDT) (beta thalassemia major, HbE/beta thalassemia, and some beta thalassemia intermedia phenotypes) wherein the genotype may be beta^0/beta^0, beta$^+$/beta^0 or beta$^+$/beta$^+$ with severely reduced beta globin production.

Non-transfusion dependent beta thalassemia (NTDT) (beta thalassemia intermedia) has individuals who are often homozygous or compound heterozygous for a beta thalassemia variant.

Thalassemia's involving delta, gamma, epsilon, and zeta chains are rare and are usually not associated with significant disease outside of the neonatal period.

Age of onset can be in utero in alpha thalassemia and, in beta thalassemia major at around 6 months after birth, as Hb switching happens after birth.

■ EPIDEMIOLOGY

Thalassemia [from the Greek word "Thalassa" (sea)] was named to this group of inherited hemoglobinopathies that arose in certain regions of the world (sub-Saharan Africa, the Asian-Indian subcontinent, Southeast Asia, Mediterranean region) in which typically malaria was found as endemic.[1-4]

Multiple registries and foundations have come into force both nationally and internationally to combat this problem. By July 2018, a total of 149 organizations from 45 countries came together as part of electronic network called ITHANET, which has been striving for dissemination of knowledge, streamline, and maintain collection of data, harmonizing treatment, and coordinate research and prevention programs for hemoglobinopathies.[5]

Worldwide, approximately 1.5% of people are β-thalassemia carriers.[6] This ever-changing epidemiology is due to various reasons such as migration, implementation of β-thalassemia prevention programs, and improved survival rates. The prevalence and carrier rates of β-thalassemia in some of countries in Southeast Asia are as follows. In India, it is 1.25–1.66% and 2.21% in China. Carrier rates are 0.5% in Myanmar 16–12.8% in Malaysia.[4-6]

IMPLICATIONS ON MATERNAL HEALTH

Women with transfusion dependant beta thalassemia presents with severe anemia. The Hb may be as low as 3–4 g/dL. There is typically marked hypochromia and microcytosis, bizarre red blood cell (RBC) morphology, and an increased RBC count. They need multiple blood transfusions and iron chelation therapy for survival. If untreated, this disease progresses to include complications of hemolysis (jaundice, gallstones, and hepatosplenomegaly), extramedullary hematopoiesis (skeletal deformities), iron overload, impaired growth, pulmonary abnormalities, thrombosis, and leg ulcers with a dramatically shortened life expectancy.[7,8]

Women with thalassemia major due to the increasing iron burden may develop new endocrinopathies, in particular, diabetes mellitus, hypothyroidism, and hypoparathyroidism.[9]

In NTDT moderate anemia in range of 7.5–10.5 g/dL is seen. These individuals can develop severe anemia during periods of erythropoietic stress such as infection or pregnancy requiring episodic transfusions. Thalassemia minor and minima are generally clinically silent.

IMPLICATIONS ON FETAL WELL-BEING

Complete lack of alpha chains to pair with gamma chains results in Hb Barts (tetramers of gamma globin) which are fatal and cause death during the late second mid-third trimester of pregnancy unless in utero transfusions are administered. In absence of normal fetal hemoglobin (HbF, alpha2 gamma2), severe anemia occurs during fetal development, with hydrops fetalis. This nonimmune hydrops may cause mirror syndrome in mother, which is equivocally lethal for her.

DIAGNOSIS AND MANAGEMENT

Diagnosis of Thalassemia

A complete blood count (CBC) with RBC indices, which shows an MCV <80 femtoliters (fL) and/or MCH <27 picogram (pg) with elevation in the RBC count in the absence of iron deficiency suggests alpha or beta thalassemia minor and further testing with hemoglobin analysis is indicated to establish a diagnosis.

It is important to note that iron deficiency should be corrected prior to hemoglobin analysis, as in setting of combined iron deficiency and beta thalassemia trait, reports can be falsely normal.

Maternal hemoglobin analysis can be performed either by high-performance liquid chromatography (HPLC) or isoelectric focusing (IEF) **(Table 1)**.

Mentzer's index which is MCV/RBC count <13 also helps in screening thalassemia.

Preconceptual Care

Multidisciplinary team involving hematologist and transfusion specialist and obstetrician should hold combined counseling sessions regarding implications of pregnancy. Prepregnancy folic acid should be initiated to prevent neural tube defects. End organs should be screened for any damage, compliance with chelation therapy and assessment of the body iron burden, and transfusion requirement should be assessed.

Aggressive chelation in the preconception stage is ideal as most of them are teratogenic.

TABLE 1: Electrophoresis patterns in hemoglobinopathies.

	Hb A (α2β2) (%)	Hb A2 (α2δ2) (%)	Hb F (α2γ2) (%)	Hb H (β4) (%)	Hb Barts (γ4) (%)
Normal	>95	2–3	<1	0	0
Alpha thal (0)	0	0	0	<10	>90
Alpha thal major	60–90	2–3	0	5–30	2–5
Alpha thal trait	95	3–4	<1	0	0
Beta thal major	0–5	0–5	>90	0	0
Beta thal intermedia	5–90	0–5	10–90	0	0
Beta thal minor	90–95	3–10	2–3	0	0

(Hb: hemoglobin)

Magnetic resonance imaging (MRI) appears to be superior to measurement of serum ferritin for estimating total body iron burden in these patients.

Deferasirox and deferiprone should ideally be discontinued 3 months before conception and women converted to desferrioxamine iron chelation. Desferrioxamine should be avoided in the first trimester owing to lack of safety data. It has been used safely after 20 weeks of gestation at low doses.[10]

Iron Chelation Indications[11]

- At the same time that a chronic transfusion program is started
- After the serum ferritin exceeds 1,000 ng/mL (1,000 μg/L)
- After the liver iron concentration exceeds 3 mg iron/g of dry weight
- After transfusion of approximately 20–25 units of RBCs.

End-organ Evaluation

Pancreas: Development of diabetes is common hence glycemic control should be well achieved with endocrinologist input. Serum fructosamine level <300 nmol/L for at least 3 months prior to conception is ideal and it is also preferred for monitoring unlike the regular glycosylated Hb (HbA1c) in thalassemia patients.

Thyroid: Euthyroid status should be achieved with thyroid supplementation.

Liver: Ultrasound might detect cholelithiasis and evidence of liver cirrhosis due to iron overload. Liver iron concentration can be checked using a FerriScan or liver T2. The liver iron is recommended to be <7 mg/g (dry weight) preconceptionally to prevent complications.

Bone density scan: Vitamin D level optimization and level of osteoporosis should be documented.

Immunization: Hepatitis B vaccine, *Pneumococcal* and *Haemophilus influenzae* type b vaccination in post-splenectomy women should be completed. Penicillin prophylaxis also is given in low dose to prevent infection in post-splenectomy women.

Rationale for Prenatal Screening, and Fetal Diagnosis

The main purpose of the prenatal hemoglobinopathy screening is to identify

> **BOX 1:** Conditions requiring counseling where the mother is affected by thalassemia.
>
> - Carrier condition in partner
> - Beta thalassemia
> - Delta beta thalassemia
> - Hb E
> - Hb S
> - Hb lepore
> - HbO Arab
> - Hb constant spring
> - Hb C
>
> (Hb: hemoglobin)

asymptomatic mothers whose offspring are at risk of an inherited hemoglobinopathy. Screening should be offered to all couples (**Box 1**) by doing a hemoglobin electrophoresis with hemogram at initial visit.[12]

Thalassemia's and hemoglobin structural variants are autosomal recessive genetic disorders. Parents who are heterozygote carriers of gene mutations that affect the same globin chain have a 25% chance of having an offspring with a hemoglobinopathy. The risk of fetal hemoglobinopathy increases to 50% if one of the parents is homozygous for the gene mutation and the other parent is a carrier. If screening is done prior to pregnancy then well and good, else better to do it in early pregnancy so that fetal diagnosis, if indicated and desired, can be performed when parents have the option of terminating the pregnancy and are considering termination. In cases with homozygous alpha thalassemia fetal diagnosis helps in reforming pregnancy plan of management by changing to close monitoring for development of fetal hydrops, serial fetal transfusions, or joining a clinical trial of in utero stem cell transplantation.

Fetal Testing

Invasive: Deoxyribonucleic acid (DNA)-based testing for hemoglobins S and C and alpha and beta thalassemia can be performed during the first trimester of pregnancy on villi obtained by chorionic villus sampling (typically performed at 10–12 weeks of gestation), or on direct or cultured cells in amniotic fluid cells obtained by amniocentesis (typically performed after 15 weeks of gestation). Celocentesis (ultrasound-guided aspiration of celomic fluid) is another technique for very early prenatal diagnosis of hemoglobinopathy. Although noninvasive prenatal testing is available for alpha and beta thalassemia, validation of this testing is ongoing.[13]

Ultrasound markers can also be used to screen fetuses of couples at risk.[14] The cardiothoracic ratio, placental thickness, and middle cerebral artery-peak systolic velocity (MCA-PSV) are most commonly used. The cardiothoracic ratio appears to be the most effective for detecting fetal alpha thalassemia major during early gestational weeks. A cardiothoracic ratio >0.5 before 17 weeks; a placental thickness >18 mm before 15 weeks or >30 mm at ≥18 weeks or greater than the mean plus 2 standard deviations for gestational age; or MCA-PSV >1.5 multiples of the median (MoM) for the gestational age after 15 weeks is suggestive of an affected fetus.[14]

Antenatal Care

Individualized plan should be chalked according to type of thalassemia and depending on the iron overload and comorbidities present. In first trimester folic acid supplementation and fetal evaluation by combined screening for aneuploidies and dietary counseling for balanced diet should be done. In post-splenectomy women with thrombocytosis of >6 lakhs low dose aspirin 75 mg/day should be commenced as antenatal thromboprophylaxis. Low molecular weight heparin is added in such mothers during period of inpatient monitoring. During second trimester iron deficiency if present in thalassemia trait, needs to be corrected after checking iron stores by oral therapy. Parenteral iron is better avoided in beta thalassemia. Targeted scan for fetal anomalies is performed at 19–20 weeks.

Monthly visits are planned till 28 weeks and there after visits every 2 weeks are planned. Fetal monitoring is done by ultrasound and serial symphysiofundal height measurement. All women with thalassemia major should be receiving blood transfusions on a regular basis aiming for a pretransfusion hemoglobin of 10 g/dL. The decision to transfuse is taken if there is worsening maternal anemia or evidence of fetal growth restriction. Mothers with cardiac dysfunction and diabetes are called for closer check-ups. At 28 weeks cardiac status of thalassemia major mother needs to be rechecked by 2D echo, electrocardiogram (ECG) with a cardiologist.

Chelation by low-dose subcutaneous desferrioxamine (20 mg/kg/day) on a minimum of 4–5 days a week under joint hematology and cardiology guidance is initiated from 20 to 24 weeks of gestation in mothers with signs of cardiac decompensation in myocardial iron overload or if liver iron >15 mg/g dry weight as measured by MRI.

Intrapartum Care

In thalassemia trait mothers, spontaneous onset of labor is awaited till 40^{+6} week. In thalassemia major timing of delivery must be individualized based on maternal hemodynamic condition and presence or absence of fetal growth restriction. Crossmatched blood (to prevent alloimmunization due to presence of red cell antibodies) should be reserved as soon as mother is admitted for delivery. Continuous intrapartum electronic fetal monitoring should be done. Active management of the third stage of labor is recommended to minimize blood loss. Peripartum chelation therapy (intravenous desferrioxamine 2 g over 24 hours during labor) is recommended in mothers who are transfusion-dependent and not on a chelating agent. Cesarean section is done for obstetric and fetal indications only. In view of maxillofacial deformities and difficult airway in TDT mothers, it is desirable to use epidural anesthesia.

Postpartum Care

Low-molecular-weight heparin should be administered for 7 days post-discharge following vaginal delivery or for 6 weeks following cesarean section. Exclusive breastfeeding is encouraged. Desferrioxamine is secreted in breast milk but is not orally absorbed and therefore safe to the new born and should be immediately started in transfusion dependent thalassemia mothers and compliance must be stressed. Bisphosphonates to be restarted after breastfeeding period is over.

Contraception with progesterone only pills and barrier methods are appropriate as intrauterine devices carry risk of infection and estrogen-containing birth control pills increase the risk of thromboembolism.

Pharmacological Interventions

Iron chelation drug in pregnancy preferred is low-dose subcutaneous desferrioxamine and should be started 20 mg/kg/day for a minimum of 4–5 days a week under joint supervision of hematologist and transfusion specialist from 20 to 24 weeks of gestation.

Thalassemia patients can have pain related to osteoporosis, splenomegaly or related to expansion of the bone marrow space due to ineffective erythropoiesis-induced erythroid expansion. Paracetamol or other opioid drugs such as tramadol, fentanyl, or pethidine can be offered for analgesia in pregnancy.

In mild-to-moderate anemia, oral ferrous sulfate formulations along with folic acid supplementation can be given to improve the hemoglobin status. Routine calcium and vitamin D supplementations should be continued.

Switching over to heparin for antenatal thromboprophylaxis if already on warfarin is recommended. Starting insulin helps in tighter glycemic control in pregnancy in comparison to oral hypoglycemic agent.

Luspatercept (previously called ACE-536) is a subcutaneous agent that improves RBC maturation was approved for the treatment of adults with transfusion-dependent beta-thalassemia in November 2019. It is given at 1–1.5 mg/kg subcutaneously once every 3 weeks. It was seen to reduce the need of transfusions by one-third but cannot be given in preconceptional period and in pregnancy as it is teratogenic.

■ CONCLUSION

Thalassemia syndromes are hereditary disorders with multiorgan involvement. Well organized and well resourced health services and emerging new therapies such as genetic interventions are beneficial for secondary prevention of the disease.

TAKE HOME MESSAGES

- Comorbidities found in beta thalassemia[15] are osteoporosis—23%. Extramedullary hematopoiesis (radiologic evidence)—21%, hypogonadism—17%, cholelithiasis (by ultrasound)—17%, thrombosis—14%, pulmonary hypertension—11%, abnormal liver function—10%, leg ulcers—8%, hypothyroidism—6%, heart failure—4%, and diabetes mellitus—2%.
- American College of Obstetricians and Gynecologists (ACOG) in 2007 stated that women with beta thalassemia major should only pursue pregnancy if they have normal cardiac function and have undergone chronic transfusion therapy with iron chelation.[16]
- When blood is requested, the blood bank should be made aware that the patient has thalassemia so that extra care can be taken and matching for Rh antigens other than RhD, such as C and E, and Kell are done which prevents alloimmunization. Red cell antibody titers should be measured along with full blood group and ABO in these patients.
- All pregnant women should be screened for hemoglobinopathies. The purpose of screening is to identify asymptomatic couples whose future offspring or current pregnancy is at high risk of an inherited hemoglobinopathy.
- Deoxyribonucleic acid-based definitive testing for fetal hemoglobinopathies should be offered during pregnancy by chorionic villus sampling at 10–12 weeks of gestation or on direct or cultured amniotic fluid cells obtained by amniocentesis (typically performed after 15 weeks of gestation) in cases where both partners are carriers of abnormal hemoglobins.
- Pregnancy in TDT has high risk of complications and multidisciplinary care in a tertiary level hospital improves outcomes.

■ REFERENCES

1. UpToDate. (2022). Diagnosis of thalassemia (adults and children). [online] Available from: https://www.uptodate.com/contents/

diagnosis-of-thalassemia-adults-and-children [Last accessed February, 2023].
2. Weatherall DJ. The definition and epidemiology of non-transfusion-dependent thalassemia. Blood Rev. 2012;26 Suppl 1:S3-6.
3. Vichinsky EP. Changing patterns of thalassemia worldwide. Ann N Y Acad Sci. 2005;1054(1):18-24.
4. Taher AT, Musallam KM, Cappellini MD. β-thalassemias. N Engl J Med. 2021; 384(8):727-43.
5. Kountouris P, Lederer CW, Fanis P, Feleki X, Old J, Kleanthous M. IthaGenes: an interactive database for haemoglobin variations and epidemiology. PloS One. 2014;9(7): e103020.
6. Colah R, Gorakshakar A, Nadkarni A. Global burden, distribution and prevention of β-thalassemias and hemoglobin E disorders. Expert Rev Hematol. 2010;3(1):103-17.
7. Modell B, Khan M, Darlison M. Survival in β-thalassaemia major in the UK: data from the UK Thalassaemia Register. Lancet. 2000;355(9220):2051-2.
8. Voskaridou E, Kattamis A, Fragodimitri C, Kourakli A, Chalkia P, Diamantidis M, et al. National registry of hemoglobinopathies in Greece: updated demographics, current trends in affected births, and causes of mortality. Ann Hematol. 201998(1):55-66.
9. Jackson LA, Hill QA, Ciantar E. The management of haemoglobinopathies in pregnancy and childbirth. Obstet Gynaecol. 2022;24(2):109-18.
10. Singer ST, Vichinsky EP. Deferoxamine treatment during pregnancy: is it harmful?. Am J Hematol. 1999;60(1):24-6.
11. Angelucci E, Barosi G, Camaschella C, Cappellini MD, Cazzola M, Galanello R, et al. Italian Society of Hematology practice guidelines for the management of iron overload in thalassemia major and related disorders. Haematologica. 2008;93(5): 741-52.
12. Committee on Genetics. Committee Opinion No. 691: Carrier Screening for Genetic Conditions. Obstet Gynecol. 2017;129:e41. Reaffirmed 2019.
13. Shaw J, Scotchman E, Chandler N, Chitty LS. Preimplantation genetic testing: non-invasive prenatal testing for aneuploidy, copy-number variants and single-gene disorders. Reproduction. 2020;160(5):A1-1.
14. Li X, Zhou Q, Zhang M, Tian X, Zhao Y. Sonographic markers of fetal α-thalassemia major. J Ultrasound Med. 2015;34(2): 197-206.
15. Taher AT, Musallam KM, Karimi M, El-Beshlawy A, Belhoul K, Daar S, et al. Overview on practices in thalassemia intermedia management aiming for lowering complication rates across a region of endemicity: the OPTIMAL CARE study. Blood. 2010;11;115(10):1886-92.
16. ACOG Committee on Obstetrics AC. ACOG Practice Bulletin No. 78: hemoglobinopathies in pregnancy. Obstet Gynecol. 2007;109(1):229-37.

CHAPTER 30

Thrombocytopenia in Pregnancy

Venigalla Rama

■ INTRODUCTION

Platelets are involved in both primary and secondary hemostasis. The normal platelet count in pregnancy is 150–400 × 10^9/L. Thrombocytopenia is defined as platelet count <150 × 10^9/L. Platelet count is arbitrarily classified as mild, if the count is 100–150 × 10^9/L, moderate if 50–100 × 10^9, and severe if <50 × 10^9/L. Thrombocytopenia may be due to an increased destruction/consumption of platelets, hemodilution or rarely also due to reduced production. Thrombocytopenia is often an incidental feature of pregnancy, but it could also be a marker of an underlying systemic or gestational disorder. It is important not only to determine the pathophysiology of thrombocytopenia, but also the associated risk to the mother and fetus. Treatment goals change with the time of diagnosis and the stage of pregnancy, especially close to delivery.[1,2]

This chapter reviews the approach to thrombocytopenia in pregnancy, maternal and neonatal implications, and their management.

■ EPIDEMIOLOGY AND MAGNITUDE OF THE PROBLEM

Thrombocytopenia is the second most common cause of hematologic abnormality encountered during pregnancy after anemia.[3] There is a reduction in the platelet count by 10% at term in all pregnancies. Platelet counts <100 × 10^9/L are seen only in 1% of pregnancies.[4] The physiological thrombocytopenia is mild and has no deleterious effects on the mother or fetus. But, a significant thrombocytopenia in the background of any medical conditions may have adverse effects on both mother and fetus and needs monitoring and timely management.

A low platelet count is seen in 8–10% of all pregnancies. Almost 75% of these cases are due to benign condition of gestational thrombocytopenia (GT); 15–20% may be associated with hypertensive disorders; 3–4% are due to immune process; and the remaining 1–2% can be attributed to rare constitutional thrombocytopenia, infections, and hematological malignancies.[1]

Platelet counts of <100 × 10^9/L need further investigation to determine a cause other than GT. Platelet counts between 100 and 150 × 10^9/L at any time during pregnancy, including the first trimester, likely have GT and may not need further evaluation.[4]

■ ETIOLOGY

The causes of thrombocytopenia are listed in **Table 1** and are elaborated in the next sections.

TABLE 1: Etiology of thrombocytopenia.

	Isolated thrombocytopenia	Thrombocytopenia secondary to systemic disorders
Pregnancy related	Gestational thrombocytopenia (GT: 70–80%)	Severe preeclampsia (15–20%) hemolysis, elevated liver enzymes, and low platelets (HELLP) syndrome (<1%)
Pregnancy unrelated	• Primary immune thrombocytopenia (ITP: 1–4%) • Secondary ITP (<1%) • Drug-induced thrombocytopenia • Type IIB von Willebrand disease (vWD) • Congenital thrombocytopenia	• Thrombotic thrombocytopenic purpura (TTP) • Hemolytic uremic syndrome (HUS) • Acute fatty liver of pregnancy (AFLP) • Systemic lupus erythematosus • Antiphospholipid syndrome • Viral infections • Bone marrow disorders • Nutritional deficiency • Splenic sequestration (liver diseases, portal vein thrombosis, storage disease, etc.) • Thyroid disorders

Causes of thrombocytopenia may be specific to pregnancy or may be unrelated to pregnancy per se, though some may occur more frequently during pregnancy.[3]

EVALUATION OF THROMBOCYTOPENIA

Many cases of thrombocytopenia in pregnancy require urgent evaluation in determining the cause and management decisions, delaying which may result in complications for the mother and the fetus. The diagnostic evaluation and interventions most of the times must be performed simultaneously. Early involvement of maternal-fetal medicine experts, hematologists, and other appropriate specialists (like nephrologist in the presence of renal failure; infectious disease specialist in suspected sepsis) is advised.

The evaluation of woman with thrombocytopenia depends on clinical history, clinical signs, and symptoms. History taking involves enquiring about the onset with respect to the trimester of pregnancy, whether new onset or chronic, presence of any mucosal bleeds, abnormal uterine bleeding, fever, medication use (frusemide, ranitidine, heparin), presence of coexisting malignancies, infections such as HIV (human immunodeficiency virus), hepatitis B, and hepatitis C virus (HCV). History of travel to endemic areas for infections such as dengue must also be recorded. Presence of symptoms for hypertensive disorders in pregnancy must be looked for.

A thorough clinical examination, for presence of fever, high blood pressure, lymphadenopathy, signs of mucosal/conjunctival hemorrhages, cardiac murmurs, organomegaly, and any signs of thrombosis should be looked for.

Table 2 shows the tests recommended by American Society of Hematology for the diagnosis of thrombocytopenia.[5]

A peripheral blood smear examination can help rule out pseudothrombocytopenia, which is recognized by platelet clumping. This can be avoided by using a citrated sample.

MATERNAL AND NEONATAL IMPLICATIONS AND THEIR MANAGEMENT

The most likely causes of thrombocytopenia in the 1st and 2nd trimester are immune

TABLE 2: Laboratory tests for thrombocytopenia.		
Recommended	Tests to be considered if clinically indicated	Tests not recommended
• Complete blood picture • Peripheral smear examination • Reticulocyte count • Liver function tests • Viral screening (HIV, hepatitis B, hepatitis C)	• Antiphospholipid antibodies • Thyroid function test • Anti-nuclear antibodies • Disseminated intravascular coagulation (DIC) testing—PT, aPTT, fibrinogen, fibrin degraded products • vWD type 2b testing • Direct antiglobulin (Coombs) test • *Helicobacter pylori* (*H. pylori*) testing • Quantitative immunoglobulin levels	• Antiplatelet antibody testing • Bone marrow biopsy • Thrombopoietin (TPO) levels

(HIV: human immunodeficiency virus; vWD: von Willebrand disease)

thrombocytopenia (ITP) and GT in the absence of history of drug intake or medical disorders. Usually, platelet count between 100×10^9/L and 149×10^9/L in an asymptomatic pregnant woman with no bleeding episodes is GT. Platelet count of $<100 \times 10^9$/L is suggestive of ITP and that <50,000/L is almost definitely ITP. In the 3rd trimester or immediate postpartum, sudden onset significant thrombocytopenia should raise the suspicion of preeclampsia, hemolytic uremic syndrome (HUS), thrombotic thrombocytopenic purpura (TTP), disseminated intravascular coagulation (DIC), or acute fatty liver of pregnancy (AFLP).[6]

GESTATIONAL THROMBOCYTOPENIA

Gestational thrombocytopenia or incidental thrombocytopenia, affects 4.4–11.6% of pregnancies. It is more common in mid-second and third trimester. Postulated mechanisms include hemodilution and accelerated platelet clearance. Usually, the platelet count is between 120×10^9/L and 149×10^9/L, platelet count between 50×10^9/L and 100×10^9/L are see in 1–5% of women. Counts $<50 \times 10^9$/L are seen rarely. Women with GT are asymptomatic, it is a diagnosis of exclusion and does not require any evaluation or treatment. Fetal thrombocytopenia is seen in <2% cases.[2] Women can be allowed to go into spontaneous labor at term. Epidural for labor analgesia can be offered if platelet count is $>70 \times 10^9$/L.[7] Cesarean section is reserved for obstetric indications. When the platelet counts are $<80 \times 10^9$, fetal scalp electrode/sampling and high/mid cavity instrumental delivery are to be avoided. Cord blood sample and neonatal day 1 and 4 samples to be checked for neonatal thrombocytopenia. GT resolves usually within 1–2 months of delivery. If the counts fail to return to normal level after 2 months of delivery evaluation for cause of thrombocytopenia is warranted. Risk of recurrence is said to be 14-fold.[1,2]

PREECLAMPSIA AND HEMOLYSIS, ELEVATED LIVER ENZYMES, AND LOW PLATELETS SYNDROME

Preeclampsia is a multisystem disorder, with systolic blood pressure at ≥140 mm Hg and/or diastolic blood pressure at ≥90 mm Hg on at least two occasions measured 4 hours apart in previously normotensive women at or after 20 weeks of gestation and accompanied by ≥1 of proteinuria, maternal organ dysfunction, and/or uteroplacental dysfunction. Thrombocytopenia is seen in 15% of women with preeclampsia out of which <5% have severe thrombocytopenia.[1,7,8]

Hemolysis, elevated liver enzymes, and low platelets (HELLP) syndrome is characterized by hemolysis, elevated liver enzymes, and low platelet count. It most commonly occurs in 3rd trimester and worsens in the initial 24–48 hours postpartum period. It is complicated by DIC in 20% and abruptio placenta in 16% of cases. Delivery is recommended when diagnosed at or after 34 weeks, after maternal stabilization. Mode of delivery is based on obstetric considerations. Platelet transfusion is recommended if the patient is undergoing cesarean and platelet count is $<50 \times 10^9$/L. Aggressive management with fresh frozen plasma with or without cryoprecipitate is needed if complicated by DIC. Neonatal thrombocytopenia is seen in 1.8% cases.[1,6]

■ IMMUNE THROMBOCYTOPENIA

Immune thrombocytopenia is an autoimmune disorder characterized by antiplatelet antibodies resulting in increased platelet destruction and reduced production. These antibodies cross the placenta and result in neonatal thrombocytopenia. It is the most common cause of severe thrombocytopenia in pregnancy ($<50 \times 10^9$/L) especially in 1st and 2nd trimester. Ideally women with ITP should have preconception counseling to review the history, previous treatments and their response, need for change of medications and vaccination status against *Haemophilus influenzae, Pneumococcus,* and *Meningococcus* in splenectomized patients. ITP itself is not a contraindication for pregnancy and there is no data on the baseline platelet count to embark on pregnancy. Need for multidisciplinary care involving maternal-fetal medicine specialist, hematologist, and anesthesiologist has to be explained. Platelet counts can be monitored 2–4 weekly in mild thrombocytopenia, if platelet count is $<80 \times 10^9$/L weekly monitoring is recommended beyond 34 weeks.[9] In an asymptomatic patient treatment is not required if platelet count is between 20 and 30×10^9/L. Treatment is recommended for women with counts $<20 \times 10^9$ or symptomatic or when close to delivery as a platelet count of 50×10^9 is recommended for delivery. A total of 15–35% women require treatment before onset of labor.[10]

Initial Treatment: Oral Corticosteroids or Intravenous Immunoglobulin

- Prednisolone 20 mg/day recommended and later adjusted to minimum dose, response is seen in 4–14 days with peak in 1–4 weeks.
- Intravenous immunoglobulin (IVIG) 0.4 g/kg/day for 5 days or 1 g/kg/day for 2 days, response is seen in 1–3 days and usually lasts for 1–3 weeks, hence delivery can be considered during this period if necessary.
- When available IV anti-D can be tried in Rh (D) positive nonsplenectomized women, but risk of maternal and neonatal hemolysis to be kept in mind.

Immune Thrombocytopenia Failing Initial Treatment with Single Agent

- Combination therapy with high dose methylprednisolone with IVIG/azathioprine.

- Rituximab can be tried in severe cases. Complications of which include prenatal and immunosuppression and risk of infection.
- Thrombopoietin receptor antagonists (TPA-RAs)—romiplostim and eltrombopag, to be considered when other treatments fail, used in 3rd trimester close to delivery. Romiplostim is preferred due to limited safety database and lesser off target effects.
- Splenectomy in 2nd trimester.

Drugs contraindicated include mycophenolate mofetil, cyclophosphamide, vinca alkaloids, and danazol.[5]

Platelet transfusions are indicated:
- If the platelet count is $<20 \times 10^9$/L or severe bleeding
- To maintain platelet count of 30×10^9/L for vaginal delivery
- To maintain platelet count 50×10^9/L for cesarean section.[11]

Women with ITP can carry pregnancy to term. Induction of labor and cesarean section are to be considered for obstetric indications. Regional axial anesthesia can be given at a platelet count of 70×10^9/L. Procedures such as fetal scalp electrode/blood sampling, ventouse or rotational forceps delivery to be avoided as they increase hemorrhagic risk to the fetus. Nonsteroidal anti-inflammatory drugs (NSAIDs) should be avoided if platelet count is $<70 \times 10^9$/L. Women at risk for thromboembolism should receive anticoagulation with caution.[6,9]

Neonatal thrombocytopenia is seen in 10–15% cases. Cord blood sample should be collected at delivery for platelet count. At birth, if platelet count is $<50 \times 10^9$/L, cranial ultrasound is indicated. IVIG is recommended if intracranial hemorrhage is detected. Previous baby with thrombocytopenia is the only reliable predictor for neonatal thrombocytopenia currently.[10]

THROMBOTIC MICROANGIOPATHIES

Thrombotic microangiopathies (TMA) can be pregnancy specific like preeclampsia and HELLP syndrome or pregnancy nonspecific like TTP and HUS. Both the conditions are associated with poor neonatal outcome in view of extensive placental ischemia.

Thrombotic thrombocytopenic purpura complicates one in 25,000 pregnancies, it is caused due to deficiency of ADAMTS 13, which is von Willebrand factor—cleaving protein resulting in formation of microthrombi in various organs, microangiopathic hemolytic anemia, and thrombocytopenia. High index of suspicion and urgent plasmapheresis is the treatment of choice. TTP has a recurrence risk of 50% in subsequent pregnancy.[1,2]

ANTICOAGULATION IN HEPATIN-INDUCED THROMBOCYTOPENIA

It is rare in pregnancy accounting for <0.1%. It is a potential life-threatening complication associated with use of heparin treatment. It occurs due to autoantibody directed against platelet factor 4 (PF4) in complex with heparin. Management includes immediate cessation of heparin and changing over to nonheparin anticoagulant, to reduce the risk of thrombosis by about 50%. Alternatives which can be used are danaparoid and fondaparinux. Danaparoid and Fondaparinux can be monitored by specific anti-Xa activity and can be given subcutaneously or intravenously. There is limited information on the use of all of these drugs in pregnancy. Fondaparinux appears to be as safer can be used in pregnancy. Limited information about the use of argatroban and bivalirudin in pregnancy refrains their use in pregnancy.[12]

CONCLUSION AND RECOMMENDATIONS

- Complete blood picture with peripheral smear is important in every trimester to diagnose an underlying ITP.
- Platelet count between 100 and 149 × 10^9/L in an asymptomatic pregnant women is most likely GT and requires no further treatment. Platelet count should be repeated after 2 months of delivery and if thrombocytopenia is persistent, further evaluation and follow-up with hematologist is recommended.
- Women with ITP should have pre-pregnancy counseling. Treatment in pregnancy is indicated if platelet count is <20 × 10^9/L or bleeding episodes or in severe thrombocytopenia close to delivery.
- Platelet counts of 30 × 10^9/L, 50 × 10^9/L, and 70 × 10^9 are recommended for vaginal delivery, cesarean section, and neuraxial anesthesia respectively.
- Invasive fetal monitoring, ventouse/rotational forceps delivery to be avoided if platelet counts are <80 × 10^9/L.
- Neonates should be monitored for neonatal thrombocytopenia by serial platelet count monitoring.

REFERENCES

1. Myers B. Thrombocytopenia in pregnancy. Obstetrician Gynaecologist. 2009;11:177-83.
2. Cines DB, Levine LD. Thrombocytopenia in pregnancy. Blood. 2017;130(21):2271-7.
3. Gernsheimer T, James AH, Stasi R. How I treat thrombocytopenia in pregnancy. Blood. 2013;121(1):38-47.
4. Reese JA, Peck JD, Deschamps DR, McIntosh JJ, Knudtson EJ, Terrell DR, et al. Platelet Counts during Pregnancy. N Engl J Med. 2018;379:32-43.
5. Rajasekhar A, Gernsheimer T, Stasi R, James AH. 2013 Clinical Practice Guide on Thrombocytopenia in Pregnancy. Washington, DC: American Society of Hematology; 2013.
6. ACOG Practical Bulletin Number 207: Thrombocytopenia in pregnancy. Obstet Gynecol. 2019;133(3):e181-93.
7. Gestational Hypertension and Preeclampsia: ACOG Practice Bulletin, Number 222. Obstet Gynecol. 2020;135(6):e237-60.
8. Brown MA, Magee LA, Kenny LC, Karumanchi SA, McCarthy FP, Saito S, et al. The hypertensive disorders of pregnancy: ISSHP classification, diagnosis and management recommendations for international practice. Pregnancy Hypertens. 2018;13:291-310.
9. Baucom AM, Kuller JA, Dotters-Katz S. Immune thrombocytopenic purpura in pregnancy. Obstet Gynecol Surv. 2019;74(8):490-6.
10. Provan D, Arnold DM, Bussel JB, Chong BH, Cooper N, Gernsheimer T, et al. Updated international consensus report on the investigation and management of primary immune thrombocytopenia. Blood Adv. 2019;3(22):3780-817.
11. Yuan S, Otrock ZK. Platelet transfusion: An update on indications and guidelines. Clin Lab Med. 2021;41(4):621-34.
12. Mauermann E, Vökt C, Tsakiris DA, Tobler D, Girard T. Heparin-induced thrombocytopenia in pregnancy: an interdisciplinary challenge—a case report and literature review. Int J Obstet Anesth. 2016;26:79-82.

Transplant Medicine

CHAPTER 31

Transplant Recipients

Malini Sukayogula

■ INTRODUCTION

The number of women considering pregnancy after solid organ transplantation is increasing as is the number of women who are receiving transplantation. Successful pregnancy outcomes in these women are possible with good care during preconception, antenatal, intrapartum, and postpartum periods.

■ MAGNITUDE OF THE PROBLEM

As per the data collected and analyzed by Transplant Pregnancy Registry International (TPRI) till 31st December 2020, there were 3,433 pregnancies in 1909 female organ transplant recipients with 3,555 outcomes (including multifetal gestations).[1]

Of these, 2,270 (66%) pregnancies were reported in 1,279 kidney transplant recipients and 724 pregnancies in 366 liver transplant recipients. Outcomes of 1,413 pregnancies fathered by 901 male transplant receipts are also documented.[1]

■ PRECONCEPTION COUNSELING

Counseling should begin ideally in the pretransplant period and continue after the transplant surgery. Obstetric considerations should be a part of pretransplant counseling and involve a return to fertility and the risks associated with an unplanned pregnancy. Discussion should also involve contraceptive options and optimal timing for conception. Both the transplant recipient and her partner should be involved in the counseling. Original disease should be considered, along with its risk of recurrence, and any pregnancy-associated comorbidities (e.g., uncontrolled diabetes adversely affecting pregnancy outcomes and antibody profile in lupus impacting the pregnancy). Delaying pregnancy for 1 year after transplantation improves maternal and fetal outcomes.[2]

American Society of Transplantation (AST) recommends that pregnancy can be safely contemplated when:
- There is no graft rejection within the past year
- Adequate and stable graft function
- There is no acute infection that may affect the fetus
- Maintenance immunosuppression in stable dosing.

A review of medications must be done, including the immunosuppressant regimen and change over to pregnancy-safe medication must be done at least 6 weeks–3 months before planning conception.[1,3] Screening and appropriate treatment of infections especially cytomegalovirus (CMV), and herpes simplex virus (HSV) should be done. Vaccination status should be checked and inactivated vaccines administered after 3–6 months of transplantation (vaccination may not generate adequate immune response during the period of intense immune suppression). Vaccination against hepatitis B virus, tetanus, and influenza can be given.[4]

■ CONTRACEPTION

Contraception should be initiated early after transplant surgery. Return of fertility and menstruation is seen as early as in the first month after transplant.

In women with uncomplicated solid organ transplants, all modes of contraception are in medical eligibility criteria (MEC) category 2 (benefits outweigh risks).

In women with complicated solid organ transplants, where there is an increased risk of graft failure, rejection or vasculopathy, estrogen-containing contraceptives are considered category 4 (having unacceptable health risk). Long-acting reversible contraceptives (LARC) – intrauterine contraceptive devices (copper-containing or progesterone-containing) are in category 3 (risks outweigh benefits) for initiation of the method, and category 2 for the continuation of the method. Progesterone-containing implants and depot medroxyprogesterone acetate (DMPA) are MEC category 2.

It is important to consider the following before prescribing a contraceptive method:
- The type of organ transplanted
- Potential interactions between the contraceptive and immunosuppressive agents
- Underlying medical comorbidities of the patient.[5,6]

■ IMMUNOSUPPRESSION

Immunosuppression medications should be reviewed by the transplant team and obstetrician before planning conception. The potential risks and benefits to the fetus as well as the allograft and any need for change in medication have to be addressed. Most of the medications used are not known to cause an increase in the incidence of birth defects. These include prednisone, azathioprine, cyclosporine, and tacrolimus.

Mycophenolate mofetil (MMF) and mycophenolic acid (MPA) exposure is associated with increased incidence of nonviable outcomes and structural anomalies. The pattern of birth defects includes microtia, cleft palate, and esophageal, cardiac, and renal anomalies.[7] A 6 weeks–3-month interval is advised before conception to allow conversion to a pregnancy-safe alternative and ensure stable disease and allograft function.[1,8]

Azathioprine is usually substituted for MMF. Azathioprine is metabolized to its active form—6-mercaptopurine, which is transported to the fetus, but, the fetal liver lacks the enzyme inosinate pyrophosphorylase that converts 6-mercaptopurine to thioinosinic acid. Hence, the fetus is protected from the harmful effects. It is advisable to monitor cell counts and liver function tests when a patient is on azathioprine.

Cyclosporine increases the production of thromboxane and endothelin, thus increasing vascular resistance and is implicated in the pathogenesis of preeclampsia and fetal growth restriction.

Calcineurin inhibitors (tacrolimus) trough level monitoring in pregnancy and adjustment of dosage are needed. Women on corticosteroids and tacrolimus must be screened for diabetes.

Sirolimus exposure during pregnancy does not appear to be associated with an increased incidence of birth defects. Data is limited regarding the safety of everolimus and belatacept in pregnancy and hence these are better avoided in pregnancy.[1,3] Benefits of eculizumab in pregnancy for organ-threatening diseases are likely to outweigh the risk.[8]

■ RENAL TRANSPLANT

Transplant Pregnancy Registry International 2020 annual report studied outcomes of 2,233 pregnancies with 2,318 outcomes (including multiples) in 1,251 female renal transplant recipients. Of these, 30% of pregnancies were unplanned. Preeclampsia was seen in 29%, and acute rejection was seen in 3%. Graft loss was seen in 5.4% within 2 years of delivery. The live birth rate was 75%, 19% had miscarriages and 2% had stillbirths. Preterm deliveries between 28 and 32 weeks were seen in 6% and 37% between 32 and 37 weeks. Low birth weight babies (<2,500 g) were 52%. Birth defects were seen in 4.6%.[1]

Prepregnancy Counseling

Conception is ideally dissuaded within the first year of transplant where the immunosuppressant medications are in high doses and graft function is difficult to assess.

Stable graft function for 1 year, well-controlled hypertension, serum creatinine <1.5 mg/dL, and nil or minimal proteinuria (<500 mg/24 hours) are associated with successful outcomes. The etiology of renal disease and comorbidities (diabetes and hypertension) also influence the outcomes. Inheritable diseases such as adult polycystic kidney disease need genetic counseling.

Immunosuppressants and antihypertensive medications should be changed to pregnancy-safe drugs. Angiotensin converting enzyme (ACE) inhibitors and angiotensin receptor blockers (ARB) are contraindicated in pregnancy. In women with significant proteinuria, these drugs can be stopped when the urine pregnancy test is positive.[3]

Effects of Renal Transplantation on Pregnancy

Pregnancy outcomes depend on the renal function, presence of hypertension, and proteinuria.

Hypertension is present prepregnancy in >50% of renal transplant recipients. An additional 16% who were normotensive before pregnancy need treatment for hypertension in pregnancy.[9] Increased rates of superimposed preeclampsia, fetal growth restriction, preterm birth, and neonatal intensive care admissions are associated with hypertension.[3,10]

The presence of proteinuria >500 mg/day is associated with adverse outcomes. Quantification of proteinuria early in pregnancy is a good practice point to help in the diagnosis of superimposed preeclampsia in later gestations.

Calcineurin inhibitors and corticosteroids predispose to gestational diabetes.

Increased rates of cesarean section are observed compared to the normal pregnant population. However, a renal transplant is not a contraindication for vaginal birth.[1]

Effect of Pregnancy on Allograft Function

Renal allografts can adapt to the physiological changes of pregnancy. An increase in creatinine clearance of approximately 30% is seen in the first trimester, with a small decrease in the second trimester and returns to prepregnancy level during the third trimester.[10,11]

Up to 20% increase in serum creatinine is seen in 38% of women with renal transplants and the most common cause for this is preeclampsia.

Acute graft rejection occurs during pregnancy in <2% of renal transplant recipients.[1,9] If graft rejection is suspected, a kidney biopsy should be undertaken.

The features of acute rejection include:
- Deteriorating renal function
- Fever
- Oliguria
- Graft swelling and tenderness
- Altered echogenicity of renal parenchyma and blurring of corticomedullary.[10]

Graft biopsy is technically easy compared to native renal biopsy, which is often performed in a prone position. Transplant rejection can be treated in pregnancy with the optimization of corticosteroids and tacrolimus and cycloserine. Biologic agents have been used in the treatment of rejection episodes. They are actively transported to the baby across the placenta.[3,12]

Antenatal Management

Women should receive multidisciplinary care, comprising of an experienced obstetrician, and a transplant team. In addition to routine investigations, renal function tests, urine routine and microscopy, urine for culture and sensitivity should be done. Proteinuria should always be quantified.

Monitoring of renal function must be done not less than monthly and frequency is influenced by the severity of renal dysfunction and the presence of hypertension.

The differential diagnosis of declining renal function includes:
- Reversible causes such as urinary tract infection, dehydration, and obstruction
- Preeclampsia
- Calcineurin inhibitor toxicity
- Acute and/or chronic rejection.[10]

Treatment with erythropoietin stimulating agents in pregnancy must be considered in iron-replete anemic women.[8]

Screening for gestational diabetes should be done early in pregnancy (16 weeks) and the test repeated at 24–28 weeks if the initial screening is negative.

Calcineurin inhibitor trough levels must be monitored at least monthly and the dose should be adjusted. Care should be taken to avoid medications that interfere with calcineurin inhibitor metabolism (erythromycin and clarithromycin).[8]

Screening for Infections

Urinary tract infections should be screened with urine for culture and sensitivity every trimester and aggressively treated.

Cytomegalovirus infection: Primary infection during pregnancy has a 40–50% transmission to the fetus. Among these, 5–18% are symptomatic at birth. Amniotic fluid culture/polymerase chain reaction (PCR) should be done to diagnose fetal infection. There are no guidelines regarding treatment with ganciclovir/CMV hyperimmune globulin to prevent fetal infection.[11]

Diagnosis of Preeclampsia

More than half the pregnant renal transplant patients have hypertension as well as proteinuria prepregnancy. Diagnosis of preeclampsia in such a cohort is difficult. New onset proteinuria after 20 weeks points to the diagnosis when there is no proteinuria in early pregnancy. An increase in blood pressure to >160/110 mm Hg, or a need to increase the treatment to maintain blood pressure to <160/110 mm Hg, or an increase in proteinuria, elevated transaminases, and low platelet count may aid the diagnosis. Low levels of placental growth factor can be considered a marker for preeclampsia as its levels are not affected by renal dysfunction.[13]

The decision to deliver in cases of severe preeclampsia is determined by the maternal condition, gestational age, and fetal growth. Magnesium sulfate can be used both for maternal and fetal indications. A loading dose of 4 g can be given irrespective of renal function, but the maintenance dose is based on maternal renal impairment and urine output. One must watch for signs and symptoms of toxicity. It is prudent to monitor serum magnesium levels every 4-6 hours when renal dysfunction is severe and aim to maintain therapeutic levels at 4-7 mEq/L.[3]

Fetal Monitoring

Fetus risks include miscarriages, prematurity, and growth restriction. Accurate dating of pregnancy in the first trimester is of paramount importance. Routine screening for chromosomal aneuploidies at 12 weeks and targeted imaging of fetal anomalies in the second trimester must be done.

Serum screening for chromosomal trisomies is affected by renal excretion of beta-human chorionic gonadotrophin (β-hCG). In women with significant renal dysfunction, high β-hCG values and a positive test for chromosomal trisomies should be followed up with a detailed ultrasound examination to look for other markers for trisomies. Non-invasive prenatal testing (NIPT) can be offered.

Serial ultrasound every 3-4 weeks for fetal growth monitoring from 26 to 28 weeks is recommended and antenatal fetal surveillance with a nonstress test (NST) may be done from 32 to 34 weeks.[3]

Labor and Delivery

Mode of delivery should be discussed early by a multidisciplinary team and a plan kept in place. The risk of intraoperative trauma to the transplanted kidney and the likely success of vaginal delivery must be considered.[8] Transplanted kidney is extraperitoneal, in the false pelvis and does not obstruct the descent of the fetal head. Inducing agents—prostaglandins and oxytocin can be safely used.

Cesarean delivery is reserved for obstetric indications.

The risk of injury to the allograft at cesarean delivery is estimated to be 1-2%. It is ideal to localize the allograft before cesarean delivery. Midline skin incision can be considered to avoid injury to the allograft. The uterine incision is a lower-segment transverse incision.

Stress dose steroids (injection hydrocortisone 50 mg IV 8th hourly during labor and for 24 hours after delivery) must be given as per recommendations.

Postpartum hemorrhage can be managed with oxytocin, carboprost, and misoprostol. Methylergometrine is a relative contraindication in patients with hypertension.[3]

Breastfeeding

Breastfeed is considered safe while taking prednisolone, hydroxychloroquine, azathioprine, ciclosporin, tacrolimus, enalapril, captopril, amlodipine, nifedipine, labetalol, atenolol, and low molecular weight heparin.[8] Breastfeeding is discouraged in women taking MMF, sirolimus, everolimus, and belatacept based on theoretical and pharmacological concerns.[1,11]

Postpartum Management

Blood pressure should be well controlled (<140/90 mm Hg). ACE inhibitors and ARBs can be safely given. Follow-up appointments with the transplant team should be made based on the condition of the woman. Contraception must be discussed. Care should be taken not to administer live vaccines for the first 6 months of life to babies exposed to biologics in utero.

LIVER TRANSPLANT

Transplant Pregnancy Registry International 2020 annual report studied 669 outcomes of 651 pregnancies in 331 liver transplant recipients—live birth rate was 71%, with 24% miscarriages and 1% stillbirths. Graft rejection during pregnancy was 4.8% and graft loss rate within 2 years of pregnancy was 2%.[1]

Pregnancy is better tolerated in recipients of a liver transplant. There is a lower incidence of preeclampsia (21%) and prematurity (37%). Cholestasis of pregnancy was observed in 17% compared to 1% in the general population.

Prepregnancy counseling involves a discussion of contraception, immunosuppression, and the ideal timing of conception. A minimum of a 2-year interval between transplant surgery and pregnancy is recommended.[14] Vaginal delivery is not a contraindication.

OTHER SOLID ORGAN TRANSPLANTS

Outcomes of pregnancies after transplant, kidney and transplant, heart, lung, and uterus are enumerated in **Table 1**.[1] Pregnancies in this cohort are rare and care should be individualized. Regular graft surveillance in pregnancy with attention to signs and symptoms of graft rejection, addressing comorbidities and fetal monitoring improves outcomes. Removing the transplanted uterus after delivery keeps the woman off immunosuppressants.

TABLE 1: Outcomes of pregnancies after kidney and pancreas, heart, lung, and uterus transplant.

	Kidney-Pancreas	Heart	Lung	Uterus
Female recipients	71	110	41	3
Pregnancies	131	187	54	3
Unplanned (%)	36%	37%	54%	
Outcomes (includes multiple pregnancies)	139	192	56	2 1-ongoing pregnancy
Live births	68%	68%	63%	2
Miscarriages	27%	26%	27%	0
Stillbirth	0	1%	0%	0
Preeclampsia	34%	27%	15%	1
Diabetes treated	2%	8%	30%	
Prematurity (<37 weeks)	63%	37%	64%	2
Low birth weight (<2,500 g)	62%	37%	66%	1
Cesarean section	70%	45%	47%	
Graft rejection during pregnancy	5%	8%	13%	
Graft loss with 2 years of delivery	11%	2.7%	5.6%	

ASSISTED REPRODUCTIVE TECHNOLOGIES

Pregnancy and transplant outcomes were studied in solid organ transplant recipients using different modalities including ovulation induction (OI) alone, intrauterine insemination (IUI) or in vitro fertilization (IVF). Impaired fecundity was found in 22% of transplant recipients compared to 11% in the general population. Successful outcomes have been reported in 70–75% of pregnancies across all modalities of assisted conception. The impact of assisted reproductive technologies (ART) on maternal health and graft function requires further studies.[1]

TAKE HOME MESSAGES

- Obstetric concerns should be a part of pre-transplant counseling.
- It is advisable to delay conception for a year after the transplant. Contraception must be discussed.
- Prepregnancy counseling must be done to assess the graft function, safety of immunosuppressants, address comorbidities and screen and treat infections.
- Pregnancy outcome is optimal in those without hypertension, proteinuria or no recent episodes of graft rejection.
- Cesarean section is only required for obstetric indications.
- Breastfeeding is encouraged with most immunosuppressants.

REFERENCES

1. Transplant Pregnancy Registry International (TPRI). Annual Report, Gift of Life Institute, Philadelphia, PA 19123; 2020.
2. Deshpande NA, Coscia LA, Gomez-Lobo V, Moritz MJ, Armenti VT. Pregnancy after solid organ transplantation: a guide for obstetric management. Rev Obstet Gynecol. 2013;6(3-4):116-25.
3. Wiles KS, Tillett AL, Harding KR. Solid organ transplantation in pregnancy. Obstet Gynaecol. 2016;18(3):189-97.
4. Danziger-Isakov L, Kumar D, The AST ID Community of Practice. Vaccination of solid organ transplant candidates and recipients: Guidelines from the American society of transplantation infectious diseases community of practice. Clin Transplant. 2019;33(9):e13563.
5. Curtis KM, Tepper NK, Jatlaoui TC, Berry-Bibee E, Horton LG, Zapata LB, et al. U.S. Medical Eligibility Criteria for Contraceptive Use, 2016. MMWR Recomm Rep. 2016;65(3):1-103.
6. World Health Organization. (2015). Medical eligibility criteria for contraceptive use [Internet]. 5th edition. [online] Available from: https://apps.who.int/iris/handle/10665/181468 [Last accessed February, 2023].
7. Klein CL, Josephson MA. Post-transplant pregnancy and contraception. Clin J Am Soc Nephrol. 2022;17(1):114-20.
8. Wiles K, Chappell L, Clark K, Elman L, Hall M, Lightstone L, et al. Clinical practice guideline on pregnancy and renal disease. BMC Nephrol. 2019;20(1):401.
9. Bramham K, Nelson-Piercy C, Gao H, Pierce M, Bush N, Spark P, et al. Pregnancy in renal transplant recipients: A UK National Cohort Study. Clin J Am Soc Nephrol. 2013;8(2):290-8.
10. Nelson-Piercy C. (2017). Handbook of Obstetric Medicine. [online] Available from: http://www.vlebooks.com/vleweb/product/openreader?id=none&isbn=9781482241938 [Last accessed February, 2023].
11. Shah S, Verma P. Overview of pregnancy in renal transplant patients. Int J Nephrol. 2016;2016:4539342.
12. Soh MC, Nelson-Piercy C. High-risk pregnancy and the rheumatologist. Rheumatology. 2015;54(4):572-87.
13. Bramham K, Seed P, Nelson-Piercy C, Lightstone L, Ashford L, Butler J, et al. Diagnostic accuracy of placental growth factor in women with chronic kidney disease or hypertension and suspected preeclampsia: A prospective cohort study. Pregnancy Hypertens Int J Womens Cardiovasc Health. 2015;5(1):21.
14. Valentin N, Guerrido I, Rozenshteyn F, Pinotti R, Wu YC, Collins K, et al. Pregnancy outcomes after liver transplantation: a systematic review and meta-analysis. Am J Gastroenterol. 2021;116(3):491-504.

SECTION 4

Procedures and Transport

32. **Cardiopulmonary Resuscitation in Obstetric Patients**
    Pradip Kumar Bhattacharya, Mohd Saif Khan

33. **Renal Replacement Therapy and Extracorporeal Membrane Oxygenation in Pregnancy**
    Kanwalpreet Sodhi, Nidhi Bhatia

34. **Transport of Critically Ill Pregnant Patients**
    Vinod K Singh, Rahul Kumar

35. **Vascular Access**
    Vinay Singhal, Arun Kumar

Cardiopulmonary Resuscitation in Obstetric Patients

Pradip Kumar Bhattacharya, Mohd Saif Khan

INTRODUCTION

Maternal cardiac arrest (MCA) is defined as the complete cessation of cardiac activity of a woman during pregnancy and up to 6 weeks postdelivery. The main causes of MCA are severe hypoxemia [due to severe pneumonia, acute respiratory distress syndrome (ARDS), and failure to tracheal intubation] and hypotension/hypoperfusion caused by hemorrhage, heart failure, amniotic fluid embolism, high spinal block, and total spinal block and sepsis.[1]

Maternal cardiac arrest is a medical emergency that is managed by a *maternal resuscitation* team (or MCA team) using a coordinated interventional approach. This approach is referred to by many as "maternal cardiopulmonary cerebral resuscitation (M-CPCR)", which has some unique differences in the steps of performing it, compared to standard (nonpregnant) adult cardiopulmonary resuscitation (CPR). There are a few important changes that occur in maternal physiology **(Table 1)**, which should be known to the maternal resuscitation team.

EPIDEMIOLOGY AND MAGNITUDE OF THE PROBLEM

Any death due to complications from pregnancy or childbirth contributes to the maternal mortality rate (MMR), which is lower in high-income group countries compared to low- or middle-income countries (*see* **Table 1**). As per the 2020 Indian Sample Registration

TABLE 1: Maternal physiological changes relevant to maternal cardiac arrest (MCA).

Changes in maternal physiology	Implications to MCA interventions
Elevated cardiac output (by 30–50%) as a result of increased stroke volume and, to a lesser extent, increased maternal heart rate (by 15–20 bpm)	Ejection fraction produced by cardiac compression during MCA is negligible to match high cardiac out state and hence chances of return of spontaneous circulation (ROSC) are very less
Physiologic anemia of pregnancy	Decreased oxygen delivery to the tissues during maternal cardiopulmonary cerebral resuscitation (M-CPCR)
Aortocaval compression resulting in reduced ejection fraction, hypotension, and decreased uteroplacental blood flow	• Left uterine displacement (LUD) using two hands by an assistant is recommended to improve the uteroplacental blood flow and also to improve venous return to heart • Perimortem cesarean delivery (PMCD) helps to relieve compression of the inferior vena cava by the gravid uterus, thereby augmenting venous return

System (SRS) data, MMR was 113 per 100,000 live births in 2016-2018. The prevalence of MCA is very low in the USA (1:12,000 hospital admissions), Canada (1:12,500), and the UK (1:36,000) compared to developing countries such as Taiwan, where it is very high (1:3,885).[2] Comorbid conditions in aging mothers could be the cause of rising global incidence of MCA. The majority of MCA occur in the intensive care units (ICUs) and operation theaters.[1]

STEPS OF MATERNAL CARDIOPULMONARY CEREBRAL RESUSCITATION

Basic Life Support

The basic life support (BLS) consists of following steps (to be initiated simultaneously):
- Check for unresponsiveness and or abnormal breathing.
- Activate maternal resuscitation team **(Box 1)** and ask for automated external defibrillator (AED).

BOX 1: Maternal resuscitation team or MCA team.

- *How to activate:* Call to a designated "number" from the nearest intercom connection. Introduce yourself to the call receiver.
- *Personnel:* Critical care physician/anesthetist, an obstetrician, a neonatologist/pediatrician, a technical assistant (OR/ICU), an obstetric nurse, and a critical care nurse.
- Most experienced anesthetist should be the part of this team due to unique airway challenges encountered during arrest.
- One team member should be dedicated for manual LUD.
- *Communication between team members:* Continuous and effective closed feedback loop type of communication between all team leaders.

(ICU: intensive care unit; LUD: left uterine displacement; MCA: maternal cardiac arrest; OR: operative room)

- Check pulse—if there is pulse → ventilate using bag at the rate of 10–12 breaths per minute (press the bag once in every 5–6 seconds) and keep checking pulse every 2 minutes.
- Check pulse—if no pulse → time of arrest to be noted and high-quality chest compression to be started by first responder (nurse/doctor/technician).
- During chest compression, one team member has to continuously perform left uterine displacement (LUD) (described later).
- Use a firm backboard during M-CPCR.
- During chest compression, continue bag mask ventilation with 100% oxygen using two-handed ventilation technique.
- Keep a compression-ventilation ratio of 30:2.
- Apply AED after maternal resuscitation team arrives and deliver shocks in shockable rhythms.

Manual Left Uterine Displacement: Techniques and Effectiveness

Endorsed by 2020 American Heart Association (AHA) guidelines for CPCR, LUD is a manual technique requiring constant presence of an assistant (healthcare provider), who performs it using either one hand or two hands.[3] So, there are two techniques which are as follows:
1. *One hand technique of performing LUD:*
   - Assistant stands on the right side of the bed
   - Dominant hand is placed over right side of the abdomen
   - Palpate the margin of gravid uterus on the right side of the abdomen
   - Constant pushing motion is applied over the uterus upward and left ward (away from assistant)
2. *Two hands technique of performing LUD:*
   - Assistant stands on the left side of the bed

- Both hands are placed over right side of the abdomen
- Palpate the margin of gravid uterus on the right side of the abdomen
- Constant pulling motion is applied over the uterus upward and left ward (toward assistant).

Effectiveness of Left Uterine Displacement versus Left-lateral Tilt

Many studies have investigated the effectiveness of CPR with manual LUD versus left-lateral tilt. Both of these techniques can effectively relieve aortocaval compression during chest compressions. Synthesizing the data from all available research on this aspect, a recent meta-analysis of eight studies showed that left-lateral tilt position resulted in lower quality chest compressions (in terms of both correct compression depth rate and correct hand position rate), therefore, LUD should be preferred over left tilt as per current evidence.[4]

Components of High-quality Chest Compression

- *Location of chest compression:* Center of lower half of sternum
- Compression rate 100–120/min
- *Depth of compression:* At least 2 inches (5 cm)
- Allow full intercompression chest recoil
- Minimize the frequency as well as the duration (<10 seconds) of interruptions during M-CPCR.

Role of Defibrillation

Most of the electrocardiogram (ECG) rhythms during MCA are nonshockable (90%). Nevertheless, defibrillation should be attempted in case of shockable rhythms [ventricular fibrillation (VF), ventricular tachycardia (VT), supraventricular tachycardia (SVT), and atrial fibrillation (AF)]. Location of application of adhesive pads/paddles is same as in nonpregnant adult (i.e., below the right collar bone and underneath the left breast). There is no difference in energy level used in pregnancy as compared to nonpregnant adult because transthoracic impedance remains the same. The first biphasic energy level should be selected between 120 and 200 J for defibrillation. Subsequently, if the first shock is ineffective, energy level may be increased provided the device allows it. If there are external or internal fetal monitors attached, no time should be wasted in removing or detaching them, rather, rapid defibrillation should be attempted if indicated. Adhesive pads are preferred over paddles for faster defibrillation with optimal energy delivery.

Advanced Cardiac Life Support

Continue high-quality chest compression along with capnography [end-tidal carbon dioxide ($ETCO_2$) monitoring] if available as to monitor the quality of effective compression. Additionally, three important interventions needed:

1. *Maternal interventions:* Advanced airway management considering difficult airway and high risk of aspiration, securing of intravenous (IV) line above the diaphragm, administer advanced cardiac life support (ACLS) drugs (epinephrine, amiodarone, etc.) along with fluids, blood, and blood products as needed. Stop magnesium infusion and administer parenteral calcium gluconate in parturient receiving magnesium infusion.
2. *Obstetric interventions:* Maintain LUD and chest compression and prepare for perimortem cesarean delivery (PMCD).

3. *Neonatal interventions:* Following PMCD, fetus has to be taken care by a neonatal team for newborn resuscitation.

Advanced Airway Management

Two important considerations regrading advanced airway placement should be followed by all care givers; first is that a pregnant status makes it difficult and second consideration is a high risk of aspiration pneumonia. Therefore, it is better to intubate the trachea early during MCA to minimize the risk of aspiration pneumonia. Endotracheal intubation should be performed preferably using a small sized (6.0–7.0 mm ID) endotracheal tube **(Box 2)**. To manage difficult airway, a video laryngoscope, gum elastic bougie, airway exchange catheter, semi-rigid stylet, supraglottic airway devices (laryngeal mask airway), and cricothyroidotomy set are useful adjuncts and hence should be kept ready. A waveform continuous capnography is must to be utilized to confirm the advanced airway placement as well as during whole period of maternal resuscitation.

Role of Continuous Waveform Capnography

If available, it is recommended to use during a cardiac arrest for the following reasons: to confirm the placement of advanced airway, to improve the quality of chest compression, and also for detecting return of spontaneous circulation (ROSC). An $ETCO_2$ level >10 mm Hg is suggestive of high-quality of chest compressions and an abrupt but sustained upsurge of $ETCO_2$ level >35–40 mm Hg suggests ROSC.

Venous Access and Medications Used during MCA

In view of reduced drug delivery to the heart secondary to aortocaval compression by a gravid uterus, the placement of an IV cannula is usually preferred above the diaphragm. First, a wide bore cannula is placed in peripheral veins if feasible, later it has to be changed to central venous access, within the internal jugular vein or subclavian vein. **Table 2** shows the list of medications used during MCA.

Perimortem Cesarean Delivery

This is a fetocentric approach to improving neonatal outcomes following MCA. Also known as resuscitative hysterotomy (RH), if performed early (within 5 minutes of MCA) versus late (after 5 minutes of MCA), has

---

BOX 2: Necessary equipment required in labor room/obstetric casualty to handle MCA.

- *Emergency cart:* All important drugs listed in **Table 2**
- *Airway equipment:* Endotracheal tubes (three sizes 6.0–7.0 for mother; 2.5–4.0 for neonates), two sets of direct laryngoscopes with all blades, gum elastic bougie, stylets, LMA, and cricothyrotomy set
- *Ambu Bag:* Both adult and manual
- *Monitoring equipment:* Capnometer with pulse oximetry
- Mechanical ventilator with breathing circuit
- Defibrillator/AED
- Suction machine with catheter
- Scalpel (with No. 10 blade), 2 Kelly clamps, sutures with suture holders, artery forceps
- Stethoscope (adult and pediatric)
- Arterial catheters (22G and 20G)
- Ultrasound with a cardiac and linear probe
- *Venous access equipment:* Peripheral cannulas (5 each, all sizes), central venous catheter (7F), tourniquet
- Heparinized 1 mL syringes for blood gas evaluations
- Equipment for monitoring core body temperature and head cooling (therapeutic hypothermia)

(AED: automated external defibrillator; LMA: laryngeal mask airway; MCA: maternal cardiac arrest)

TABLE 2: List of medications used during MCA.

Name of medications	Indicated in	Doses
Adrenaline/epinephrine	MCA during ACLS to attain ROSC and cardiac activity	1 mg IV every 3–5 minutes
Amiodarone	Ventricular fibrillation or pulseless ventricular tachycardia that is unresponsive to CPR, defibrillation, and epinephrine	300 mg rapid IV infusion and repeat doses of 150 mg
Calcium gluconate	Antidote for magnesium toxicity	10 mL of 10% calcium gluconate/chloride IV
Atropine	Symptomatic bradycardia	1 mg IV push and may repeat every 3–5 minutes
Lipid emulsion 20%	Suspected local anesthetic toxicity	1.5 mL/kg IV over 1 minute
Naloxone	Narcotic-induced respiratory depression/arrest	0.4 mg IV as a bolus followed by infusion (0.2–0.6 mg/h) in case of unresponsive
Tranexamic acid	Within 3 hours of birth of postpartum hemorrhage	1 g IV at 1 mL/min repeat the same dose if bleeding continues after 30 minutes, or if bleeding restarts after 24 hours of the first dose
High concentration dextrose solution (25–50%)	For hypoglycemia detected in peri-arrest period	Dose is 0.5 to 1 g/kg 25% solution contains 25 g dextrose in 100 mL

Note: Oxytocin should be used cautiously because it can trigger MCA by virtue of its vasodilatory property. Lower dose may be used.
(ACLS: advanced cardiac life support; CPR: cardiopulmonary resuscitation; IV: intravenous; MCA: maternal cardiac arrest; ROSC: return of spontaneous circulation)

shown an improvement in maternal survival (61% vs. 35%) and neonatal survival (96% vs. 70%).[5] Two main contraindications to PMCD are ROSC within two cycles of M-CPCR and the gestational age of <20 weeks. PMCD should be performed at the site of the resuscitation only to avoid unnecessary delay to reach operative room (OR). An on-spot PMCD (RH) is better in terms of survival compared to shifting to OR (72% vs. 36%).[6] Surgeon should not wait for full set of surgical instruments, and commence the PMCD with a surgical knife and clamps. Maintain LUD while surgeon performs PMCD.

POST-MATERNAL CARDIAC ARREST CARE

Main goals of post-MCA care are to prevent further cardiac arrest by treating reversible causes of cardiac arrest, prevent further organ damage and to predict nonsurvivor and neurological outcome **(Table 3)**.

The intensity of post-MCA care depends on temporal relationship of ROSC and delivery status of parturient. In cases where ROSC is achieved postdelivery, extracorporeal membrane oxygenation (ECMO) or cardiac bypass may be instituted. If ROSC is achieved predelivery, put parturient in full left lateral

TABLE 3: Reversible and treatable causes of maternal cardiac arrest (MCA)-mnemonic ABCDEFGH.

Categories of etiologies	Factors
Anesthetic issues	Hypoxia/anoxia (due to pulmonary aspiration, difficult airway, loss of airway, and equipment failure) and hypotension
Bleeding issues	Coagulopathy [disseminated intravascular coagulation (DIC)/liver failure induced], uterine problems (atony and rupture), placental issues (abruption, previa, and accreta), and retained product of conception
Cardiovascular causes	Acute myocardial ischemia, congenital heart defects, valvular heart diseases, aortic dissection, peripartum cardiomyopathy, and fatal arrhythmias
Drug related	Medication overdose, anaphylaxis, medication error, overdose of oxytocin, magnesium sulfate, opioid, insulin and wrong drug administration, and interactions
Embolic causes	Amniotic fluid embolism and pulmonary thromboembolism
Fever (high grade)	Sepsis and blood transfusion reactions
General issues	• *5Ts:* Thrombosis (coronary and pulmonary), tension pneumothorax, tamponade-cardiac, and toxins • *5Hs:* Hypoxia, hypovolemia, hydrogen ions (acidosis), hyper/hypokalemia, and hypothermia
Hypertension	Pregnancy-induced hypertension and severe preeclampsia

decubitus position, and transfer to ICU. In case of recurrent life-threatening arrhythmias consider the placement of an implantable cardioverter-defibrillator or beta blocker (metoprolol) or amiodarone. Rule out and correct thyroid dysfunction, adverse drug effects, electrolyte disturbances, cardiac ischemia, and heart failure. To prevent further organ damage, adequate perfusion pressure [by targeting mean arterial pressure (MAP) >70 mm Hg] and oxygenation [oxygen saturation (SpO_2) target 94–98%] and ventilation [target partial pressure of arterial carbon dioxide ($PaCO_2$) 35–45 mm Hg] by applying hemodynamic support (fluid vasopressors and inotropes) and protective mechanical ventilation, respectively. If patient is unconscious following ROSC, targeted temperature management (TTM) or therapeutic euthermia should be applied despite scant evidence of its effectiveness in post-MCA care. Core body temperature should be monitored and fever should be actively treated and prevented. Any seizure must be detected and controlled using antiepileptic medication.

ROLE OF TRANSESOPHAGEAL ECHO AND EXTRACORPOREAL CARDIOPULMONARY RESUSCITATION

There is a definite role of resuscitative transesophageal echo (TEE) during cardiac arrest, in terms of improving the CPR quality, and finding out the cause of arrest. Evidence is available in the form of case reports.[7,8] There is a scope of further research on the role of TEE in this subset of patients.

Extracorporeal CPR may be used as a rescue intervention in MCA with potentially reversible etiologies, provided absolute contraindications have been ruled out such as massive hemorrhage or disseminated intravascular coagulation (DIC). As per findings of a systematic review, extracorporeal life support (ECLS) was indicated in 15.9% of MCA cases and associated with survival of 87.7% which was higher than any other indications of ECLS (ARDS, cardiac failure, peripartum cardiomyopathy, etc.).[9]

IMPLICATIONS FOR MATERNAL HEALTH

Maternal cardiac arrest may have a good survival rate, provided that M-CPCR is started timely. The maternal survival-to-discharge rates have been reported in the literature from 13 to 71%.[1,10-12]

IMPLICATIONS FOR FETAL WELL-BEING

The greatest optimism for fetal well being depends on the time to achieve ROSC in mother and timing of PMCD. According to a large prospective and descriptive study using the UK Obstetric Surveillance System (UKOSS), fetal survival was higher when PMCD was performed within 5 minutes after cardiac arrest (96% vs. 70%; $p = 0.059$).

CONCLUSION

Maternal cardiac arrest, a consequence of complications from pregnancy or childbirth, is a medical emergency managed by a multi-professional resuscitation team using M-CPCR, which is slightly different from standard adult CPCR. It essentially incorporates manual left uterine displacement and if needed, a timely perimortem caesarean delivery, with demonstrated improvement in fetomaternal survival especially if performed at the site of the M-CPCR. In majority of cases, a good survival rate is noted, provided that M-CPCR is started timely.

TAKE HOME MESSAGES

- Maternal CPCR is a set of coordinated interventions performed by a maternal resuscitation team.
- Manual left uterine displacement is an important part of maternal CPCR, which can be maintained using either one hand or two hands and should be preferred over left lateral tilt as per current evidence.
- Location of chest compression is at center of lower half of sternum.
- Perimortem cesarean delivery, also known as RH, helps to relieve compression of the inferior vena cava by the gravid uterus, thereby augmenting venous return.
- Two main contraindications to PMCD are ROSC within two cycles of M-CPCR and the gestational age of <20 weeks.
- An on-spot PMCD (RH) is better in terms of survival compared to shifting to operative room.
- Reversible and treatable causes of maternal cardiac arrest (MCA)-should be actively searched using various investigations and treated in a timely fashion to prevent re-arrest situations.
- Extracorporeal CPR may be used as a rescue intervention in MCA with potentially reversible etiologies.

REFERENCES

1. Nivatpumin P, Lertbunnaphong T, Dittharuk D. A ten-year retrospective review of maternal cardiac arrest: Incidence, characteristics, causes, and outcomes in a tertiary-care hospital in a developing country. Taiwan J Obstet Gynecol. 2021; 60(6):999-1004.
2. Pandya ST, Jain K, Grewal A, Parikh KS, Sharma K, Gupta AK, et al. The association of obstetric anesthesiologists, India–An expert committee consensus statement and recommendations for the management of maternal cardiac arrest. J Obstet Anaesth Crit Care. 2022;12(2):85.
3. Panchal AR, Bartos JA, Cabanas JG, Donnino MW, Drennan IR, Hirsch KG, et al. Part 3: adult basic and advanced life support: 2020 American Heart Association guidelines

for cardiopulmonary resuscitation and emergency cardiovascular care. Circulation. 2020;142(16_suppl_2):S366-468.
4. Enomoto N, Yamashita T, Furuta M, Tanaka H, Ng ESW, Matsunaga S, et al. Effect of maternal positioning during cardiopulmonary resuscitation: a systematic review and meta-analyses. BMC Pregnancy Childbirth. 2022;22(1):1-21.
5. Beckett V, Knight M, Sharpe P. The CAPS study: Incidence, management and outcomes of cardiac arrest in pregnancy in the UK: A prospective, descriptive study. BJOG. 2017;124:1374-81.
6. Fischer C, Bonnet MP, Girault A, Le Ray C. Update: Focus in-hospital maternal cardiac arrest. J Gynecol Obstet Hum Reprod. 2019; 48:309-14.
7. Oh CS, Kwak SW, Kim TY, Woo NS, Sohn IS, Chee HK. Transesophageal Echocardiographic Diagnosis of Pulmonary Thromboembolism during Cesarean Delivery: A case report. Korean J Anesthesiol. 2008;54(1):117-22.
8. Brown H, Barrett HL, Lee J, Pincus JM, Kimble RM, Eley VA. Successful resuscitation of maternal cardiac arrest with disseminated intravascular coagulation guided by rotational thromboelastometry and transesophageal echocardiography: A Case Report. AA Practice. 2018;10(6):139-43.
9. Naoum EE, Chalupka A, Haft J, MacEachern M, Vandeven CJM, Easter SR, et al. Extracorporeal Life Support in Pregnancy: A Systematic Review. J Am Heart Assoc. 2020; 9(13):e016072.
10. Zelop CM, Einav S, Mhyre JM, Lipman SS, Arafeh J, Shaw RE, et al. Characteristics and outcomes of maternal cardiac arrest: a descriptive analysis of get with the guidelines data. Resuscitation. 2018;132:17-20.
11. Mhyre JM, Tsen LC, Einav S, Kuklina EV, Leffert LR, Bateman BT. Cardiac arrest during hospitalization for delivery in the United States, 1998–2011. Anaesthesiology. 2014;120(4):810-8.
12. Balki M, Liu S, León JA, Baghirzada L. Epidemiology of cardiac arrest during hospitalization for delivery in Canada: a nationwide study. Anesth Analg. 2017; 124(3):890-7.

CHAPTER 33

Renal Replacement Therapy and Extracorporeal Membrane Oxygenation in Pregnancy

Kanwalpreet Sodhi, Nidhi Bhatia

■ INTRODUCTION

Pregnancy is a physiological condition associated with significant changes in the mother. Superimposed comorbidities and systemic diseases can pose significant challenges. Pregnancy-related acute kidney injury (PRAKI) is an important obstetric complication seen in critically ill patients that is associated with significant maternal as well as fetal morbidity and mortality, with almost 10% of these patients requiring renal replacement therapy (RRT). Majority of maternal deaths being preventable during the peripartum period, the intensive care physicians need to be well-versed with the challenges faced during the management of PRAKI patients, especially those requiring RRT. Also, we need to be aware of salvage therapies like extracorporeal membrane oxygenation (ECMO), that can be used during severe cardiopulmonary failure.

■ RENAL REPLACEMENT THERAPY IN PREGNANCY

Pregnancy-related acute kidney injury is a significant cause of fetal and maternal morbidity and mortality. It mainly results from decreased renal perfusion or ischemic acute tubular necrosis, arising from physiological disturbances, like hyperemesis gravidarum or pathological conditions, like puerperal sepsis. The incidence of PRAKI is varying, ranging from 1 in 20,000 pregnancies to as high as 1 in 50 pregnancies.[1,2] PRAKI requiring dialysis usually occurs in women with major pregnancy-related medical comorbidities **(Box 1)**, with a reported incidence of RRT in 10% of PRAKI patients.[2] These patients often have complex health concerns, making their management during RRT significantly challenging. Intensivists involved in care for this high-risk population should be familiar with the current evidence-based practices that guide their management.[3]

BOX 1: Risk factors for developing dialysis-dependent pregnancy-related acute kidney injury.

- Pre-pregnancy hypertension, diabetes, chronic kidney disease, and systemic lupus erythematosus
- Preeclampsia
- Thrombotic microangiopathy
- Sepsis
- Heart failure
- Abruptio placentae
- Postpartum hemorrhage
- Pyelonephritis

Physiological Considerations in Obstetric Patients Requiring RRT[3,4]

Effect of Gravid Uterus

The mechanical effect of gravid uterus in the third trimester can cause patient discomfort and respiratory insufficiency. It is preferable to place the dialysis catheter in semi-Fowler, dorsal decubitus position. The enlarged gravid uterus also limits the use of peritoneal dialysis in pregnant patients, especially in the last trimester.

Changes in Renal System

- Pregnancy results in 80% increase in renal blood flow and 50% increase in glomerular filtration rate (GFR), resulting in increased renal clearance. Thus, during pregnancy the renal system works to its maximum capacity of functional reserve. Any further compromise in the renal function makes it difficult to accommodate the aggravated volume and metabolic load of pregnancy. Hence, to meet these increased demands, RRT regimen needs to be intensified.
- Increased GFR also causes a fall in serum creatinine values. Thus, GFR estimation from serum creatinine values is grossly underestimated and not validated in pregnancy.

Changes in Hematological System

- Blood volume increases by almost 45% in pregnancy and total body water increases by 6–8 liters. Prescribing ultrafiltration should be individualized to account for this maternal blood volume expansion and weight gain, keeping in mind that rapid withdrawal of large amounts of fluid can result in reduced fetoplacental blood flow, with resultant deleterious effects.
- Greater increase in plasma volume as compared to red blood cell mass produces physiological anemia of pregnancy. This is compounded in pregnant patients with chronic kidney disease (CKD) requiring dialysis. So, patients should be intensively monitored for anemia and managed with adequate supplementation.
- The dose of erythropoietin might need to be increased due to circulatory blood volume expansion and resistance to the effect of erythropoietin, as a result of increased cytokine production during pregnancy.

Changes in Coagulation System

Pregnancy produces a physiological hypercoagulable state, with an increase in certain clotting factors and decrease in anticoagulants. The risk of clotting within the tubing and membrane used for RRT should be balanced with the type and dose of anticoagulant. Unfractionated heparin (UFH) is the preferred anticoagulant, as it does not cross the placental barrier and has no teratogenic potential. The extended half-life of heparin in renal failure should be kept in mind.

Indications for Initiating RRT

The decision to initiate RRT in a pregnant patient is clinical and depends on the patients' overall profile as well as the expected chances of renal recovery. However, in order to decrease the unwanted effects of uremia on the fetus (developmental delay and preterm birth), threshold for initiating the same should be lower than in the general population and may need to be repeated with higher frequency. Indications for initiating RRT in pregnant population are listed in **Box 2**.[2,4]

> **BOX 2:** Indications of renal replacement therapy in pregnant patients.
>
> - Symptomatic uremia (associated with pericarditis/encephalopathy/neuropathy)
> - Maternal blood urea nitrogen >18 mmol/L
> - Refractory metabolic acidosis
> - Refractory hyperkalemia
> - Fluid overload unresponsive to diuretic therapy
> - Intoxication with dialyzable toxins
> - Oliguria/anuria

Timing for Initiating RRT

Various randomized controlled trials, conducted in general population, have put forth conflicting data with regards to the timing of initiation of RRT. However, pregnant patients behave differently having special requirements, with the renal system already working at its maximum capacity. Early or late RRT is not known to affect maternal morbidity or mortality, though fetal outcome is reported to be better in patients started on early RRT. Thus, it is advisable to keep a low threshold to initiate dialysis in a pregnant patient and start dialysis early.[3]

Modes of RRT

In pregnant patients with renal disease, all modes of RRT including intermittent hemodialysis and peritoneal dialysis have been used.[2,5]

Continuous Renal Replacement Therapy

Continuous renal replacement therapy (CRRT), which avoids excessive fluid shifts and hypotension, that can influence fetal well being, is advantageous in pregnancy, more so in hemodynamically unstable and critically ill patients.

Peritoneal Dialysis

Though peritoneal dialysis is not associated with large fluctuations in blood volume, electrolytes, solutes, and blood pressure (BP), however, it can result in increased risk of intra-abdominal infections and peritonitis. Further, use of this mode is technically challenging in pregnant patients, especially in the third trimester.

Intermittent Hemodialysis

This is the gold standard modality for substitution of renal function in pregnant women with acute kidney injury (AKI). Hemodialysis technique needs to be modified to meet the demands of pregnancy. The live birth rate as well as median gestational age at delivery and the birth weight are reported to be greater in pregnant women with CKD receiving 37–56 hours/week of dialysis as compared to fewer than 20 hours/week.[2,5]

Renal Replacement Therapy Protocol

The main objectives of RRT during pregnancy are to cause the least possible hemodynamic instability and volume depletion, which can have deleterious effects on the fetus. Thus, certain changes need to be made in RRT so as to improve dialysis adequacy and tolerability in pregnant patients **(Box 3)**.[6-8]

Additional Considerations for Pregnant Patients on RRT[8]

Nutritional Concerns

- It is important to optimize the nutritional status of pregnant patients on dialysis. They should have access to dietary counseling and nutritional assessment. Total calorie and protein intake should be increased,

BOX 3: Modifications in renal replacement therapy prescription during pregnancy.

Technique modifications:
- Dialysis intensification for at least 24–36 hours/week (6–7 sessions/week)
- Use high blood flows (400–500 mL/min) and high dialysis flow rate (600–800 mL/min)
- Use biocompatible, preferably steam sterilized dialyzers
- Recommended levels in dialysate: Potassium: 3–3.5 mmol/L; calcium: 1.5 mmol/L; and bicarbonate: Lower dose of 25 mmol/L (instead of 28–32 mmol/L)
- Administer lowest possible dose of unfractionated heparin

Targets:
- Goal currently is to initiate at blood urea nitrogen <18 mmol/L
- Dry weight increase of 0.3–0.5 kg every week beyond 20 weeks of gestation
- Maintain stable conditions in relation to maternal circulating volume, blood pressure (BP) and interdialytic weight gain (target BP after the dialysis session: 120–140/70–90 mm Hg)
- Avoid hypocalcemia
- Target lower ultrafiltration/treatment, allowing better fluid management

Maternal monitoring during dialysis:
- Vital signs
- Arterial blood gas analysis
- Hemoglobin and platelet levels
- Blood urea, blood urea nitrogen, and serum creatinine
- Serum potassium, calcium, and phosphorus
- Blood glucose levels
- A weekly clinical assessment of ultrafiltration target should be done so as to accommodate anticipated weight gain in pregnancy

Fetal monitoring during dialysis:
- Fetal heart rate monitoring
- Regular fetal ultrasound monitoring
- Umbilical artery Doppler flowmetry
- Cardiotocography

Recommendations for peritoneal dialysis:
- Increase exchange frequency and reduce volumes to <1.5 L
- Add continuous outpatient peritoneal dialysis and automatic peritoneal dialysis

so as to compensate for intensified dialysis-induced protein loss. Daily energy needs should be calculated based on the patient's pregestational weight and pregnancy needs, while keeping a check on interdialytic weight gain.

- Dialysate concentrations of calcium, potassium, and phosphate may require an increase, with increased dietary supplementation of electrolytes, folic acid, and water-soluble vitamins, to account for dialysate losses.

Anemia

It is advisable to keep the hematocrit levels between 30 and 35%, with transferrin saturation higher than 30%. Regular supplementation with folic acid and erythropoietin, if required, is recommended.

Hypertension

Hypertension is commonly associated with complicated PRAKI patients on RRT. Antihypertensives commonly used in patients with renal insufficiency, such as angiotensin-converting enzyme inhibitors and angiotensin-receptor blockers are teratogenic; while others may cross the placenta and adversely affect the fetus. Drugs such as labetalol, methyldopa, and nifedipine are the safe choices.

Postpartum Concerns

In the postpartum period, aggressive ultrafiltration should be avoided to prevent volume depletion.

Potential Fetal and Maternal Risks[1,9]

The major complications of RRT are listed in **Box 4**. The potential risks include:
- *Fetal risks*:
  - Increased risk of preterm birth
  - Fetal growth restriction
  - Fetal death in early pregnancy
  - Increased rates of intensive care admissions
- *Maternal risks*:
  - Maternal perinatal mortality rate in patients on RRT is 0.4%
  - Hypertensive disorders of pregnancy occur in almost 52.6% of the pregnant women on dialysis
  - More prone to infections and anemia
  - Increased risk of polyhydramnios and premature rupture of membranes
  - Increased risk of hemorrhage.

Intradialytic Hypotension

Intradialytic hypotension (IDH), the end result of the interaction between ultrafiltration rate, cardiac output, and arteriolar tone, is defined as a decrease in either the systolic BP of ≥20 mm Hg or mean arterial BP of ≥10 mm Hg leading to symptoms. The various measures that can be taken to prevent IDH are enumerated in **Box 5**.

Conclusion

With recent advancement in technology and knowledge, there has been a significant improvement in maternal and fetal outcome of pregnant patients on dialysis, attributed to intensive dialysis regimes, advanced monitoring and collaborative efforts of a multidisciplinary team and thereby, better patient care.

BOX 4: Complications of renal replacement therapy.

Peritoneal dialysis:
- Catheter malposition
- Catheter site infections
- Peritonitis
- Uterine trauma and placental abruption due to peritoneal dialysis catheter
- Premature rupture of membranes and preterm deliveries in association with peritonitis

Hemodialysis:
- Infection
- Hemodynamic instability/intradialytic hypotension
- Metabolic derangements
- Acidosis
- Coagulation abnormalities

BOX 5: Measures to prevent intradialytic hypotension during pregnancy.

- Cool dialysate (temperature below the core body temperature)
- Slower ultrafiltration rate (<13 mL/kg/h)
- Sodium profiling (maintaining high sodium concentrations during beginning of dialysis session, with gradual decrease as waste solutes are cleared from plasma)
- High flux hemodiafiltration
- Avoidance of antihypertensive medication prior to dialysis
- Prolong dialysis time or increase frequency
- Infuse fluids preferably blood/colloids
- Analyze patient's dry weight at regular intervals

EXTRACORPOREAL MEMBRANE OXYGENATION IN PREGNANCY

During the peripartum period, up to 40% of maternal deaths are potentially preventable, so clinicians are getting aware of the salvage therapies available for severe cardiopulmonary failure including extracorporeal membrane oxygenation (ECMO). The past decade has seen increasing use of venoarterial ECMO (VA-ECMO) or venovenous ECMO (VV-ECMO) respectively for complex cardiac problems and refractory respiratory diseases in critically ill pregnant and postpartum patients. The literature is flooded with case reports and series on the use of ECMO in obstetric patients attesting to favorable maternal and fetal outcomes with ECMO.[10-12] However, the altered physiology in pregnancy, interactions with ECMO, and the fetal oxygenation and perfusion being the prime objective for fetal safety, ECMO in obstetric patients requires meticulous planning and adaptation.

Indications for ECMO

There are certain indications of ECMO in obstetrics beyond the routine ECMO indications **(Box 6)**.[12]

Physiological Changes in Obstetric Patients Relevant to ECMO

The normal physiological changes of pregnancy and the postpartum period put the pregnant women at risk for complications that need considerations for a patient on ECMO.[13]

Hematologic System Changes

Plasma volume increases up to 50%; there occurs a decrease in hemoglobin, hematocrit,

---

BOX 6: Indications of ECMO in obstetrics.

Potential indications for VV-ECMO support during pregnancy and postpartum:
- Severe, potentially reversible, respiratory failure
- *Refractory ARDS:* PaO$_2$/FiO$_2$ ratio <100 with inspired fraction of oxygen ≥0.9 and PEEP ≥10 cmH$_2$O, despite optimal ventilator support and use of adjunctive methods including recruitment maneuvers, prone ventilation, and optimal PEEP
- Hypercapnia with severe respiratory acidosis despite optimal conventional mechanical ventilation with increased respiratory rate and high I:E ratio

Potential indications for VA-ECMO support during pregnancy and postpartum:
- Refractory left ventricular failure from peripartum cardiomyopathy, myocardial infarction, and myocarditis
- Women with severe pulmonary artery hypertension
- Eisenmenger syndrome
- Massive pulmonary embolism with refractory right ventricular failure
- Need for prolonged cardiopulmonary resuscitation (at least 10 minutes) with a potentially reversible precipitating condition
- Inability to wean from cardiopulmonary bypass after heart surgery
- Bupivacaine intoxication requiring prolonged cardiopulmonary resuscitation
- Refractory right or left ventricular failure in suspected cases of amniotic fluid embolism

(ARDS: acute respiratory distress syndrome; ECMO: extracorporeal membrane oxygenation; FiO$_2$: fraction of inspired oxygen; PaO$_2$: partial pressure of arterial oxygen; PEEP: positive end-expiratory pressure; VA-ECMO: venoarterial ECMO; VV-ECMO: venovenous ECMO)

and red blood cell count; a decrease in platelet count potentially increasing the risk of bleeding.

Coagulation System Changes

Levels of certain clotting factors increase; endogenous anticoagulants decrease, making anticoagulant management for ECMO treatment during pregnancy difficult; potential risk of bleeding to be balanced with a hypercoagulable state in which clotting of circuits is more likely; also increased risk for venous thromboembolism.

Cardiovascular System Changes

Peripheral vasodilation leads to increase in overall plasma volume; BP decreases in the first and second trimesters of pregnancy; systemic vascular resistance decreases by as much as 30%, and cardiac output increases by 40%, caused by enhanced stroke volume and increased heart rate; higher initial ECMO flow rates may be required (5–6 L/m^2/min as compared to normal 3–4 L/m^2/min).

Respiratory System Changes

In pregnancy, there occurs around 15% increase in metabolic rate, a 20% increase in oxygen consumption, and a reduction in functional residual capacity by 10–25% leading to a profound increase in the demand for oxygen and profound hypoxia due to hypoventilation, apnea, or impaired gas exchange. Higher maternal partial pressure of arterial oxygen (PaO$_2$) >70 mm Hg and oxygen saturation (SaO$_2$) >90% is aimed for adequate fetal oxygenation. Additional venous drainage cannula placement might be considered when the flow is limited by the cannula size and oxygenation goals are not met. Beta-blockade may be required to reduce metabolic demand and reduce the circulation of deoxygenated blood.

Increased intra-abdominal pressure and decreased chest wall compliance during pregnancy affect the lung protective ventilation strategy during ECMO.

Immune System Changes

The maternal immune system is usually downregulated to tolerate paternally derived fetal antigens: increased susceptibility to infections, more so during ECMO: thereby, more stringent infection control measures are required for pregnant patients on ECMO.

Specific Considerations for ECMO in Pregnancy

Pregnant women who are at high risk of requiring ECMO, should be transferred to an ECMO center, i.e., a level IV center. A delivery plan should be prepared for all potential pregnant patients likely to receive ECMO considering both the maternal and fetal condition. Early consultation with a maternal-fetal medicine specialist should be done to ensure adequate fetal support, identify signs of physiologic stress or fetal decompensation and optimize the fetus for potential premature delivery. ECMO can be used in the delivery room as standby for extremely high-risk deliveries. As of date, there are no guidelines recommending ECMO procedure for pregnant patients. We have formulated a broad protocol that may be modified as per individual center's need (**Box 7**).

There are specific issues which need to be addressed for pregnant patients during ECMO.[13,14]

Issues with Cannulation

- *Likely difficult due to aortocaval compression:* Left uterine displacement might ease out guidewire advancement.
- Ultrasonography can be used to confirm cannula placement.

BOX 7: Extracorporeal membrane oxygenation (ECMO) protocol in pregnancy.
- Cannulation with special considerations; preferably avoid femoral vessels
- Circuit priming with crystalloid routinely; if hemoglobin (Hb) <8.0 g/dL, blood might be used for priming
- *ECMO flow rate:* 100–120 mL/kg/min (5–6 L/m^2/min) (to compensate for elevated cardiac output and improve oxygenation)

Monitoring targets:
- PaO_2 >70 mm Hg (for fetal oxygenation)
- SaO_2 >90–95 mm Hg (for fetal oxygenation)
- pH >7.40 (maternal acidosis poorly tolerated by fetus)
- $PaCO_2$ @ 28–32 mm Hg (maternal hypercapnia and hypocapnia associated with fetal hypoxemia and acidosis)
- HCO_3 @ 18–21 mmol/L (compensation for chronic respiratory alkalosis)
- Continuous fetal heart rate tracing as a "fifth vital sign"
- MAP >70 mm Hg

Ventilation during ECMO:
- Modified lung-protective ventilation with somewhat higher tidal volumes and airway pressures (up to 35 cmH$_2$O) might be needed
- Driving pressure to be kept <15–20 cm
- Airway pressure release ventilation (APRV) with P-high <30 cmH$_2$O may also be used; to reduce the risk of barotrauma
- Proning with special considerations for up to 16 hours/day

Anticoagulation: Unfractionated heparin (UFH) preferred
During cannulation: 50–100 units/kg; then continuous infusion titrated as per laboratory testing and clinical evaluation:
- aPTT goal is 60–80 seconds in VA-ECMO; 45–55 seconds in VV-ECMO; a higher goal of 60–80 seconds in COVID-19 pregnant patients
- ACT goal is 160–220 s
- Anti-Xa 0.3–0.7 U/mL (most closely reflects UFH effect)
- TEG/ROTEM (expertise required for interpretation)

Blood/products: Maintain hematocrit >40%
- Hb >13 g/dL
- Platelet count >80,000 × 10^9/L during ECMO (ELSO guidelines)

Weaning: Commenced once there is clinical evidence of native organ recovery
- ECMO settings (sweep gas flow, sweep FiO$_2$, and ECMO flow) are progressively reduced
- ECMO flow is usually decreased by 500 mL every 5–10 minutes until a minimum flow of 500 mL/hour is reached
- A trial off ECMO is attempted along with fetal heart rate monitoring
- Decannulation: At the bedside for VV-ECMO after the patient tolerates a minimal sweep gas flow (i.e., 0–1 L/min) and on acceptable ventilator settings
- For VA-ECMO, decannulation is performed in the operating room along with echocardiographic assessment of ventricular and valvular function

(ACT: activated clotting time; aPTT: activated partial thromboplastin time; COVID-19: coronavirus disease-2019; ELSO: Extracorporeal Life Support Organization; FiO$_2$: fraction of inspired oxygen; MAP: mean arterial pressure; PaO$_2$: partial pressure of arterial oxygen; ROTEM: rotational thromboelastometry; SaO$_2$: oxygen saturation; TEG: thromboelastography; VA-ECMO: venoarterial ECMO; VV-ECMO: venovenous ECMO)

- Uterine stimulation might occur with femoral catheterization.
- Preferential selection of a dual-lumen cannula for catheterization; through the distant jugular vein to avoid trauma to the uterus and reduce the impact of drugs on the fetus.
- Fetal heart rate monitoring during cannulation may provide early indication of impaired uterine blood flow during cannulation. Maintain physiologic uteroplacental perfusion at all times.

Issues with Positioning

- Aortocaval compression always has to be kept in mind while positioning pregnant female: Left uterine displacement is recommended while supine.
- Logistic issues with proning a pregnant female.
- Proning requires careful padding around gravid abdomen.
- Fetal compromise might occur during proning; fetal monitoring is mandatory during prone positioning
- If resources are limited, lateral decubitus positioning may be preferred to prone.

Anticoagulation Issues

- Concern with regards to anticoagulation practices due to potential bleeding diatheses in obstetric ECMO patients.
- Anticoagulation level has to be judicially adjusted considering all complex factors affecting it: the severity of illness, underlying pathology and circuit components.
- Unfractionated heparin being inexpensive, reversible, clinical benefit of inability to cross the placenta, and no potential for congenital malformations is preferred for anticoagulation; special attention is required in monitoring for heparin-induced thrombocytopenia (HIT), reported in up to 8% of pregnancies.
- Thromboelastography/rotational thromboelastometry (TEG/ROTEM) may be better options for anticoagulation monitoring due to complex coagulation factors abnormalities during pregnancy.
- Anticoagulation might have to be discontinued for patients with significant bleeding diatheses.

Psychosocial Considerations

- Interruption of the emotional connection, i.e., maternal-newborn bonding: touching and cuddling, can be difficult; innovative strategies like facetime or video conferencing can allow for visualization of the newborn and other children at home.
- Anxiety, depression, or post-traumatic stress during the postpartum period: Empathetic and compassionate behavior of healthcare workers and appropriate drug therapy are required.
- Breastfeeding after birth for obstetric patients on ECMO is usually not possible; breasts can become engorged and painful and comfort measures including ice packs, assisting with breastfeeding or pumping and snug-fitting bras or wraps should be provided.

Complications of ECMO

In mother:

- Hemorrhagic complications: Most frequently reported ECMO-related complication; fatal intracranial bleeding, nonfatal vaginal or upper gastrointestinal bleeding, disseminated intravascular coagulation, hemothorax, and bleeding from the cannulation sites.

- Thrombosis, pulmonary embolism, and limb ischemia
- Infections
- AKI
- Atrial fibrillation
- Severe right heart failure
- Multiorgan failure

In fetus:
- Central nervous system hemorrhage
- Low birth weight fetus
- Fetal mortality.

Outcomes

Literature has reported good clinical outcomes for both mother and fetus with minimal major complications during ECMO for obstetric patients. The reported maternal survival varies from 60 to up to 91% with varying factors affecting the maternal outcomes.[10-12] The most common causes of maternal deaths included bleeding including obstetric hemorrhage and intracranial hemorrhage, pulmonary embolism, infection, multiorgan failure, and severe right heart failure.

Maternal Outcomes

- Obstetric patients with cardiac indications had lower mortality than those needing ECMO for respiratory indications
- Peripartum patients needing VV-ECMO needed ECMO for longer duration and had lower mortality as compared to VA-ECMO
- Corticosteroid use prior to initiation of ECMO was associated with higher maternal mortality.

Fetal Outcomes

- Fetal survival vary from 60 to 83%
- Hypoxia prior to the start of ECMO

- *Fetal heart rate variability*: Round-the-clock, continuous external fetal monitoring with a dedicated labor nurse at the patient's bedside for fetal heart rate interpretation and appropriate intervention; reversible causes of variability including maternal hypoxia, aortocaval compression, hypotension, cannula malposition, inadequate ECMO settings, or circuit thrombosis must be quickly identified and treated. Persistent maternal cardiopulmonary instability usually warrants emergent delivery. Do consider that sedative-hypnotic medications in mother reduce fetal heart rate variability.
- Potential adverse effects of the contrast agents used for imaging
- Adverse effects of drugs used during ECMO which potentially cross the uteroplacental circulation including analgesia/sedatives, muscle relaxants, and the antibiotics required during the ECMO intervention.

Extracorporeal Cardiopulmonary Resuscitation

Extracorporeal cardiopulmonary resuscitation (ECPR) is the VA-ECMO during cardiac arrest. Cardiac arrest in pregnancy is a complex situation and the current scientific data is limited with regards to the use of ECPR in maternal cardiac arrest. ECPR has been used for varied etiologies leading to maternal cardiac arrest, including amniotic fluid embolism, postpartum hemorrhage, and severe cardiomyopathy. Although ECPR has been applied for a variety of gestational ages, it is more commonly used after resuscitative hysterotomy in second half of pregnancy. It is recommended to consider using ECPR following maternal cardiac arrest when there is no return of spontaneous circulation after resuscitative hysterotomy or in cases of refractory CPR in patients of <20 weeks of gestational age.

Conclusion

In the last decade, ECMO has come up as an effective rescue therapy for obstetric patients with severe cardiopulmonary dysfunction. Given the complex interplay of maternal and ECMO physiology, a multidisciplinary team approach is the best for good maternal and fetal outcomes. Survival can be drastically improved by early recognition of high-risk maternal critical illness likely to require ECMO and timely referral to a specialized center with expertise in ECMO.

■ REFERENCES

1. Wiles K, Chappell L, Clark K, Elman L, Hall M, Lightstone L, et al. Clinical practice guideline on pregnancy and renal disease. BMC Nephrol. 2019;20:401.
2. Acharya A. Management of acute kidney injury in pregnancy for the obstetrician. Obstet Gynecol Clin N Am. 2016;43:747-65.
3. Banerjee A, Mehrotra G. Comparison of Standard Conservative Treatment and Early Initiation of Renal Replacement Therapy in Pregnancy-related Acute Kidney Injury: A Single-center Prospective Study. Indian J Crit Care Med. 2020;24:688-94.
4. Lobo VA. Renal Replacement Therapy in Pregnancy-related Acute Kidney Injury: Getting the Timing Right. Indian J Crit Care Med. 2020;24:624-5.
5. Wiles K, de Oliveira L. Dialysis in pregnancy. Best Pract Res Clin Obstet Gynaecol. 2019;57:33-46.
6. Cabiddu G, Castellino S, Gernone G, Santoro D, Giacchino F, Credendino O, et al. Kidney and Pregnancy Study Group of Italian Society of Nephrology. Best practices on pregnancy on dialysis: The Italian Study Group on Kidney and Pregnancy. J Nephrol. 2015;28:279-88.
7. Krane NK. Peritoneal dialysis and hemodialysis in pregnancy. Hemodial Int. 2001;5:97-101.
8. Ribeiro CI, Silva N. Pregnancy and dialysis. J Bras Nefrol. 2020;42:349-56.
9. Hirano H, Ueda T, Tani H, Kosaka K, Nakatani E, Hawke P, et al. Pregnancy and delivery in women receiving maintenance hemodialysis in Japan: Analysis of potential risk factors for neonatal and maternal complications. J Nephrol. 2021;34:1599-609.
10. Naoum EE, Chalupka A, Haft J, MacEachern M, Vandeven CJM, Easter SR, et al. Extracorporeal Life Support in Pregnancy: A Systematic Review. J Am Heart Assoc. 2020;9:e016072.
11. Webster CM, Smith KA, Manuck TA. Extracorporeal membrane oxygenation in pregnant and postpartum women: a ten-year case series. Am J Obstet Gynecol MFM. 2020;2:100108.
12. Ong J, Zhang JJY, Lorusso R, MacLaren G, Ramanathan K. Extracorporeal membrane oxygenation in pregnancy and the postpartum period: a systematic review of case reports. Int J Obst Anes. 2020;43:106-13.
13. Wong MJ, Bharadwaj S, Galey JL, Lankford AS, Galvagno S, Kodali BS. Extracorporeal Membrane Oxygenation for Pregnant and Postpartum Patients. Anaesth Analg. 2022; 135(2):277-89.
14. Tonna JE, Abrams D, Brodie D, Greenwood JC, Mateo-Sidron JAR, Usman A, et al. Management of Adult Patients Supported with Venovenous Extracorporeal Membrane Oxygenation (VV ECMO): Guideline from the Extracorporeal Life Support Organization (ELSO). ASAIO J. 2021;67(6):601-10.

CHAPTER 34

Transport of Critically Ill Pregnant Patients

Vinod K Singh, Rahul Kumar

■ INTRODUCTION

The maternal transport system is an important component of modern perinatal care which focus on institutional delivery of high-risk pregnancies and providing timely emergency obstetric care (EmOC). It is a process of transferring a pregnant woman under the supervision of skilled emergency medical services (EMS) personnel either from home to a medical institution or from one hospital to a higher center (level III institution) when available local resources are inadequate to manage anticipated maternal or neonatal complications.

It is estimated that 15% of all pregnancies will encounter complications and 7% will be serious enough to require referral to a higher center.[1] India has made a significant improvement in achieving United Nations Sustainable Development Goals which target a maternal mortality rate of <70 per 100,000 live births by 2030. Over the last two decades maternal mortality rate in India has declined by 70% from 398/100,000 live births (1997–1998) to 99/100,000 live births (2020).[2] The majority of deaths have occurred in rural and tribal areas of poorer states with obstetric hemorrhage (47%), pregnancy-related infections (12%), and hypertensive disorders of pregnancy (7%) being the most common causes. Most maternal deaths can be prevented if women are assisted by skilled attendants at birth and those experiencing complications could reach quality EmOC on time.

Because of poor transport system many high-risk pregnancies or patients with obstetric complications fail to reach quality EmOC. Studies in India reveal that about one-third to one-half of reported maternal deaths occurred at home or on the way to care.[3-6] The Indian government has started many schemes to improve basic transport and ambulances for pregnant women such as Janani Suraksha Yojana, sate run call center-based ambulance systems ("108" and "102"), district-level public-private partnerships such as Janani Express, and local community-based innovations. The "108" call center-based ambulance system is a free of cost emergency response system functioning in 20 states and 2 union territories and aims to reach patients/sites within 20 minutes in urban and 40 minutes in rural areas and reach the nearest health facility within 20 minutes following pick-up. Though India has achieved a high institutional delivery rate of 88.6% (2019–2021) maternal and neonatal mortality rate have not improved at the same rate indicating the need to further improve the quality of the maternal transport system.

The decision regarding the antenatal transport should be made jointly by the referring physician or midwife, accepting physician and transport personnel after discussing with the family members and the process should be explained to the patient. Early consultation and referral to the appropriate center is always preferred over emergency transport if prelabor complications are anticipated. Mode of transport [private vehicle, advanced cardiac life support (ACLS) ambulance, and air ambulance] to the most appropriate accepting center depends on the condition of the mother and the fetus and on the distance, travel time, and climate. In case of life-threatening emergencies, pregnant woman should be transported to the nearest hospital skilled in providing EmOC.

Institutions providing obstetric and neonatal care should develop effective regional referral and transport system with focus on following components:
- 24-hour availability of the referral and transport system
- Early identification and referral of the high-risk pregnancies
- Providing a continuum of care during transport with well-equipped ACLS ambulances and skilled EMS personnel
- Inter-hospital communication and collaboration.

Emergency medical services personnel involved in maternal transport should have the experience and skill to assess maternal and fetal well-being, and if required they should be able to conduct emergency delivery, provide intravenous (IV) therapy, and ACLS (adult and neonatal).

INDICATIONS AND CONTRAINDICATIONS OF MATERNAL TRANSPORT

Indications and contraindications of maternal transport are presented in **Table 1**.

TIMING OF MATERNAL TRANSPORT

When possible, referral should be made while the woman and fetus are stable and birth is not expected to occur within a reasonable time frame that transport could occur. Patients in early labor can be transported if the woman condition is stable, the time of transport is <2 hours, birth is not anticipated for 4–6 hours, and a professional attendant (nurse, physician, or trained EMS personnel) can accompany the woman during the transport. In high-risk transport situations (unstable woman with unpredictable time

TABLE 1: Indications and contraindications of maternal transport.

Indications for maternal transport	Contraindications to maternal transport
• Preterm labor • Preterm rupture of membranes • Hypertensive disorders of pregnancy • Antepartum hemorrhage • Medical complications of pregnancy such as diabetes, renal disease, and hepatitis • Multiple gestations • Intrauterine growth retardation or fetal anomalies • Inadequate progress of labor • Malpresentation • Maternal trauma	• Mother's condition too unstable for transport such as actively bleeding placenta previa or abruption placentae • Rapidly deteriorating fetal condition • Delivery is imminent (such as cervical dilatation of >5 cm) • Skilled emergency medical services (EMS) person not available to accompany the woman • Hazardous weather or geographic conditions

of birth), the referring physician or designate and a neonatologist or a nurse with skill and experience to provide neonatal resuscitation should accompany the woman during transport.

Transfer of patients in early labor is recommended in the following circumstances:
- Time for transport will take <2 hours
- The woman's condition is stable
- Birth is not anticipated for 4–6 hours
- A professional attendant, such as a nurse, physician, or trained emergency medical technician, should accompany the woman.

Well-established communication among the referring hospital personnel, referral hospital personnel, transport personnel, family members, and the patient is fundamentally important for safe and effective maternal transport system. Perinatal care personnel must be familiar with mechanisms in place for initiating transport and confirming the ability of the receiving hospital to provide the necessary care. The need for transport must be communicated and discussed with the woman and her family to clear all the doubts. The reason, time, mode, and duration of transport along with destination hospital and transport personnel details must be informed to the woman and her family. Decisions regarding the mode of transport (road or air ambulance), need for accompanying personnel, and the required skill set are usually made by referring center with input from the receiving center. Following documents should accompany the patient—maternal transfer form, photocopies of antenatal records, the pertinent hospital records, and ultrasound reports.

An IV access should be established and interventions required to stabilize the patient must be completed prior to initiation of transport. Availability and functioning of all transport equipment must be checked prior to departure. Sufficient oxygen availability during transport must be ensured. During high-altitude flights supplemental oxygen therapy should be considered. During transit pregnant woman are usually nursed in left lateral decubitus position to minimize the risk of supine hypotension and subsequent fetal hypoxia. Both mother and fetus need to be monitored during transport. Assessments should include uterine activity, maternal vital signs, and fetal heart rate and documented on maternal transport form. Transport personnel should also pay attention to the emotional needs of the woman.

PLANNING AND LOGISTICS— KEY COMPONENTS

Providers at the transferring facility should initiate stabilization and treatment efforts prior to transport. The screening examination should include ongoing evaluation of fetal heart rate; frequency, strength, and duration of uterine contractions; fetal position and station; cervical dilation; and status of the membranes. All patients should have IV access with at least an 18-gauge catheter (if possible), and oral intake should not be permitted. Placement of a bladder catheter should be considered, depending on the patient's condition (e.g., ability to use a bedpan and need for information on hourly urine output) and anticipated duration of transport.

The receiving facility should be able to provide the appropriate level of care for both the mother and the newborn.

The transport team should be able to provide a timely response and should have the training and experience to assess the patient's status, determine the appropriateness of transfer, and provide appropriate monitoring and care during transport.

TYPES OF EQUIPMENT FOR MATERNAL TRANSPORT

- External fetal heart tracing monitor (or intermittent documentation of fetal heart tones by Doppler)
- Tocolytic and antihypertensive medications
- IV infusion pumps with a minimum three line capability
- Neonatal resuscitation equipment and supplies
- Pulse oximeter
- Emergency airway management
- Blood pressure measurement device
- IV fluids and maternal medications
- Emergency birth sterile kit
- Infant resuscitation equipment
- Adult resuscitation equipment.

CONCLUSION

Maternal transport should be considered if the facility does not have sufficient resources to meet maternal and/or neonatal medical needs, and there is low probability for clinical deterioration of mother and fetus during transport.

When possible, a referral should be made while the woman and fetus are in a stable condition, and birth is not expected to occur within a reasonable time frame that transport could occur. This presents a low risk for transferring the woman and fetus.

Good communication between the referring facility, transport team, and receiving facility is important. The decision regarding the type of vehicle depends on the condition of the pregnant woman and fetus as well as distance and travel time. It is a decision that should be shared jointly by the referring care provider and flight personnel or receiving physician.

TAKE HOME MESSAGES

Key components of maternal transport system include:
- Early identification and referral of high risk pregnancy.
- 24 hours availability of well-equipped ambulances and skilled EMS personnel.
- Stabilize maternal and feral condition and rule out imminent delivery before initiating transport.
- Decision to transport the patient should be made jointly by the referring hospital, accepting hospital, transport team and family members.

REFERENCES

1. World Health Organization. The World Health Report 2005: Make Every Mother and Child Count. Geneva: World Health Organization; 2005.
2. Meh C, Sharma A, Ram U, Fadel S, Correa N, Snelgrove JW, et al. Trends in maternal mortality in India over two decades in nationally representative surveys. BJOG. 2022;129:550-61.
3. Ganatra BR, Coyaji KJ, Rao VN. Too far, too little, too late: a community-based case-control study of maternal mortality in rural west Maharashtra, India. Bull World Health Organ. 1998;76(6):591-8.
4. Iyengar K, Iyengar SD, Suhalka V, Dashora K. Pregnancy-related deaths in rural Rajasthan, India: exploring causes, context, and care-seeking through verbal autopsy. J Health Popul Nutr. 2009;27(2):293-302.
5. Singh S, Murthy GV, Thippaiah AT, Upadhyaya S, Krishna M, Shukla R, et al. Community Based Maternal Death Review: Lessons Learned from Ten Districts in Andhra Pradesh, India. Matern Child Health J. 2015;19(7):1447-54.
6. Lee SK, McMillan DD, Ohlsson A, Boulton J, Lee DS, Ting S, et al. The benefit of preterm birth at tertiary care centres is related to gestational age. Am J Obstet Gynecol. 2003;188(3):617-22.

CHAPTER 35

Vascular Access

Vinay Singhal, Arun Kumar

INTRODUCTION

The incidence of intensive care unit (ICU) admissions with obstetric or maternal critical illness has been found to range from 0.3 to 0.24% of all deliveries. Leading causes of ICU admission include hemorrhage, hypertensive disorders of pregnancy, and sepsis.

A well-secured/reliable vascular access is a prerequisite for the safe care of admitted pregnant patients. The technique involves the insertion of a flexible and sterile catheter, into the blood vessel to provide an effective method of delivering medications, infusions, blood products, or nutrition.

There are varied options available and the device selection needs to be tailored to individual patient needs and the clinical context.

The key to successful cannulation not only requires clinical experience but is confounded by factors such as obesity, length of hospital stay, and critical illness. An obstetrical patient, by virtue of a higher body mass index, would easily qualify for difficult peripheral intravenous cannulation.

Early referral to a vascular access specialist team (VAST) with advanced knowledge and skills in catheter insertion and care, or interventions putting into practice the recommendations of experts in the management of vascular catheters, can help to avoid the adverse events associated with cannulation and their associated costs.[1]

PREGNANCY PHYSIOLOGY AND VENOUS ACCESS

The normal course of pregnancy is marked by major physiological changes. This includes weight gain and edema. Peripheral intravenous access is a challenge in advanced pregnancy and especially in those with complicated clinical situations.

Pregnancy alters the anatomic landmarks for internal jugular vein (IJV) cannulation. The IJV overlies the carotid artery to a greater extent in pregnant patients than in nonpregnant patients. Thus, a landmark approach for IJV cannulation might expose pregnant women to a greater risk of carotid puncture.[2]

Table 1 provides a simplistic approach to the decision on the selection of invasive devices and has been adopted from the royal college hospital reference guidelines available on their web page.[3]

The Michigan Appropriateness Guide for Intravenous Catheters (MAGIC)[4] presents an algorithm for the selection of venous access devices based upon the risk versus benefit of the device. The algorithm is helpful and prevents the unnecessary placement of devices. The avid reader is advised to use the

TABLE 1: The selection of intravenous (IV) access.

Duration of IV access	Selection of cannula
<7 days	Peripheral IV access (use forearm, hand, cubital fossa)
7–14 days	Upper arm midline, peripherally inserted central catheter (PICC), or central venous access device (CVAD)
>14 days	PICC, percutaneous CVAD, tunneled CVAD or port

same for the reference in easing the decision making in difficult situations.

■ PERIPHERAL VENOUS ACCESS

The peripheral catheters are preferred when IV access is required for shorter periods especially when the direct access to the central circulation is unnecessary. Peripheral access is generally safer, easier to obtain, and less painful than central access.

The access site for peripheral cannulation can be selected based on the clinical circumstances, anticipated duration of treatment, and the condition of the extremities. The ease of cannulation and potential complications too vary depending upon the size selected.

Veins of the upper extremity are preferred over the lower extremities due to the increased risk of thrombosis and thrombophlebitis with venous cannulation of the latter. Peripheral access is preferable in patients with coagulopathy or on anticoagulants due to the ease of direct compression of the puncture site. The risk of hematoma formation is also lower as compared to central cannulation.

According to observational data, factors associated with difficulty placing a peripheral IV catheter in an adult include obesity, being underweight, clinician inexperience, and clinician judgement of poor peripheral venous access.[5,6]

When veins are not easily visible, illumination devices can be helpful for vein location. The available technology includes infrared light, which reflects the tissues surrounding the veins. Brandt et al. have suggested that ultrasound-guided peripheral access could be considered a first-line choice to guide peripheral intravenous access in morbidly obese patients especially when there are no detectable veins.[7]

Doppler ultrasound is a valuable aid for situations where veins are not easily seen.[8] The flow rates seen with different catheters are represented in **Table 2**.[9]

TABLE 2: Intravenous catheter flow rates.

Catheter size (diameter, length)	Flow rate with gravity	Flow rate with pressure
22 gauge, 25 mm	35.7 mL/min	71.4 mL/min
20 gauge, 33 mm	64.4 mL/min	105 mL/min
18 gauge, 45 mm	98.1 mL/min	153 mL/min
16 gauge, 50 mm	155 mL/min	334 mL/min
14 gauge, 50 mm	236 mL/min	384 mL/min

■ CENTRAL VENOUS ACCESS

The use of central venous access would be considered in a patient with limited peripheral access or access requirement for >7 days. Additional indications include infusion of concentrated solutions and hemodynamic monitoring. Central venous catheters (CVC) can be placed either peripherally through deep veins in upper limb (peripherally inserted central catheters—PICC) **(Fig. 1)** or through the internal jugular, subclavian, or femoral venous route **(Fig. 2)**. The coagulation parameters should be corrected whenever feasible before CVC insertion, and the subclavian approach should not be used in patients with uncorrected coagulopathy because the venepuncture site cannot be monitored or compressed. Chest X-ray is a must for the confirmation of CVC tip position for the internal jugular and subclavian access **(Fig. 3)**. CVCs can be kept in situ for 2–4 weeks.

The use of ultrasound guidance is recommended especially in patients with coagulopathy, as it has been shown to decrease the number of attempts needed for cannulation and reduces complication rates. The real-time ultrasound guidance is especially helpful in pregnancy considering the anatomical variation induced by pregnancy and as discussed above.

Central venous catheters are usually available as single or multi-lumen catheters. They are also available as high flow catheters. Although the type of catheter and site have chosen are often determined by individual clinical and patient characteristics, a jugular CVC is usually preferred to a subclavian CVC (associated with a higher risk of bleeding and pneumothorax) or femoral CVC (associated with a higher risk of infection). During cardiac arrest, while cardiopulmonary resuscitation (CPR) is going on, femoral access may be the most preferred option because of ease of cannulation.

The CVC are available as chlorhexidine-silver sulfadiazine (CHSS)-coated and minocycline-rifampin (MR) coated catheters. The rationale for these coating is the prevention of catheter-related bloodstream infection (CRBSI), however, the efficacy of these devices is uncertain.[10] These coated catheters may be preferred when the catheter-related infection rates have not reduced despite the implementation of routine infection prevention measures.

The risk of complications associated with central venous catheter insertion is noted in approximately 1% of the patients and is

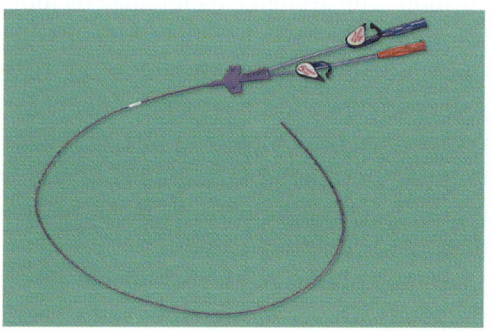

Fig. 1: Peripherally inserted central catheters line.

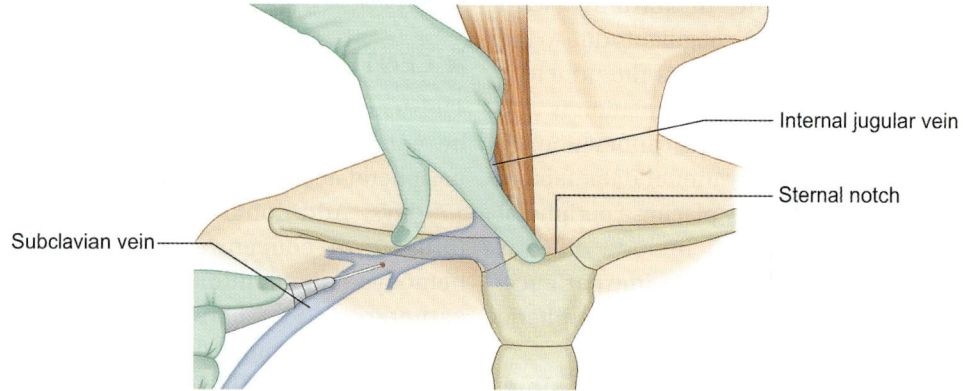

Fig. 2: Anatomy of internal jugular vein and subclavian vein.

documented in **Table 3**. Rhythm disturbances are usually noted with jugular and subclavian approaches especially related to too deep insertion of a guidewire. The same can be prevented by graded wire insertion and continued monitoring of vital parameters during line insertion. It is equally important to follow the World Health Organization (WHO)/ Centers for Disease Control and Prevention (CDC) recommended maintenance bundles to prevent the risks of secondary infections.[11] A daily assessment for removal is strongly recommended. The invasive device needs to be withdrawn as soon as the clinical indication for insertion ceases to exist.

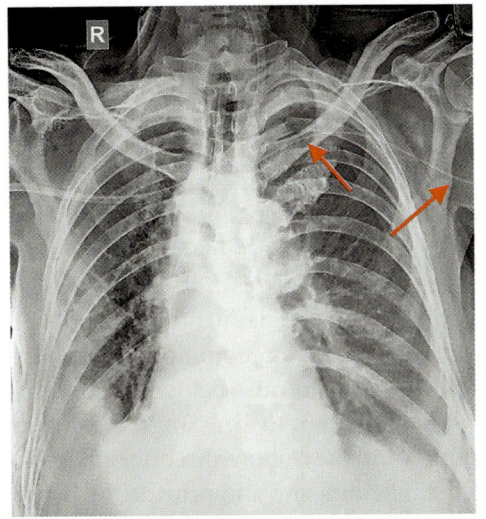

Fig. 3: Chest X-ray showing the course of peripherally inserted central catheters line (arrows).

■ MIDLINE PERIPHERAL CATHETERS

Midline catheters (MC) are usually 8–20 cm in length (*see* **Fig. 1**), have a single or double lumen, and are placed peripherally 1.5 cm above or below the antecubital fossa, into the basilic, cephalic, or brachial vein. They are usually inserted in the deep veins of the upper limb under sonographic guidance. Thus, X-ray confirmation of the correct placement of the MC tip is not necessary. They can be kept for 2–4 weeks in situ. They are not CVC as their tip is away from the axillary vein.

TABLE 3: Complications associated with central venous catheters.

Complications	Possible sequelae
Common	
Carotid artery injury	Bleeding, respiratory compromise, neurologic complications
Subclavian artery injury	Hemothorax, hemodynamic compromise
Femoral artery injury	Bleeding, hemodynamic compromise
Puncture of the vein resulting in a leak	Bleeding, extravasation of fluid
Puncture of pleura or lung	Pneumothorax
Thrombosis	Limb edema, pulmonary embolism
Less common	
Air embolism	Cardiac arrest
Arrhythmias	Cardiac arrest
Brachial plexus injury	Weakness of limb
Infection	Sepsis, catheter-related bloodstream infection (CRBSI)
Lymphatic injury	Chylothorax

These catheters are usually used for a patient requiring long-term intravenous access and frequent blood sampling. These lines are, however, considered to be more thrombogenic due to insertion in veins, which have nearly the same diameter.

■ ARTERIAL ACCESS

Arterial catheterization is usually needed to monitor intra-arterial blood pressure monitoring in patients who are hemodynamically unstable requiring vasopressors or dilators, patients requiring arterial blood gas sampling at frequent intervals or patients where a pressure monitoring cuff cannot be placed. The most common site for intra-arterial access is a radial artery, followed by the femoral and rarely dorsalis pedis or posterior tibial arteries. Arterial catheters are usually placed under sonographic guidance.

One of the most common contraindications for arterial cannulation is anticoagulation. Other contraindications include coagulopathy, arterial atherosclerosis, insufficient collateral perfusion, partial or full-thickness burns over the cannulation site, synthetic arterial or vascular grafts, or infection at the proposed site of cannulation. Absolute contraindications for arterial cannulation are absent pulse and Raynaud syndrome.

■ ANTISEPTIC SOLUTIONS, SITE PREPARATION, AND DRESSINGS

The use of an antiseptic solution for skin disinfection at the insertion site reduces the risk of infection. The available data shows the superiority of chlorhexidine-containing antiseptic solutions over iodine solutions or 70% alcohol, particularly for the reduction of the risk of catheter colonization and CRBSIs.[12]

If chlorhexidine is not available, povidone-iodine is considered superior to alcohol (it is both an antiseptic and detergent) and should be left to dry for 2 full minutes before starting procedures. Shaving is not recommended as it can promote colonization. The use of clippers is recommended.

The use of local anesthetic (lidocaine 1-2%) for skin infiltration is strongly recommended. The use of lignocaine with adrenaline is useful for the placement of a tunneled catheter to reduce the incidence of bleed from the subcutaneous tunnel.

The use of antibiotic prophylaxis before catheter placement is not recommended. There was no difference in the rate of infection in a meta-analysis comparing antibiotic versus no antibiotic use before insertion.[13]

The transparent dressings are recommended as they allow direct visualization of the insertion site and provide the earliest indication of removal if any localized erythema or tenderness is noted. The dressing needs to be replaced in the event of it getting damp, loose, or visibly soiled. The gauge dressing may be used as an alternative if the patient is diaphoretic or bleed is present at the insertion site. There is no role in the application of topical antimicrobial ointments at the catheter exit site.

Catheter Management

Proper catheter management involves minimizing the duration of a catheter by daily assessment for the need, routine assessment for catheter site infections, use of the aseptic technique for handling and catheter change at the earliest indication of infection.

■ CONCLUSION

Obtaining venous access in an obstetric patient is a routine with a certain unique set of challenges. The intervention must be planned in a manner to improve the efficacy of the first puncture by selecting the most appropriate catheter and site, thus minimizing its adverse effects. The involvement of the hospital vascular access team can be a beneficial intervention in reducing adverse events.

■ REFERENCES

1. Au AK, Rotte MJ, Grzybowski RJ, Ku BS, Fields JM. Decrease in central venous catheter placement due to use of ultrasound guidance for peripheral intravenous catheters. Am J Emerg Med. 2012;30:1950-4.
2. Siddiqui N, Goldszmidt E, Haque SU, Carvalho JC. Ultrasound simulation of internal jugular vein cannulation in pregnant and non-pregnant women. Can J Anaesth. 2010;57(11):966-72.
3. The Royal Children's Hospital Melbourne. (2019). [online] Available from: https://www.rch.org.au/clinicalguide/guideline_index/Intravenous_access_Peripheral/ [Last accessed February, 2023].
4. Chopra V, Flanders SA, Saint S, Woller SC, O'Grady NP, Safdar N, et al. The Michigan Appropriateness Guide for Intravenous Catheters (MAGIC): Results From a Multispecialty Panel Using the RAND/UCLA Appropriateness Method. Ann Intern Med. 2015;163(6 Suppl):S1-40.
5. Sebbane M, Claret PG, Lefebvre S, Mercier G, Rubenovitch J, Jreige R, et al. Predicting peripheral venous access difficulty in the emergency department using body mass index and a clinical evaluation of venous accessibility. J Emerg Med. 2013;44(2):299-305.
6. Jacobson AF, Winslow EH. Variables influencing intravenous catheter insertion difficulty and failure: an analysis of 339 intravenous catheter insertions. Heart Lung. 2005;34(5):345-59.
7. Brandt HG, Jepsen CH, Hendriksen OM, Lindekær A, Skjønnemand M. The use of ultrasound to identify veins for peripheral venous access in morbidly obese patients. Dan Med J. 2016;63(2):A5191.
8. Whiteley MS, Chang BY, Marsh HP, Williams AR, Manton HC, Horrocks M. Use of hand-held Doppler to identify 'difficult' forearm veins for cannulation. Ann R Coll Surg Engl. 1995;77(3):224-6.
9. Reddick AD, Ronald J, Morrison WG. Intravenous fluid resuscitation: Was Poiseuille right?. Emerg Med J. 2011;28(3):201-2.
10. O'Grady NP, Alexander M, Burns LA, Dellinger EP, Garland J, Heard SO, et al. Guidelines for the prevention of intravascular catheter-related infections. Clin Infect Dis. 2011;52(9):e162-93.
11. O'Neil C, Ball K, Wood H, McMullen K, Kremer P, Jafarzadeh SR, et al. Central line care maintenance bundle for the prevention of central line-associated bloodstream infection in non-intensive care unit settings. Infect Control Hosp Epidemiol. 2016;37(6):692-8.
12. Mimoz O, Pieroni L, Lawrence C, Edouard A, Costa Y, Samii K, et al. Prospective, randomized trial of two antiseptic solutions for prevention of central venous or arterial catheter colonization and infection in intensive care unit patients. Crit Care Med. 1996;24(11):1818-23.
13. Johnson E, Babb J, Sridhar D. Routine antibiotic prophylaxis for totally implantable venous access device placement: meta-analysis of 2,154 patients. J Vasc Interv Radiol. 2016;27(3):339-43.

SECTION 5

Syndromic Approach

36. **Hypoxia in Pregnancy**
    Priteema Chanana, Kesari Masaipeta, Arindam Kar

37. **Altered Sensorium in Pregnancy**
    Mithilesh Raut, Ganshyam Jagathkar

38. **Fulminant Hepatic Failure in Pregnancy**
    Lalita Gouri Mitra, Sunaina Tejpal Karna

39. **Sepsis in Full Term Pregnancy**
    Rajesh Mishra, Maneendra Singarapu

40. **Noncardiogenic Pulmonary Edema in Pregnancy**
    Sharmili Sinha, Neeraj Kumar

41. **Acute Disseminated Encephalomyelitis**
    Simant Kumar Jha, Sameer Bhuwania, Bhumika Sambyal

42. **Neuromuscular Disorders in Pregnancy**
    Saurabh Taneja, Asish Kumar Sahoo

43. **Posterior Reversible Encephalopathy Syndrome**
    Nithya CA, Ajith Kumar AK

44. **Management of Obstetric Shock with Emphasis on Fluids and Vasopressors**
    Rajesh Pande, Maitree Pandey, Jitin Sharma

45. **Hematological Cancers in Pregnancy**
    Suresh Kumar Sundaramurthy, Raymond Dominic Savio

46. **Airway Management in Critically Ill Obstetric Patients**
    Anirban Hom Choudhuri, Deepika Jain

47. **Status Epilepticus in Pregnancy**
    Bhuvna Ahuja, Ahsina Jahan Lopa, Sabina Regmi

48. **Pyrexia of Unknown Origin during Pregnancy**
    Jay Prakash, Tushar Kumar, Bhawesh Upreti

49. **Anaphylaxis in Pregnancy**
    Aklesh Tandekar, Suvadeep Sen, Sachin Narayan Rathore

CHAPTER 36

Hypoxia in Pregnancy

Priteema Chanana, Kesari Masaipeta, Arindam Kar

INTRODUCTION

Anatomical and physiological changes take place throughout pregnancy to accommodate the body's higher metabolic demands, allow for the fetus' proper development, and get the body ready for giving birth. In healthy females, these alterations are well tolerated, but they might exacerbate or reveal an underlying illness or pregnancy-related pathology. The secret to managing both obstetric and non-obstetric interventions during pregnancy is easy if treating physician has thorough knowledge of the physiological changes in pregnancy. The alterations start early in the first trimester, peak during labor or term, and return to prepregnancy levels a few weeks after delivery.

A healthy mother and a normal placenta are necessary for a normal pregnancy to develop. Vital organs in the mother and fetus may suffer serious harm as a result of maternal exposure to hypoxic incidents. There are many causes of hypoxia during pregnancy.[1] Evidence suggests that a number of pregnancy problems are linked to hypoxia. However, mid- to late gestation is when hypoxia's negative consequences are most prevalent. In reality, due to poor blood flow in the uterus during the early stages of a healthy pregnancy, oxygen (O_2) availability is typically low. The trophoblast stem cells, or progenitor cells, require this hypoxic microenvironment in order to maintain homeostasis, prevent deoxyribonucleic acid (DNA) damage, and differentiate in a targeted manner.[2]

PHYSIOLOGICAL CHANGES WITH PREGNANCY

In order to provide care for and accommodate the growing fetus, the pregnant woman goes through considerable anatomical and physiological changes. These changes start soon after conception and impact every organ system in the body. For the majority of women who had an easy pregnancy, these alterations disappear after delivery with no lasting impact. It is essential to understand the typical physiological changes that take place during pregnancy in order to differentiate between normal and pathological adaptations.

In nonpregnant women, uteroplacental blood flow is <50 mL/min, which increases to 350 mL/min by a full-term pregnancy. Due to the increase in demand for uteroplacental blood flow (20% of the total maternal cardiac output), pregnancy requires huge physiological changes.[3]

In pregnancy, the cardiac output increases to meet the demand for uteroplacental blood flow. The cardiac output increases by 20–25% in the first trimester, followed by 30–40% in the third trimester.

The stroke volume, heart rate, and cardiac output increase progressively to reach around

45% higher than prepregnancy levels with the effects of gestational hormones, circulating prostaglandins, the excessive release of human placental growth factors (PLGF), and the low-resistance uteroplacental unit.[4,5]

The total number of red blood cells will increase, but not as much as the plasma volume expansion, which will result in relative anemia. Because of these changes, the hemoglobin-oxygen dissociation curve will shift rightward,[6-9] increasing the risk of hypoxic episodes compared to nonpregnant women.

Oxygen consumption also increases around 25-30% above prepregnancy levels to meet the increasing maternal and fetal requirements. The metabolic rate also increases by 15%. The increase in maternal O_2 consumption during pregnancy and the lower functional residual capacity means that pregnant women have lower reserves of O_2 and are more susceptible to becoming hypoxic.

The arteriovenous oxygen ($A-VO_2$) gradient is low in early pregnancy but widens in late pregnancy.

Pregnancy-induced hyperventilation is the result of complex interactions between changes in acid-base balance, chemo response drives, metabolic rate, and cerebral blood flow.

Due to changes in respiratory physiology, partial pressure of oxygen (PaO_2) levels increase to 13-14 kPa and alveolar and arterial carbon dioxide tension ($PaCO_2$) levels decrease to plateau around 27 and 32 mm Hg, respectively. The higher the PaO_2 in the maternal circulation, the easier it is to transfer O_2 from the maternal to the fetal circulation, and the lower the $PaCO_2$ in the maternal circulation, the easier it is to transfer carbon dioxide in the opposite direction. The lower $PaCO_2$ in the maternal circulation results in a state of respiratory alkalosis. To maintain the maternal pH in the range of 7.40-7.45, there is an increase in the excretion of bicarbonate, resulting in lower bicarbonate levels in pregnant women.

This decrease in bicarbonate levels shifts the maternal O_2 dissociation curve to the right, lowering maternal hemoglobin's affinity for O_2 and allowing O_2 to be released from maternal hemoglobin for transfer to fetal circulation.

PLACENTAL DEVELOPMENT AND OXYGEN

During the development of the human placenta, cytotrophoblasts (CTBs) produce two distinct placental subtypes: a multinucleated syncytiotrophoblast (STB) and a migratory extravillous trophoblast (EVT). The initial epithelial breach and implantation within the uterine wall are facilitated by STBs. Following implantation, the junctional zone, also known as the maternal-fetal interface, is finally established by the growth of fetal trophoblasts. Anatomically defined, the junctional zone is made up of two sections: (1) the "placental bed," which remains connected to the uterus, and (2) the "basal plate," which is expelled together with the placenta after birth. The "floating villi," which are made of STB, are the primary hub of maternal-fetal exchange. The "anchoring villi" that anchor the villi to the basal plate are made of EVT and are also known as "cell columns."[10-14]

In normal placental development, O_2 is a key regulator of trophoblast differentiation, proliferation, and migration.[10] According to measurements made in the intervillous space and endometrial tissue in humans, trophoblast invasion happens during the first trimester of pregnancy at a relatively low partial pressure of O_2 of 18-40 mm Hg.[15-17] However, after spiral artery remodeling and improved placental perfusion, this partial pressure rises to 60–80 mm Hg. A low-oxygen environment is necessary for the placenta's growth. Hypoxia-inducible factors (HIFs), among other transcription factors, are stabilized by low O_2 levels. To activate the gene expression of angiogenic factors such as vascular endothelial growth factor (VEGF), PLGF, and angiopoietins 1 and 2, which increase blood vessel formation in endometrial tissue, HIF1 and HIF2 proteins can bind to consensus DNA recognition sequences.

The key purpose of EVT is the formation of plugs that occlude capillaries in the stroma of the endometrial gland and prevent disruption of the conceptus by stopping maternal hemorrhage and entering maternal blood in the lacunar spaces of the trophoblastic shell, which is called the plugging mechanism.

Up to 8–9 weeks of gestation, the embryonic development and the embryonic placental villi are shielded from oxidative damage by the "plugging" mechanism.[18,19]

Up to 10 weeks of pregnancy, embryogenesis occurs in a hypoxic environment because the placenta's O_2 tension is significantly lower than that of the endometrial glands.[17,20-22]

Between 11 and 13 weeks, endothelial cells of spiral arteries are replaced, and vascular smooth cells die with the help of angiogenesis, which leads to an increase in the diameter of the lumen and finally placental perfusion.[17,23-25]

■ HYPOXIA IN PREGNANCY

A mismatch between tissue O_2 supply and demand is referred to as hypoxia. Intrauterine hypoxia is defined as a drop in the PaO_2 in the maternal, placental, or fetal compartments due to a disruption in the supply/demand ratio for O_2. As the placenta and the fetus grow throughout pregnancy, O_2 delivery fluctuates, and metabolic demand increases.

Placental Hypoxia: The Role of Oxidative Stress

- Oxidative stress can occur in hypoxic conditions or due to reoxygenation injury when the production of reactive O_2 species (superoxide anions, hydrogen peroxides, and hydroxyl radicals) outpaces the antioxidant capacity of the cell (superoxide dismutase, catalase, glutathione peroxidase, and/or peroxiredoxins).[26-29]
- Along with that, the formation of peroxynitrite interferes with membrane and enzyme function, which forms with the interaction between superoxide anions and nitric oxide.[30,31]
- Oxidized lipids, proinflammatory cytokines (interleukin-6, tumor necrosis factor-α), and reactive O_2 species are elevated in the hypoxic placenta, interfering with trophoblast invasion and resulting in abnormal spiral artery remodeling, tissue inflammation, trophoblast apoptosis, and the release of surface membrane microparticles[32,33] into the maternal circulation.
- Reduced endovascular invasion, abnormal spiral artery remodeling, and membrane fragment release are thought to be important risk factors for preeclampsia.

Intrauterine Hypoxia

Numerous maternal, placental, and fetal disorders are linked to intrauterine hypoxia; these conditions might present differently and result in various outcomes. Three categories of hypoxic pregnancy conditions were proposed by Kingdom and Kaufmann:[34-36]

1. Preplacental hypoxia **(Flowchart 1)**, a condition in which both the mother and the fetus are hypoxic (e.g., high altitude, cyanotic maternal heart disease, etc.).
2. Uteroplacental hypoxia **(Flowchart 2)** occurs when the uteroplacental circulation

Flowchart 1: Preplacental hypoxia.

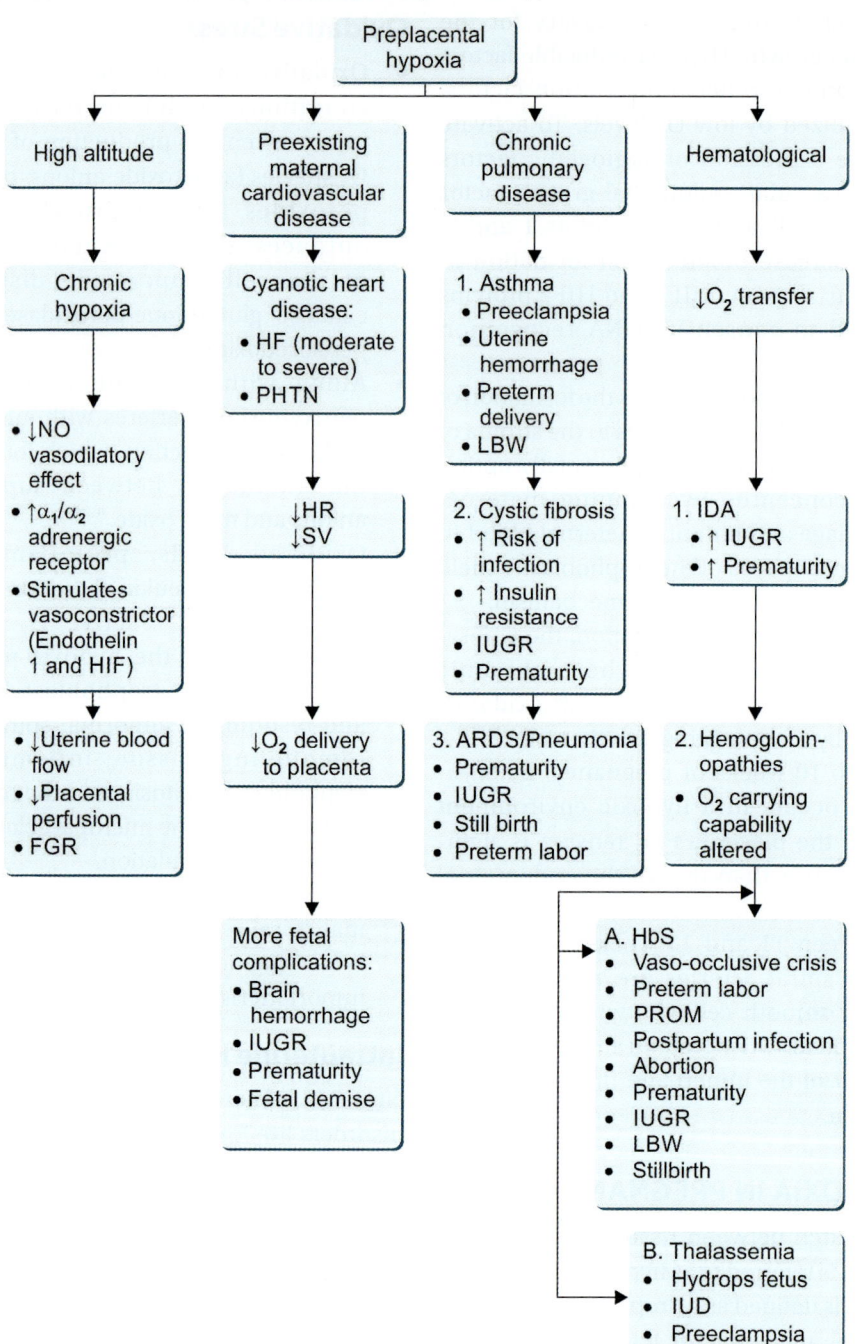

(ARDS: acute respiratory distress syndrome; FGR: fetal growth restriction; HbS: hemoglobin S (Sickle cell disease); HF: heart failure; HIF: hypoxia-inducible factor; IDA: iron-deficiency anemia; IUGR: intrauterine growth restriction; LBW: low birth weight; PHTN: pulmonary hypertension; PROM: premature rupture of membranes)

Flowchart 2: Uteroplacental hypoxia.

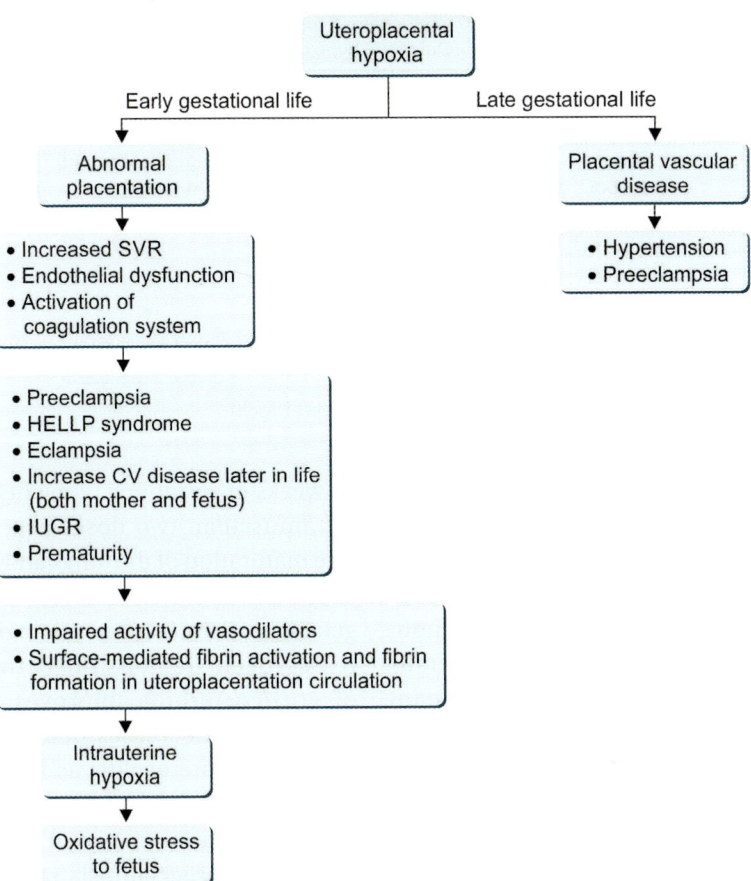

(CV: cardiovascular; HELLP: hemolysis, elevated liver enzymes, and low platelets; IUGR: intrauterine growth restriction; SVR: systemic vascular resistance)

is compromised but the maternal oxygenation is normal (i.e., preeclampsia, placental insufficiency, etc.).
3. Postplacental hypoxia **(Flowchart 3)**, in which only the fetus is hypoxic.

CLINICAL MANAGEMENT OF PREGNANT MOTHER

With careful antenatal Doppler US monitoring, intrauterine hypoxia-related pregnancy problems can be avoided. Because fetal growth restriction (FGR) is a significant problem, the goal of care should be to restore fetal health when there is intrauterine hypoxia.[35] The best testing methods for determining or categorizing the level of FGR are fetal Doppler US and biophysical profiles.

Preeclampsia

The maternal status will dictate the clinical care of a preeclampsia-complicated pregnancy. In this situation, the mother is observed very closely for any indications or symptoms of preeclampsia or worsening hypertension. Once preeclampsia is identified, delivery is

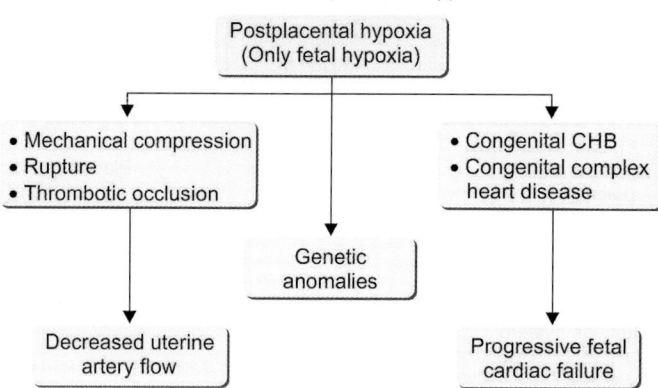

Flowchart 3: Postplacental hypoxia.

(CHB: congenital heart block)

the only curative option. The date of delivery is determined by two interconnected factors:
1. The gestational age at diagnosis
2. The severity of preeclampsia.

Preeclampsia can be controlled without delivery up to 37 weeks or until serious symptoms start to show. When a pregnant woman has hypoxia, delivery should begin as soon as the fetus is >34 weeks old. When the fetus is <32 weeks gestation, antenatal steroids are administered, and vaginal delivery is suggested unless there is a maternal contraindication.

The following are some severe maternal warning signs:[37]
- Eclampsia
- Hemolysis, elevated liver enzymes, and low platelets (HELLP) syndrome
- Abruptio placentae
- Severe, uncontrolled hypertension
- Pulmonary edema.

If FGR is caused by placental insufficiency, fetuses have few therapeutic options, and delivery is the recommended treatment. To lower infant morbidity and mortality, the mother receives one course of prenatal corticosteroids between 24 and 34 weeks of gestation (12 mg betamethasone intramuscular, two doses every 24 hours). The maturation of the lungs and other tissues is caused by corticosteroid stimulation of gene expression and physiologic processes. It has been demonstrated that a course of corticosteroids improves infant lung growth and decreases neonatal mortality, necrotizing enterocolitis, and interventricular hemorrhage.

The mother is treated in one of two ways if maternal preeclampsia is the underlying cause of FGR. Antihypertensive treatment is used to lower blood pressure to prevent brain hemorrhage and/or pulmonary edema [aim for systolic blood pressure (SBP) of 160 mm Hg and diastolic blood pressure (DBP) of 110 mm Hg]. The methods through which magnesium sulfate normalizes blood pressure and prevents seizures are complex yet still unknown. Magnesium sulfate may act as a vasodilator, lowering peripheral vascular resistance, protecting the blood-brain barrier, and preventing cerebral edema. Treatment of preeclampsia with antihypertensive drugs and magnesium sulfate has the immediate benefit of extending pregnancy. Magnesium sulfate may act as a vasodilator, lowering peripheral vascular resistance, protecting the blood-brain barrier, and preventing cerebral edema.

MANAGEMENT OF PREGNANT FEMALE IN SPECIFIC CONDITIONS

- *Asthma:* The consequences of asthma itself on the placenta are more harmful than those of its therapy. Inhaled corticosteroids (ICS) containing budesonide are thought to be safe during pregnancy. Salbutamol is a preferred short-acting beta agonist (SABA) because of its safety record in pregnant women with asthma. Formoterol, salmeterol, and long-acting beta-agonists (LABA) are examples of prohibited substances. Theophylline at low doses is being examined as a potential substitute for moderately persistent asthma during pregnancy, and there have been no reports of teratogenic effects. Only patients who responded well to leukotriene receptor antagonists (LTRAs) before becoming pregnant are advised to use them. Due to the unknown danger of anaphylaxis and the minor benefits that seem to accompany allergic immunotherapy (AIT), it is not advised to begin AIT during pregnancy. Keeping away from infections and triggers is a key step in reducing asthma episodes.
- *Obstructive sleep apnea (OSA):* Predisposing factors for OSA in pregnancy include lower functional residual capacity and airway edema. Continuous positive airway pressure (CPAP) is typically used to manage this.
- *Smoking:* Smoking during pregnancy is associated with abruption, placenta previa, stillbirth, miscarriage, early delivery, low birth weight, and spontaneous pregnancy loss. O_2 transport to the fetus is compromised due to altered placental anatomy, nicotine-induced vasospasm, and increased amounts of circulating carboxyhemoglobin.
- *Neuromuscular and spinal deformities:* These individuals may have respiratory failure during pregnancy because of their reduced reserve capacity and changed lung volumes. Maintenance of saturation in these individuals is aided by O_2 supplementation and pain avoidance. In some circumstances, mechanical ventilation may be necessary.
- *Cardiovascular disorders:* Cyanosis (arterial oxygenation of <80%) is associated with a bad prognosis for both the mother and the fetus. Chronic lung illness, hypoxia, OSA, and chronic thrombotic disease are all linked to pulmonary hypertension. Avoiding hypoxia, hypercarbia, and acidemia can help to prevent the worsening of pulmonary hypertension. Mechanical ventilation and O_2 supplementation are required to prevent hypercarbia and hypoxia, respectively. It is best to prevent hypovolemia. Pain should be minimized since the right ventricular afterload is increased by catecholamine-mediated tachycardia.
- *Trauma:* To avoid fetal hypoxia, pregnant trauma victims should never be given hypotensive resuscitation.

CONCLUSION

Since early embryogenesis already occurs in anaerobic environments during the first trimester, hypoxia does not significantly affect this stage of development. Only during the second and third trimesters does O_2 become increasingly important for proper fetal organogenesis and development. Intrauterine hypoxia, which can happen in circumstances of placental insufficiency, high-altitude settings, and exposure to toxic chemicals, is one of the most prevalent clinical concerns in obstetric critical care. Preeclampsia is a maternal outcome associated with placental dysfunction and defective spiral artery development that has an impact on the health of both the mother and fetus. Understanding the underlying processes of the placental dysfunction brought on by intrauterine hypoxia is crucial to enhancing therapy techniques for the clinical management of the condition.[35] Future treatments for preeclampsia and other placental diseases should be more successful as we learn more about the factors that regulate trophoblast invasion of the placenta and its spiral arteries and how regulatory mechanisms are changed during placental hypoxia.

TAKE HOME MESSAGES

- Hypoxia during pregnancy causes harmful effects on pregnancy and embryo growth.
- Presence of hypoxia in early pregnancy is very important for blastocyst implantation, trophoblast cell anchoring, decidual development, spiral artery remodeling, immune tolerance, and angiogenesis/vasculogenesis.
- After 14 weeks, intrauterine hypoxia can lead to maternal, placental and fetal problems out of which FGR is a significant problem.
- With careful antenatal Doppler US monitoring, intrauterine hypoxia-related pregnancy problems can be avoided.
- Understanding the underlying disease process of specific conditions and their impact on pregnancy is crucial in enhancing therapy techniques for the clinical management of the condition.

REFERENCES

1. Borghi C, Spadaro S, Lombana Mariño MG, Bianchi B, Morano D, Bianchi B, et al. Hypoxic events during non-obstetric abdominal surgery in pregnant women. Eur Rev Med Pharmacol Sci. 2020;24(6):2795-801.
2. Spencer JA, Ferraro F, Roussakis E, Klein A, Wu J, Runnels JM, et al. Direct measurement of local oxygen concentration in the bone marrow of live animals. Nature. 2014;508:269-73.
3. Palmer SK, Zamudio S, Coffin C, Parker S, Stamm E, Moore LG. Quantitative estimation of human uterine artery blood flow and pelvic blood flow redistribution in pregnancy. Obstet Gynecol. 1992;80(6):1000-6.
4. Kitanaka T, Gilbert RD, Longo LD. Maternal responses to long-term hypoxemia in sheep. Am J Physiol. 1989;256(6 Pt 2):R1340-7.
5. Kametas NA, McAuliffe F, Krampl E, Chambers J, Nicolaides KH. Maternal cardiac function during pregnancy at high altitude. BJOG. 2004;111(10):1051-8.
6. Magness RR. Maternal cardiovascular and other physiologic responses to the endocrinology of pregnancy. In: FW Bazer (Ed). The Endocrinology of Pregnancy. Totowas, NJ, USA: Humana Press; 1998. pp. 507-39.
7. Abbas AE, Lester SJ, Connolly H. Pregnancy and the cardiovascular system. Int J Cardiol. 2005;98(2):179-89.
8. Miller RD. Anesthesia, 5th edition. Philadelphia, PA, USA: Churchill Livingston; 2000.
9. Siu SC, Colman JM. Congenital heart disease: heart disease and pregnancy. Heart. 2001;85(6):710-5.
10. Ji L, Brkić J, Liu M, Fu G, Peng C, Wang YL. Placental trophoblast cell differentiation: physiological regulation and pathological relevance to preeclampsia. Mol Aspects Med. 2013;34:981-1023.
11. Kaufmann P, Black S, Huppertz B. Endovascular trophoblast invasion: implications for the pathogenesis of intrauterine growth retardation and preeclampsia. Biol Reprod. 2003;69:1-7.

12. Zhao H, Wong RJ, Stevenson DK. The impact of hypoxia in early pregnancy on placental cells. Int J Mol Sci. 2021;22(18):9675.
13. Lyall F. Primary and remodeling of human placenta bed spiral arteries during pregnancy – a review. Placenta. 2005;26 Suppl A:S31-6.
14. Knöfler M. Critical growth factors and signaling pathways controlling human trophoblast invasion. Int J Dev Biol. 2010;54(2-3):269-80.
15. Rooth G, Sjostedt S, Caligara F. Hydrogen concentration, carbon dioxide tension and acid base balance in blood of human umbilical cord and intervillous space of placenta. Arch Dis Child. 1961;36:278-85.
16. Jauniaux E, Watson A, Ozturk O, Quick D, Burton G. In-vivo measurement of intrauterine gases and acid-base values early in human pregnancy. Hum Reprod. 1999;14(11):2901-4.
17. Rodesch F, Simon P, Donner C, Jauniaux E. Oxygen measurement in endometrial and trophoblastic tissues during early pregnancy. Obstet Gynecol. 1992;80(2):283-5.
18. Jauniaux E, Watson AL, Hempstock J, Bao Y-P, Skepper JN, Burton GJ. Onset of maternal arterial blood flow and placental oxidative stress: a possible factor in human early pregnancy failure. Am J Pathol. 2000;157(6):2111-22.
19. Watson AL, Skepper JN, Jauniaux E, Burton GJ. Susceptibility of human placental syncytiotrophoblastic mitochondria to oxygen-mediated damage in relation to gestational age. J Clin Endocrinol Metabol. 1998;83(5):1697-705.
20. Burton GJ, Jauniaux E, Watson AL. Maternal arterial connections to the placental intervillous space during the first trimester of human pregnancy: the Boyd collection revisited. Am J Obstet Gynecol. 1999;181(3):718-24.
21. Jauniaux E, Greenwold N, Hempstock J, Burton GJ. Comparison of ultrasonographic and Doppler mapping of the intervillous circulation in normal and abnormal early pregnancies. Fertil Steril. 2003;79(1):100-6.
22. Jauniaux E, Jurkovic D, Campbell S, Hustin J. Doppler ultrasonographic features of the developing placental circulation: correlation with anatomic findings. Am J Obstet Gynecol. 1992;166(2):585-7.
23. Robertson WB, Brosens I, Dixon G. Maternal uterine vascular lesions in the hypertensive complications of pregnancy. Perspect Nephrol Hypertens. 1976;5:115-27.
24. Hirano H, Imai Y, Ito H. Spiral artery of placenta: development and pathology-immunohistochemical microscopical, and electromicroscopic study. Kobe J Med Sci. 2002;48:13-23.
25. Robertson WB, Manning PJ. Elastic tissue in uterine blood vessels. J Pathol. 1974;112(4):237-43.
26. Burton GJ. Oxygen, the Janus gas; its effects on human placental development and function. J Anat. 2009;215:27-35.
27. Wang Y, Walsh SW. Increased superoxide generation is associated with decreased superoxide dismutase activity and mRNA expression in placental trophoblast cells in pre-eclampsia. Placenta. 2001;22(2-3):206-12.
28. Guzy RD, Hoyos B, Robin E, Chen H, Liu L, Mansfield KD, et al. Mitochondrial complex III is required for hypoxia-induced ROS production and cellular oxygen sensing. Cell Metab. 2005;1:401-8.
29. Wilcox CR, Trudinger BJ. Fetal platelet consumption: a feature of placental insufficiency. Obstet Gynecol. 1991;77(4):616-21.
30. Myatt L. Review: Reactive oxygen and nitrogen species and functional adaptation of the placenta. Placenta. 2010;31 Suppl(Suppl):S66-9.
31. Webster RP, Roberts VH, Myatt L. Protein nitration in placenta – functional significance. Placenta. 2008;29(12):985-94.
32. Laresgoiti-Servitje E, Gomez-Lopez N. The pathophysiology of preeclampsia involves altered levels of angiogenic factors promoted by hypoxia and autoantibody-mediated mechanisms. Biol Reprod. 2012;87(2):36.

33. Huppertz B, Kingdom J, Caniggia I, Desoye G, Black S, Korr H, et al. Hypoxia favours necrotic versus apoptotic shedding of placental syncytiotrophoblast into the maternal circulation. Placenta. 2003;24(2-3): 181-90.
34. Kingdom JC, Kaufmann P. Oxygen and placental villous development: origins of fetal hypoxia. Placenta. 1997;18(8):613–21.
35. Thompson LP, Crimmins S, Telugu BP, Turan S. Intrauterine hypoxia: clinical consequences and therapeutic perspectives. Res Rep Neonatol. 2015(default):79.
36. Hutter D, Kingdom J, Jaeggi E. Causes and mechanisms of intrauterine hypoxia and its impact on the fetal cardiovascular system: A review. Int J Pediatr. 2010;2010:401323.
37. Haukkamaa L, Salminen M, Laivuori H, Leinonen H, Hiilesmaa V, Kaaja R. Risk for subsequent coronary artery disease after preeclampsia. Am J Cardiol. 2004;93(6): 805-8.

CHAPTER 37

Altered Sensorium in Pregnancy

Mithilesh Raut, Ganshyam Jagathkar

INTRODUCTION

Pregnancy is a state of normal maternal anatomical and physiological changes to meet increased metabolic demands, fetal development, and childbirth. The major changes are increase in plasma volume, cardiac output, and reduction in systemic vascular resistance. There is procoagulant state with increase in clotting factors. The immune responses are reduced, leading to impaired pathogen clearance and increased susceptibility to infections. Deranged physiological response can lead to several pathological states which may present with altered sensorium. A systematic multisystem approach is required for diagnosis and early treatment to reduce risk to mother and fetus **(Flowchart 1)**. Causes of altered sensorium in pregnancy are given in **Table 1**.

HYPERTENSIVE DISORDERS OF PREGNANCY

Criteria for Hypertension during Pregnancy

Systolic blood pressure (BP) ≥140 mm Hg and/or diastolic BP ≥90 mm Hg. Severe hypertension is defined BP ≥160/110 mm Hg.

Preeclampsia is defined as newly diagnosed hypertension in a previously normotensive pregnant patient after 20 weeks of gestation with or without organ dysfunction and proteinuria. The incidence of preeclampsia is around 5% across the world.[1,2] Hemolysis, elevated liver enzymes, and low platelets (HELLP) syndrome is a severe form of preeclampsia.

Eclampsia is defined as occurrence of a seizure in a woman with preeclampsia in the absence of other neurologic conditions which may cause seizures.[5]

Risk Factors for Pregnancy-induced Hypertension

It includes nulliparity, increased age of pregnancy, artificial reproductive techniques, multiple pregnancy, previous history of preeclampsia chronic hypertension, and diabetes mellitus.[3]

Pathophysiology

Preeclampsia is characterized by abnormal placentation resulting in chronic placental insufficiency, oxidative stress, and endothelial dysfunction.[4]

Clinical Presentation

The most common presentation in preeclampsia may be headache, visual abnormalities, upper abdominal, or epigastric pain, altered mental status (confusion and

Flowchart 1: Approach to altered sensorium in pregnancy.

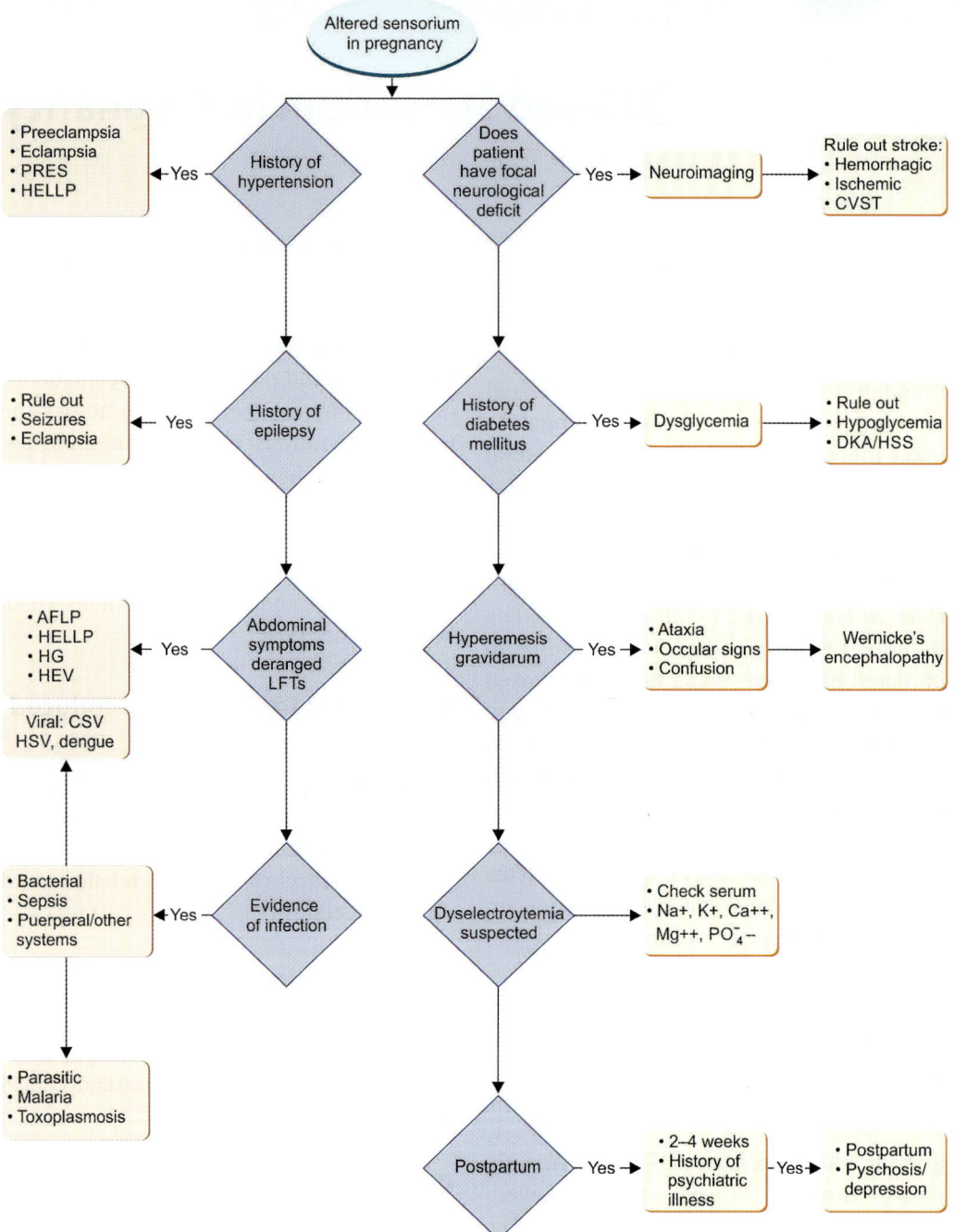

(AFLP: acute fatty liver of pregnancy; CVST: cerebral venous sinus thrombosis; DKA: diabetic ketoacidosis; HELLP: hemolysis, elevated liver enzymes, and low platelets; HEV: hepatitis E virus; HSS: hyperosmolar hyperglycemic state; HSV: herpes simplex virus; LFTs: liver function tests; PRES: posterior reversible encephalopathy syndrome)

TABLE 1: Causes of altered sensorium in pregnancy.	
Pregnancy related	Preeclampsia, eclampsia, PRES, HELLP
Neurological	Ischemic stroke, hemorrhagic stroke, CVST
Infection	HSV, CMV, toxoplasmosis, malaria, dengue, bacterial sepsis
Hepatic/GIT	Hyperemesis gravidarum, AFLP, HELLP
Postpartum	Postpartum—blues, depression, psychosis
Miscellaneous	Dyselectrolytemia, dysglycemia, drug overdose/poisoning

(AFLP: acute fatty liver of pregnancy; CMV: cytomegalovirus; CVST: cerebral venous sinus thrombosis; GIT: gastrointestinal tract; HELLP: hemolysis, elevated liver enzymes, and low platelets; HSV: herpes simplex virus; PRES: posterior reversible encephalopathy syndrome)

agitation) new onset dyspnea, or orthopnea. These symptoms can present up to 6 weeks post delivery.

Management

Principles of management involve the control of BP, fetal monitoring, early delivery, anticipating, and treating complications.[5] Regular BP monitoring, assessments for proteinuria twice weekly and blood tests for hemoglobin, platelet count, and tests of liver and renal function.

Aspirin 100 mg is used to reduce the risk of preeclampsia.

Goal of BP reduction is 15–25% of admission BP, with drugs with good safety profile as:
- Labetalol, 100 mg BD titrated to control BP (400 mg BD)
- Alpha-methyldopa, 0.5–3 g in two to four divided dosage
- Intravenous hydralazine, 5 mg IV repeat 30 minutes to maximum 30 mg or infusion 0.5–10 mg/h
- Magnesium sulfate, if neurological signs are present[6]
- Avoid angiotensin-converting enzyme (ACEI) and angiotensin receptor blockers (ARBs) for the risk of teratogenicity in fetus.[5]

Women with preeclampsia should be delivered at 37 weeks of gestation or as soon as possible if they develop any of the following:[7]
- Severe hypertension despite treatment with antihypertensive agents
- Altered mental status
- Thrombocytopenia
- Worsening renal or liver enzyme tests
- Pulmonary edema.

Treatment of Severe Hypertension
- Labetalol 20 mg IV over 2 minutes repeat doses (40, 80, 80, and 80 mg) every 10 minutes up to a maximum dose of 300 mg. A continuous infusion at 1–2 mg/min can be used as an alternative to intermittent therapy.
- Hydralazine is added 5 mg IV stat, if the BP is not controlled give bolus 5–10 mg.
- If BP is not controlled, nicardipine 5–15 mg/h or esmolol 250–500 µg/h infusion can be used.[7]

Management of Seizures[8]
- Initial management of airway, breathing, and circulation
- Magnesium sulfate 4 g over 20 minutes then infusion at 1–2 g/h (24 hours post delivery)

- Magnesium sulfate 2 g can be repeated in recurrent seizure with clinical and drug level monitoring
- Benzodiazepines can be administered
- Fluid assessment and adequate resuscitation.

POSTERIOR REVERSIBLE ENCEPHALOPATHY SYNDROME

Hypertensive disorders of pregnancy (preeclampsia and eclampsia) may manifest with acute neurological symptoms and can range from headache and visual disturbances to altered levels of consciousness and seizure.[9] Rapid increase in BP overcomes the autoregulatory capabilities of the cerebral vasculature leading to vascular leakage and resulting in vasogenic edema. This leads to blood–brain barrier (BBB) dysfunction with proteins leaking through the tight junction mainly in areas supplied by the posterior circulation.

The clinical presentation depends on the involved areas of the brain. For example, primary involvement of the occipital lobes may result in visual disturbances or hallucinations. About 5–15% of patients may present with focal neurological deficits.[10]

Vasogenic edema in the setting of posterior reversible encephalopathy syndrome (PRES) may be bilateral and show hyperintense signals on diffusion-weighted imaging (DWI) which may not be accompanied by a corresponding decreased signal on apparent diffusion coefficient (ADC). Early finding of PRES includes mild sulcal fluid-attenuated inversion recovery (FLAIR) hyperintensity and leptomeningeal enhancement on postcontrast T1 later followed by typical parieto occipital edema, while in case of ischemia may be unilateral and there is corresponding decreased signal on ADC.[11]

Findings related to PRES are usually reversible as name suggests with normalization of clinical and imaging findings once the issue is addressed. It may rarely progress to necrosis or hemorrhage in some patients.[12]

Maternal outcome for PRES are better in eclampsia patients but had a higher perinatal mortality.[13]

Treatment

Nonrapid reduction in BP is sought to avoid the risk of causing cerebral ischemia. In preeclampsia and eclampsia patients treatment is aimed at the timely delivery of the fetus as well as BP management and magnesium sulfate for seizure.[14]

STROKE IN PREGNANCY

The incidence of pregnancy-related strokes is 30 per 100,000 pregnancies, with ischemic, hemorrhagic, and venous thrombosis having a similar contribution.[15] Clinical examination and early evaluation is similar to nonpregnant patient. Hemorrhagic stroke is more commonly associated with hypertensive disorders of pregnancy and has higher fatality and disability rate. The risk of ischemic stroke is more in hyperstimulation syndrome, hyperemesis gravidarum, antiphospholipid syndrome, and preeclampsia.[16] Initial non-contrast CT brain to rule out bleed and decide about thrombolysis. IV thrombolysis with recombinant tissue plasminogen activator (rtPA) within 4.5 hours improves stroke outcomes. The American Heart Association has advised to weigh risk of uterine bleed versus benefit of stroke outcomes.[17] CT angiography is safe and has less exposure than CT perfusion in patients where mechanical thrombectomy is planned.[18] Mechanical thrombectomy is superior to thrombolysis and can be done till 24 hours.[19] Management principles are similar to a nonpregnant patient with emphasis on BP control and other neurosupportive measures.

CENTRAL VENOUS SINUS THROMBOSIS (CVST) IN PREGNANCY

Not an uncommon finding with an incidence of 4.5/1,000 pregnancies. More often occurs during puerperium. Outcomes are usually favorable with low mortality.

Inherited prothrombotic tendencies such as factor V Leiden mutation, protein S and C, and antithrombin III deficiencies are important causes. Headache is most common presentation; other symptoms are nausea, vomiting, altered consciousness, and visual disturbances.[20] Initial CT scan may show venous infarct or bleed, magnetic resonance imaging (MRI) with magnetic resonance venography (MRV) is imaging modality of choice.[21]

Treatment option is with anticoagulation with low-molecular-weight heparin. Local intravenous thrombolysis and surgical thrombectomy can be considered for patients who have poor response to anticoagulation. Vitamin K antagonists are used for long-term anticoagulation.[22]

LIVER DISORDERS IN PREGNANCY

Hyperemesis Gravidarum

Hyperemesis gravidarum occurs in approximately 1% of pregnant patients usually during the first trimester and presents as nausea and intractable vomiting that results in dehydration, weight loss >5% of body weight, and ketosis.[23]

It may be associated with abnormal liver tests with elevated serum aminotransferases, however the abdominal ultrasound may show normal liver parenchyma and no biliary obstruction.[24]

Some patients with severe hyperemesis gravidarum can land up with Wernicke's encephalopathy. Common presentation is with acute mental confusion, encephalopathy, and ophthalmoplegia. MRI of the brain is diagnostic. The recommend treatment is intravenous thiamine 200 mg tid started before any carbohydrate administration.[25]

Acute Fatty Liver of Pregnancy

Acute fatty liver of pregnancy (AFLP) is a rare condition, usually occurring in the third trimester. Clinical presentation includes nonspecific symptoms such as nausea, vomiting, abdominal pain, headache, and malaise. It may rapidly progress to acute liver failure and present with encephalopathy, jaundice, and coagulopathy which may progress to disseminated intravascular coagulation (DIC).[26] Early diagnosis and supportive treatment like correction of coagulopathy, hypoglycemia, if needed plasma exchange and continuous renal replacement therapy (CRRT) may be done. Liver transplantation is the last alternative in management. Prompt delivery of fetus is mainstay of treatment.[27,28]

Hemolysis, Elevated Liver Function Tests, and Low Platelet Counts Syndrome

Another clinical condition resembling AFLP is HELLP which presents in third trimester (antepartum or postpartum) with preeclampsia (12% patients).[29] Diagnosis is based on clinical features and laboratory findings. It presents as epigastric or right upper quadrant pain, nausea, vomiting, and malaise. Arterial hypertension and proteinuria are noted, microangiopathic hemolytic anemia results in increased unconjugated bilirubin and lactate dehydrogenase (LDH).

Liver enzymes are moderately elevated alanine transaminase (ALT) 2–30-fold low haptoglobin due to hemolysis is present.[30] Delivery of fetus is definitive treatment.[30,31]

The HELLP syndrome is associated with preeclampsia and usually has hypertension proteinuria and reduced platelets. AFLP is comparatively rare but presents in third trimester with more severe liver disease manifestations, increased ALT and bilirubin as compared to HELLP. It may progress to liver failure. It is more commonly associated with coagulopathy and DIC.[32]

■ INFECTION IN PREGNANCY

Pregnancy induces significant physiological changes including a modified immune response and thus predisposing to severe infections which could lead to an altered sensorium.[33-35]

Herpes Simplex Virus in Pregnancy

Herpes simplex virus (HSV) is the leading cause of encephalitis, predominantly due to type-1 HSV. HSV infections are usually common during the third trimester due to a rise in estrogen and progesterone concentrations leading to a modulation of the immune response.[37] HSV-1 encephalitis in a pregnant woman presents with headaches, fever, altered mental status, and seizures. MRI of the brain is the preferred imaging method if maternal meningoencephalitis suspected, as it is safe throughout pregnancy. Classical MRI findings are temporal hyperintensities. Intravenous acyclovir at a dose of 10 mg per kg q8h for 14–21 days is the treatment of choice. Acyclovir crosses the placenta, with similar drug levels between mother and fetus.[37] Cesarean delivery is recommended in the presence of genital lesions. Infants with disseminated HSV infection should be treated with intravenous acyclovir 20 mg/kg every 8 hours for 21 days.[36,38]

Cytomegalovirus Infection in Pregnancy

Primary cytomegalovirus (CMV) infection (2%) and reactivation in seropositive (10%) in pregnant women is seen. Usual clinical presentation is with flu-like symptoms, but in immunocompromised women it may present with encephalitis or as an acute confusional state.[36] CMV is diagnosed with immunoglobulin M (IgM) antibodies which may persist for months. First and early second trimester transmission increases the risk of sensory neural hearing loss or neurologic manifestations in fetus.[36,39] Asymptomatic pregnant women with normal fetal ultrasound needs no treatment. In fetus with abnormal cerebral ultrasound findings in utero, maternal treatment with valacyclovir (8 g daily) decreases fetal CMV viral loads with improved neonatal outcomes.[40]

Toxoplasmosis

Toxoplasmosis is a rare parasitic disease in pregnancy, mostly asymptomatic caused by the *Toxoplasma gondii*, placental transmission can cause severe fetal infection. In an immunosuppressed patient, it may present with necrotizing encephalitis in the brain commonly presents with headache, fever, focal neurological deficits, seizures, altered sensorium ataxia, and visual alterations.[41] On MRI brain the lesions that appear as T2 hyperintensity with ring enhancement and perilesional edema. Diagnosis of an acute infection is done by IgM and IgG antibody level. Treatment with spiramycin 1 g (3 million U) every 8 hours, early diagnosis, and treatment have shown good outcomes.[42]

Malaria

Pregnant women have a higher risk of severe malaria. Cerebral malaria may present as encephalopathy, seizures, status epilepticus, hypertonicity, and coma. Demonstration of malarial parasite on peripheral smear is gold standard for diagnosis, other tests are antigens or polymerase chain reaction (PCR)-based techniques. MRI brain may suggest cerebral edema, infarction, or bleed.[36,43]

Treatment

Mefloquine and quinine with clindamycin are prescribed to treat uncomplicated malaria in pregnancy. Cerebral malaria in pregnant women is considered life-threatening and treated with intravenous artesunate 2.4 mg/kg body weight, at 12 and 24 hours, then once a day for 7 days. Artesunate has adverse outcomes in pregnancy but recommended by the WHO due to severe nature of disease.[36,44]

Epilepsy

Pregnancy can have variable effects on seizure frequency.[45] Risk of seizures is the highest during delivery. Status epilepticus can happen in <1% of patients. The risk of fetal congenital malformations in women on anticonvulsant treatment ranges from 4 to 9%.[46] Antiepileptic drugs are enzyme inducers and reduce the levels of folate. Periconceptional folic acid supplementation is associated with better neurodevelopment scores in children.[47] Antiepileptic drugs having lowest rates of major congenital malformations are lamotrigine, levetiracetam, and oxcarbazepine and commonly used in pregnancy. Valproate and polytherapy have higher risk of congenital malformations and should be avoided.[48,49]

Sudden cessation of anticonvulsant therapy should be avoided as status epilepticus can occur up to 1.8% of pregnancies in women with epilepsy.[50] Treatment includes airway management including intubation and mechanical ventilation whenever necessary, fluid resuscitation, and antiepileptic agents such as lorazepam 2-4 mg intravenously which can be repeated in 15 minutes, diazepam 5-10 mg to a maximum of 30 mg, and phenytoin 15-20 mg/kg IV administration. Signs of fetal distress should prompt exclusion of abruption placentae and immediate delivery of fetus to be considered.[51,52]

Dyselectrolytemia in Pregnancy

Hyponatremia

During pregnancy, sodium is generally decreased by 5 mmol/L and serum osmolality is reduced by 10 mOsmol/kg. Arginine–vasopressin receptors cause water absorption in the collecting ducts and resets osmoreceptors to 275–285 mOsmol/kg.[53] The hyponatremia causes in pregnancy are nausea, vomiting in the first trimester, and pain stimulating arginine vasopressin (AVP) secretion in third trimester. Symptoms can range from headache, nausea, drowsiness, coma, seizures, respiratory arrest, and death. These patients should be treated with the standard protocol of hyponatremia management as in nonpregnant patients. The management of euvolemic hyponatremia with fluid restriction can be relatively harmful in pregnancy as it may result in oligohydramnios and dehydration.[2] Irrespective of etiology, acute severe hyponatremia below 120 mEq/L is corrected by infusion of hypertonic saline to reduce the risk of seizures. The prescribed increase in sodium level is 8-10 mEq/L in 24 hours.[54]

Hypocalcemia

Hypocalcemia in pregnancy occurs in cases of hypoparathyroidism and in mothers with severe dietary inadequacy. Low calcium and magnesium levels are associated with hypertensive pregnancy disorders.[55] The fall in albumin leads to fall in total serum calcium, check the ionized calcium (Ca) to confirm true hypocalcemia.[56] Clinical presentation is variable with neuromuscular irritability, acroparesthesias (perioral, fingers, and toes), and tetany (Trousseau's and Chvostek's signs). It may also cause carpopedal spasm and laryngeal spasm which may be life-threatening. Confusion, seizures, muscle stiffness, myalgias, and QT interval prolongation on electrocardiogram (ECG) can also been frequently seen. Pregnant patients with acute symptomatic hypocalcemia with cardiac arrhythmias or tetany, preeclampsia, and serum ionized calcium level <0.8 mmol/L should be treated with intravenous calcium. Goal is to maintain serum calcium in the low-normal range 8.0 mg/dL and maintaining serum phosphorus within a normal range. Supplemental vitamin D should be administered. In patients with hypoparathyroidism, daily calcitriol dose is up to 2 µg/day and up to 9 g/day for daily doses of calcium.[57]

Dysglycemia in Pregnancy

Pregnant diabetic patient with altered sensorium should be evaluated for hypoglycemia which is a reversible cause but if not corrected may be associated with adverse maternal and fetal outcomes. The occurrence of diabetic ketoacidosis (DKA) during pregnancy is rare, with an estimated incidence of 1–3%[58] of all diabetic gestations. DKA occurs more commonly in third trimester due to increased glucose utilization by fetus, insulin resistant state, noncompliance, or skip dose of insulin or infection. Clinical presentation is nausea, vomiting, abdominal pain, dehydration, tachycardia, hyperventilation, and altered sensorium. Principles of treatment are similar to routine nonpregnant patients, adequate volume replacement to correct dehydration, correction of dyselectrolytemia, insulin therapy, and treatment of precipitating factor.[59]

POSTPARTUM MOOD DISORDERS

Decrease in the levels of progesterone and estrogen levels drop suddenly following delivery affects the serotonin and dopamine; influencing affective and psychotic symptoms.[60] They are mainly classified as:

- *Postpartum blues*: It is a phase of emotional lability following delivery of baby, such as crying, irritability, confusion, and anxiety. Treatment is social support.
- *Postpartum depression*: It is seen in 10–15% patients. Negative thoughts are mainly related to the newborn. Symptoms are depressed mood, disturbed sleep, reduced appetite, and suicidal ideation.[61]
- *Postpartum psychosis*: It is considered as obstetric emergency observed within the first 2 weeks following delivery. History of schizophrenia and bipolar disorders are risk factors.[62] Symptoms such as elation, mood changes, rambling speech, and hallucinations or delusions that infant is possessed, divine, and special are seen. A careful neurological evaluation and neuroimaging is done to rule out other pathologies. Treatment options are psychotherapy and avoid sleep disruption. In moderate depression and postpartum psychosis, medical treatment is necessary. Sertraline, paroxetine, and nortriptyline are antidepressants of choice in nursing women. Atypical antipsychotics (olanzapine and quetiapine) are drugs of choice in patients with symptoms of

psychosis and mania. Lorazepam and haloperidol are used to achieve rapid tranquilization.[62]

The prognosis of postpartum disorders is generally good if diagnosed and treated early.

■ CONCLUSION

Altered sensorium in pregnancy is not an uncommon occurrence. A systematic approach can help in early diagnosis and treatment to reduce morbidity and mortality in pregnant women.

TAKE HOME MESSAGES

- Pregnancy is a state of altered physiology which if uncontrolled may present with altered sensorium.
- A systematic multisystem approach to infective and noninfective etiology is required for early diagnosis and management.
- Hypertensive disorders of pregnancy and its extended spectrum (PRES, HELLP) are important causes of altered sensorium.
- Procoagulant state in pregnancy may lead to CVST and present with altrered sensorium.
- MRI is the neuroimaging modality of choice in pregnant patients with altered sensorium.
- Postpartum mood disorders are an important cause for altered sensorium and should be evaluated and treated appropriately.

■ REFERENCES

1. Gestational Hypertension and Preeclampsia: ACOG Practice Bulletin, Number 222. Obstet Gynecol. 2020;135:e237-60.
2. Abalos E, Cuesta C, Grosso AL, Chou D, Say L. Global and regional estimates of preeclampsia and eclampsia: a systematic review. Eur J Obstet Gynecol Reprod Biol. 2013;170:1-7.
3. Bartsch E, Medcalf KE, Park AL, Ray JG; High Risk of Pre-eclampsia Identification Group. Clinical risk factors for pre-eclampsia determined in early pregnancy: systematic review and meta-analysis of large cohort studies. BMJ. 2016;353:i1753.
4. Meekins JW, Pijnenborg R, Hanssens M, McFadyen IR, van Asshe A. A study of placental bed spiral arteries and trophoblast invasion in normal and severe pre-eclamptic pregnancies. Br J Obstet Gynaecol. 1994;101:669-74.
5. American College of Obstetricians and Gynecologists' Committee on Practice Bulletins—Obstetrics. ACOG Practice Bulletin No. 203: Chronic Hypertension in Pregnancy. Obstet Gynecol. 2019;133:e26-50.
6. Duley L, Gulmezoglu AM, Henderson-Smart DJ, Chou D. Magnesium sulphate and other anticonvulsants for women with pre-eclampsia. Cochrane Database Syst Rev. 2010;11:CD000025.
7. Report of the National High Blood Pressure Education Program Working Group on High Blood Pressure in Pregnancy. Am J Obstet Gynecol. 2000;183(1):S1-22.
8. Sibai BM. Magnesium sulfate prophylaxis in preeclampsia: Lessons learned from recent trials. Am J Obstet Gynecol. 2004;190:1520-6.
9. Bartynski WS. Posterior reversible encephalopathy syndrome, Part 1: fundamental imaging and clinical features. Am J Neuroradiol. 2008;29:1036-42.
10. McKinney AM, Short J, Truwit CL, McKinney ZJ, Kozak OS, SantaCruz KS, et al. Posterior reversible encephalopathy syndrome: incidence of atypical regions of involvement and imaging findings. Am J Roentgenol. 2007;189:904-12.
11. Doelken M, Lanz S, Rennert J, Alibek S, Richter G, Doerfler A, et al. Differentiation of cytotoxic and vasogenic edema in a patient with reversible posterior leukoencephalopathy syndrome using diffusion-weighted MRI. Diagn Interv Radiol. 2007;13:125-8.
12. Aracki-Trenkić A, Stojanov D, Trenkić M, Radovanović Z, Ignjatović J, Ristić S, et al. Atypical presentation of posterior reversible encephalopathy syndrome: clinical and radiological characteristics in eclamptic patients. Bosn J Basic Med Sci. 2016;16:180-6.
13. Bembalgi S, Kamate V, Shruthi KR. A study of eclampsia cases associated with posterior

13. reversible encephalopathy syndrome. J Clin Diagn Res. 2015;9(7):QC05-7.
14. Cozzolino M, Bianchi C, Mariani G, Marchi L, Fambrini M, Mecacci F. Therapy and differential diagnosis of posterior reversible encephalopathy syndrome (PRES) during pregnancy and postpartum. Arch Gynecol Obstet. 2015;292:1217-23.
15. Swartz RH, Cayley ML, Foley N, Ladhani NNN, Leffert L, Bushnell C, et al. The incidence of pregnancy-related stroke: a systematic review and meta-analysis. Int J Stroke. 2017;12:687-97.
16. Cauldwell M, Rudd A, Nelson-Piercy C. Management of stroke and pregnancy. Eur Stroke J. 2018;3:227-36.
17. Powers WJ, Rabinstein AA, Ackerson T, Adeoye OM, Bambakidis NC, Becker K, et al. 2018 Guidelines for the early management of patients with acute ischemic stroke: a guideline for healthcare professionals from the American Heart Association/American Stroke Association. Stroke. 2018;49:e46-110.
18. Gartman EJ. The use of thrombolytic therapy in pregnancy. Obstet Med. 2013;6:105-11.
19. Campbell BCV, Mitchell PJ, Kleinig TJ, Dewey HM, Churilov L, Yaassi N, et al. Endovascular therapy for ischemic stroke with perfusion-imaging selection. N Engl J Med. 2015;372:1009-18.
20. Nie Q, Guo P, Ge J, Qiu Y. Cerebral venous sinus thrombosis with cerebral haemorrhage during early pregnancy. Neurosciences. 2015;20(1):48-51.
21. Thammishetti V, Dharanipragada S, Basu D, Ananthakrishnan R, Surendiran D. A prospective study of the clinical profile, outcome and evaluation of D-dimer in Cerebral Venous Thrombosis. J Clin Diagn Res. 2016;10(6):OC07-10.
22. Einhaupla K, Stamb J, Bousserc MG, Bruijnd SFTM, Ferroe JM, Martinellif I, et al. Guideline on the treatment of cerebral venous and sinus thrombosis in adult patients. Eur J Neurol. 2010;17:1229-35.
23. Kamimura K, Abe H, Kawai H, Kamimura H, Kobayashi Y, Nomoto M, et al. Advances in understanding and treating liver diseases during pregnancy: A review. World J Gastroenterol. 2015;21:5183-90.
24. Italian Association for the Study of the Liver (AISF); Italian Association for the Study of the Liver AISF. AISF position paper on liver disease and pregnancy. Dig Liver Dis. 2016;48:120-37.
25. Galvin R, Brathen G, Ivashynka A, Hillbom M, Tanasescu R, Leone MA. EFNS guidelines for diagnosis, therapy and prevention of Wernicke encephalopathy. Eur J Neurol. 2010;17:1408-18.
26. Shekhar S, Diddi G. Liver disease in pregnancy. Taiwan J Obstet Gynecol. 2015;54:475-82.
27. Liu J, Ghaziani TT, Wolf JL. Acute fatty liver disease of pregnancy: Updates in pathogenesis, diagnosis and management. Am J Gastroenterol. 2017;112:838-46.
28. Yu CB, Chen JJ, Du WB, Chen P, Huang JR, Chen YM, et al. Effects of plasma exchange combined with continuous renal replacement therapy on acute fatty liver of pregnancy. Hepatobiliary Pancreat Dis Int. 2014;13:179-83.
29. Ahmed KT, Almashhrawi AA, Rahman RN, Hammoud GM, Ibdah JA. Liver diseases in pregnancy: Diseases unique to pregnancy. World J Gastroenterol. 2013;19:7639-46.
30. Haram K, Svendsen E, Abildgaard U. The HELLP syndrome: Clinical issues and management. A Review. BMC Pregnancy Childbirth. 2009;9:8.
31. Goel A, Jamwal KD, Ramachandran A, Balasubramanian KA, Eapen CE. Pregnancy-related liver disorders. J Clin Exp Hepatol. 2014;4:151-62.
32. Mikolasevic I, Filipec-Kanizaj T, Jakopcic I, Majurec I, Brncic-Fischer A, Sobocan N, et al. Liver Disease During Pregnancy: A Challenging Clinical Issue. Med Sci Monit. 2018;24:4080-90.
33. Zoller AL, Schnell FJ, Kersh GJ. Murine pregnancy leads to reduced proliferation of maternal thymocytes and decreased thymic emigration. Immunology. 2007;121:207-15.
34. Kraus TA, Engel SM, Sperling RS, Kellerman L, Lo Y, Wallenstein S, et al. Characterizing the pregnancy immune phenotype: results of the viral immunity and pregnancy (VIP) study. J Clin Immunol. 2012;32:300-11.

35. Sappenfield E, Jamieson DJ, Kourtis AP. Pregnancy and susceptibility to infectious diseases. Infect Dis Obstet Gynecol. 2013;2013:752852.
36. Curcio AM, Shekhawat P, Reynolds AS, Thakur KT. Neurologic infections during pregnancy. In: Steegers EAP, Cipolla MJ, Miller EC (Eds). Handbook of Clinical Neurology, 3rd edition. Amsterdam, Netherlands: Elsevier; 2020. pp. 79-104.
37. Dodd KC, Michael BD, Ziso B, Williams B, Borrow R, Krishnan A, et al. Herpes simplex virus encephalitis in pregnancy—a case report and review of reported patients in the literature. BMC Res Notes. 2015;8:118.
38. Corey L, Wald A. Maternal and neonatal herpes simplex virus infections. N Engl J Med. 2009;361:1376-85.
39. Silasi M, Cardenas I, Kwon JY, Racicot K, Aldo P, Mor G. Viral infections during pregnancy. Am J Reprod Immunol. 2015;73:199-213.
40. Codaccioni C, Vauloup-Fellous C, Letamendia E, Saada J, Benachi A, Vivanti AJ. Case report on early treatment with valaciclovir after maternal primary cytomegalovirus infection. J Gynecol Obstet Hum Reprod. 2019;48:287-9.
41. Halonen SK, Weiss LM. Toxoplasmosis. Handb Clin Neurol. 2013;114:125-45.
42. Paquet C, Yudin MH. No. 285-toxoplasmosis in pregnancy: prevention, screening, and treatment. J Obstet Gynaecol Can. 2018;40:e687-93.
43. Murthy JM, Dastur FD, Khadilkar SV, Kochar DK. Rabies, tetanus, leprosy, and malaria. Handb Clin Neurol. 2014;121:1501-20.
44. Bauserman M, Conroy AL, North K. An overview of malaria in pregnancy. Semin Perinatol. 2019;43:282-90.
45. EURAP Study Group. Seizure control and treatment in pregnancy: Observations from the EURAP epilepsy pregnancy registry. Neurology. 2006;66:354-60.
46. Holmes LB, Harvey EA, Coull BA, Huntington KB, Khoshbin S, Hayes AM, et al. The teratogenicity of anticonvulsant drugs. N Engl J Med. 2001;344(15):1132-8.
47. Marrow J, Russell A, Guthrie E, Parsons L, Robertson I, Waddell R, et al. Malformation risks of antiepileptic drugs in pregnancy: a prospective study from the UK epilepsy and pregnancy register. J Neurol Neurosurg Psychiatry. 2006;77(2):193-8.
48. Bromley R, Weston J, Adab N, Greenhalgh J, Sanniti A, McKay AJ, et al. Treatment for epilepsy in pregnancy: neurodevelopmental outcomes in the child. Cochrane Database Syst Rev. 2014;2014(10):CD010236.
49. Harden C, Hopp J, Ting T, Pennell PB, French JA, Hauser WA, et al. Practice parameter update: management issues for women with epilepsy–focus on pregnancy (an evidence-based review): obstetrical complications and change in seizure frequency: report of the Quality Standards Subcommittee and Therapeutics and Technology Assessment Subcommittee of the American Academy of Neurology and American Epilepsy Society. Neurology. 2009;73(2):126-32.
50. Aminoff MJ, Douglas VC. Neurologic disorders. In: Creasy RK, Resnik R, Iams JD (Eds). Creasy and Resnik's Maternal-Fetal Medicine: Principles and Practice, 7th edition. Philadelphia: Elsevier; 2014. pp. 1100-3.
51. Indian Epilepsy Society. (2008). Guidelines for Management of Epilepsy in India. [online] Available from: http://clinicalestablishments.gov.in/WriteReadData/epilepsy-guidelines.pdf. [Last accessed February, 2023].
52. Royal College of Obstetricians and Gynaecologists. (2016). Epilepsy in Pregnancy (Green-top Guideline No. 68). [online] Available from: https://www.rcog.org.uk/globalassets/documents/guidelines/green-top-guidelines/gtg68_epilepsy.pdf. [Last accessed February, 2023].
53. Belzile M, Pouliot A, Cumyn A, Côté AM. Renal physiology and fluid and electrolyte disorders in pregnancy. Best Pract Res Clin Obstet Gynaecol. 2019;57:1-14.
54. Pazhayattil GS, Rastegar A, Brewster UC. Approach to the diagnosis and treatment of hyponatremia in pregnancy. Am J Kidney Dis. 2015;65(4):623-7.
55. Ladipo OA. Nutrition in pregnancy: mineral and vitamin supplements. Am J Clin Nutr. 2000;72(1 Suppl):280S-90S.
56. Schafer AL, Shoback DM, Feingold KR, Anawalt B, Blackman MR, Boyce A. Hypocalcemia: diagnosis and treatment.

South Dartmouth (MA): MDText.com, Inc; 2000.
57. Bilezikian JP, Khan A, Potts JT Jr, Brandi ML, Clarke BL, Shoback D, et al. Hypoparathyroidism in the adult: epidemiology, diagnosis, pathophysiology, target-organ involvement, treatment, and challenges for future research. J Bone Miner Res. 2011;26(10):2317-37.
58. Veciana M. Diabetes ketoacidosis in pregnancy. Sem Perinatol. 2013;37:267-73.
59. Carroll M, Yeomans E. Diabetic ketoacidosis in pregnancy. Crit Care Med. 2005;33:347-53.
60. Shah LP, Parkar S, Pandit AS. Handbook of Postgraduate Psychiatry. 1999. pp. 369-75. Vora Medical Publication Mumbai.
61. Henshaw C. Mood disturbance in the early puerperium: A review. Arch Womens Ment Health. 2003;6(Suppl 2):S33-42.
62. Nonacs R, Cohen LS. Postpartum mood disorders: Diagnosis and treatment guidelines. J Clin Psychiatry. 1998;59(Suppl 2):34-40.

CHAPTER 38

Fulminant Hepatic Failure in Pregnancy

Lalita Gouri Mitra, Sunaina Tejpal Karna

INTRODUCTION

The diagnosis and clinical care in pregnant women with liver failure is challenging with the spectrum of liver disease ranging from mild asymptomatic transaminitis to fatal and irreversible deterioration of the liver function leading to significant morbidity and mortality.

Fulminant hepatic failure (FHF), a rare and frightening event is defined as a sudden, severe impairment of hepatic function leading to encephalopathy, which occurs within 8 weeks of appearance of first symptoms in the absence of preexisting liver disease.[1] FHF is associated with massive necrosis of the hepatocytes and can be lethal when associated with pregnancy. It is frightening because of its abrupt onset, and possibly fatal outcome.

Diagnosis of liver alterations is difficult in pregnancy due to the different physiological changes already occurring in the liver in pregnancy. Hepatic failure in pregnancy may be classified into three categories: (1) Specific to pregnancy, (2) Coincidental with pregnancy, and (3) Unrelated to pregnancy. Pregnancy-related conditions are preeclampsia and eclampsia, HELLP (hemolysis, elevated liver enzymes and low platelets) syndrome, acute fatty liver of pregnancy (AFLP). Hepatic diseases coincidental with pregnancy include viral hepatitis (VH), biliary diseases such as gallstones and primary sclerosing cholangitis, vascular alterations such as Budd-Chiari syndrome (BCS). Hepatic failure may be unrelated to pregnancy like in drug-induced hepatotoxicity, shock, trauma, decompensation of preexisting hepatic cirrhosis (hepatitis-B, C, nonalcoholic fatty liver disease, autoimmune liver diseases, metabolic disorders and Wilson's disease).[2]

This chapter will focus on pregnancy associated and coincidental liver disease leading to FHF. The fatality rate among pregnant women with acute liver failure (ALF) is reported to be high at 22.2%, with the maximum severity in third trimester.

EPIDEMIOLOGY AND MAGNITUDE OF THE PROBLEM

About 3–5% of pregnancies have an accompanying hepatic derangement, due to coincidental liver pathology or an underlying chronic liver disease (CLD). In a study by U.S. Acute Liver Failure Study Group of 33 tertiary care centers, 70/3,155 (2.2%) patients developed acute liver injury or failure during pregnancy. Only half of these cases were pregnancy associated acute liver diseases (PAALD) attributed to HELLP or AFLP while the rest were due to paracetamol poisoning and other etiologies including exacerbation of preexisting liver diseases.[3] The prevalence of CLD in women between 15 and 39 years of age has increased from 10.4% during 1988–1994 to 24.9% during 2007–2012 in this subpopulation. Such epidemiologic data suggest that women who are pregnant and of childbearing age are at risk of significant morbidity and mortality due to liver disease.

The course of acute VH is unaffected by pregnancy except in patients with hepatitis-E, which is endemic in most third world countries and can cause very high maternal and fetal mortality. In India, 95% of ALF is virus-related, with hepatitis-E virus (HEV) and hepatitis-B virus (HBV) contributing to 40% and 30%, respectively.[4] The reasons for this increased maternal morbidity and mortality during pregnancy are not clear, however it is possible that malnutrition and pregnancy appear to be a potential risk factors for viral replication and low immune status in Indian/Asian pregnant women.

IMPLICATIONS FOR MATERNAL HEALTH (ANTENATAL AND TRIMESTER SPECIFIC)

Maternal outcome depends upon the type of liver disease, the degree of impaired synthetic, metabolic, and excretory liver function, and timing of delivery. There is a specific trimester occurrence for pregnancy related liver diseases while nonpregnancy related liver disease can occur at any time.

Pregnancy-associated Acute Liver Diseases

With a mortality rate of 0–25%, pregnancy-specific disorders are the leading cause of abnormal liver function tests (LFTs) during pregnancy, particularly in the third trimester. It is important to rule out benign causes of liver alterations such as hyperemesis gravidarum (HG) and intrahepatic cholestasis of pregnancy (IHCP). Any increase in transaminases, bilirubin, fasting total bile acids, or the prothrombin time (PT) above normal values during pregnancy is abnormal and requires prompt evaluation. PAALD is frequently recognized but distinguishing specific etiologies is challenging due to non-specific common clinical symptoms and tests **(Table 1)**. Aminotransferases levels being very high in HELLP as compared to AFLP are of diagnostic importance. Imaging may be used to rule out extra and intrahepatic hemorrhage.[3] Usually, the patient is referred to a liver unit after delivery.

First trimester: Acute liver failure in first trimester is unlikely to be related to pregnancy.
- *Hyperemesis gravidarum* is the only condition causing raised LFTs in half of the parturients, with no reported case of ALF, hence no specific liver management is needed. Presenting with severe nausea, untreatable vomiting, resulting in dehydration, ketosis, weight loss >5% body weight, HG starts before the 9th week and disappears by 20th week gestation. The aminotransferases may rise to 200 U/L with raised lipase, amylase, increased renal values, electrolyte abnormalities, metabolic alkalosis, and erythrocytosis due to dehydration. Ruling out multiple or molar pregnancy is essential by ultrasound. HG is a diagnosis of exclusion and treatment is based on correcting electrolytes, preventing dehydration, and general medical support.

Second trimester: Raised aminotransferases in second trimester may be pregnancy associated in the following two conditions, with risk of liver failure in the latter.

TABLE 1: Prevalence, differential diagnosis, and characteristics of liver disease in pregnancy.

	Prevalence	Trimester	Protein-uria	Hypo-glycemia	Uric acid/creatinine	Platelets	Hemo-lysis	Clotting	LDH	Imaging	Treatment	Complication	Recurrence
HG	0.3–3.6%	1st/2nd	N	N	N	N	N	N	N	Normal	Supportive, rehydration, antiemetics, and vitamin supplementation	Hyponatremia and encephalopathy	15–81%
IHCP	0.1–5%	2nd/3rd	N	N	N	N	N	May be prolonged	N	Exclude cholelithiasis	Ursodeoxycholic acid, antihistamines, aqueous cream, and consider delivery at 37 weeks (or sometimes before this if bile acids are >100 µmol/L)	Preterm labor and stillbirth	45–90%
PET with liver dysfunction	5–10%	>20 weeks	Y	N	Increase	Decrease	Y	Risk of disseminated intravascular coagulation	Increase	Hepatic rupture/hematoma/infarcts	Antihypertensives, consider IV magnesium sulfate and consider delivery if deterioration in maternal or fetal condition	Eclampsia, maternal/fetal mortality	16–52%

Contd...

Contd...

	Prevalence	Trimester	Proteinuria	Hypoglycemia	Uric acid/ creatinine	Platelets	Hemolysis	Clotting	LDH	Imaging	Treatment	Complication	Recurrence
HELLP	0.2–0.6%	2nd/3rd/ postnatal	Y	N	Increase	Decrease	Y	Risk of disseminated intravascular coagulation	≥600 IU/L	Hepatic rupture/ hematoma/ infarcts	As per PET and urgent discussion with obstetricians regarding delivery	Liver rupture and maternal/ fetal mortality	2–19%
AFLP	0.01%	2nd/3rd/ postnatal	Y	Y	Increase	Decrease	N	Prolonged (PT >14 seconds or a APTT >34 seconds)	Increase	Often normal, may look bright NB fatty infiltration on US is a sign of MACROvesicular steatosis (NAFLD) not MICROvesicular steatosis (AFLP)	Correct coagulopathy, treat hypoglycemia and expedite delivery	Fulminant liver failure and maternal/ fetal mortality	Rare; 25% in defect of fatty acid beta-oxidation

(AFLP: acute fatty liver of pregnancy; APTT: activated partial thromboplastin time; HELLP: hemolysis, elevated liver enzymes, and low platelets; HG: hyperemesis gravidarum; IHCP: intrahepatic cholestasis of pregnancy; IV: intravenous; LDH: lactate dehydrogenase; N: absent or negative; NAFLD: non-alcoholic fatty liver disease; PET: preeclamptic toxemia; PT: prothrombin time; Y: present or positive)

- *Intrahepatic cholestasis of pregnancy/ Obstetric cholestasis* is seen in 0.1–5% of parturients. It occurs in the late second and third trimester of pregnancy. It presents with intense pruritus (palms and soles), followed by jaundice in 25% women. History may be suggestive of dyslipidemia, gestational diabetes, with history of IHCP in previous pregnancies. The LFTs are abnormal with raised bilirubin levels (<5 mg/dL), bile acids (30–100 times) and aminotransferases (1–5 times), in absence of any preexisting liver disease. Hepatocellular bile and canalicular bile plugs, cholestasis without parenchymal inflammation is seen on liver biopsy (LB). Maternal outcomes are usually excellent in IHCP, with no reported cases of ALF.
- *Preeclampsia* with liver dysfunction manifests after 20 weeks of gestation with a frequency of 5–10%. Preeclampsia/ eclampsia is a multisystemic, multifactorial disorder characterized by abnormal vascular response to placental growth associated with vasoconstriction, endothelial dysfunction, metabolic changes, and increased inflammatory responses. Patient presents with severe headache with vomiting, blurred vision/ diplopia, peripheral edema, abdominal epigastric pain, and proteinuria. The aminotransferases may rise 10 times the normal value along with increase in ALP, lactate dehydrogenase (LDH), uric acid levels, and creatinine. Bilirubin levels are rarely increased. Liver rupture and necrosis can prove fatal and is associated with ALF. LB shows platelet and fibrin deposition in hepatic sinusoids causing hepatocellular necrosis and hemorrhage in zone 1 initially, which progresses to zone 3 once shock intervenes in severe cases but is usually not indicated.[5]

Third trimester: Two potentially life-threatening pregnancy-related liver diseases may be associated with FHF in the third trimester. Severe liver dysfunction in late pregnancy is a dramatic event because it can progress very rapidly to fulminating disease and the lives of both the mother and fetus are at stake.

- *Hemolysis, elevated liver enzymes and low platelets syndrome* may occur with and without preeclampsia. However, all three components of hemolysis, elevated liver enzymes, and low platelets need to be present for definitive diagnosis to be made. Usually seen between 28 and 36 weeks gestation, the incidence is preterm (53%), term (18%), or postpartum (30%), with high maternal (5%), and fetal (30%) mortality if not treated in time. Risk factors include multiparity, advanced maternal age, family history of HELLP, preeclampsia in previous pregnancies and white ethnic origin.

The diagnosis is challenging as the symptoms such as abdominal pain, vomiting, headache, and peripheral edema vary in type and severity and mimic other diseases. Severe complications include liver infarction, large hematoma, liver rupture, hemoperitoneum, and acute liver failure. There is a higher risk of acute kidney injury, pulmonary edema, retinal detachment, disseminated intravascular coagulopathy (DIC), and abruptio placentae.[5,6]

A complete blood count and transaminase levels is mandatory. If platelet count <50,000/μL, DIC work-up should be done. On investigation, intravascular hemolysis (raised LDH >600 IU/L, schistocytes on peripheral smear), low platelets, raised bilirubin (<5 mg/dL, with unconjugated hyperbilirubinemia), and aminotransferases (ALT >10 times ALP) may be seen. Diagnosis and grading of HELLP syndrome may be done as shown in **Table 2**. Imaging may show hepatic infarcts, hematoma, or liver rupture. LB shows fibrin deposition, hemorrhage, and hepatocellular necrosis.[6,7]

- *Acute fatty liver of pregnancy* is a rare, potentially catastrophic liver disease diagnosed in the third trimester, associated with high fetal (45%) and maternal mortality (10%). The likely mechanism is defective long chain fatty acid oxidation leading to mitochondrial dysfunction. Risk factors include nulliparity, male offspring, and twin pregnancy. AFLP should be considered after ruling out preeclampsia, HELLP syndrome and fulfilment of at least six Swansea criteria **(Table 3)** on clinical evaluation. Most Swansea criteria are also present in pregnant patients with ALF of any cause, so it is specific to presence of ALF.[5,7,9] LB is nonessential but confirms AFLP with presence of centrilobular microvesicular steatosis. The treatment of choice is interruption of pregnancy.

Sometimes it is difficult to differentiate between HELLP and AFLP based on clinical and biochemical tests. A LB may be attempted despite risk of bleeding. Once the pregnancy is terminated, the management does not differ.

TABLE 2: Diagnosis and grading of HELLP syndrome.

Tennessee criteria	Mississippi criteria
2/3 partial HELLP, 3/3 full HELLP	
PC <1 lakh/mm^3	*Class 1 severe:* Low platelet count ≤50,000/L and AST/ALT ≥70 IU/L, LDH >600 IU/L
AST >70 IU/L and LDH >600 IU/L	*Class 2 moderate:* PC between 50,000–100,000/L and AST/ALT ≥70 IU/L, LDH >600 IU/L
Hemolysis on peripheral smear	*Class 3 mild:* PC between 100,000–150,000/L and AST/ALT ≥40 IU/L, LDH >600 IU/L

(ALT: alanine transaminase; AST: aspartate transaminase; LDH: lactate dehydrogenase; PC: platelet count)

TABLE 3: Swansea criteria for acute fatty liver of pregnancy.

Signs and symptoms	Nausea, vomiting, polyuria/polydipsia/abdominal pain, anorexia, encephalopathy
USG abdomen	Ascites or bright-appearing liver
Investigations	• Elevated bilirubin (>0.8 mg/dL) • Transaminases (AST/ALT >42 U/L) • Ammonia (>66 micromol/l) • Coagulopathy (PT >14 sec or aPTT >34 sec) • Hypoglycemia (<72 mg/dL) • Urea (>950 mg/dL) • Renal impairment (Creatinine >1.7 mg/dL) • Leukocytosis (>11 × 10^9/L) • Micro-vesicular steatosis on liver biopsy

(ALT: alanine transaminase; AST: aspartate transaminase; PT: prothrombin time; USG: ultrasonography)

Acute Liver Failure Coincidental with Pregnancy

Preexisting liver disease may be exacerbated by physiological hepatic changes seen in pregnancy. Infection, toxins, veno-occlusive diseases, and decompensation of hereditary diseases such as Wilson's disease, in pregnancy, may cause liver failure.

Viral hepatitis due to hepatitis-A, B, C, and D virus, is the most frequent cause of jaundice in pregnancy with the course of illness unaltered by pregnancy. A severe course with fulminant liver failure is seen in HEV and herpes simplex virus (HSV) with significant maternal mortality ranging from 20 to 25%, and 50%, respectively, usually in third trimester. Reduced expression of progesterone receptor or a mutation of the human methylene-tetra hydro folate reductase (MTHFR) gene might be associated with FHF.[7,10,11]

A total of 70% of pregnant women with acute hepatitis-E progress to ALF with a short pre-encephalopathy period due to rapid development of cerebral edema with DIC.[8] Patients are anicteric with normal bilirubin, LFTs are severely deranged, with 50% having mucocutaneous manifestations. Disseminated HSV infection is associated with prodromal systemic illness, vesicular skin rash, and leukopenia.[6,8]

Viral hepatitis and AFLP are difficult to differentiate at presentation. AFLP has a poorer prognosis. Factors predictive of poor prognosis include non-HEV etiology (CFR 84, 2% vs. 51.9% in HEV-ALF), PT >30 sec, grade of coma >2, and age >40 years and a low platelet count at admission.[10-12] Pregnancy per se does not contribute to higher mortality.

Drug-induced liver disease in pregnancy is underreported. Most common agents include antibiotics and antihypertensives. Immediate termination of the toxic agent and monitoring synthetic function is essential.

Veno-occlusive disease such as BCS can be exacerbated as pregnancy is a procoagulant state. Patient presents with right upper quadrant pain, jaundice, and ascites. Doppler ultrasonography is essential for diagnosis. Treatment involves anticoagulation, shunting, and in extreme cases, liver transplantation.[6,7]

Acute liver failure may also be associated with Wilson's disease, an autosomal recessive hereditary disease with defective copper excretion and copper deposition in brain, liver, and kidneys. Patient presents with hyperbilirubinemia, raised aminotransferases, Coombs negative hemolytic anemia and low serum ALP. In 50% of cases, Kayser–Fleischer rings in cornea are present. In pregnant patients, it is easily confused with HELLP. Serum copper levels and ceruloplasmin levels may help in diagnosis.

IMPLICATIONS FOR FETAL WELL-BEING

Pregnancy associated acute liver diseases is associated with a fetal survival of 88.9% and 88.6% overall maternal survival.[3] Because of the need to consider both maternal and fetal health, there are special considerations for the implementation of diagnostic strategies and pharmacologic therapies for liver disease that occurs in pregnancy.

- *Hyperemesis gravidarum:* It is rarely associated with premature low-birth-weight babies.
- *Intrahepatic cholestasis of pregnancy:* Adverse outcomes associated with IHCP include premature labor, fetal distress, and stillbirth/intrauterine death (IUD). Data from a large Swedish cohort

demonstrated that the likelihood of the development of meconium-stained fluid, spontaneous preterm birth, and fetal asphyxia increased by 1–2% for every µmol/L of bile acids. Such complications develop when bile acid levels are >40 µmol/L.[7,9] The reason for fetal distress and stillbirths in IHCP is unclear. A cardiac source of these adverse events is possible as fetal tachyarrhythmia with atrial flutter and left ventricular dysfunction has been observed.

More recent data from a multicenter, randomized, placebo-controlled trial investigating the effect of ursodeoxycholic acid (UDCA) on perinatal outcomes concluded that UDCA does not significantly reduce the incidence of fetal death, preterm delivery, or fetal distress.[8] Early delivery at 37 weeks must be considered in severe cases. IUD is most common in the last month of pregnancy.

- *Preeclampsia:* Fetal/obstetric complications include intrauterine growth retardation (IUGR) (10–25%), placental abruption, preterm delivery (15–65%), and IUD.
- *Acute fatty liver of pregnancy:* It occurs in the third trimester and the incidence is reported to be 1/7,000–1/16,000 pregnancies. There is a significant increase in maternal and fetal mortality rates ranging from 1 to 20%.[9]
- *Autoimmune hepatitis:* It can flare in pregnancy in 20% of women and disease activity should ideally be controlled prior to conception. Disease flares can increase the risk of adverse fetal outcomes, such as prematurity and preeclampsia.[5]
- *Viral hepatitis:* Abortion, premature rupture of membranes, still birth, IUD, and coagulopathy-associated bleeding are documented in HEV-ALF and must be managed by standard obstetric practice. Termination of pregnancy is not advocated in pregnant women with HEV-ALF.[5] However, in case of lower grades of encephalopathy, termination of pregnancy was observed to be associated with better maternal outcomes.[10-12]
- *Drugs:* Use of azathioprine for treatment of autoimmune hepatitis has been associated with side effects of lymphopenia, hypogammaglobulinemia, and thymic hypoplasia.

■ IMAGING-RELATED ISSUES

Greatest risk of radiation exposure is at 8–15 weeks of gestation; hence CT scan and X-rays are avoided. Since gadolinium is associated with teratogenicity and it crosses the placenta (it has been found in amniotic fluid and fetal circulation), contrast magnetic resonance imaging (MRI) is not recommended. Transjugular LB confers radiation exposure. Ensure proper informed consent with discussion about fetal risks prior to any endoscopic procedure, which is ideally recommended in the second trimester **(Table 4)**.

■ MANAGEMENT

Pregnant women presenting with FHF often poses a diagnostic dilemma. Alteration in liver function with coagulopathy and change in mental status should raise suspicion and recognition of PAALD is the first step in the diagnosis and management **(Tables 1 and 5, Fig. 1)**. Treatment decision for FHF in pregnancy is complicated by the diverse clinical presentations. A multidisciplinary team effort involving the obstetrician, anesthetist, intensivist, hepatologist, neonatologist, and even the liver transplant team may be necessary.[5,6,12-14]

TABLE 4: Diagnostic modalities for liver disease in pregnancy.

Modality	Ultrasound	CT	MRI	Liver biopsy	Transient elastography	Endoscopy
Pregnancy considerations	Acceptable modality	Risk of ionizing radiation exposure to fetus during pregnancy	Acceptable modality when performed without contrast	Can be performed in pregnancy	Not approved by the FDA for use in pregnancy	Upper endoscopy is acceptable in pregnancy and typically recommended to occur in the second trimester. Consideration of compatibility of sedating medications with pregnancy
Lactation considerations	Acceptable modality	Acceptable modality	Acceptable modality with and without contrast	Acceptable modality	Not contraindicated in lactation	Acceptable modality with consideration of compatibility of sedating medications with lactation
Other issues	No available data on contrasted ultrasound in pregnancy and lactation	• Greatest risk of radiation exposure is at 8–15 weeks of gestation • Oral and iodinated contrast not teratogenic. Less than 1% of iodinated contrast is excreted in breast milk	Gadolinium is associated with teratogenicity; crosses the placenta and is found in amniotic fluid and fetal circulation. Less than 0.04% is excreted into breast milk	Limited data on preterm births seen when performed during pregnancy		• Ensure proper informed consent with discussion about fetal risk. • Ensure adequate oxygenation and hemodynamic stability during procedure. • Ensure left lateral decubitus position to avoid IVC compression

(CT: computed tomography; FDA: Food and Drug Administration; IVC: inferior vena cava; MRI: magnetic resonance imaging)

TABLE 5: Common causes of acute liver failure and investigations.

Etiology	Investigation
Drug related	History of drug intake (ATT or CAM are common)
Acute viral hepatitis	anti-HAV IgM and anti-HEV IgM. If above mentioned are negative test for anti-HSV IgM, anti-VZV IgM, CMV, HSV, EBV, parvovirus and VZV PCR
Budd-Chiari syndrome	Doppler will show absent hepatic venous outflow
Autoimmune	ANA, ASMA, anti-soluble liver antigen, globulin profile, ANCA IgG
HBV reactivation	HBsAg, anti-HBc IgM (HBV DNA)
Fulminant presentation of Wilson's disease	Coombs negative hemolytic anemia, and high bilirubin to alkaline phosphatase ratio. In 50% of cases, Kayser-Fleischer rings are present. Serum and urinary copper are markedly increased

(ANCA: anti-neutrophil cytoplasmic antibody; ANA: anti-nuclear antibodies; ASMA: anti-smooth muscle antibodies; ATT: anti-tubercular treatment; CAM: complimentary and alternative medication; CMV: cytomegalovirus; EBV: Epstein-Barr virus; HBV: hepatitis-B virus; HSV: herpes simplex virus; PCR: polymerase chain reaction; VZV: varicella zoster virus)

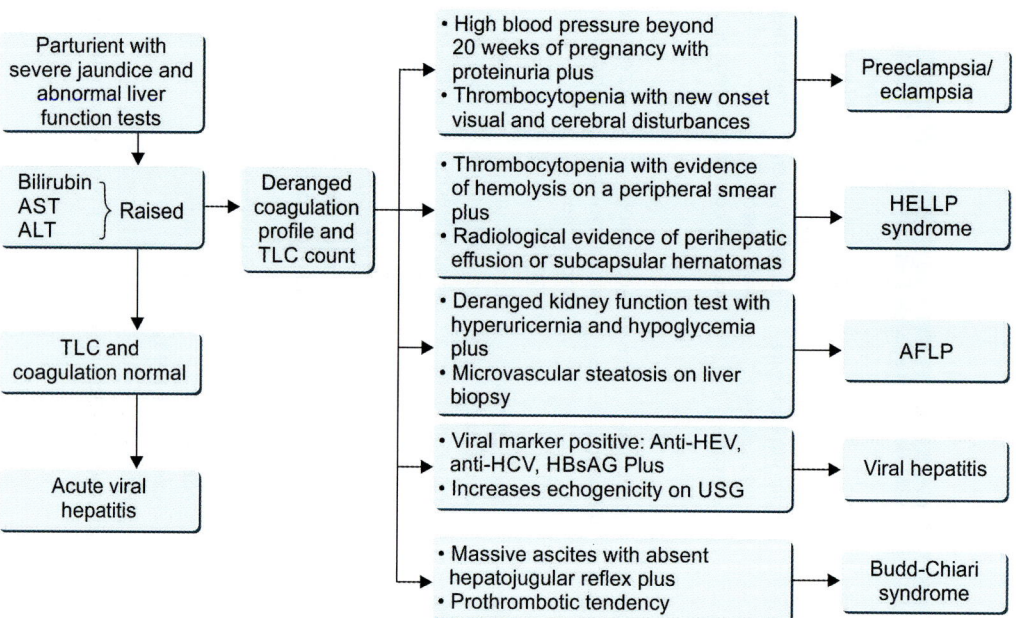

Fig. 1: Clinical diagnostic approach to a parturient with fulminant hepatic failure.

General Supportive Management

Irrespective of the cause, the general management which has been summarized in **Table 6**, remains the same. Impending signs of liver failure are shrinking liver, rising INR, rapid rise in serum bilirubin, ascites, or coagulopathy, hence ICU management (preferably in a liver unit) is related to the prevention and complications of encephalopathy, cerebral edema, hypoglycemia, coagulopathy,

CHAPTER 38: Fulminant Hepatic Failure in Pregnancy

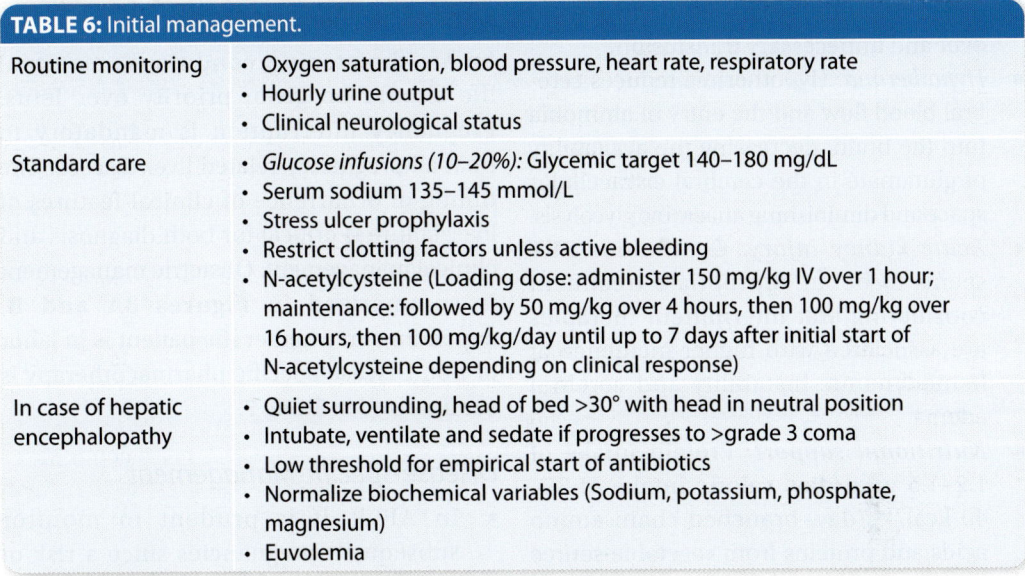

TABLE 6: Initial management.

Routine monitoring	• Oxygen saturation, blood pressure, heart rate, respiratory rate • Hourly urine output • Clinical neurological status
Standard care	• *Glucose infusions (10–20%):* Glycemic target 140–180 mg/dL • Serum sodium 135–145 mmol/L • Stress ulcer prophylaxis • Restrict clotting factors unless active bleeding • N-acetylcysteine (Loading dose: administer 150 mg/kg IV over 1 hour; maintenance: followed by 50 mg/kg over 4 hours, then 100 mg/kg over 16 hours, then 100 mg/kg/day until up to 7 days after initial start of N-acetylcysteine depending on clinical response)
In case of hepatic encephalopathy	• Quiet surrounding, head of bed >30° with head in neutral position • Intubate, ventilate and sedate if progresses to >grade 3 coma • Low threshold for empirical start of antibiotics • Normalize biochemical variables (Sodium, potassium, phosphate, magnesium) • Euvolemia

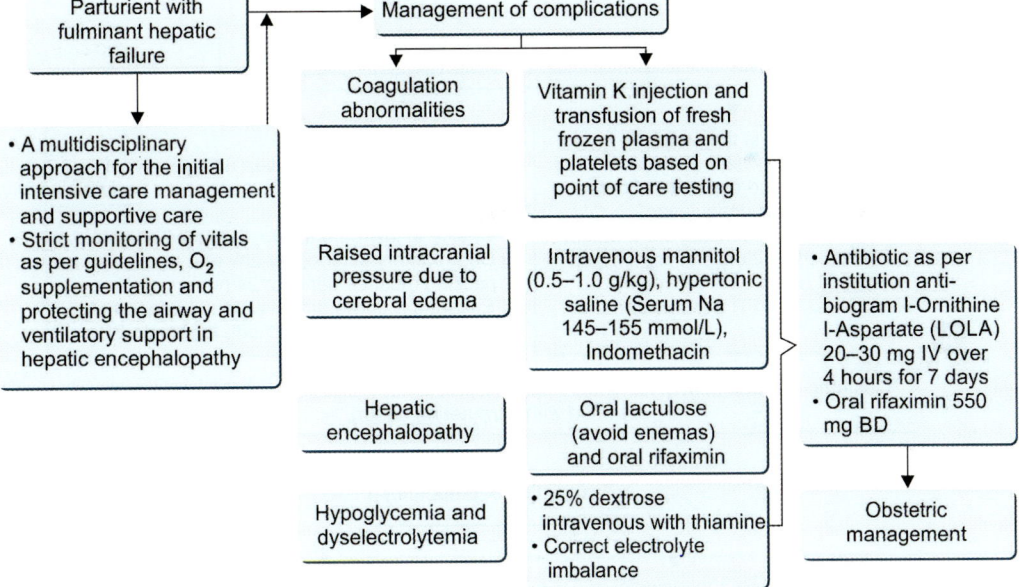

Fig. 2: Medical management of fulminant hepatic failure in a parturient.

DIC, GI bleed, sepsis, and renal failure. Surveillance of infections, strict asepsis, and prompt antimicrobial therapy should be implemented. **Figure 2** summarizes the medical management of FHF in a parturient.

Other issues to remember are:
- *Coagulation:* Coagulation disturbance may continue for days or weeks even after termination of pregnancy in some cases such as AFLP. Management is ongoing

based on point of care testing to avoid over and unnecessary transfusion.
- *Hypothermia:* Hypothermia reduces cerebral blood flow and the entry of ammonia into the brain, decreasing the availability of glutamate in the cerebral extracellular space and diminishing anaerobic glycolysis.
- *Acute kidney injury:* Continuous RRT seems to be an appropriate treatment considering that intermittent therapies are associated with higher incidence of hemodynamic instability and cerebral edema.
- *Nutritional support:* Protein intake of 1.2–1.5 g/kg/day, caloric intake of 35–40 kcal/kg/day, branched chain amino acids and proteins from vegetable source are recommended.

Obstetric Management

In life-threatening conditions, maternal life should be given priority over fetus. Pregnancy interruption is mandatory to treat all pregnancy-related liver disease. The timing of occurrence of clinical features of liver failure is critical for both diagnosis and clinical management. Obstetric management is summarized in **Figures 3A and B**, depending on whether the patient is in labor or not. Disease-specific pharmacotherapy is summarized in **Table 7**.

Disease-specific Management

- In AFLP, it is prudent to monitor subsequent pregnancies since a risk of recurrence is present in patients with

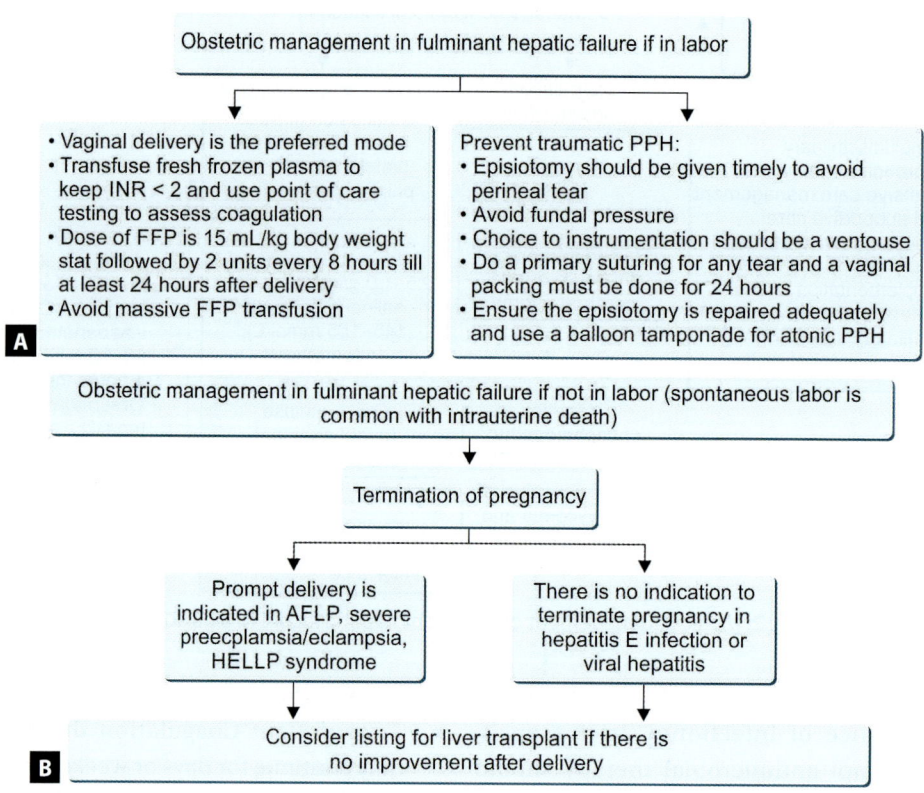

Figs. 3A and B: (A) Obstetric management in FHF (in labor); (B) Obstetric management in FHF (not in labor).
(AFLP: acute fatty liver of pregnancy; FHF: fulminant hepatic failure; HELLP: hemolysis, elevated liver enzymes and low platelets; PPH: postpostpartum hemorrhage)

TABLE 7: Pharmacotherapy in liver failure in pregnancy.

Disease	Drug/Therapy	Comment
HEV	Entecavir, lamivudine, adefovir and interferon	• No specific therapy • Rest, high caloric diet, and UDCA/Cholestyramine in presence of cholestatic symptoms
	Ribavirin	Teratogenic
Wilson's disease	Penicillamine, trientine or zinc	Dose reduction to avoid fetal harm Monitoring of hepatic and neurological symptoms
Autoimmune hepatitis	Corticosteroids	
Early disseminated HSV infection	Intravenous acyclovir	
HBV hepatitis	Telbivudine and tenofovir	
Budd-Chiari	Anticoagulation with heparin is recommended, unless contraindicated	Placement of TIPS or shunt surgery is technically difficult due to the gravid uterus

(HBV: hepatitis-B virus; HEV: hepatitis-E virus; HSV: herpes simplex virus; TIPS: transjugular intrahepatic portosystemic shunt; UDCA: ursodeoxycholic acid)

defects of fatty acid β-oxidation. Liver transplantation is warranted in cases of failure of recovery of liver function and severe encephalopathy.

- In preeclampsia, urgent control of hypertension (labetalol, hydralazine, and modified release nifedipine), seizure prophylaxis and treatment (intravenous magnesium sulfate) and urgent delivery is a must to avoid eclampsia. In eclampsia with ALF, the target systolic and diastolic arterial pressure of 90 and 65 mm Hg should be kept to maintain cerebral perfusion pressure (CPP). Liver dysfunction usually normalizes 2 weeks after delivery, though hypertension may persist. Measurement of platelet count, transaminases, and serum creatinine 48–72 hours postdelivery is recommended.
- In HELLP, supportive management with antihypertensives and magnesium sulfate should be considered for the mother. Early delivery should be done at 34 weeks. If there is evidence of renal/hepatic failure, intensive care admission is warranted. Further, liver rupture in HELLP syndrome is life-threatening with 39% mortality. Immediate exploratory laparotomy, packing, hematoma evacuation, hepatic artery embolization or ligation and suturing of laceration may be needed along with maintenance of hemodynamics and correction of coagulation disturbances associated with massive blood loss.

Extracorporeal support systems: These are usually used as bridge to liver transplantation.

High-volume plasma exchange can improve transplant-free survival. The mechanisms involved seems to be reduced activation of the innate immune system secondary to the elimination of cytokines and toxic molecules and the administration of physiological substances contained in fresh frozen plasma. The benefit has been seen in patients with acetaminophen overdose, but its usefulness in a different cohort of patients remains to be elucidated.

Molecular adsorbent recirculating system (MARS) significantly reduces the levels of both water soluble, and albumin-bound substances and improves the hemodynamics, clotting, hepatic, renal, neural, and pulmonary function, as is reported in patients with AFLP.

Liver transplantation: The King's College Criteria (KCC), the model for end stage liver disease (MELD) score, the acute physiology and chronic health evaluation (APACHE) II score and the sequential organ failure assessment (SOFA) score are the commonly used prognostic scoring systems to predict mortality and the need for LT. KCC seem to be more accurate in paracetamol-induced ALF and the MELD score can be a better predictor in non-paracetamol-induced ALF. The SOFA score is a useful prognostic tool in ALF. However, these scores have not been validated in pregnant patients with ALF/FHF.

Deceased and live donor liver transplantation for ALF during pregnancy has been reported in the second and third trimester, the cause being hepatitis viral infection, drug associated, autoimmune hepatitis, AFLP, and unknown etiology.[14,15] A favorable survival rate of 83% is reported in liver transplant for HELLP syndrome, the main indications being ALF, liver necrosis after rupture, and uncontrollable bleeding. LT done for ALF in BCS has been shown to be effective in 88% patients combined with anticoagulation.

TAKE HOME MESSAGES

- Liver disease in pregnancy can be difficult to diagnose and manage due to varied presentation ranging from subtle biochemical liver alterations to frank FHF. It is trimester specific or could be coincidental.
- Safety of both the mother and the fetus needs to be ensured. However, maternal outcome takes precedence over fetal well-being in life-threatening situations. Stress should be given to educate regarding preventable diseases such as hepatitis-E.
- A pregnant woman with FHF with altered sensorium, will require multidisciplinary approach in tertiary care center with intensive monitoring and frequent reviews of maternal-fetal status by experts to decide on the best course of action. Intensive care management of such a patient should be focused on cardiovascular, hemodynamic, and respiratory support.
- Aim would be to stabilize the patient, maintain optimum hemodynamics, treat cerebral edema/intracranial hypertension, evaluate, and treat any infections, correct coagulopathy, hypoglycemia, dyselectrolytemia, maintain nutrition, give volume replacement, and vasopressor support if needed and ensure adequate renal perfusion.
- Once patient meets criteria for transplantation, the chance of spontaneous survival is hardly 10%, hence is the way forward in this cohort of patients.

REFERENCES

1. Wendon J, Cordoba J, Dhawan A, Larsen F, Manns M, Nevens F, et al. EASL Clinical Practical Guidelines on the management of acute (fulminant) liver failure. J Hepatol. 2017;66(5):1047-81.
2. Lim E, Mouyis M, MacKillop L. Liver diseases in pregnancy. Clin Med (Lond). 2021;21(5):e441-5.
3. Casey LC, Fontana RJ, Aday A, Nelson DB, Rule JA, Gottfried M, et al. Acute Liver Failure (ALF) in pregnancy: how much is pregnancy related? Hepatology. 2020;72(4):1366-77.
4. Kar P, Karna R. A review of the diagnosis and management of hepatitis. E Curr Treat Options Infect Dis. 2020;12:1-11.
5. Tran TT, Ahn J, Reau NS. ACG clinical guideline: liver disease and pregnancy. Am J Gastroenterol. 2016;111(2):176-94.
6. Brady CW. Liver disease in pregnancy: what's new. Hepatol Commun. 2020;4:145-56.

7. Byrne T. Acute liver failure in pregnancy. SOJ Gynecol Obstet Womens Health. 2016; 2(2):7.
8. Chappell L, Bell J, Smith A, Linsell L, Juszczak E, Dixon PH, et al. Ursodeoxycholic acid versus placebo in women with intrahepatic cholestasis of pregnancy (PITCHES): a randomised controlled trial. Lancet. 209;394(10201):849-60.
9. Wand S, Waeschle RM, Von Ahsen N, Hawighorst T, Bräuer A, Quintel M. Acute liver failure due to acute fatty liver of pregnancy. Minerva Anestesiol. 2012;78:503-6.
10. Khuroo MS, Kamili S. Aetiology, clinical course and outcome of sporadic acute viral hepatitis in pregnancy. J Viral Hepat. 2003;10:61-9.
11. Kumar RM, Uduman S, Rana S, Kochiyil JK, Usmani A, Thomas L. Sero-prevalence and mother-to-infant transmission of hepatitis E virus among pregnant women in the United Arab Emirates. Eur J Obstet Gynecol Reprod Biol. 2001;100(1):9-15.
12. Pandey CK, Karna ST, Pandey VK, Tandon M. Acute liver failure in pregnancy: Challenges and management. Indian J Anaesth. 2015; 59(3):144-9.
13. Bhatia V, Singhal A, Panda SK, Acharya SK. A 20-year single-center experience with acute liver failure during pregnancy: is the prognosis really worse? Hepatology. 2008;48:1577-85.
14. Kanogawa N, Kanda T, Ohtsuka M, Nakamura M, Miyamura T, Yasui S, et al. Acute Liver Failure Occurring during the First Trimester of Pregnancy Successfully Treated with Living Donor Liver Transplantation. Case Rep Transplant. 2013;2013:309545.
15. Babu R, Kanianchalil K, Sahadevan S, Nambiar R, Kumar A. Liver transplantation for acute liver failure due to hepatitis E in a pregnant patient. Indian J Anaesth. 2018;62:908-10.

CHAPTER 39

Sepsis in Full Term Pregnancy

Rajesh Mishra, Maneendra Singarapu

■ INTRODUCTION

World Health Organization (WHO) in 2017 has defined maternal sepsis as "organ dysfunction resulting from infection during pregnancy, childbirth, postabortion, or postpartum period" which includes 42 days after the pregnancy has been terminated, irrespective of the cause.[1]

Pregnant women are more susceptible not only to bacterial infections but also tropical diseases such as malaria and listeriosis and unfortunately severity of the diseases is also worse. There are multiple reasons for increase in severity and susceptibility, which are as follows:[2]

- Modifications in the immune system
- Pressure effects of fetus causing increased urinary stasis
- Predisposition to develop conditions like gestational diabetes which decreases immunity
- Infections specific to pregnancy, i.e., chorioamnionitis
- Infections secondary to procedures like amniocentesis.

Factors that increase the risk of sepsis in pregnancy can be broadly classified into three categories **(Table 1)**.[3,4]

There are lot of physiological changes which happen in pregnancy which result in adverse outcomes on various organ systems making them more vulnerable to develop sepsis and septic shock with various infections **(Table 2)**.[5]

Due to these multiple physiological changes in pregnancy scoring system such as sequential organ failure assessment (SOFA) and quick sequential organ failure assessment (qSOFA) have been modified by Society of Obstetric Medicine of Australia and New Zealand specific to pregnancy.[6]

In qSOFA respiratory rate targets have been changed from 22 to 25 breaths/min and systolic pressure has been reduced to 90 from 100 mm Hg as tachypnea and hypotension are physiological in pregnancy.

A qSOFA score ≥2 is associated with an increased risk of mortality.

Obstetrically modified qSOFA is enumerated in **Table 3**.

Obstetrically modified SOFA is enumerated in **Table 4**.

■ EPIDEMIOLOGY AND MAGNITUDE OF PROBLEM

The prevalence of only puerperal sepsis as per WHO in live births is 4.4% with higher incidence in low-/middle-income countries (LMICs) (7%) than in high-income countries (HICs) (1–2%).[7]

Major sites for pregnancy related sepsis constitute:
- Urinary tract (pyelonephritis)

TABLE 1: Factors that increase the risk of sepsis in pregnancy.

Social factors	Medical factors	Childbirth factors
• Poverty • Long distance to health facilities • Ethnic minority population groups • Extremes of age • Lower educational attainment • Unsafe abortion practices • Reduced access to family planning services • Reduced autonomy of women	• Primiparity • Previous miscarriage • Anemia • Untreated HIV • Untreated TB • Cardiac diseases • Obesity • Diabetes/Impairment glucose tolerance • Malnutrition • Malaria • Assisted fertility • Impaired immunity or immunosuppressant treatment • Previous pelvic infection • Previous Group B streptococcal infection • Amniocentesis • Cervical circlage • Group A streptococcal infection in close contact	• Induction of labor • PROM • Prolong labor • More than five vaginal exam during labor • Cesarean section (especially when prophylactic antibiotics are not used) • Multiple birth • Instrumental labor • Use of unskilled health workers • Unhygienic home births • Vaginal trauma • Wound hematoma • Retained hematoma

(HIV: human immunodeficiency virus; PROM: premature rupture of membranes; TB: tuberculosis)

TABLE 2: Adverse effects of physiological changes on various organs.

Cardiovascular	Respiratory	Renal	Coagulation
Rapid hemodynamic collapse	Susceptibility to pulmonary edema	Acute kidney injury	Increased microvascular thrombus formation
	Rapid decrease in oxygenation		Microcirculation dysregulation
	Adult respiratory distress syndrome		Tissue hypoperfusion
	Decreased ability to compensate for metabolic acidosis		End-organ dysfunction

TABLE 3: Obstetrically modified quick sequential organ failure assessment.

Parameter	Score 0	Score 1
Systolic blood pressure (mm Hg)	≥90	<90
Respiratory rate	<25 breaths/min	≥25 breaths/min
Altered mentation	Alert	Not alert

TABLE 4: Obstetrically modified sequential organ failure assessment.

System parameter	Score		
	0	1	2
Respiration			
PaO$_2$/FiO$_2$	≥400	300 to <400	<300
Coagulation			
Platelets (×10^6/L)	≥150	100–150	<100
Liver			
Bilirubin (μmol/L)	≤20	20–32	>32
Cardiovascular			
Mean arterial pressure (mm Hg)	≥70	<70	Vasopressors required
Central nervous system	Alert	Rousable by voice	Rousable by pain
Renal			
Creatinine (μmol/L)	≤90	91–120	>120

- Pelvic structures (chorioamnionitis and endometritis)
- Surgical wounds (cesarean section and perineal laceration)
- Breast (mastitis).

Major Pathogens

- Group A β-hemolytic streptococci (GAS), also known as *Streptococcus pyogenes*
- Group B *Streptococcus*
- *Escherichia coli*
- *Klebsiella*
- *Staphylococcus aureus*
- *Anaerobes*: Peptostreptococci, peptocicci, *Bacteroides*, *Clostridium* species, and *Listeria monocytogenes* are less common
- Viral causes, e.g., influenza, varicella, hepatitis, and herpes simplex
- Malaria and other tropical infections.

IMPLICATIONS FOR MATERNAL HEALTH

Third most common cause of maternal death is maternal sepsis following postpartum hemorrhage and preeclampsia.

Common infections such as genitourinary tract, surgical site, and mastitis that contributes to maternal mortality of around 11%.[8]

When all the sites are evaluated, it contributes to 25–40% of maternal deaths worldwide.[9]

IMPLICATIONS FOR FETAL HEALTH

These patients need continuous electronic fetal monitoring.

Worsening maternal organ perfusion is demonstrated by changes in baseline variability and new onset fetal decelerations.

Incidence of preterm birth, stillbirth, and miscarriage are higher in this subset of patients.

Maternal infections are associated with 10–25% of cases of stillbirth in HICs and as 50% in LMICs.[10]

Intrauterine infection is associated with increased risk of neonatal encephalopathy and cerebral palsy hence emergency delivery is compulsory especially in this condition.

There is increased risk of neonatal sepsis in this subset of patients due to maternal transmission which can manifest as decreased intake, irritability, pallor, tachycardia, and increased work of breathing.

In presence of risk factors for early-onset neonatal infections or any clinical indicators as mentioned above early assessment should be done for need of antibiotics.

■ MANAGEMENT

Three components are discussed under this:
1. Diagnosis
2. Treatment
3. Prevention.

Diagnosis

Early diagnosis improves outcomes:
- *Detailed history and clinical examination*: Clinical manifestations depend on source of infection which has been clearly detailed in the **Table 5**.[11,12]

- *Blood cultures*: It is gold standard for identifying bloodstream infections, but the positivity is <50% mainly due to inadequate number of samples, inadequate volume of sample, and prior antibiotic usage.

At least two sets (1 aerobic and 1 anaerobic) each sample containing a volume of 10 mL each helps improving the sensitivity to 90%.

The Clinical and Laboratory Standards Institute (CLSI) guidelines recommend paired culture sets to help discriminate between contaminant organisms and true pathogens; four 10 mL bottles (2 sets) should be used for the initial evaluation to detect about 90–95% of bacteremias and six 10 mL bottles (3 sets) should be used to detect about 95–99% of bacteremias.

TABLE 5: Clinical manifestations of infections and their features.

Infection	Features
Breast abscess/mastitis	Breast pain and tenderness, erythema, painful induration, and nipple discharge
Chorioamnionitis	Abdominal pain, vaginal bleeding, offensive vaginal discharge or lochia, uterine tenderness, delayed uterine involution, fetal tachycardia >160 beats/min, and fever
Endometritis/septic abortion	Abdominal pain, vaginal bleeding, and offensive cervical
Infected wound (perineal or abdominal)	Discharge from wound, pain, erythema, and swelling around wound
Malaria	Fever, headache, muscle/joint pain, jaundice, and anemia
Meningitis	Headache, rash, photophobia, neck stiffness, confusion, fever, nausea, and vomiting
Respiratory tract infection	Productive cough, sore throat, shortness of breathing/difficulty breathing, chest, and fever
Toxic shock syndrome (streptococcal and staphylococcal)	Nausea, vomiting, diarrhea, watery vaginal discharge, generalized maculopapular rash, and conjunctival suffusion
Urinary tract infection	Dysuria, increased frequency, urgency, abdominal/flank/back pain, rigors, fever, nausea, and vomiting
Nonspecific features of infection	Lethargy, reduced appetite, fever, nausea, and vomiting

- *Localization of source*: Throat swabs, midstream urine, high vaginal swab, or cerebrospinal fluid sample should be obtained prior to starting antibiotic therapy based on symptoms of the patient.

  Immediate imaging based on symptoms helps to identify the source of the infection and treat accordingly.

  Imaging should not be delayed on grounds of pregnancy as maternal well-being always scores over fetal well being.
- *Biomarkers*: White cell count (WCC), C-reactive protein (CRP), procalcitonin (PCT), and lactate are commonly used biomarkers in sepsis.

  White cell count and CRP can be elevated in inflammation and infection.

  Procalcitonin is more specific for bacterial infection but all clinical trials show its efficacy mainly in de-escalation and stopping of antibiotics but not in initiation and its normal range of PCT in pregnancy and postoperative period is not clear.

Treatment

They may be treated in intensive care unit (ICU) or ward based on following criterion:
- If the patient needs any organ support **(Table 6)**.
- If sepsis in obstetrics score score >6 patient needs ICU admission **(Table 7)**:[13] Sepsis bundles have been changed from 6 to 1 hour now this can be used even in maternal sepsis or FAST-M is one more bundle which is being used exclusively in pregnancy the components include **(Table 8)**.[14-16]
- *Fluid resuscitation*: As per surviving sepsis guidelines initial rate of recommendation for initial intravenous fluid resuscitation is 30 mL/kg.

  In pregnancy colloid oncotic pressure is reduced so there is high risk of extravasation of fluid so it is reduced to 20 mL/kg.[17-19]

  Lactate >4 mmol/L indicates impaired organ perfusion and shock so fluid resuscitation is initiated immediately to target mean arterial pressure (MAP) >65 mm Hg.

  Crystalloids are preferred over colloids due to the increased risk of acute kidney injury and coagulopathy with colloids with no additional clinical benefit.

  Passive leg raising test (PLR) can be used in spontaneously breathing patients to assess fluid responsiveness. Patients in whom there is a rise of cardiac output

TABLE 6: Indication for transfer to the intensive care unit.

System	Indication
Cardiovascular	Hypotension or raised serum lactate persisting despite fluid resuscitation, suggesting the need for inotrope support
Respiratory	• Pulmonary edema • Mechanical ventilation • Airway protection
Renal	Renal dialysis
Neurological	Significantly decreased conscious level
Miscellaneous	• Multiorgan failure • Uncorrected acidosis • Hypothermia

TABLE 7: The sepsis in obstetrics score a model to identity risk of morbidity from sepsis in pregnancy.

Variable score	Value +4	+3	+2	+1	0 (normal)	+1	+2	+3	+4
Temp (°C)	>40.9	39–40.9	–	38.5–38.9	36–38.4	34–35.9	32–33.9	30–31.9	<30
SBP	–	–	–	–	>90	–	70–90	–	<70
HR (bpm)	>179	150–179	130–149	120–129	≤119	–	–	–	–
RR (breaths/min)	>49	35–49	–	25–34	–	12–24	10–11	6–9	–
SpO$_2$ (%)	–	–	–	–	>92	90–91	–	85–89	<85
Leucocytes (number/μL)	>39.9	–	25–39.9	17–24.9	5.7–16.9	3–5.6	1–2.9	–	<1
Immature neutrophils (%)	–	–	>10%	–	<10%	–	–	–	–
Lactic acid (mmol/L)	–	–	>4	–	<4	–	–	–	–

(HR: heart rate; RR: respiration rate; SBP: systolic blood pressure; SpO$_2$: oxygen saturation)

TABLE 8: FAST-M.

F	Fluids
A	Antibiotics
S	Source identification and control
T	Transfer to higher center
M	Monitoring

after 2–3 minutes are considered as fluid responders and those with no change in cardiac output are considered fluid non responders.

Passive leg raising test is not reliable in the third trimester due to inferior vena cava (IVC) compression. Instead small boluses of 250 mL is administered which if associated with increase in cardiac output, further fluid administration can be done otherwise vasopressors should be initiated.

Lactate normalization can also be used to guide fluid resuscitation in pregnancy.

After adequate fluid resuscitation, vasopressor should be started to target MAP >65 mm Hg.[15,20,21]

First line vasopressor recommended for use in maternal sepsis is norepinephrine.

- *Antibiotics*: Corner stone for sepsis management is choosing the correct antibiotic **(Table 9)**.[17,18]

Appropriate antibiotic always remember 5Ds diagnosis, drug, dose, duration and de-escalation.

Diagnosing the site of infection properly with symptomatic and laboratory assessment, chose an empirical antibiotic based on possible causative organism with good tissue penetration, dose it based on hemodynamics, renal and liver functions, duration based on site of infection and finally de-escalation if we find a susceptible organism in cultures to prevent development of resistance.

Every hour delay in antibiotic administration increases mortality risk.

TABLE 9: Antibiotic selection-based on source of infection.

Source of sepsis	Organisms	Antimicrobial	In case of allergy	Notes
Mastitis OR cesarean section wound infection OR intravenous cannula site infection	• MSSA • MRSA • Streptococci	• Flucloxacillin* + clindamycin • *If MRSA use vancomycin instead of flucloxacillin	• Vancomycin + clindamycin • Clindamycin/teicoplanin are alternatives in MRSA	• Trough level • Vancomycin 5–20 mg/L needed for mastitis cases
Endometritis	• Gram-negative anaerobes • Streptococci	Cefotaxime + metronidazole + gentamicin (gentamicin immediately and once only)	Gentamicin + clindamycin + ciprofloxacin	
Acute pyelonephritis	• Gram-negatives • Occasionally caused by staphylococci and streptococci	Cefotaxime + gentamicin (gentamicin once only)	Gentamicin + ciprofloxacin	*ESBLs:* Gentamicin + meropenem
Unknown origin	• MRSA • Streptococci • Gram-negatives • Anaerobes	Meropenem + clindamycin + gentamicin (gentamicin usually once only)	Clindamycin + gentamicin + metronidazole + ciprofloxacin	• Gram-negative organism possibilities include ESBL producers and *Pseudomonas* • Carbapenems contraindicated in severe penicillin allergy
Toxic shock syndrome	• Staphylococci • Streptococci	Flucloxacillin* + clindamycin + gentamicin (gentamicin once only) *For MRSA use vancomycin instead of flucloxacillin	Vancomycin+ clindamycin + gentamicin (gentamicin Immediately and once only) OR Linezolid + gentamicin (gentamicin once only)	• Essential to include an antitoxin agent; i.e., clindamycin or linezolid • Consider intravenous immunoglobulin

(ESBL: extended-spectrum beta-lactamase; MRSA: methicillin-resistant *Staphylococcus aureus*; MSSA: methicillin-susceptible *Staphylococcus aureus*)

Source: Royal College of Obstetricians and Gynaecologists. (2012). Bacterial Sepsis following pregnancy. [online] Available from: https://www.rcog.org.uk/guidance/browse-all-guidance/green-top-guidelines/bacterial-sepsis-following-pregnancy-green-top-guideline-no-64b/ [Last accessed February, 2023].
Adapted from RCOG Green Top Guidelines No. 64b.

Most crucial step is microbiological diagnosis of the causative agent to optimize the antibiotic and minimize potential antibiotic resistance.

Prior to administration of antibiotics blood cultures should be taken; however this should not delay administration of antibiotics.[19]

De-escalation is then implemented in accordance with culture results.

- *Source identification control*: Surviving sepsis guidelines also clearly demonstrates any delay in source control is associated with considerable increase in 28-day mortality rates, hence, every effort should be made to identify the source of infection, e.g., retained products of conception, indwelling catheters, and intra-abdominal collections. Once identified source should be removed immediately.

  Next most crucial decision in source control is delivery timing which again depends on maternal condition, gestational age, and fetal condition.

  Preterm delivery is attempted only if there is high suspicion of intrauterine infection,[11] general anesthesia should be preferred over regional anesthesia.[22]
- *Transfer to higher center*: Indications for transfer: As per RCOG **(Box 1)**.[16]
- *Monitoring*: Patients with maternal sepsis should have continuous monitoring of their vital signs to evaluate their response to treatment and early recognition of clinical worsening and upgradation of antibiotics.[15]

  In patient's being treated for maternal sepsis during the intrapartum period, fetal monitoring is also recommended.

Other Treatments

- *Steroids*: There is no role of steroid in sepsis in pregnancy except in preterm pregnancy for fetal lung maturity. But it should be avoided if suspected chorioamnionitis or ongoing systemic infection like tuberculosis even for fetal lung maturity.

  Maternal outcome is always important than fetal outcome so stress dose steroid can be used if patient is in septic shock and steroids may need to be given for pregnant patients with severe asthma and connective tissue disease based on their requirement.
- *Intravenous immune globulin (IVIG)*:
  - In exotoxin mediated severe invasive staphylococcal and streptococcal sepsis support use of IVIG causing toxic shock syndrome.[11]
  - But surviving sepsis guidelines say no role of IVIG.
  - Role in maternal sepsis and septic shock is questionable.

> **BOX 1:** Indications for transfer—as per RCOG.
> - A case of maternal sepsis presenting outside of an acute hospital setting, e.g., in a health center
> - The patient requires higher level of care than the facility can provide (e.g., radiological investigations, the need for surgical intervention, etc.)
> - Persistent maternal hypotension or a non-improving serum lactate despite adequate fluid resuscitation requiring vasopressor support
> - Decreased levels of consciousness requiring airway protection or mechanical ventilation
> - Multiorgan failure

Prevention

- *Water, sanitation, and hygiene infrastructure*: In pregnant and nonpregnant patients; water, sanitation, and hygiene of infrastructure are important for prevention of infections in any healthcare setting.
- *Hand hygiene*: Five key moments for hand hygiene are—(1) before touching patient, (2) before aseptic procedures, (3) after contact with body fluids, (4) after touching a patient, and (5) after touching the patient's surroundings.

TABLE 10: World Health Organization guidelines for antibiotics.

Is antibiotic prophylaxis recommended?		Yes	No
First trimester	Abortion or miscarriage surgery (MVA/EVAC/D and C)	√	
	Preterm labor with intact amniotic membranes		√
	Prelabor rupture of membranes (PROM) at or near term		√
First and second stage of labor	Vaginal group B *Streptococcus* (GBS) colonization	√	
	Meconium-stained amniotic fluid		√
	Normal vaginal birth		√
	Operative vaginal birth (forceps or vacuum-assisted delivery)		√
Third stage of labor	Manual removal of placenta	√	
	Third or fourth degree perineal tears (torn anal sphincter, anus, or rectum)	√	
	Episiotomy		√
Cesarean section	Effective or emergency cesarean section (antibiotics should be given before skin incision)	√	

(EVA: electric vacuum aspiration; MVA: manual vacuum aspiration)

If visibly soiled, or after toileting hands should be cleaned with soap and water, otherwise, it is appropriate to use alcohol-based hand rub.

- *Antibiotic prophylaxis (Table 10):* WHO guidelines for antibiotics are described in **Table 10**.[23,24]

- *Antenatal care:* Screening activities and preventative measures for infections that are endemic to the region are important components of antenatal care. Oral iron and folic acid prevent maternal sepsis. A summary of the approach to maternal sepsis is presented in **Flowchart 1**.

TAKE HOME MESSAGES

- Maternal sepsis is defined as organ dysfunction resulting from infection during pregnancy, childbirth, postabortion, or postpartum period.
- Due to the various physiological changes there is a higher possibility of clinical worsening in maternal sepsis so early identification based on clinical manifestations and appropriate investigations are most important.
- In qSOFA respiratory rate targets have been changed from 22 to 25 and systolic pressure has been reduced to 90 from 100 as tachypnea and hypotension are physiological in pregnancy and score of >2 is associated with poor prognosis.
- Initial fluid resuscitation should be restricted to 20 mL/kg unlike 30 mL/kg in routine population due to higher risk of interstitial and pulmonary edema.
- Passive leg raising test which is used regularly for fluid assessment cannot be used in third trimester due to uterine compression.
- Early appropriate antibiotics and source control are the core elements of the treatment.
- Delivery should be done only after maternal hemodynamic stabilization.
- Preterm delivery only if strong suspicion of maternal genital infections.
- Steroids are again compulsory in all preterm deliveries unless its chorioamnionitis or maternal TB where its contraindicated.
- Proper hand hygiene and antibiotic prophylaxis is important to prevent maternal sepsis.

Flowchart 1: Maternal sepsis.

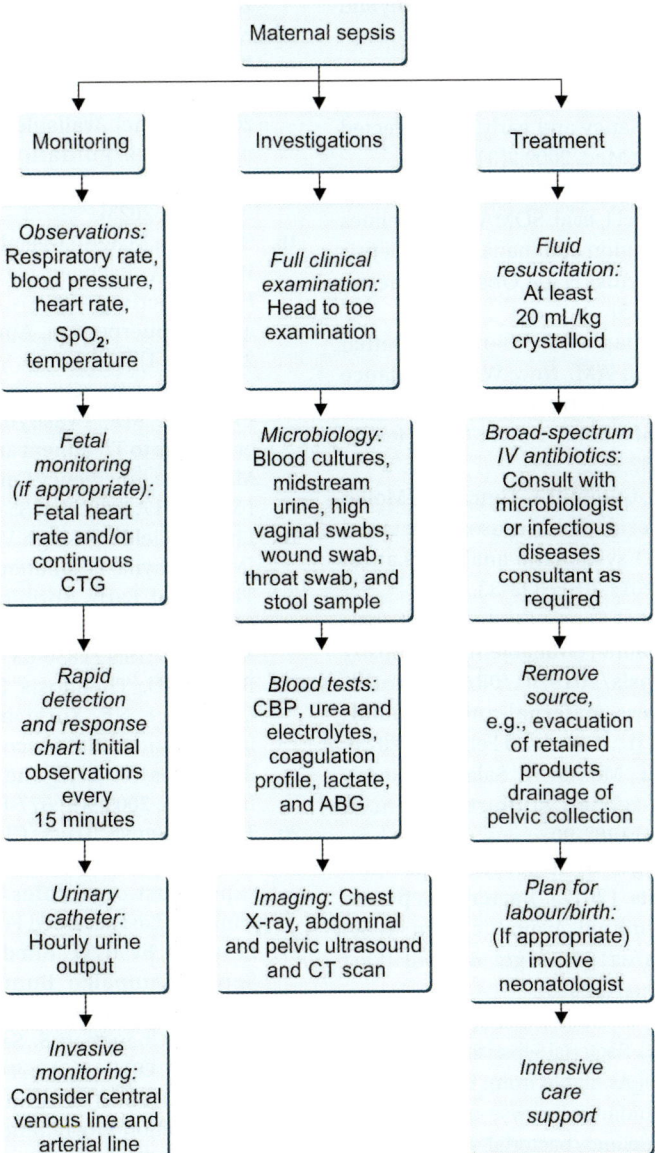

(ABG: arterial blood gas; CT: computed tomography; CTG: cardiotocography; IV: intravenous; SpO$_2$: oxygen saturation)
Source: World Health Organization, Human Reproduction Programme. WHO recommendations for prevention and treatment of maternal peripartum infections, 2015.

REFERENCES

1. Bonet M, Nogueira Pileggi V, Rijken MJ, Coomarasamy A, Lissauer D, Souza JP, et al. Towards a consensus definition of maternal sepsis: results of a systematic review and expert consultation. Reprod Health. 2017;14(1):67.
2. Kourtis AP, Read JS, Jamieson DJ. Pregnancy and infection. N Engl J Med. 2014;370(23):2211-8.
3. van Dillen J, Zwart J, Schutte J, van Roosmalen J. Maternal sepsis: epidemiology, etiology and outcome. Curr Opin Infect Dis. 2010;23(3):249-54.

4. Acosta CD, Harrison DA, Rowan K, Lucas DN, Kurinczuk JJ, Knight M. Maternal morbidity and mortality from severe sepsis: a national cohort study. BMJ Open Access. 2016;6:e012323.
5. Joseph J, Sinha A, Paech M, Walters BNJ. Sepsis in pregnancy and early goal-directed therapy. Obstet Med. 2009;2(3):93-9.
6. Bowyer L, Robinson HL, Barrett H, Crozier TM, Giles M, Idel I, et al. SOMANZ guidelines for the investigation and management sepsis in pregnancy. Aust N Z J Obstet Gynaecol. 2017;57(5):540-51.
7. Bonet M, Oladapo OT, Khan DN, Mathai M, Gulmezoglu AM. New WHO guidance on prevention and treatment of maternal peripartum infections. Lancet Glob Health. 2015;3(11):e667-8.
8. Say L, Chou D, Gemmill A, Tuncalp O, Moller AB, Daniels J, et al. Global causes of maternal death: a WHO systematic analysis. Lancet Glob Health. 2014;2(6):e323-33.
9. Global Maternal Sepsis Study. Stop Sepsis Campaign. [online] Available from: https://srhr.org/se psis/2019/01/08/2nd-world-sepsis-congress-maternal-and-neonatal-sepsissession/ [Last accessed February, 2023].
10. Goldenberg RL, McClure E, Saleem S, Reddy U. Infection-related stillbirths. Lancet. 2010;375(9724):1482-90.
11. Royal College of Obstetricians and Gynaecologists. (2012). Bacterial Sepsis in pregnancy. [online] Available from: rcog.org.uk/media/ea1p1r4h/gtg_64a.pdf [Last accessed February, 2023].
12. Royal College of Obstetricians and Gynaecologists. (2012). Bacterial Sepsis following pregnancy. [online] Available from: https://www.rcog.org.uk/guidance/browse-all-guidance/green-top-guidelines/bacterial-sepsis-following-pregnancy-green-top-guideline-no-64b/ [Last accessed February, 2023].
13. Albright CM, Ali TN, Lopes V, Rouse DJ, Anderson BL. The Sepsis in Obstetrics Score: a model to identify risk of morbidity from sepsis in pregnancy. Am J Obstet Gynecol. 2014;211:39.e1-8.
14. Rhodes A, Evans LE, Alhazzani W, Levy MM, Antonelli M, Ferrer R, et al. Surviving Sepsis Campaign: International Guidelines for Management of Sepsis and Septic Shock: 2016. Intensive Care Med. 2017;43(3):304-77.
15. National Institute for Health and Care Excellence (NICE). (2016). Sepsis: recognition, assessment and early management, 2016. [online] Available from: https://www.nice.org.uk/guidance/ng51/evidence/full-guideline-2551523297 [Last accessed February, 2023].
16. Society for Maternal-Fetal Medicine (SMFM); Plante LA, Pacheco LD, Louis JM. SMFM Consult Series #47: Sepsis during pregnancy and the puerperium. Am J Obstet Gynecol. 2019;220(4):B2-10.
17. Seymour CW, Gesten F, Prescott HC, Friedrich ME, Iwashyna TJ, Phillips GS, et al. Time to Treatment and Mortality during Mandated Emergency Care for Sepsis. N Engl J Med. 2017;376(23):2235-44.
18. Liu VX, Fielding-Singh V, Greene JD, Baker JM, Iwashyna TJ, Bhattacharya J, et al. The Timing of Early Antibiotics and Hospital Mortality in Sepsis. Am J Respir Crit Care Med. 2017;196(7):856-63.
19. Becker JU, Theodosis C, Jacob ST, Wira CR, Groce NE. Surviving sepsis in low-income and middle-income countries: new directions for care and research. Lancet Infect Dis. 2009;9(9):577-82.
20. The UK Sepsis Trust. Clinical Professional Resources. [online] Available from: https://sepsistrust.org/professional-resources/clinical/ [Last accessed February, 2023].
21. Levy MM, Evans LE, Rhodes A. The Surviving Sepsis Campaign Bundle: 2018 update. Intensive Care Med. 2018;44(6):925-8.
22. Elton R, Chaudhari S. Sepsis in Obstetrics. BJA Educ. 2015;15(5):259-64.
23. World Health Organization, Human Reproduction Programme. (2015). WHO recommendations for prevention and treatment of maternal peripartum infections. [online] Available from: https://apps.who.int/iris/bitstream/handle/10665/186171/9789241549363_eng.pdf;jsessionid=06112336E0E6E67991C66E40C0C8B0E9?sequence=1 [Last accessed February, 2023].
24. Lissauer D, Wilson A, Hewitt C, Middleton L, Bishop JRB, Daniels J, et al. A Randomized Trial of Prophylactic Antibiotics for Miscarriage Surgery. N Engl J Med. 2019;380:1012-21.

CHAPTER 40

Noncardiogenic Pulmonary Edema in Pregnancy

Sharmili Sinha, Neeraj Kumar

INTRODUCTION

Noncardiogenic pulmonary edema (NCPE) appears due to increased vascular permeability secondary to direct or indirect lung damage.[1] Sudden deterioration in respiratory condition following acute hypoxia results in NCPE. Pulmonary edema is very uncommon in the setting of pregnancy, and it mainly appears in the antepartum, intrapartum, and postpartum phases of pregnancy. NCPE is mostly seen in the last trimester of pregnancy.[2]

The physiological changes of pregnancy lead to diminished pulmonary reserve and the fetus is more liable for sudden hypoxemia. There are multiple etiological factors for this disease process and early recognition and intervention are primarily important. The main mechanism for NCPE is due to the difference in pressure gradient inside the pulmonary vasculature and due to increased alveolar-capillary permeability and decreased alveolar fluid clearance. In NCPE, the pulmonary capillary wedge pressure is <18 mm Hg whereas in cardiogenic pulmonary edema (CPE) it is ≥18 mm Hg.[3,4]

So, several times its management depends upon the capillary wedge pressure also. The retained alveolar fluid is very difficult to be removed and this retained alveolar fluid has a very high protein content which primarily affects the lung compliance and damages the alveolar epithelial lining. This makes the management of pulmonary edema even more challenging. In NCPE there should be an absence of peripheral edema, no history of acute cardiac diseases, and flat neck veins.[5] The initial chest roentgenogram of NCPE shows the classical picture of peripherally distributed bilaterally infiltrates and air bronchogram without pulmonary congestion and cardiomegaly. Even a bedside echocardiogram (2D-Echo) may show no evidence of acute systolic or diastolic dysfunction. However, acute respiratory distress syndrome (ARDS) is better identified as NCPE and it may be due to several inflammatory factors such as sepsis, pneumonia, aspiration pneumonitis, following transfusion of blood products, and acute pancreatitis, drug toxicity, and acute trauma. The scope of NCPE is much larger and widened than ARDS.

ETIOLOGY

As there are various etiological factors associated with the development of NCPE and they are:
- Due to increasing alveolar-capillary permeability and decreased alveolar fluid clearance:
  - ARDS
  - Neurogenic pulmonary edema (NPE) following traumatic brain injury, seizures, and electrocution

- Preeclampsia
■ Due to drug abuse and toxic inhalation:
  - Overdose of opioids
  - Salicylate poisoning
  - Radiocontrast-related pulmonary edema
  - Tricyclic antidepressant overdose
  - Environmental and toxic inhalation
■ Due to an imbalance in alveolar capillary pressure:
  - Perioperative pulmonary edema (PPE)
■ Due to increased alveolar-capillary pressure:
  - Peripartum pulmonary edema
  - Polycystic ovarian syndrome
  - Pulmonary edema following exertion
■ Due to hypoxia:
  - High-altitude pulmonary edema (HAPE)
■ Due to sudden change in thoracic pressure in the postoperative period:
  - Post upper airway obstruction
  - Post pneumonectomy
  - Post evacuation of pleural effusion
  - Post evacuation of pericardial effusion.

EPIDEMIOLOGY AND MAGNITUDE OF PROBLEM

About 0.08–0.5% of pregnancies are complicated due to acute pulmonary edema. Because of the adaptations in physiological changes of pregnancy, pregnant patients have an increased propensity to develop pulmonary edema. Some of the common causes like tocolytics use (25%), underlying cardiac disease (25%), fluid overload (21%), and preeclampsia (18%) lead to pulmonary edema in pregnancy.[6] The presence of preterm labor complicates about 11–14% of pregnancies. Preterm delivery (birth before 37 weeks of gestation) is the leading cause of neonatal morbidity and mortality.[2] The previous practice of using tocolytics for suppressing labor is been not followed and now calcium channel blockers and indomethacin are more commonly used which has reduced the incidence of pulmonary edema in pregnancy.[7] ARDS is one of the important etiologies of NCPE responsible for 10% of intensive care unit (ICU) admissions globally.[3]

Noncardiogenic pulmonary edema is less common than CPE. The incidence of ARDS incidence is uncertain. But the mortality depends on various factors such as age, cause of ARDS, and involvement of organs and it varies from 50 to 75%. The predictive outcome of the patient does not depend upon a single variable. Even the degree of hypoxemia has not been found valuable. If ascent to an altitude of >2,200 meters increases the risk for development of acute mountain sickness or HAPE.[8] Within 6 hours of blood transfusion products presence of respiratory deterioration and hypoxia confirms transfusion-related acute lung injury (TRALI).[9] The incidence of TRALI is more with blood products with a higher ratio of plasma content, with 1 in 2,000 plasma containing components and 1 in 400 whole blood products. Pregnant female donors have a higher incidence of TRALI due to human leukocyte antigen (HLA) antibodies.[10] Mendelson's syndrome is another well-recognized cause of lung injury and pulmonary edema secondary to aspiration of gastric contents into the tracheobronchial tree.

IMPLICATIONS OF MATERNAL HEALTH

Development of Pulmonary Edema following Physiologic Adaptations to Pregnancy

There is a rapid physiological change in the entire organ system of pregnant women to support the developing fetus. The changes which may lead to increased risks of

pulmonary edema in pregnant patients are as follows:
- *Changes in blood volume:* At 5-6 weeks of gestation, the plasma volume started to increase and will reach 45-50% above prepregnancy values by 32 weeks. With an increase in plasma volume, a 20-30% increase in erythrocytic cell mass is also observed. These patients have physiological anemia during pregnancy due to a larger increase in plasma volume than red cell mass increase.
- *Peripheral resistance changes*: Systemic vascular resistance is decreased due to a progesterone-mediated increase in venous dilatation. By 7 weeks of pregnancy blood pressure begin to fall, so this period is often defined as a high flow and low resistance state.
- *Changes in cardiac output*: Due to the resultant increase in ventricular wall mass and end-diastolic volume, cardiac output is increased. By 32 weeks of gestation maternal heart rate increased by 15–20% of its prepregnant values. Maternal oxygen consumption is also increased.
- *Changes in colloid oncotic pressure*: Albumin is responsible for creating 75–80% of colloid oncotic pressure during pregnancy. As a central dogma of life protein will attract water. However, due to hemodilution colloid oncotic pressures fall by 3–5 mm Hg in pregnancy following decreased albumin concentration. So, pregnant patients are more prone to develop pulmonary edema as they have a less intravascular fluid reserve.

■ MANAGEMENT STEPS

The management part includes supportive care and treatment of the underlying pathophysiological cause of NCPE till the complete improvement of acute lung conditions **(Flowchart 1)**.

However, various treatment strategies such as prostacyclin (PGI2), inhaled nitric oxide, high-frequency oscillatory ventilation (HFOV), and anti-inflammatory therapy were tried but were not found effective.[11] Similarly, other causes of NCPE were managed with oxygen therapy or using the noninvasive or invasive mode of ventilation depending upon the inciting cause. The causes of CPE as a differential diagnosis should be excluded. Other diagnoses like ARDS needs evaluation. The goal of treatment is to keep the partial pressure of arterial oxygen (PaO_2) >60 mm Hg without injuring the lungs with excessive O_2 or volutrauma/barotrauma. Lowering the pulmonary artery wedge pressure with diuretics and fluid restriction may improve pulmonary function in ARDS. If a history of quick ascent in altitude is present, diagnosis of HAPE should be considered. Specific drug and medication history should be reviewed, especially for salicylate toxicity and opioid overdose.[12] If a pregnant patient has a sudden onset of shortness of breath, tachycardia along with signs of hemodynamic instability diagnosis of pulmonary embolism should be considered. Re-expansion and reperfusion pulmonary edema should be kept in differential, and the development of pulmonary edema with hypoxia within 6 hours of a blood transfusion should raise the suspicion of TRALI.[13]

■ PROGNOSIS

Several causes such as major obstetric hemorrhage, preeclampsia, septic shock, abruptio placentae, and trophoblastic disease during pregnancy can cause capillary leak leading to pulmonary edema. Maternal mortality due to severe ARDS is common and has an incidence of 40%. If a patient has a previous diagnosis of HAPE, the chance of recurrence is about 50–60% of patients if these patients ascend above 4,500 meters.[14]

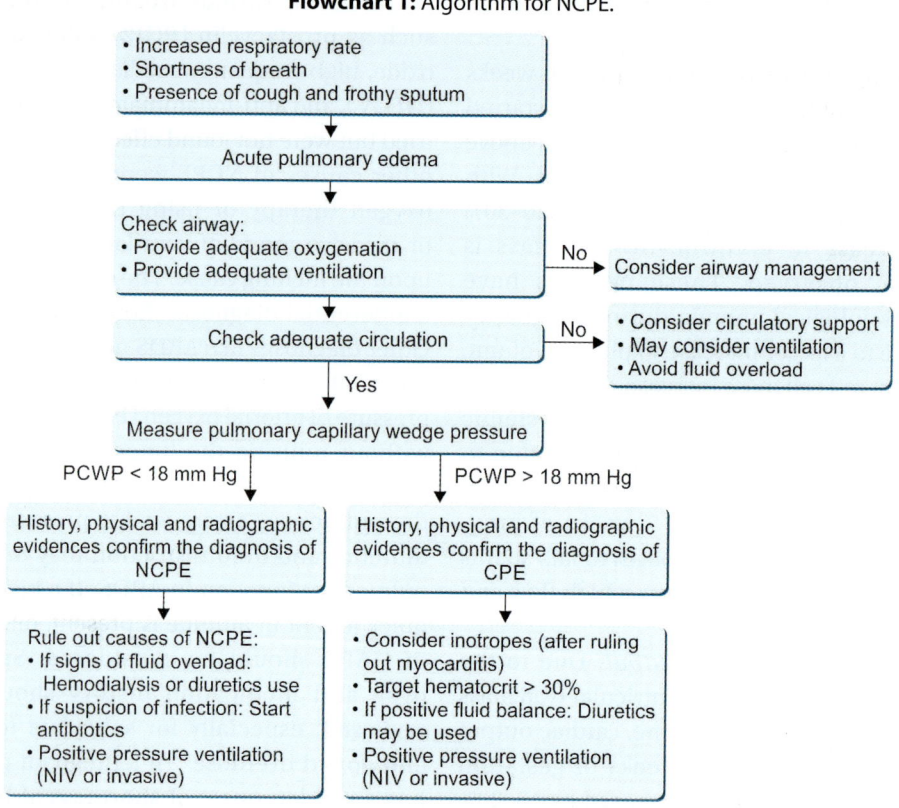

Flowchart 1: Algorithm for NCPE.

(CPE: cardiogenic pulmonary edema; NCPE: noncardiogenic pulmonary edema; NIV: noninvasive ventilation; PCWP: pulmonary capillary wedge pressure)

Even NPE has a very poor prognosis and it primarily insults the central nervous system (CNS). About 60–70% of intracranial hemorrhages were associated with NPE. However, there are no statistics related to NPE in association with epilepsy.[15] Mortality from TRALI is 5–10%; however, it can reach 47% in critically ill patients.[16]

■ CONCLUSION

Noncardiogenic pulmonary edema appears due to increased vascular permeability secondary to direct or indirect lung damage. NCPE can occur without pathologic cardiac disease and an elevation in left atrial pressure. NCPE has a very close similarity with CPE. So initial management of both these illnesses would be similar and mainly focuses on supporting oxygenation to and reducing preload.

TAKE HOME MESSAGES

- There are various etiologies of NCPE that include ARDS, HAPE, NPE, reperfusion pulmonary edema, and re-expansion pulmonary edema.
- NCPE commonly develops within 24 hours of the onset of the initial insult and its presentation may be delayed for 5 days. It usually begins with mild signs and symptoms that may progress rapidly to hypoxic respiratory failure.

- Unlike CPE, it is not caused by high pulmonary capillary pressure and the most common mechanism is an increase in pulmonary capillary permeability and elevated intravascular pressure.
- Clinically NCPE is characterized by a bilateral alveolar infiltrates "butterfly" pattern causing hypoxemia in the absence of pneumonia or congestive heart failure or cardiomegaly.
- NCPE has a very close similarity with CPE. So initial management of both these illnesses would be similar and mainly focuses on supporting oxygenation to and reducing preload.
- In pregnancy, NCPE is less common and is often associated with higher maternal and fetal adverse outcomes.

REFERENCES

1. Kakouros NS, Kakouros SN. Non-cardiogenic pulmonary edema. Hellenic J Cardiol. 2003;44:385-91.
2. Murray JF, Nadel JA, Flick MR. The lungs and gynecologic and obstetric disease. In: Murray JF, Nadel JA (Eds). Textbook of Respiratory Medicine, 2nd edition. Philadelphia: WB Saunders; 1994. pp. 2475-88.
3. Dries DJ. ARDS: From syndrome to disease: prevention and genomics. Air Med J. 2019;38(1):7-9.
4. Skalická H, Bělohlávek J. Non-cardiogenic pulmonary edema, acute respiratory distress syndrome. Cas Lek Cesk. 2015;154(6):273-9.
5. Akunov AC, Sartmyrzaeva MA, Maripov AM, Muratali Uulu K, Mamazhakypov AT, Sydykov AS, et al. High altitude pulmonary edema in a mining worker with an abnormal rise in pulmonary artery pressure in response to acute hypoxia without prior history of high altitude pulmonary edema. Wilderness Environ Med. 2017;28(3):234-8.
6. Sciscione AC, Ivester T, Largoza J, Manley J, Shlossman P, Colmorgen GHC. Acute pulmonary edema in pregnancy. Obstet Gynecol. 2003;101(3):511-5.
7. Amorim MM, Katz L, Ávila MB, Araújo DE, Valença M, da Mata Albuquerque CJ, et al. Admission profile in an obstetric intensive care unit in a maternity hospital in Brazil. Rev Bras Saude Matern Infant. 2006;6(suppl 1):s55-62.
8. Luks AM, Swenson ER, Bärtsch P. Acute high-altitude sickness. Eur Respir Rev. 2017;26(143):160096.
9. Fernandes Júnior CJ, Hidal JT, Barbas CS, Akamine N, Knobel E. Noncardiogenic pulmonary edema complicating diabetic ketoacidosis. Endocr Pract. 1996;2(6):379-81.
10. Cho MS, Modi P, Sharma S. Transfusion-related acute lung injury. Treasure Island (FL): StatPearls Publishing; 2021.
11. Malhotra A, Drazen JM. High-frequency oscillatory ventilation on shaky ground. N Engl J Med. 2013;368(9):863-5.
12. Radke JB, Owen KP, Sutter ME, Ford JB, Albertson TE. The effects of opioids on the lung. Clin Rev Allergy Immunol. 2014;46(1):54-64.
13. Tank S, Sputtek A, Kiefmann R. Transfusion-related acute lung injury. Anaesthesist. 2013;62(4):254-60.
14. Korzeniewski K, Nitsch-Osuch A, Guzek A, Juszczak D. High altitude pulmonary edema in mountain climbers. Respir Physiol Neurobiol. 2015;209:33-8.
15. Romero Osorio OM, Abaunza Camacho JF, Sandoval Briceño D, Lasalvia P, Narino Gonzalez D. Postictal neurogenic pulmonary edema: Case report and brief literature review. Epilepsy Behav Case Rep. 2018;9:49-50.
16. Kim J, Na S. Transfusion-related acute lung injury; clinical perspectives. Korean J Anesthesiol. 2015;68(2):101-5.

An electroencephalogram (EEG) may reveal disturbed sleep pattern with a focal or generalized slowing of electrical activity of the brain.[1]

Ultimately Magnetic resonance imaging (MRI) is done which can reveal single or multiple confluent lesions throughout the white and gray matter of the brain. Characteristically they are seen as multiple, asymmetric, and diffuse bilateral lesions in the brain, brainstem, cerebellum, and spinal cord. There lesions may not visualized on T1-weighted sequences but show hyperintensity on T2-weighted, fluid-attenuated inversion recovery (FLAIR), proton density, and echo-planar trace diffusion MRI sequences.[9]

Very rarely, MRI can be normal as well during presentation of the disease and the lesions appear few days later in the course of illness.

■ DIAGNOSIS

With the help of history and clinical examination we can arrive at a syndromic diagnosis and localize the site of lesion. There are no well-defined criteria in adults for ADEM but studies done in children have formulated a diagnostic criterion which can be used to diagnose these cases **(Table 2)**.[10]

A list of differential diagnosis **(Box 1)** should be kept as these findings are not exclusive for ADEM. In case the patient

Clinical features	Characteristics on MRI FLAIR and T2-weighted images
First clinical attack of inflammatory or demyelinating disease in the CNS	Large (>1–2 cm in size) multifocal, hyperintense, bilateral, asymmetric lesions in the supratentorial or infratentorial white matter. Rarely, brain MRI shows a single large (≥1–2 cm) lesion predominantly affecting white matter
Acute or subacute onset	Gray matter, especially basal ganglia and thalamus, may be involved
Affects multifocal areas of the CNS	Spinal cord MRI may show confluent intramedullary lesion(s) with variable enhancement, in addition to the abnormalities on brain MRI
Polysymptomatic presentation	No radiologic evidence of previous destructive white matter changes
Must include encephalopathy: Acute behavioral change such as confusion or irritability and/or Alteration in consciousness ranging from somnolence or coma	Large (>1–2 cm in size) multifocal, hyperintense, bilateral, asymmetric lesions in the supratentorial or infratentorial white matter. Rarely, brain MRI shows a single large (≥1 to 2 cm) lesion predominantly affecting white matter
Attack should be followed by improvement on clinical and/or neuroradiologic (MRI) measures	
Sequelae may include residual deficits	
No other etiologies can explain the event	

TABLE 2: Diagnostic criteria of ADEM.[10]

Note: ADEM relapses within 3 months of the inciting episode are considered part of the same event. In addition, ADEM relapses occurring during a steroid taper or within four weeks of therapy completion are considered part of the initial episode.
(ADEM: acute disseminated encephalomyelitis; CNS: central nervous system; FLAIR: fluid-attenuated inversion recovery; MRI: magnetic resonance imaging)

deteriorate further, it is always helpful to reassess the case later.

■ TREATMENT[11]

No specific therapy has been established for management of ADEM. Controlled trials done on patients with multiple sclerosis have shown benefit with the use of immunomodulators. Being a similar demyelinating illness, these agents have been useful in ADEM as well.

Treatment of ADEM has been divided into the following:
- Supportive therapy
- Specific therapy
- Physical and rehabilitation therapy.

Supportive Care

This includes antiseizure medication, fluid and electrolyte balance, nutritional support, prophylactic anticoagulation, and other supportive care.

Airway protection is provided in unconscious/comatose cases, prophylactic pressure sore care and regular limb physiotherapy. Patients with associated cervical myelitis may also require mechanical ventilatory support.

Obstetric consult needs to be taken for pregnant cases. Therapy to delay delivery or rapid maturation of fetal lung maybe required based on the condition of the patient.

Specific Therapy (Flowchart 1)

There are no randomized trials done in pregnant females with ADEM and most patients are provided with supportive care. Anecdotal studies done in pregnant females have suggested the use of following therapy.

Immunomodulation

Intravenous methylprednisolone is the drug of choice at dosage of 10–30 mg/kg/day (maximum 1 g/day) for 3–5 days followed by oral prednisolone with gradual tapering over 6 weeks to reduce the risk of relapses.[12] Full recovery has been reported in 50–80% of patients with this regime.

If patient fails to respond to corticosteroids, plasma exchange (PE) should be tried to remove the culprit antibodies attacking

BOX 1: Various differentials for a case of acute disseminated encephalomyelitis.[1]

Differential diagnosis:
- Multiple sclerosis
- Neuromyelitis optica spectrum disorders
- Aseptic meningitis
- Brain metastasis
- Cardioembolic stroke
- Cauda equina and conus medullaris syndrome
- Cavernous sinus syndromes
- Cerebral venous thrombosis

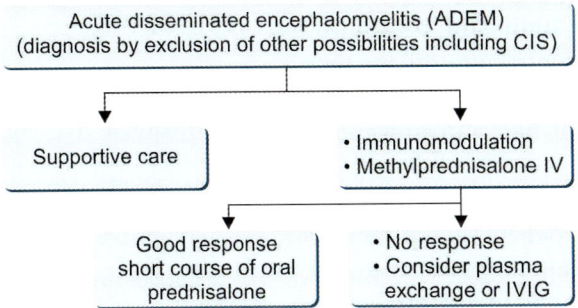

Flowchart 1: Treatment algorithm for ADEM.[11]

(CIS: clinically isolated syndrome; IV: intravenous; IVIG: intravenous immunoglobulin)

the nerurons.[13] A course of four to six PE over 2 weeks has shown marked and sustained symptomatic improvement.[13]

Intravenous immunoglobulin (IVIG) at dose of 0.4 g/kg/day for 5 days is another option which has been tried by few authors.[14] It helps to bind and remove preformed antibodies and provide symptomatic relief. The improvement is seen within 2–3 days in the neurological and general condition of the patient. The power and sensation of the limbs improve gradually overtime.

The choice to start with second-line agent should be individualized depending on the severity of the disease, complications, and comorbidities of the patient. A hyperacute onset, severe neurologic deficits as a result of aggressive disease, multifocal extensive lesions on MRI, and unresponsiveness to steroids are poor prognostic indicators.[11] There are no written guidelines on this to help us decide but if early recovery is not expected in a patient with severe disease, a decision to start on second-line therapy may be fruitful.

Other second-line therapies[11] include use of cyclophosphamide, hypothermia, or decompressive hemicraniectomy in patients with massive fulminant ADEM and life-threatening cerebral edema. These patients have a very poor overall outcome even in the best of the setup with all kinds of therapy.

Physical and Rehabilitation Therapy

This includes giving physiotherapy to the affected paralyzed limb and preventing the development of contractures till the time full recovery occurs. It includes mobilization of the patient out of bed and preventing pressure sores.

This is very important as it provides rehabilitation to the patient, equip them to be self-reliant and help in speedy recovery. It gives both physical and mental strength to deal with stress in life.

■ PROGNOSIS[11]

Long-term prognosis depends on the cause of ADEM. Postmeasles ADEM patients have significant morbidity and higher mortality as compared to others. The prognosis of nonmeasles ADEM is favorable with full recovery in 50–75% of patients over 6 months of therapy.[11]

Mortality rates of up to 20% have been reported in ADEM.[15] Now with early diagnosis, investigation, imaging facilities along with immunomodulator therapy, the mortality rates have drastically reduced and outcomes have become favorable.

■ CONCLUSION

- ADEM should always be on our differential list whenever we encounter a neurological case.
- History of definite infection or vaccination may not always be available but a thorough clinical examination is a must to arrive at a diagnosis.
- Once a diagnosis is suspected, focused investigation to rule out other causes should be done and therapy initiated.
- In neurological cases, CSF and MRI form the basis of diagnosis and prognosis. We should avoid skipping steps if the facilities are available at your center because these also help us rule out other diseases.
- Early initiation of therapy can help prevent long-term sequelae in these young patients.

■ REFERENCES

1. Anilkumar AC, Foris LA, Tadi P. Acute Disseminated Encephalomyelitis. Treasure Island (FL): StatPearls; 2022.
2. Nishiyama M, Nagase H, Tomioka K, Tanaka T, Yamaguchi H, Ishida Y, et al. Clinical time course of pediatric acute disseminated encephalomyelitis. Brain Dev. 2019;41(6):531-7.

3. Shah AK, Tselis A, Mason B. Acute disseminated encephalomyelitis in a pregnant woman successfully treated with plasmapheresis. J Neurol Sci. 2000; 174(2):147-51.
4. Tenembaum S, Chitnis T, Ness J, Hahn JS. Acute disseminated encephalomyelitis. Neurology. 2007;68(16 Suppl 2):S23-36.
5. Marchioni E, Ravaglia S, Montomoli C, Tavazzi E, Minoli L, Baldanti F, et al. Postinfectious neurologic syndromes: a prospective cohort study. Neurology. 2013;80:882-9.
6. Menge T, Kieseier BC, Nessler S, Hemmer B, Hartung HP, Stuve O. Acute disseminated encephalomyelitis: an acute hit against the brain. Curr Opin Neurol. 2007;20:247-54.
7. Alper G. Acute disseminated encephalomyelitis. J Child Neurol. 2012;27:1408-25.
8. Svensson-Arvelund J, Ernerudh J, Buse E, Cline JM, Haeger JD, Dixon D, et al. The placenta in toxicology. Part II: Systemic and local immune adaptations in pregnancy. Toxicol Pathol. 2014;42(2):327-38.
9. Kawanaka Y, Ando K, Ishikura R, Katsuura T, Wakata Y, Kodama H, et al. Delayed appearance of transient hyperintensity foci on T1-weighted magnetic resonance imaging in acute disseminated encephalomyelitis. Jpn J Radiol. 2019;37(4):277-82.
10. Krupp LB, Banwell B, Tenembaum S; International Pediatric MS Study Group. Consensus definitions proposed for pediatric multiple sclerosis and related disorders. Neurology. 2007;68(16 Suppl 2):S7-12.
11. Alexander M, Murthy J. Acute disseminated encephalomyelitis: Treatment guidelines. Ann Indian Acad Neurol. 2011;14:60-4.
12. Wingerchuk DM. Current Evidence and Therapeutic Strategies in Multiple Sclerosis. Semin Neurol. 2008;28:56-68.
13. Miyazawa R, Hikima A, Takano Y, Arakawa H, Tomomasa T, Morikawa A. Plasmapheresis in fulminant acute disseminated encephalomyelitis. Brain Dev. 2001;23:424-6.
14. Brekke OH, Sandlie I. Therapeutic antibodies for human diseases at the dawn of the twenty-first century. Nat Rev Drug Disc. 2003;2:52-62.
15. Anlar B, Basaran C, Kose G, Guven A, Haspolat S, Yakut A, et al. Acute disseminated Encephalomyelitis in Children: Outcome and Prognosis. Neuropediatrics. 2003;34:194-9.

CHAPTER 42

Neuromuscular Disorders in Pregnancy

Saurabh Taneja, Asish Kumar Sahoo

■ INTRODUCTION

Females in peripartum period may develop various neuromuscular disorders. Few of these may be precipitated by pregnancy and might require careful monitoring throughout the peripartum period. Many hereditary disorders affecting neuromuscular functions are also unmasked during pregnancy for the first time affecting both maternal and fetal health. Disorders may range from focal neuropathies such as Bell's palsy, carpal tunnel syndrome, etc., to more generalized and serious conditions such as myasthenia gravis (MG), muscle diseases (hereditary and acquired), inflammatory neuropathy (acute and chronic), spinal muscular atrophy, amyotrophic lateral sclerosis (ALS), autonomic neuropathy, channelopathies, and other neuromuscular junction disorders. Many conditions affect the skeletal muscles while sparing the uterine smooth muscles. Both, anesthetic management for delivery and critical care management of these disorders in the peripartum period are challenging. Special precautions need to be taken while avoiding certain complications. We will be enumerating the conditions and their management strategies.

COMPRESSIVE NERVE AND ROOT DISORDERS (ACQUIRED) DURING PREGNANCY AND DELIVERY

Various focal neuropathies occur throughout the pregnancy period. These may happen due to the stretch during the child birth or increased tissue swelling and fluid retention under the effect of hormones. Other reasons may include malposition during labor, using forceps for assisted delivery and during cesarean section.[1] These conditions do not seem to affect the fetal well-being but careful consideration needs to be given to the pharmaceutical therapies used to manage these conditions as some medications might indirectly affect the fetus **(Table 1)**. Most of the conditions are self-limiting and subside with the conservative management.

Agents used should be carefully chosen. Antiepileptics and tricyclic antidepressants (TCA) traditionally used for pain management are avoided in pregnancy due to safety issues. Use of nonsteroidal anti-inflammatory agents (NSAIDs) carries risk of miscarriage and malformation, hence, caution is advised.

Treatment of carpel tunnel syndrome may be tried by bracing and splinting or local dexamethasone injections.

TABLE 1: US FDA category for commonly used neuromuscular disease treatments.

Drug	Category
Duloxetine	C
Eculizumab	NA
Edaravone	NA
Fludrocortisone	C
Gabapentin	C
Intravenous immunoglobulin	C
Mycophenolate mofetil	D
Methotrexate	X
Midodrine	C
Pregabalin	C
Pyridostigmine	C
Riluzole	C
Rituximab	NA

(A) Adequate and well-controlled studies found no increased risk.
(B) No risk found in animal studies but insufficient human studies.
(C) Adverse fetal animal studies but no adequate human studies; treatment benefits may warrant use despite potential risk.
(D) Evidence of human fetal risk based on studies or marketing experience but benefit may outweigh risk.
(X) Animal or human studies or other experience find fetal abnormalities so that potential benefit in pregnancy is outweighed by risk.

(FDA: Food and Drug Administration; NA: not assigned)

Low back pain is very common and it usually responds to conservative management. Activity modification, physical therapy, pain relief by analgesics, and use of muscle relaxants (after checking their safety profile) are often helpful. Some patients require epidural injections and only few require surgical treatment in case of no response in 6–8 weeks.[2]

INFLAMMATORY NERVE AND MUSCLE CONDITIONS (ACQUIRED) DURING PREGNANCY

Guillain–Barré syndrome (GBS) or acute inflammatory demyelinating polyneuropathy: The characteristic features are sensory disturbances such as pain and tingling, progressive weakness, and a loss of deep tendon reflexes (DTR). It may lead to respiratory involvement requiring ventilatory support, which may lead to complications in the pregnancy. In severe cases, facial, cranial, and autonomic nerves are involved. Respiratory insufficiency and autonomic instability are the main causes of ICU admission. Various reports suggest that pregnant state does not increase the risk of GBS in women, however the incidence increases up to thrice in a month after delivery.[2] It is usually triggered by infections such as *Campylobacter jejuni* and cytomegalovirus (CMV).[3] Although not yet proven, novel coronavirus COVID-19 may also have an association of GBS. There are reports associating Zika virus with GBS,[4] though actual causation requires further studies. Pregnant patients with GBS and concurrent CMV infections are found to have adverse fetal outcome such as sensorineural hearing loss, microcephaly, and even fetal demise. Due to associations with adverse fetal outcome, it is reasonable to screen pregnant GBS patients for CMV and Zika virus. Management of GBS in pregnancy is almost same as in nonpregnant state. It consists of either plasmapheresis or intravenous immune globulin (IVIg).[2,3] Both are effective modalities and are considered safe in pregnancy. Plasmapheresis should be done with caution as it can cause fluid shift and trigger hypotension, which may lead to adverse fetal outcome. However, various large studies have found no added risk with plasmapheresis. There are few notable adverse effects of IVIg during pregnancy namely, hyperviscosity, hypercoagulability, and volume overload. There is no additional benefit in terms of maternal or fetal outcome with termination of pregnancy. Even with complete maternal paralysis, normal fetal movements have been demonstrated, supporting a lack of transplacental transmission in most cases of the causative agents. As GBS does not affect the uterine muscle, normal vaginal delivery is preferred. In pregnant patients with GBS, cesarean section should be reserved mainly for obstetric indications. It is safe to give epidural anesthesia and in case, general anesthesia is given, succinylcholine should be avoided.

Chronic inflammatory demyelinating polyneuropathy (CIDP): This is a chronic immune-mediated neuropathy and the characteristic features are proximal and distal muscle weakness along with sensory loss, and reduced DTR. There has been a tendency for patients to worsen during the third trimester or immediate postpartum period. Treatment is similar to acute inflammatory demyelinating polyneuropathy (AIDP).

Autoimmune MG: This is a neuromuscular disease causing fluctuating and fatigable weakness in skeletal muscles, ptosis, diplopia, dysarthria, and dysphagia. Bulbar and ocular muscle involvement is very common. Autoantibodies are formed against the nicotinic acetylcholine postsynaptic receptors. Myasthenic crisis is an emergency in which there is worsening of muscle weakness leading to severe dysphagia, respiratory failure, and increased risk of aspiration. These patients may require urgent airway and ventilator support. Most of the women with controlled MG can have uneventful pregnancy. Exact course of disease during the pregnancy is difficult to ascertain and can impact the maternal and fetal outcome. In general, 30–50% of patients worsen during pregnancy. There is a paradoxically improvement in 30% of patients, and no change in the remainder.[5] The exacerbation of the disease is most commonly in first trimester, third trimester, and in postpartum period especially 6–8 weeks after delivery. Careful adjustment of medical treatment is essential. It is prudent to have a multidisciplinary team approach consisting of neurologist, an obstetrician, and an obstetric anesthetist. Patients whose disease is not well-controlled should be counselled to avoid pregnancy because of the possible need for teratogenic drugs. Infection, emotional stress, some medications may act as triggers. Most patients have antibodies to acetylcholine receptor (AChR), muscle-specific kinase (MuSK), or lipoprotein receptor-related 4 (LRP4). Diagnostic studies such as single fiber electromyography (EMG) and repetitive nerve stimulation are safe in pregnancy. Treatment options include acetylcholinesterase inhibitors such as pyridostigmine, corticosteroids, immunosuppressive agents, intravenous immunoglobulins, plasma exchange, and thymectomy.[2,3]

The first line of management in all trimesters of pregnancy is oral pyridostigmine. Its efficacy and safety has been demonstrated in various studies.[2,3] In patients who require immune modulation, corticosteroids at the lowest effective dose can be started and are found to be relatively safe. Few earlier studies[2,3] demonstrated the risk of cleft lip and plate but recent reports have not found any association. Corticosteroids use might increase the risk of gestational diabetes, and adrenal suppression during pregnancy. Stress dose of steroids need to be supplemented during labor and delivery in patients taking corticosteroids during pregnancy. Other immunosuppressive agents are usually avoided due to lack of sufficient data, although recent consensus guidelines suggest that azathioprine and cyclosporine are relatively safe when corticosteroids are not effective or tolerated.[6] Methotrexate and mycophenolate mofetil are contraindicated in pregnancy as they are considered teratogenic. A subset of patients having anti-MuSK antibodies might respond to rituximab but it is better avoided due to lack of safety data.[6]

In the case of a myasthenic crisis, patients should be admitted to a critical care unit and given respiratory support to maintain normocarbia and prevent hypoxia. Fetal monitoring is also required. Intravenous immunoglobulins and plasma exchange can be used to treat pregnant patients in the crisis period, and thymectomy may be considered after a stable postpartum period. Both intravenous immunoglobulins, plasma exchange therapies are tolerated well by pregnant patients.

Managing hypertensive disorders of pregnancy in MG patients can be challenging due to the risk of exacerbating the disease. Methyldopa and hydralazine can be considered for managing hypertension, while other drugs such as magnesium, beta blockers, calcium channel blockers, and lidocaine may exacerbate MG **(Box 1)**. Commonly used drugs to treat urinary tract infections like aminoglycosides and fluoroquinolones have a risk of aggravating the weakness and hence, are avoided in pregnant MG patients.

Patients of MG should be planned for normal spontaneous delivery. They should preferably be treated in centers with intensive care facilities. Epidural labor analgesia should be encouraged because it protects against prolonged overexertion. For cesarean section, regional anesthesia is preferred over general anesthesia. Narcotics and non-depolarizing muscle relaxants should be avoided as much as possible. Overall, a careful and individualized approach is necessary to manage MG during pregnancy, in order to ensure the best possible outcome for both the mother and the baby.

> **BOX 1:** Commonly used medications that may unmask or exacerbate myasthenia gravis.
>
> - Antiarrhythmic agents—including lidocaine, quinidine, quinine and procainamide
> - Antimicrobial agents—including aminoglycosides, fluoroquinolones, macrolides
> - Beta-blockers
> - Calcium channel blockers
> - Corticosteroids
> - Iodinated contrast agents
> - Magnesium
> - Neuromuscular blocking agents—including succinylcholine, vecuronium, and botulinum

Transient neonatal MG: This is an important complication in neonates born to myasthenic mother. Neonates have a generalized hypotonia, poor suck reflex, a weak cry and may suffer from respiratory difficulties. Incidence ranges from 10 to 30%, so such child should be screened by a neonatologist. It is due to transplacental passage of antibodies during pregnancy, but it is not related to severity of maternal disease. It may even happen in sero negative mothers. Management is usually supportive and consists of ventilatory support and nasogastric feeding. Acetylcholinesterase inhibitors are used and some severe cases, may require intravenous immunoglobulins or plasma exchange. It usually resolves within 7 days.

Inflammatory muscle disease: These include polymyositis (PM) and dermatomyositis

(DM). The usual presenting features are symmetric proximal limb weakness but severe disease may present with dysphagia or respiratory failure.[7] Elevated creatine kinase is the hallmark laboratory finding. The incidence is 0.5–2 cases per 100,000 population.

Dermatomyositis: This presents with muscle and characteristic skin manifestations. Pregnant females with active disease have higher risk of fetal complications, although the effect of pregnant female is minimal. Treatment is similar to MG and the disease is not known to affect the uterine muscles. Severe disease should be treated with intravenous immunoglobulins or plasma exchange.

Necrotizing myositis is a rare but aggressive form of muscle disease that requires immune treatment. Normal term, spontaneous delivery should be aimed for.

INHERITED DISORDERS OF NERVE AND MUSCLE COMPLICATING PREGNANCY

Inherited neuropathies like Charcot-Marie-Tooth disease (CMT): This is the most common hereditary motor sensory neuropathy. Females with symptoms of CMT since childhood have an almost 50% chance of exacerbating the disease during pregnancy. Epidural anesthesia is safe in these patients but succinylcholine is to be avoided while giving general anesthesia due to the risk of hyperkalemia. Risk of postpartum bleeding is considered high in pregnant CMT patients, so needs careful planning.[3]

Inherited myopathies include a variety of conditions that impact pregnancy **(Table 2)**.

The myotonic dystrophies are autosomal dominant disorders, which usually affects multiple organ systems. The common presentations are muscle weakness and stiffness, endocrine dysfunctions, cataracts, and cardiac symptoms. There are two types—myotonic dystrophies type 1 (DM1) and type 2 (DM2). The genetic defect in DM1 is expansion of a cytosine-thymine-guanine (CTG) repeat in the dystrophia myotonica protein kinase (*DMPK*) gene.

If a mother has this condition, her children may have more severe disease and expanded repeats that can present at birth as congenital myotonic dystrophy. This is characterized by severe symptoms such as respiratory failure, hypotonia, generalized weakness, poor feeding, and mental retardation. Only three-fourth live up to 18 months and half reach adulthood. Risk of maternal complications during pregnancy such as miscarriage, preterm labor, preeclampsia, and peripartum hemorrhage is very high.[8] DM2 also called proximal myotonic myopathy is a less severe condition though systemic involvement might be present. Risk of fetal and maternal complications is also less compared to DM1. Smooth muscles are affected in these patients, hence, affecting the uterine contractions. These patients may require assisted delivery and there is increased risk of hemorrhage. It is better to avoid depolarizing muscle relaxants due to the risk of triggering severe and dangerous myotonic spasms. Only few females with DM1 or DM2 are aware of the diagnosis prior to pregnancy. Although there are few reports of malignant hyperthermia with patients of DM1 and DM2, the causation is not established.

Facioscapulohumeral muscular dystrophy (FSHD): This is characterized by weakness and progressive wasting of the facial and shoulder-girdle muscles. The inheritance pattern is autosomal dominant. In FSHD, weakness is often asymmetric or selective. It is usually not associated with adverse maternal

TABLE 2: Common neuromuscular diseases in pregnancy.

Condition	Timing in pregnancy
Lumbosacral radiculopathy	Throughout pregnancy
Meralgia paresthetica	Third trimester and during delivery
Femoral neuropathy	Third trimester and during delivery
Postpartum foot drop	Third trimester and during delivery
Bell's palsy	Third trimester and early puerperium
Acute and chronic inflammatory demyelinating polyneuropathies	First 14 days postpartum
Myasthenia gravis	Throughout pregnancy
Inflammatory muscle disease in pregnancy [Polymyositis (PM) and dermatomyositis (DM)]	Throughout pregnancy and puerperium
Inherited neuropathies [Charcot–Marie–Tooth disease (CMT)]	Third trimester
<ul><li>Inherited myopathies</li><li>Myotonic dystrophy type 1 (DM1)</li><li>Myotonic dystrophy type 2 (DM2)</li><li>Facioscapulohumeral muscular dystrophy</li><li>McArdle's disease or myophosphorylase deficiency</li><li>Familial hypokalemic periodic paralysis</li><li>Mitochondrial myopathies</li></ul>	Throughout pregnancy
<ul><li>Motor neuron disease</li><li>Spinal muscular atrophy amyotrophic lateral sclerosis</li></ul>	

and fetal outcome. Muscle weakness may be exacerbated during pregnancy and this may persist postdelivery. Risk of malignant hyperthermia is present as with other hereditary myopathies.[9]

McArdle's disease: This is also known as glycogen storage disease type V or myophosphorylase deficiency. Although, there are no reports of rhabdomyolysis during delivery but creatinine kinase levels have found to be raised during labor. Exercise tolerance is improved with increasing blood glucose levels in patients and some reports have suggested using intravenous dextrose during labor.[10]

Familial hypokalemic periodic paralysis: This is characterized by hypokalemia provoked repeated episodes of weakness. The inheritance pattern is autosomal-dominant. The common triggers are stress, both psychologic and physical, medications that cause intracellular shift of potassium like beta-agonists and insulin and carbohydrate load. It can be triggered in pregnant patients for first time after the 1-hour glucose tolerance test. Severe weakness may necessitate strict monitoring and supplementation of potassium intravenously during labor and postpartum period. Strict monitoring of serum potassium and acid-base status is warranted.[1,2]

Mitochondrial myopathies: Mutations of mitochondrial or nuclear deoxyribonucleic acid (DNA) lead to defects in electron transport chain and finally adenosine triphosphate (ATP) production. The patients suffering from mitochondrial myopathies may experience an aggravation of symptoms during pregnancy[3] due to increase in metabolic demands and physiological hemodynamic changes in pregnancy.

Motor neuron disease like spinal muscular atrophy and ALS, though rare, can complicate the pregnancy in such patients. As like other myopathies, depolarizing muscle relaxants should be avoided and spinal and epidural anesthesia is preferred.

Spinal muscular atrophies: Mutations in the *SMN1* gene lead to selective degradation of anterior horn cells. The inheritance pattern is autosomal recessive. Severe progressive weakness is seen in most patients. A higher rate of cesarean section, preterm delivery and instrument-assisted delivery was seen in these patients although few patients undergo successful normal vaginal deliveries too. Progression of weakness during pregnancy is seen in patients and this weakness persist postdelivery in almost 50% of cases.[11] Recently Food and Drug Administration (FDA) has approved two drugs—an intrathecal infusion named nusinersen, which is approved for all age groups and a single dose adenovirus vector gene therapy named onasemnogene abeparvovec-xioi. Use of these therapies is not studied in pregnant patients.

Amyotrophic lateral sclerosis: Patients suffering from ALS have progressive weakness of the limbs, bulbar muscles, and respiratory muscles. It is an extremely rare disorder in women of childbearing age group. It affects both upper and lower motor neurons. It is still not clear if the disease causes obstetric complications. Riluzole, a benzothiazole, routinely used for its treatment is listed as the US FDA category C,[12] and data on its use in pregnancy are lacking.

■ CONCLUSION

- Neuromuscular disorders, though not very common during pregnancy, do offer specific management challenges.
- Many drugs used in general population cannot be used due to lack of safety data and teratogenic effects.
- Early diagnosis and optimization are of utmost importance for maternal and fetal safety.
- Well-designed anesthetic plan for labor and cesarean delivery is required.
- These patients will benefit from multidisciplinary management in setup with availability of intensive care facilities.

■ REFERENCES

1. Sax TW, Rosenbaum RB. Neuromuscular disorders in pregnancy. Muscle Nerve. 2006; 34(5):559-71.
2. Weimer LH. Neuromuscular disorders in pregnancy. Handb Clin Neurol. 2020; 172:201-18.
3. Edmundson C, Guidon AC. Neuromuscular disorders in pregnancy. Semin Neurol. 2017; 37(6):643-52.
4. Krauer F, Riesen M, Reveiz L, Oladapo OT, Martínez-Vega R, Porgo TV, et al. Zika virus infection as a cause of congenital brain abnormalities and Guillain-Barré syndrome: systematic review. PLoS Med. 2017;14(1):e1002203.
5. Ducci RD, Lorenzoni PJ, Kay CSK. Clinical follow-up of pregnancy in myasthenia gravis patients. Neuromuscul Disord. 2017; 27(4):352-7.

6. Sanders DB, Wolfe GI, Benatar M, Evoli A, Gilhus NE, Illa I, et al. International consensus guidance for management of myasthenia gravis: executive summary. Neurology. 2016;87(4):419-25.
7. Munira S, Christopher-Stine L. Pregnancy in myositis and scleroderma. Best Pract Res Clin Obstet Gynaecol. 2020;64:59-67.
8. Johnson NE, Hung M, Nasser E. The impact of pregnancy on myotonic dystrophy: a registry-based study. J Neuromuscul Dis. 2015;2:447-52.
9. Ciafaloni E, Pressman EK, Loi AM, Smirnow AM, Guntrum DJ, Dilek N, et al. Pregnancy and birth outcomes in women with facioscapulohumeral muscular dystrophy. Neurology. 2006;67:1887-9.
10. Vissing J, Haller RG. The effect of oral sucrose on exercise tolerance in patients with McArdle's disease. N Engl J Med. 2003; 349(26):2503-9.
11. Abati E, Corti S. Pregnancy outcomes in women with spinal muscular atrophy: a review. J Neurol Sci. 2018;388:50-60.
12. Kawamichi Y, Makino Y, Matsuda Y. Riluzole use during pregnancy in a patient with amyotrophic lateral sclerosis: a case report. J Int Med Res. 2010;38(2):720-6.

CHAPTER 43

Posterior Reversible Encephalopathy Syndrome

Nithya CA, Ajith Kumar AK

■ INTRODUCTION

Posterior reversible encephalopathy syndrome (PRES), also known as reversible posterior leukoencephalopathy syndrome (RPLS), is a neurological disorder characterized by headache, confusion, visual disturbances, or seizures. PRES is a clinicoradiological diagnosis.

It was first described by Hinchey et al. in 1996 and called reversible posterior leukoencephalopathy.[1] They described reversible white matter changes in 15 patients, out of whom three had eclampsia, seven were receiving immunosuppressive therapy, four had hypertensive encephalopathy associated with renal disease, and one was receiving interferon for melanoma.

■ PATHOPHYSIOLOGY

Several theories have been described regarding the pathophysiology of PRES, the most common being the vasogenic theory and endothelial dysfunction.

Vasogenic Theory/Cerebral Autoregulatory Failure

Cerebral autoregulation maintains a constant blood flow to the brain over a range of systemic blood pressure by causing arteriolar constriction and dilatation. When there is hypertension with systolic blood pressure above the upper limit of cerebral autoregulation, there is arteriolar dilatation and hyperperfusion to the brain.[2] This may result in the breakdown of the blood-brain barrier, especially in the watershed zones, resulting in vasogenic edema which results in PRES. The relative lack of sympathetic innervation in the posterior circulation makes it prone to these changes when there is a sudden fluctuation in blood pressure'.

Endothelial Dysfunction

This is postulated as the pathophysiology of PRES associated with preeclampsia and cytotoxic therapies. This addresses the fact that 30% of the patients with PRES have normal blood pressure.[3] Circulating toxins either endogenous or exogenous cause vascular endothelial damage. This in turn results in the release of vasoconstrictive and immunogenic agents which may cause vasospasm and increased vascular permeability. The resulting vasogenic edema is the driving factor behind PRES.

■ ETIOLOGY

Posterior reversible encephalopathy syndrome is associated with a host of entities, common ones being eclampsia, hypertension, and immunosuppressive treatment **(Box 1)**.

> **BOX 1:** Etiology of posterior reversible encephalopathy syndrome.
>
> - Hypertension
> - Eclampsia/preeclampsia
> - Immunosuppressive agents or cytotoxic medications—bevacizumab, cisplatin, cyclosporine A, methotrexate, and rituximab
> - Autoimmune disorders—systemic lupus erythematosus, scleroderma, and thrombotic thrombocytopenic purpura
> - Hypomagnesemia and hypercalcemia
> - Sepsis
> - Others—renal disease and iodide contrast media exposure

Hypertension is frequent but not mandatory for the diagnosis of PRES.

CLINICAL FEATURES

Posterior reversible encephalopathy syndrome is associated with a myriad of symptoms. Common presentations are headaches, impairment in the level of consciousness, seizures, visual disturbances, nausea, vomiting, and focal neurological deficits.

The clinical manifestations depend on the area of the brain involved. Involvement of the occipital lobe results in visual disturbances and hallucinations. Focal neurological deficits depend on the site of the focal lesions.

ANATOMIC DISTRIBUTION

Parietal and occipital lobes are commonly involved, and findings are usually bilateral and symmetrical. The possible reason for preferential involvement of posterior circulation is reduced sympathetic innervation of the arterioles of the posterior circulation. This results in reduced protection of this area from fluctuations in blood pressure.

POSTERIOR REVERSIBLE ENCEPHALOPATHY SYNDROME AND PREGNANCY

Preeclampsia, eclampsia, and hemolysis, elevated liver enzymes and low platelets (HELLP) syndrome are the obstetric conditions related to PRES. The exact incidence of PRES in preeclampsia and eclampsia is not known. Brewer et al. observed that 98% (46 out of 47) of patients with eclampsia had PRES.[4] In a separate study, of 39 patients with eclampsia and preeclampsia with neurologic symptoms, magnetic resonance imaging (MRI) revealed that 92.3% of eclampsia patients had PRES; however, only 19.2% of preeclampsia patients had PRES.[5] Fisher et al. observed that out of 46 patients, 9 developed PRES. The predisposing factors were younger age, proteinuria, thrombocytopenia, and higher peak systolic and diastolic blood pressures.[6] There is wide variability in literature as to the incidence of PRES (10–90%) in preeclampsia/eclampsia, probably since most of the patients do not undergo neuroimaging and this may result in underdiagnosis.

Roth et al. studied 21 patients with PRES and found that headache was reported by 87.5% of pregnant patients versus 30.8% of nonpregnant patients, and visual disturbance was reported in 75% of pregnant patients versus 46.2% of nonpregnant patients. There was no difference between the groups with regard to symptoms, cerebral imaging, or outcome, apart from a difference in age, premedical history, and a significantly higher occurrence of headache and visual disturbances in the pregnant group.[7]

DIAGNOSIS

Posterior reversible encephalopathy syndrome presents as bilateral symmetrical vasogenic edema mainly in the parietal and occipital region in up to 70–90% of the patients. However, watershed areas, including the frontal, inferior temporal, cerebellar, and brainstem regions can be involved. Both cortical and subcortical locations are affected.[8] McKinney et al. reported that in 67 patients with PRES, the incidence of involvement of regions was parieto-occipital (98.7%), posterior frontal (78.9%), temporal (68.4%), thalamus (30.3%), cerebellum (34.2%), brain stem (18.4%), and basal ganglia (11.8%).[9]

The abnormalities are usually apparent on CT scans but are best depicted by MRI.

Computed Tomography Brain

Hypoattenuation is seen in the CT brain in the earlier-mentioned areas.

Magnetic Resonance Imaging Brain

An MRI shows high signal intensity on T2-weighted and fluid-attenuated inversion recovery (FLAIR) sequences **(Fig. 1)**. Diffusion-weighted imaging (DWI) shows a hypo- or isointense signal with an increased signal on apparent diffusion coefficient (ADC).

■ TREATMENT

- Prompt recognition is crucial as it is usually reversible with appropriate treatment.
- *Control of hypertension*: Gradual lowering of blood pressure by 25% from baseline is recommended. Nicardipine, hydralazine, and labetalol are the drugs of choice.
- *Seizure*: In the setting of eclampsia, magnesium sulfate is the agent of choice for seizures. In other settings, any antiseizure medication such as levetiracetam, lacosamide, or phenytoin can be used as per the patient's underlying condition and comorbidities. Electroencephalography (EEG) should be done in all patients with altered consciousness to rule out seizures.
- Discontinue all inciting agents like cytotoxic or immunosuppressive drugs. It is still a controversy if complete discontinuation of the agent is required or if reduction of the drug dose with strict therapeutic monitoring is sufficient.
- *Pregnancy*: In the setting of pregnancy with preeclampsia/eclampsia, delivery of the baby is the first mode of treatment.
- Hypomagnesemia should be avoided and serum level of magnesium should be maintained at a high normal range.

■ PROGNOSIS

The prognosis is usually benign with a complete reversal of symptoms within days to weeks. Around 70% of the patients show near complete resolution in neuroimaging. In a series of follow-up neuroimaging in 74 patients with PRES, an improvement in the imaging features was noted in 65 (88%) cases with a complete or near-complete resolution

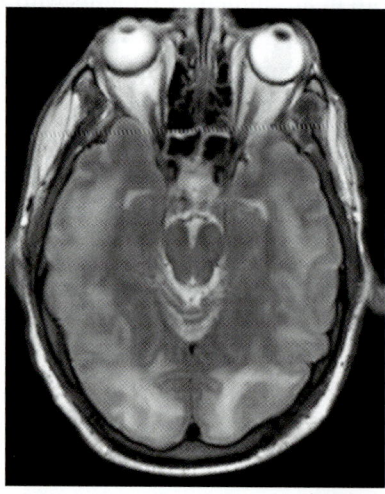

Fig. 1: T2-weighted image showing hyperintensity in the bilateral parieto-occipital region.

of abnormalities in 52 (70%) of them. This series included seven patients with eclampsia/preeclampsia and a complete resolution was seen in all seven of them.[10]

However, death and permanent neurological deficits have been reported. Death can occur due to cerebral edema and intracranial hemorrhage or as a complication of the underlying condition.

■ CONCLUSION

Posterior reversible encephalopathy syndrome is a neurological syndrome with a clinicoradiological diagnosis. The pathophysiology behind PRES requires further research though the commonly accepted theories are a cerebral autoregulatory failure and endothelial dysfunction. Parieto-occipital regions are mainly involved even though atypical features can also be seen. Treatment involves control of blood pressure and management of seizures.

Posterior reversible encephalopathy syndrome associated with pregnancy is commonly seen in preeclampsia/eclampsia. Studies have not shown any major difference as compared with nonpregnant patients except a higher incidence of headache and visual disturbances in pregnant patients. Treatment involves the delivery of the baby and magnesium sulfate for treatment of seizures when associated with preeclampsia/eclampsia.

■ REFERENCES

1. Hinchey J, Chaves C, Appignani B, Breen J, Pao L, Wang A, et al. A reversible posterior leukoencephalopathy syndrome. N Engl J Med. 1996;334:494-500.
2. Paulson OB, Waldemar G, Schmidt JF, Strandgaard S. Cerebral circulation under normal and pathologic conditions. Am J Cardiol. 1989;63:2C-5C.
3. Feske SK. Posterior reversible encephalopathy syndrome: a review. Semin Neurol. 2011;31(2):202-15.
4. Brewer J, Owens MY, Wallace K, Reeves AA, Morris R, Khan M, et al. Posterior reversible encephalopathy syndrome in 46 of 47 patients with eclampsia. Am J Obstet Gynecol. 2013;208:468.e1-6.
5. Mayama M, Uno K, Tano S, Yoshihara M, Ukai M, Kishigami Y, et al. Incidence of posterior reversible encephalopathy syndrome in eclamptic and patients with preeclampsia with neurologic symptoms. Am J Obstet Gynecol. 2016;215:239.e1-5.
6. Fisher N, Saraf S, Egbert N, Homel P, Stein EG, Minkoff H. Clinical correlates of posterior reversible encephalopathy syndrome in pregnancy. J Clin Hypertens. 2016;18:522-7.
7. Roth C, Ferbert A. Posterior reversible encephalopathy syndrome: is there a difference between pregnant and non-pregnant patients? Eur Neurol. 2009;62:142-8.
8. Bartynski WS, Boardman JF. Distinct imaging patterns and lesion distribution in posterior reversible encephalopathy syndrome. AJNR Am J Neuroradiol. 2007;28(7):1320-7.
9. McKinney AM, Short J, Truwit CL, McKinney ZJ, Kozak OS, SantaCruz KS, et al. Posterior reversible encephalopathy syndrome: incidence of atypical regions of involvement and imaging findings. Am J Roentgenol. 2007;189(4):904-12.
10. Fugate JE, Claassen DO, Cloft HJ, Kallmes DF, Kozak OS, Rabinstein AA. Posterior reversible encephalopathy syndrome: Associated clinical and radiologic findings. Mayo Clin Proc. 2010;85:427-32.

CHAPTER 44

Management of Obstetric Shock with Emphasis on Fluids and Vasopressors

Rajesh Pande, Maitree Pandey, Jitin Sharma

INTRODUCTION

Shock is diagnosed based on clinical criteria, signs of impaired perfusion (depressed levels of consciousness, oliguria, and peripheral cyanosis), and signs reflecting compensatory mechanisms such as hypotension, tachycardia, tachypnea, diaphoresis, and mental obtundation **(Table 1)**. Hypotension in shock occurs when normal compensatory afferent or efferent reflexes have failed, and the heart cannot further increase its output or the peripheral vasculature is inappropriately vasodilated, or unresponsive. The reversible causes of hypotension such as loss of intravascular volume, cardiac tamponade, tension pneumothorax, weakness of the heart muscle [acute myocardial infarction (MI)], valvular lesions, and peripheral circulatory failure should be excluded. Patient may also develop frank disseminated intravascular coagulation (DIC), especially in cases where shock is due to sepsis, amniotic fluid embolism (AFE), or retained placenta.

Obstetric shock is defined as a life-threatening cardiovascular collapse associated with pregnancy, childbirth, and puerperal, and is generally due to hemorrhage. It is the most common significant cause of high maternal mortality. Other nonhemorrhagic causes may also result in shock, with either obstetric specific causes or sepsis and septic shock.[1]

Types of obstetric shock presenting to intensive care unit (ICU) may be broadly divided based into hemorrhagic and nonhemorrhagic. The nonhemorrhagic causes include septic (distributive) 62%, nonseptic (distributive) 4%, cardiogenic 16%, hypovolemic 16%, and obstructive 2%.[2] The obstetric causes are septic shock which include pneumonia, pyelonephritis, appendicitis, septic abortion, chorioamnionitis, postpartum endometritis, incisional infection, and pelvic thrombophlebitis **(Table 2)**.

TABLE 1: Identification of shock.

Mental status	Anxious to severe obtundation
Heart rate	>100
Respiratory rate	>22
Hypotension	(SBP < 90 mm Hg) or 30 mm Hg fall in baseline BP
Urine output	<0.5 mL/kg/hour
Lactate	>3 mmol/L (27 mg/dL)
Base deficit	<−4 mEq/L
$PaCO_2$	<32 mm Hg

(BP: blood pressure; $PaCO_2$: partial pressure of carbon dioxide in blood; SBP: systolic blood pressure)

POSTPARTUM HEMORRHAGE

Hemorrhage is among the major causes of maternal deaths worldwide and a major contributor to maternal deaths in developing countries.[3,4] Postpartum hemorrhage (PPH) is defined as blood loss of ≥500 mL following vaginal delivery or ≥1,000 mL following cesarean delivery. It is classified as early/primary PPH, when it occurs within 24 hours of delivery, and late/secondary PPH when it occurs after 24 hours of delivery. Massive obstetric bleed is defined as very rapid loss at 150 mL/min or >50% blood volume (≈3 L) within 3 hours. There may not be any major physiological response until ~5–25% total blood volume lost (1,000–1,500 mL blood). The classification of hemorrhagic shock is described in **Table 3**.

Postpartum hemorrhage is responsible for one-fourth of all maternal deaths with an incidence of 5–6% in pregnancy. Severe blood loss results in hypovolemic shock, organ dysfunction, coagulopathy, and significantly high morbidity and mortality. Severe complications such as organ dysfunction and death can occur due to hypovolemic shock and coagulopathy from substantial blood loss.[2] Early diagnosis is sometimes difficult as the symptoms are often attributed to hemodynamic changes of pregnancy. The causes of PPH are listed in **Table 4**.[5] Hemorrhagic shock is a form of hypovolemic shock in which severe blood loss leads to hypotension and inadequate oxygen delivery at the cellular level. If hemorrhage continues unchecked, death quickly follows. The obstetric causes of hemorrhagic shock are discussed here.

TABLE 2: Types of obstetric shock.

Types of obstetric shock	Conditions
Hemorrhagic—antepartum	Placental abruption
	Placenta previa
	Placenta accreta
Hemorrhagic—postpartum	Retained placenta
	Failure of uterine contraction
	Trauma
	Coagulopathy
Nonhemorrhagic	Pulmonary thromboembolism
	Amniotic fluid embolism
	Acute uterine inversion
	Septic shock—chorioamnionitis, endometriosis, and generalized sepsis
	Peripartum cardiomyopathy

TABLE 3: Classification of hemorrhagic shock (American College of Surgeons Committee on Trauma).

Class	Blood loss (mL, %)	Heart rate (Beats/min)	Blood Pressure (mm Hg)	Pulse pressure	Respiratory rate (Breaths/min)	Mental status
I	<750 (15)	<100	Normal	Normal	14–20	Slightly anxious
II	750–1,500 (15–30)	100–120	Normal	Narrowed	20–30	Mildly anxious
III	1,500–2,000 (30–40)	120–140	Decreased	Narrowed	30–40	• Anxious • Confused
IV	>2,000 (>40%)	>140	Decreased	Narrowed	>35	• Confused • Lethargic

TABLE 4: Four Ts mnemonic for causes of postpartum hemorrhage.[5]

Four Ts	Cause	Approximate incidence (%)
Tone	Atonic uterus	70
Trauma	Lacerations, hematomas, inversion, rupture	20
Tissue	Retained tissue, invasive placenta	10
Thrombin	Coagulopathies	1

Uterine Atony

Uterine atony is the most common cause of PPH and may be treated with oxytocin, bimanual massage, and the use of other uterotonic agents such as ergometrine, carboprost (15-methyl prostaglandin F2α), and misoprostol (prostaglandin E1). Oxytocin is the initial drug of choice, after a 5 U intravenous bolus, an infusion of 20 U in 1 L of normal saline (NS) intravenously is run as fast as possible. For giving bimanual massage, a hand is placed on the fundus, and the second hand is placed anterior to the cervix in the vagina and the uterus is raised from the pelvis, pivoted anteriorly, and compressed between the two hands. Ergonovine (or Ergotrate) is given as an initial dose of 100 or 125 μg intravenously or intramyometrially or 200 or 250 μg intramuscular (IM), up to a maximum dose of 1.25 mg. IM carboprost is the second-line agent when it is available. The recommended dose is 250 μg intramuscularly or intramyometrially, not to exceed 2 mg (eight doses).

Retained placental products can be removed manually after exploration or intrauterine catheterization followed by bimanual massage. Any trauma can be repaired directly after exploration. The coagulopathy should be corrected and the precipitating cause in DIC identified and treated. The refractory PPH may require uterine artery ligation, uterine artery embolization, or abdominal hysterectomy. The management of major hemorrhage requires a multidisciplinary system wide approach, where transfusion is only one aspect of complex management. As logistics can be a major limitation, a management plan is required. Early identification is the key and can be achieved by taking history of prehospital major blood loss, use of anticoagulants or antiplatelets, X-ray and ultrasonography (USG), and laboratory test such as arterial blood gas with lactate, complete blood count, electrolytes, coagulation studies, thromboelastography (TEG) or rotational thromboelastometry (ROTEM), and blood group. Major blood loss may require immediate resuscitation with crystalloids, blood and blood products with the use of rapid infusers and fluid warmer. Preventative strategies and evidence-based therapies are needed. Specific drugs to aid hemostasis (e.g., rFVIIa and tranexamic acid) may have roles in clinical practice.[4] As the patient may require massive blood transfusion, one should be watchful for transfusion reactions and other complications. The principles of management of postpartum bleeding are listed in **Table 5**.

Chances of fluid overload, pulmonary edema, and organ dysfunction are high if fluid therapy is not controlled and properly guided. Wherever possible, massive blood transfusion protocols should be used and any necessary surgical, endoscopic or angioembolization should not be delayed. The concept of deresuscitation, achieving a net negative fluid balance and weaning from vasopressors in 5–6 days

TABLE 5: Principles of management of postpartum bleeding.

Identify the problem	Uterine atony, retained placenta, placental abruption, amniotic fluid embolism, sepsis, and genital tract trauma
Immediate resuscitation	Maintain circulating blood volume, use packed red cells, and crystalloids
Blood and blood products replacement	Platelets, PT, aPTT, fibrinogen levels to be done (ROTEM, may be helpful). Restore normal homeostasis. In addition to red cells, FFP, cryoprecipitate, and platelets may be used
Definitive clinical intervention	Uterotonic agents and tamponade, arterial ligation, embolization, hysterectomy, factor VIIa, etc.

(aPTT: activated partial thromboplastin time; FFP: fresh frozen plasma; PT: prothrombin time; ROTEM: rotational thromboelastometry)

TABLE 6: Four phases in treatment of shock (SOSD approach).[6]

Salvage	Optimization	Stabilization	De-escalation
Get minimal acceptable blood pressure (BP)	Ensure adequate O_2 availability	Provide organ support	Taper the vasopressors
Perform lifesaving measures	Optimize cardiac output, lactate, and SVO_2	Minimize complications	Achieve a net negative fluid balance

TABLE 7: Phases of ROSE approach.[7]

Resuscitation	Optimization	Salvage	Evacuation
The ebb phase: • Low MAP • Low CO	Occurs within hours. It is the phase of ischemia and reperfusion	• Evolves over days • Fluid is needed for maintenance and replacement • Monitor daily weight and organ function • Maintain neutral or negative fluid balance	Some patients do not transition from the "ebb" to "flow" phase
Resuscitation targets: • MAP > 65 mm Hg • CI > 2.5 L/min/m² • PPV 8 cm/m	Targets: • MAP > 65 mm Hg • CI > 2.5 L/min/m² • PPV <12% • GEDVI 640–800 mL/m²	Targets: • MAP > 65 mm Hg • CI > 2.5 L/min/m², PPV < 14% • IAP < 15 mm Hg • APP > 55 mm Hg • GEDVI-640–800 mL/m²	Target: • Deresuscitation to negative fluid balance • Diuretics and albumin may be used

(APP: abdominal perfusion pressure; CI: cardiac index; CO: cardiac output; GEDVI: global end-diastolic volume index; IAP: intra-abdominal pressure; MAP: mean arterial pressure; PPV: pulse pressure variation; ROSE: resuscitation optimise stabilisation evacuation)

after initial aggressive resuscitation is gaining popularity and should be practiced. Two such approaches are described in **Tables 6 and 7**, respectively.

■ AMNIOTIC FLUID EMBOLISM

Amniotic fluid embolism (AFE) is a rare but significant cause of maternal mortality. Risk factors for development include advanced age multiparity, instrumentation during labor, amniotomy, C-section, etc. AFE has been reported to occur during labor/within 8 minutes of delivery resulting in hypotension and fetal distress. Complications included respiratory failure—acute respiratory distress syndrome (ARDS), pulmonary edema, and about 90% patients developed coagulopathy and suffered cardiac arrest, resulting in high mortality (61%). Almost 85% patients either died or survived with permanent neurological sequelae.

Amniotic fluid embolism may occur during first and second trimester abortions/trauma, abrupt onset of respiratory distress, cardiovascular collapse, and coagulopathy during labor or postpartum.

Amniotic fluid includes particulates such as squames, lanugo hairs, mucin, bile from meconium, prostaglandin E2, F2a, leukotriene B4, and thrombokinase-like element. Exact mechanism is unclear/controversial but this is postulated that amniotic fluid enters mother's circulation by disruption of uterine wall and rupture of the placental membranes. The amniotic fluid elements produce pulmonary artery obstruction, activation of inflammation, and coagulation. It is also known as anaphylactoid syndrome of pregnancy. The response to AFE may be biphasic—initial pulmonary hypertension followed by myocardial depression caused by cytokines and hypoxia. The left heart failure may cause pulmonary edema, shock, or cardiac arrest. Neurologic dysfunction may manifest as seizures and coma. For survivors, there is high chance of neurological dysfunction. Nearly all patients who survive will develop DIC in few hours. There is coagulopathy and histology demonstrates foreign material in pulmonary capillaries, arterioles, and arteries. Management is primarily supportive.

■ PULMONARY EMBOLISM

Venous thromboembolism (VTE) complicates 0.06% of pregnancies. VTE may occur throughout pregnancy but the highest incidence in the immediate postpartum period. The risk factors are prior VTE, recent surgery, older age, obesity, and thrombophilia.

Pregnancy favors venous stasis, endothelial injury, and increase in coagulation. Progesterone causes increase in venous capacitance and promotes stasis. The pregnant uterus causes venous obstruction and vascular injury may occur at uteroplacental surface occurs at delivery. There is increase in factor I, II, VII, VIII, X, increase in resistance to activated protein C, decrease in coagulation inhibitor protein S, and impaired fibrinolysis.

The clinical findings are dyspnea, chest pain, and acute respiratory failure. Massive embolism may cause shock due to embolic obstruction to right ventricle cardiac output. It may lead to cardiac ischemia and impaired myocardial function. D-dimer is of no use as the levels are raised in pregnancy. The investigations include chest X-ray (CXR) to rule our other pathologies, a lower extremity compression ultrasound and a 2D echo, which may reveal right ventricular (RV) dilatation and hypokinesia, paradoxical septal motion, and compression of left ventricle. Deep vein thrombosis occurs on the left side in majority of pregnant patients. It is more likely to occur higher in the pelvis and so USG is sensitive. Chest imaging is an important complement to leg ultrasound. Fetal exposure to radiation should be <5 rads and the CXR: <0.001 rad, ventilation-perfusion (V/Q) scan: <0.011 rad, pulmonary angiography: <0.05 rad, and chest CT scan: <0.016 rad. Fetal studies show both V/Q scan and computed tomography pulmonary angiography (CTPA) are safe with no higher spontaneous fetal loss, congenital abnormalities, or malignancies. It is safe to use heparin as it does not cross placental barrier; however, warfarin is contraindicated as it is teratogenic, but may be used postpartum. Low-molecular-weight heparin (LMWH) is safe and dopamine is a good agent in case of severe pulmonary embolism (PE) causing shock. Thrombolytic therapy with TPA may be considered for massive PE.

PERIPARTUM CARDIOMYOPATHY

It is generally defined as heart failure of unknown cause toward the end of pregnancy or in the months after delivery (5 months), in patients with no previous cardiac dysfunction. The incidence is 1 in 3,000–4,000 live births with a morbidity and mortality of about 20%. The prognosis depends on normalization of left ventricular (LV) function. Diagnosis is difficult as symptoms are similar to those expected in the last trimester. There is absence of any other cause of heart failure, and a 2D echo shows LV dysfunction with left ventricular ejection fraction (LVEF) <45% and/or M mode fractional shortening <30% with >2.7 cm/m^2 end-diastolic dimension. The clinical features are cough, orthopnea, paroxysmal nocturnal dyspnea, fatigue, palpitations, and hemoptysis.

Management includes delivery of the fetus which may significantly improve symptoms. Vaginal delivery with low-dose epidural and close monitoring of blood pressure (BP) and fluid status should be priority.[8] Treating the chronic heart failure (CHF) with salt restriction, loop diuretics, vasodilators (nitroglycerine), digoxin for arrhythmias, and inotropy dopamine or dobutamine, milirinone, and anticoagulation but LVEF <25% carries a poor prognosis. Afterload may be reduced with hydralazine and nitrates [angiotensin-converting enzyme (ACE) inhibitors should be avoided). Once stabilized, can be put on oral hydralazine and isosorbide dinitrate or agents suitable for lactating mothers.

SEPSIS AND SEPTIC SHOCK

Septic shock in pregnant women may occur due to nonobstetric infectious causes such as pneumonia, pyelonephritis, and appendicitis or due to obstetric causes such as septic abortion, chorioamnionitis, postpartum endometritis, incisional infection, and pelvic thrombophlebitis. Wherever sepsis is suspected based on clinical signs such as fever, tachycardia, tachypnea, hypotension, and diagnostic criteria like leukocytosis, and positive body fluid cultures, an attempt should be made to identify the source and start with appropriate broad-spectrum antibiotic therapy. Aminoglycosides should be avoided to avoid fetal ototoxicity and nephrotoxicity. Chorioamnionitis generally requires fetal delivery. Patient's fluid status should be maintained, and resuscitation may be guided by USG. The principles of sepsis and septic shock management are no different in obstetric patients and the sepsis bundles should be followed. Sometimes, delivery of fetus results in dramatic improvement and makes management easier.

Uterine vessels are maximally dilated at term and contain mostly α receptors. Ephedrine as a short-term bolus agent is used for brief episodes of hypotension. Dopamine has been used most extensively in obstetric patients, and the animal data suggests that it increases muscular tone of uterus and blood vessels, raises mean arterial pressure (MAP) with a varying effect on heart rate (HR). Vasopressin may cause significant uterine contraction and has been studied only for diabetes insipidus in pregnant patients. Noradrenaline and adrenaline cause considerable vasoconstriction of maternal and placental circulation. Their effect on α and β receptors may vary. Because of uterine relaxation, α effect results in uterine contraction. The vasopressors and their doses are given in **Table 8**.

TABLE 8: Vasopressors and their doses.

Name	Classification	Pharmacological action on different receptors				HR	CO	SVR	Dose
		Dopaminergic	α1	β1	β2				
Noradrenaline	Vasoconstrictor	–	+++	++	–	↔	↔	↑↑	0.5–30 µg/min
Vasopressin	Vasoconstrictor	–	–	–	–	↔	↔↓	↑↑	0.01–0.05 U/min
Phenylephrine	Vasoconstrictor	–	+++	–	–	↔	↔	↑↑	40–180 µg/min
Dopamine	Inoconstrictor	++	–	++	–	↔	↔	↔	1–5 µg/min
Dopamine	Inoconstrictor	+++	–	–	–	↑	↑↑	↔↑	5–10 µg/min
Dopamine	Inoconstrictor	++	+++	++	–	↑↑	↔↑	↑↑	10–20 µg/min
Adrenaline	Inoconstrictor	–	+++	++	++	↑↑	↑	↑↑	1–10 µg/min
Dobutamine	Inodilator	–	+	+++	++	↔↑	↑↑	↓	2.5–20 µg/min

(CO: cardiac output; HR: heart rate; SVR: systemic vascular resistance)

Hydroxyethyl starch is not recommended in septic patients as its use in various studies was associated with increased risk of death and higher requirement of renal replacement therapy. A protocolized approach like early goal directed therapy has not been found to result in better outcomes when compared to usual physician directed care and was associated with a higher hospitalization cost in septic shock patients.[9] Resuscitation with intravenous fluids is a common intervention to restore fluid balance in septic patients as well as in hypovolemic shock. Crystalloids are the preferred solution in septic patients, where colloids are contraindicated due to loss of glycocalyx in the leaky blood capillaries. Crystalloids are mainly distributed to interstitial space (75%) and only 1/4th amount goes to intravascular compartment. Therefore, large volume may be required in septic shock and the beneficial effect also lasts for a shorter time. Large volume resuscitation with 0.9% sodium chloride solution may cause hyperchloremic metabolic acidosis and is also associated with development of acute kidney injury. Although balanced crystalloids are being used more commonly as their composition and osmolality is like plasma, a recent major study has not shown any difference between balanced crystalloids and NS in terms of risk of death or acute kidney injury.[10-12]

CARDIAC ARREST IN PREGNANCY

Cardiac arrest in pregnancy may be caused by hemorrhage VTE, pregnancy-induced hypertension, sepsis, aspiration pneumonia, amniotic fluid embolism, trauma and cardiac disease (preexisting cardiac disorders, MI, and peripartum cardiomyopathy), and iatrogenic causes (hypermagnesemia). The oxygen reserves are limited, and airway should be achieved immediately. The American Heart Association-advanced cardiac life support (AHA-ACLS) guidelines should be followed. If the pregnant woman with a fundus height at or above the umbilicus has not achieved return of spontaneous circulation (ROSC) with usual resuscitation measures plus manual left uterine displacement (LUD), it is advisable to prepare to evacuate the uterus while resuscitation continues. In situations such as nonsurvivable maternal trauma or prolonged pulselessness, in which maternal resuscitative efforts are obviously futile, there is no reason to delay performing perimortem cesarean delivery (PMCD). PMCD should be considered at 4 minutes after onset of maternal cardiac arrest or resuscitative efforts (for the unwitnessed arrest) if there is no ROSC.

CONCLUSION

The cardiovascular collapse associated with obstetric shock requires urgent attention to avoid high mortality. Obstetric hemorrhagic shock should be recognized early and treated in a protocolized manner, including bimanual massage, use of other uterotonic agents, fluid resuscitation, treatment of coagulopathy and blood and blood product transfusion. In some situations, exploration may be required for retained placental products or uncontrolled bleeding. Specific hemostatic drugs may be used in diffuse uncontrollable bleeding. Massive blood transfusion may expose the patient to develop transfusion related complicated requiring immediate recognition and management. The nonhomorganic obstetric shock may require echocardiographic assessment of heart, special imaging to detect pulmonary embolism or assessment for sepsis and septic shock. These critical obstetric patients should be managed in the ICU by a multidisciplinary team with intensivist playing a lead role.

REFERENCES

1. Cerovac A, Habek D, Cerovac E, Čerkez Habek J. Obstetric shock and shock in obstetrics – steady obstetrical syndrome. Med Glas (Zenica). 2022;19(2).
2. Thomson AJ, Greer IA. Non-haemorrhagic obstetric shock. Baillieres Best Pract Res Clin Obstet Gynaecol. 2000;14(1):19-41.
3. Zwart JJ, Dupuis JRO, Richters A, Ory F, Roosmalen JV. Obstetric intensive care unit admission: a 2-year nationwide population-based cohort study. Intensive Care Med. 2010;36:256-63.
4. Mehdi M, Chandraharan E. (2021). Diagnosis and Management of Shock in Postpartum Hemorrhage. [online] Available from: https://www.glowm.com/article/heading/vol-13-Obstetric Emergencies-diagnosis and management of shock in postpartum hemorrhage/id/409603#. [Last accessed February 2023].
5. Anderson JM, Etches D. Prevention and management of postpartum hemorrhage. Am Fam Physician. 2007;75:875-82.
6. Vincent JL, Backer, DD. Circulatory shock. N Engl J Med. 2013;369:1726-34.
7. Monteiro JN, Goraksha SU. 'ROSE concept' of fluid management: Relevance in neuroanaesthesia and neurocritical care. J Neuroanaesthesiol Crit Care. 2017;4:10-6.
8. Tsang W, Bales AC, Lang RM (2016). Peripartum cardiomyopathy: Treatment and prognosis. [online] Available from: https://www.medilib.ir/uptodate/show/95071. [Last accessed February 2023].
9. PRISM Investigators; Rowan KM, Angus DC, Bailey M, Barnato AE, Bellomo R, et al. Early, goal-directed therapy for septic shock—a patient-level meta-analysis. N Engl J Med. 2017;376:2223-34.
10. Myburgh JA, Mythen MG. Resuscitation fluids. N Eng J Med. 2013;369:1243-5.
11. Zayed YZM, Aburahma AMY, Barbarawi MO, Hamid K, Banifadel MRN, Rashdan L, et al. Balanced crystalloids versus isotonic saline in critically ill patients: systematic review and meta-analysis. J Intensive Care. 2018;6:51.
12. Semler MW, Wanderer JP, Ehrenfeld JM, Stollings JL, Self WH, Siew ED, et al. Balanced crystalloids versus saline in the intensive care unit. The SALT randomized trial. Am J Respir Crit Care Med. 2017;195:1362-72.

CHAPTER 45

Hematological Cancers in Pregnancy

Suresh Kumar Sundaramurthy, Raymond Dominic Savio

■ INTRODUCTION

Although malignancy is the second leading cause of mortality during the reproductive age group, fortunately it is uncommon in pregnancy. Hematological malignancies are even rarer during pregnancy with an incidence of 0.02%.[1] This rarity explains the paucity of randomized controlled trials to address this issue and most of the available data are extrapolated from retrospective analysis, case studies, or expert opinions. Albeit uncommon, the diagnosis of a hematological malignancy during pregnancy not only puts the family in distress but also becomes a delicate challenge for the treating physician, as the implications of diagnosis and treatment on two lives have to be considered with every step. It is, therefore, essential to balance the treatment of cancer based on the type and stage with its potential detrimental effects on the development of fetus.

■ IMPLICATIONS IN PREGNANCY

Multiple theories exist trying to establish a causal relationship between hematological cancers and pregnancy-related physiological changes such as the immuno suppressive effects of pregnancy and higher titers of female gonadal steroids. However, none of these have managed to establish a clear association between the two medical conditions, thus failing to prove any increased occurrence or recurrence of blood cancers due to pregnancy.[2]

It is unfortunate that the diagnosis of hematological cancers is often delayed in pregnancy, as early diagnosis may enable prompt treatment and thus improve outcome. One of the main reasons for this delay could be the similarity of clinical manifestations such as tiredness, abdominal discomfort/pain, back pain, and shortness of breath, between the two conditions. Furthermore, there is an understandable hesitancy to undergo diagnostic modalities such as imaging and invasive diagnostic procedures during pregnancy, which further delays the diagnosis.

The treatment of hematological cancers also poses a significant challenge in pregnancy. Chemotherapy and radiotherapy, both of which form the main modalities of treatment, have significant adverse effects on the mother and fetus. Although the chemotherapy-related adverse effects on mother are not very different from that of a nonpregnant woman, altered drug metabolism (delayed gastric emptying, decreased albumin level, enhanced hepatic metabolism/renal clearance) has to be kept in mind while treating these patients.[3,4]

The lethal effects of antineoplastic drugs and radiation on fetus also are to be kept in mind, and this depends on the gestational age.

While exposure to chemotherapy during first trimester can cause abortion or congenital abnormalities, it can also result in impaired fetal growth and functional abnormalities when administered after the first trimester.[5] Similarly, the risk of radiation-induced fetal malformations are greatest when it is instituted during organogenesis in first trimester.[5]

COMMON HEMATOLOGICAL MALIGNANCIES DURING PREGNANCY

Due to its prevalence in young age, lymphoma, especially Hodgkin's lymphoma is the most common hematological malignancy during pregnancy with an incidence of 1/6,000. Chronic myeloid leukemia (CML), multiple myeloma (MM), and myeloproliferative neoplasms (MPN), which are considered to be malignancies of old age, are being reported in pregnancy recently due to rising median age of pregnancy. **Figure 1** shows the common hematological malignancies encountered in pregnancy and **Table 1** provides an overview about the same.

SALIENT FEATURES OF THESE CANCERS IN PREGNANCY

Diagnosis and staging depend on invasive procedures and imaging. Core needle or open excisional biopsies are considered safe during pregnancy. Imaging techniques such as chest X-ray with abdominal shield, ultrasound, and magnetic resonance imaging (MRI) need to be considered where appropriate.

Majority of the chemotherapeutic agents cross placenta and cause major morphological abnormalities during first trimester and hence termination of pregnancy is recommended during this period in case of aggressive malignancy necessitating immediate management. Administration of antineoplastic agent after 1st trimester is not without risk, as it can still result in intrauterine growth restriction, premature birth, stillbirth, and impaired functional/intellectual

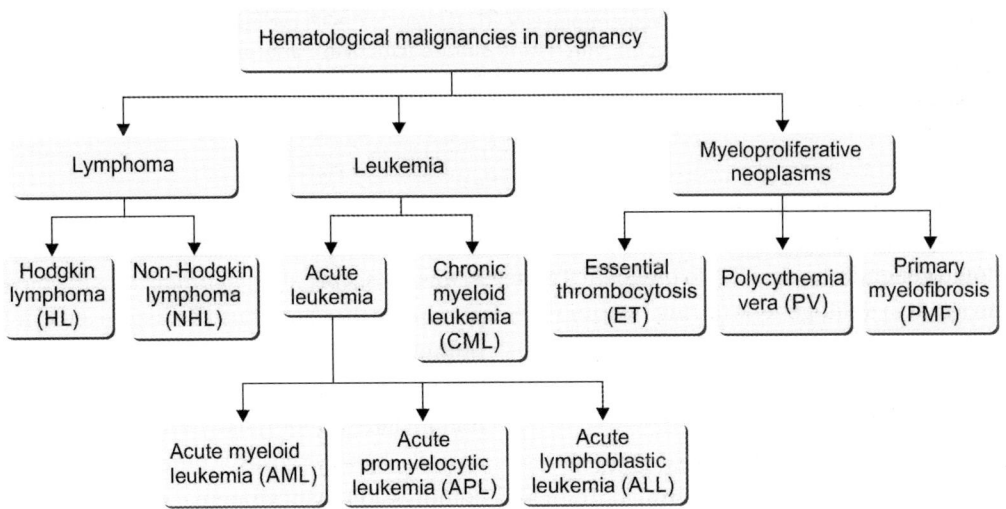

Fig. 1: Hematological malignancies in pregnancy.

TABLE 1: Features of common hematological malignancies in pregnancy.[6-8]

Malignancy	Incidence in pregnancy	Subtypes	Nature	Treatment 1st trimester	Treatment 2nd/3rd trimester
Lymphoma	1 in 6,000	HL	Aggressive but curable	Advanced-pregnancy termination*	ABVD
		NHL	Indolent/Aggressive	Aggressive-pregnancy termination	CHOP
Leukemia	Acute: 1 in 75,000–100,000	AML	Aggressive	Pregnancy termination	Cytarabine-doxorubicin
		APL	Aggressive	Pregnancy termination	Cytarabine-doxorubicin
		ALL	Aggressive	Pregnancy termination	Cytarabine-doxorubicin
	Chronic: <1 in 100,000	CML	Not aggressive	Interferon-alpha	Interferon-alpha
Myeloproliferative neoplasm	Not ascertained	ET	Variable	Low risk: Aspirin OD	High risk: INF-α + aspirin/LMWH
		PV	Variable	Aspirin OD + Phlebotomy	Phlebotomy + INF-α + aspirin/LMWH

*Pregnancy termination followed by definitive therapy.
(ABVD: adriamycin (doxorubicin), bleomycin, vinblastine, and dacarbazine; ALL: acute lymphocytic leukemia; AML: acute myeloid leukemia; APL: acute promyelocytic leukemia; CHOP: cyclophosphamide, doxorubicin hydrochloride (hydroxydaunorubicin), vincristine sulfate (Oncovin), and prednisone; CML: chronic myelogenous leukemia; ET: essential thrombocythemia; HL: Hodgkin's lymphoma; INF-α: interferon-alpha; LMWH: low molecular weight heparin; NHL: non-Hodgkin's lymphoma; PV: polycythemia vera)

development. Radiotherapy, which is occasionally required in hematological cancers, should generally be avoided in pregnancy as it can result in teratogenesis during 1st trimester and carcinogenesis during any trimester.

■ COMPLICATIONS

Pregnant patients already have certain hematological changes such as physiological anemia, neutrophilia, mild thrombocytopenia, increased procoagulant factors, and diminished fibrinolysis. Hematological malignancy in this subset of patients complicates the blood picture further and thus predisposes them to unique set of adverse events. Some of these, which warrant hospitalization to a critical care unit include tumor lysis syndrome (TLS), leukostasis, hyperviscosity syndrome, spinal cord compression, pancytopenia, thrombosis, and disseminated intravascular coagulation (DIC).

Tumor Lysis Syndrome

It is a constellation of signs and symptoms due to sudden release of intracellular contents from the tumor cells. Albeit it can occur with any type of cancer, it is more common with rapidly proliferating, bulky, therapy responsive tumors such as Burkitt lymphoma and acute leukemia.[9] It can occur either spontaneously or 48–72 hours after initiation of therapy. Its occurrence in pregnancy is extremely rare. Till date, only one case of acute spontaneous tumor lysis syndrome has been reported in a pregnant patient with non-Hodgkin's lymphoma (NHL).[10]

Patients usually present with metabolic abnormalities such as hyperkalemia, hyperphosphatemia (both directly due to rapid cell lysis), hypocalcemia (due to acute hyperphosphatemia), hyperuricemia (due to nucleic acid metabolism), uremia, and raised lactate dehydrogenase levels. The diagnosis can be based on the Cairo–Bishop criteria **(Table 2)** for TLS, which requires a combination of laboratory and clinical parameters.[11]

Treatment of TLS is the same as in a non-pregnant patient. Hyperuricemia is addressed with hydration, allopurinol, rasburicase, and febuxostat. Aggressive volume replacement at a rate of 200–300 mL/h to target a urine output of 80–100 mL/m^2/h (4–6 mL/kg/h). Extra caution should be taken in patients with cardiac and renal dysfunction during volume replacement. Diuretics and alkalinization of urine are not routinely recommended. In high-risk patients and those with uric acid level above 8 mg/dL, rasburicase is preferred over allopurinol. If the patient is hypersensitive to allopurinol, febuxostat may be used. They should be cautiously observed for methemoglobinemia and hemolysis. No clear data is available regarding the use of rasburicase in pregnancy as just one case report exists, that has documented the safe use of rasburicase in a pregnant woman with acute lymphocytic leukemia (ALL) and imminent TLS.[12]

Routine antihyperkalemia measures including intravenous calcium gluconate, glucose with insulin infusion, salbutamol nebulization or hemodialysis (in severe cases) can be instituted in these patients. Hyperphosphatemia is managed with oral phosphate binders or dialysis (in severe cases). Unless severe symptoms such as neuromuscular irritability exists, hypocalcemia need not be treated as this gets normalized with correction of hyperphosphatemia.

Leukostasis

It is an oncological medical emergency, which can occur in both acute and chronic leukemia, more commonly with acute myeloid leukemia, where it occurs even at lower white blood cells (WBC) counts as compared to other leukemias.

These patients usually present with pulmonary (tachypnea, dyspnea, hypoxia, and

TABLE 2: Cairo–Bishop criteria for diagnosis of tumor lysis syndrome (TLS).

Laboratory TLS: Two or more of the below abnormalities within 3 days or 7 days after initiation of treatment
- Uric acid ≥8 mg/dL or 25% increase from baseline
- Potassium ≥6 mEq/L or 25% increase from baseline
- Phosphate ≥4.5 mg/dL or 25% increase from baseline
- Calcium ≤7 mg/dL or 25% decrease from baseline

Clinical TLS: Laboratory TLS + 1 or more of the following:
- Creatinine >1.5 times upper limit of age-adjusted reference range
- Cardiac dysrhythmia or sudden death
- Seizure

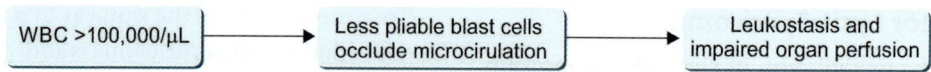

Fig. 2: Pathogenesis of organ dysfunction in leukostasis.

pulmonary hemorrhage) and central nervous system (CNS) manifestations (headache, mental status changes, seizures, and papilledema) due to pulmonary and cerebral microcirculatory dysfunction **(Fig. 2)**. These may sometimes be mistaken for other pregnancy-related complications such as preeclampsia. Other reported manifestations include GI bleeding, abdominal pain, and renal insufficiency. Leukostasis may also result in impaired placental perfusion leading to abnormal fetal development.

Symptoms can be mitigated by hydration, allopurinol (due to high risk of TLS) and avoidance of red blood cell (RBC) transfusion. Patients may need cytoreduction with chemotherapy and leukopheresis or exchange transfusion procedures, similar to the non-pregnant situation. Though leukopheresis can be considered for significant leukostasis irrespective of the gestational age, it can be associated with detrimental effects such as infection, bleeding, and thrombosis (both pregnancy and malignancy being hypercoagulable states).[13]

Hyperviscosity Syndrome

It is a group of clinical manifestations arising from an increase in the viscosity of the blood. It can occur due to increase in either cellular or non-cellular components of blood. While it occurs more commonly due to non-cellular components in non-pregnant patients, e.g., plasma cell dyscrasias, increase in cellular fraction as occurs in myeloproliferative neoplasms such as polycythemia vera and essential thrombocytosis are more commonly described in pregnancy. This elevated viscosity leads to sluggish blood flow, especially in the microvascular circulation and thus impairing the perfusion of tissues. Hyperviscosity can affect aggregation of platelets, leading to prolongation of bleeding time.

The severity of clinical manifestations is directly proportional to the level of serum viscosity. The presenting features consist of a triad of mucocutaneous hemorrhage (GI bleed, epistaxis, gum bleed), neurological disturbances (headache, dizziness, ataxia, seizures, stupor, coma), and visual disturbances (diplopia, blurring of vision, fundoscopy showing papilledema, "boxcar" engorgement of retinal veins). In pregnancy, this syndrome can result in decreased villous perfusion, leading to fetal hypoxia and intrauterine growth restriction (IUGR). These symptoms can be exaggerated in preeclampsia as this is in itself a hyperviscous state from increased plasma fibrinogen and decreased erythrocyte deformability.[14]

Hyperviscosity syndrome is another oncological medical emergency, in which absence of timely intervention can result in life-threatening complications such as stroke, myocardial infarction, and other vital organ ischemia leading to multiple organ failures. Treatment consists of supportive therapy, hydration, plasmapheresis or exchange transfusion (definitive treatment), and chemotherapy. In those circumstances where timely plasmapheresis cannot be done, phlebotomy can be considered as a temporary measure.

Spinal Cord Compression

Malignant spinal cord compression (SCC), one of the life-threatening complications and the second most frequent neurological complication of cancer, can sometimes occur in hematological cancers like lymphoma, although it is more common in breast, prostate, lung, or renal cancers with metastasis. It occurs either due to indentation or encasement of the thecal sac of spinal cord by locally advanced or metastatic neoplasms.

These patients can present with sensory or motor symptoms. Sensory deficits include paresthesia, local pain, and radicular pain. Motor disturbances include paraplegia, quadriplegia (depending on the site of compression) and bowel and bladder dysfunction. Some of the symptoms like pain can be confused to represent a common feature in pregnancy. Diagnosis is based on clinical features and imaging studies. Among imaging modalities, usage of CT for staging is not recommended due to radiation. Although there is no clarity regarding the appropriateness of contrast-enhanced MRI and its teratogenicity, it is the most sensitive and preferred imaging technique for this purpose as there is no sufficient evidence to prove its harmful effects.

There are significant implications of all treatment modalities namely, surgery, steroids, and radiotherapy, in pregnancy. Although spinal surgery is a reasonable treatment option with techniques varying from percutaneous to open spinal cord decompression and fixation, surgery carries severe obstetrical risks such as miscarriage, preterm delivery, and fetal distress.[15] Surgical issues such as prone positioning, significant blood loss hampering fetoplacental perfusion, and anesthesia-related issues such as effects of anesthetic drugs have to be considered in these pregnant patients. As already mentioned, the biological effects of radiotherapy on the fetus are incompatible with its survival especially during organogenesis. The role of steroid in these patients is controversial as there is still doubt around their causative relationship with preterm delivery and congenital abnormalities.

Superior Vena Cava Syndrome

This is a medical condition caused by the obstruction of superior vena cava (SVC) (extra luminal or intraluminal). Although extremely rare in pregnancy, it can occur as a complication in patients with lymphoma. Patients present with cardiorespiratory and neurological manifestations, which can sometimes be mistaken with systemic physiological changes that occur in pregnancy. While dyspnea is the most common symptom, others such as hoarseness of voice, stridor, chest pain, orthopnea, facial swelling, headache, nasal stuffiness, nausea and visual disturbances may also be the presenting complaint.

Apart from clinical features, imaging modalities such as CT scan of chest (with risk of fetal radiation exposure) or MRI (with inconclusive safety in pregnancy) would be required for diagnosis. Furthermore, contrast venography which is the most conclusive diagnostic technique to delineate the etiology of obstruction, comes with the risk of both radiation and contrast exposure.

Treatment involves cardiorespiratory support, prevention and treatment of cerebral edema, and definitive measures. Definitive therapy includes radiotherapy (standard treatment) and surgical procedures such as surgical bypass, endovascular stent or percutaneous transluminal angioplasty. Radiation, surgery, and anesthesia-related fetomaternal risk should be considered before planning treatment.

OTHER NOTABLE COMPLICATIONS

In case of thrombosis, DIC and pancytopenia, the clinical symptoms, diagnostic tests, and treatment are almost similar to that of nonpregnant patients. Pregnancy, being a hypercoagulable state, necessitates the initiation of prophylactic antiplatelet or anticoagulant medication in patients with severely elevated cell count. Low molecular weight heparin is the preferred anticoagulant. Warfarin is contraindicated during 1st trimester due to its teratogenic potential.

Granulocyte-colony stimulating factor can be safely used in pregnancy though strong evidence is lacking. Certain antibiotics such as aminoglycosides, tetracyclines, trimethoprim should be avoided due to their potential teratogenicity.

CONCLUSION

Multidisciplinary approach is essential to address the critical illnesses in this subset of patients with a team consisting of intensivist, obstetrician, oncologist, neonatologist, anesthesiologist, nurse, and other concerned specialists. It is imperative to ensure the same quality of therapy as that provided to a non-pregnant patient while limiting any harm to the developing fetus at the same time.

TAKE HOME MESSAGES

- A multidisciplinary approach is paramount while managing such patients.
- Definitive management depends on the nature of the tumor and the gestational age.
- An aggressive tumor during the first trimester requires termination of pregnancy followed by definitive therapy.
- Definitive therapy can be initiated during the second and third trimester without terminating pregnancy, however, with close monitoring for complications.

- Hematological malignancy related complications such as hyperviscosity, leukostasis, tumor lysis syndrome and complications due to cancer therapy can manifest during any of the trimesters and warrants a high index of suspicion.

REFERENCES

1. Pavlidis NA. Coexistence of pregnancy and malignancy. Oncologist. 2002;7:279-87.
2. Lishner M, Avivi I, Apperley JF, Dierickx D, Evens AM, Fumagalli M, et al. Hematologic malignancies in pregnancy: Management guidelines from an international consensus meeting. J Clin Oncol. 2016;34:501-8.
3. Davison JS, Davison MC, Hay DM. Gastric emptying time in late pregnancy and labour. Br J Obstet Gynaecol. 1970;77:37-41.
4. Parry E, Shields R, Turnbull AC. Transit time in the small intestine in pregnancy. Br J Obstet Gynaecol. 1970;77:900-1.
5. Beeley L. Adverse effects of drugs in the first trimester of pregnancy. Clin Obstet Gynaecol 1986;13:177-195.
6. Mahmoud HK, Samra MA, Fathy GM. Hematologic malignancies during pregnancy: a review. J Adv Res. 2016;7:589-96.
7. Barzilai M, Avivi I, Amit O. Diagnosis and management of hematological malignancies in pregnancy (review). Mol Clin Oncol. 2019;10(1):3-9.
8. Sakri NAM, Nusee Z, Mustafa AMA, Roziah Husin. A review of hematological malignancy in pregnancy. Eur J Med Health Sci. 2021;3:67-71.
9. Mirrakhimov AE, Voore P, Khan M, Ali AM. Tumor lysis syndrome: a clinical review. World J Crit Care Med. 2015; 4(2):130-8.
10. El-Sonbaty MR, Bitar Z, Abdulrazak A. Acute spontaneous tumor-lysis syndrome in a pregnant woman with non-Hodgkin's lymphoma. Int J Hematol. 2001;73:386-9.
11. Cairo MS. Bishop M. Tumour lysis syndrome: new therapeutic strategies and classification. Br J Haematol. 2004;127(1):3-11.

12. Middeke JM, Bruck N, Parmentier S, Bornhauser M, Schetelig J. Use of rasburicase in a pregnant woman with acute lymphoblastic leukaemia and imminent tumour lysis syndrome. Ann Hematol. 2014;93(3):531-2.
13. Staley EM, Simmons SC, Feldman AZ, Lorenz RG, Marques MB, Williams LA 3rd, et al. Management of chronic myeloid leukemia in the setting of pregnancy: when is leukocytapheresis appropriate? A case report and review of the literature. Transfusion. 2018;58(2):456-60.
14. Fahraeus R. Eclampsia: a disease of the checked microcirculation. Acta Obstet Gynecol Scand. 1962;41:101-14.
15. Vandenbroucke T, Verheecke M, Fumagalli M, Lok C, Amant F. Effects of cancer treatment during pregnancy on fetal and child development. Lancet Child Adolesc Health. 2017;1(4):302-10.

CHAPTER 46

Airway Management in Critically Ill Obstetric Patients

Anirban Hom Choudhuri, Deepika Jain

■ INTRODUCTION

It is estimated that around 0.5–15% of critically ill obstetric patients are admitted in the intensive care units (ICUs) and their mortality is about 5%. Acute respiratory failure (ARF) is the leading cause for ICU admission and also the main cause of death. Thus, airway management in these patients is not only important in preventing respiratory failure and death but also in minimizing the inadvertent complications during airway manipulations causing an increased morbidity. The clinical skill and knowledge of the intensivist becomes paramount in overcoming the challenges posed by the anatomical and physiological alterations of the respiratory system during pregnancy. The widespread use of neuraxial blockade during cesarean section reduces the scope of detection of difficult airway in the intraoperative period thereby increasing its detection in the ICUs during emergency intubation. The skill and experience of the intensivist in handling a difficult airway becomes valuable in saving the life of the patient. It needs to be remembered that the incidence of difficult/failed intubation in an obstetric patient is almost eight times higher than a nonobstetric patient. Since there are no different guidelines for airway management in obstetric patients, the guidelines for difficult airway management hold true here as well. But some modifications may be necessary as a consequence to the anatomical and physiological changes to minimize risks and maximize benefits. The unique nature of two (or more) lives at risk warrants a team approach involving the intensivist, obstetrician, and neonatologist to ensure that the best outcome can be achieved.[1-3]

The obstetric ICU admission falls under one of the following categories:
- *Pregnancy-induced complications:* Preeclampsia, eclampsia, hemorrhage, amniotic fluid embolism, aspiration syndrome, acute fatty liver of pregnancy, cardiomyopathy of pregnancy, etc.
- *Underlying diseases aggravated by pregnancy:* Heart diseases, autoimmune disorders, anemia, etc.
- *Occurrence of diseases unrelated with pregnancy:* Asthma, trauma, etc.

The initial stabilization of these patients in the ICU involves the same sequence of airway, breathing, and circulation management. Fetal monitoring is an additional essential and intricate part of patient care. The patients who are admitted beyond 24 weeks of gestation should be considered as potential candidates for emergency cesarean delivery.

FACTORS AFFECTING AIRWAY MANAGEMENT IN OBSTETRIC PATIENTS

- First and foremost, the oxygen requirement in an obstetric patient is increased several folds in comparison to a non-obstetric patient due to increased metabolic demand. This along with a reduced functional residual capacity (FRC) increases the risk of early hypoxia. Hypoxic spells in the mother can lead to hypoxia in the fetus. Therefore strict vigil is necessary to prevent hypoxia by monitoring the oxygen saturation.
- Weight gain and water retention during pregnancy can cause edema of the airway. This can cause difficulty in visualizing the vocal cords during laryngoscopy. Moreover, capillary engorgement makes the airway more prone to bleeding during airway manipulations. So all airway manipulations, viz., laryngoscopy, passage of bougie, stylet, etc., should be performed very gently and with extra care. All these changes are further aggravated in hypertensive patients. At times, it is better to insert a smaller endotracheal tube (ETT) to prevent airway trauma and bleeding.
- Enlarged breasts often hinder laryngoscope handle insertion in the form of mechanical barrier.
- The decreased tone of lower esophageal sphincter; increased residual gastric volume and acidity and delayed gastric emptying increases the risk of pulmonary aspiration and the subsequent complications.
- The application of cricoid pressure (CP) for rapid sequence induction (RSI) can make mask ventilation/laryngoscopy/supraglottic airway device insertion difficult.[3,4]

MECHANICAL VENTILATION IN OBSTETRIC PATIENTS

The decision to start mechanical ventilation in obstetric patient should be made keeping in mind the physiological changes occurring during pregnancy. Pregnant females are in a state of compensated respiratory alkalosis with lower partial pressure of arterial carbon dioxide ($PaCO_2$) (28–32 mm Hg) levels. Also, partial pressure of arterial oxygen (PaO_2) levels above 70 mm Hg are desirable at all times for fetal well-being. So, though noninvasive ventilation has its place in cases such as cardiogenic pulmonary edema and type 2 respiratory failure, a low threshold should be kept for intubation and initiation of invasive ventilation. Prone ventilation and extracorporeal membrane oxygenation, though initially considered contraindicated in pregnancy, have been tried during coronavirus disease (COVID) times and found to be beneficial. Nonetheless, the associated complications should be anticipated and strict vigil and timely intervention executed for the same. Aggressive fetal monitoring is required. The following goals for mechanical ventilation should be maintained: PaO_2 60–100 mm Hg, $PaCO_2$ 28–32 mm Hg, peak inspiratory pressure (PIP) <35 cmH_2O, and plateau pressure (Pplat) <27 cmH_2O.

MEASURES TO MINIMIZE PROBLEMS LEADING TO EVENTUAL COMPLICATIONS

- A quick yet thorough airway assessment. Look for predictors of difficult mask ventilation, laryngoscopy/intubation, supraglottic airway device (SAD) insertion, and front of neck access (FONA). Age, body mass index (BMI), and a higher Mallampati score are found

- to be independent risk factors for failed obstetric tracheal intubation.
- Reducing the risk and complications of pulmonary aspiration. Confirm the fasting status of the patient, aspiration prophylaxis with H_2 receptor antagonist like ranitidine and sodium citrate antacid should be administered. RSI with CP should be used.
- Difficult airway trolley with the equipment for difficult mask ventilation (oropharyngeal airway and SADs), difficult laryngoscopy, and intubation aids such as bougie/stylet to be kept ready. Short handle laryngoscope, video laryngoscope best familiarized to the attending anesthesiologist, smaller size ETTs form integral part of the difficult airway cart. Equipment for FONA be it cricothyroidotomy set or jet ventilation kit should be available and the anesthesiologist trained to perform the same. Second-generation SAD with conduit for gastric drainage are preferred as there is higher risk of aspiration in these patients. SAD can also serve as conduit for intubation in event of failed intubation. Fiberoptic bronchoscopy is the gold standard modality for anticipated difficult when planned electively.
- Optimal position the patient either in "sniffing" or "heat escape lessening posture (HELP)" position depending on the built. A slight head up tilt in either setting improves FRC.
- All obstetric patients should be considered to be with full stomach and should be induced with RSI with sustained CP till airway is secured. In case CP interferes with mask ventilation/laryngoscopy view/SAD insertion, it can be momentarily released as oxygenation/ventilation takes precedence in such circumstances.

Flowchart 1 guides for safe intubation practices.

FAILED INTUBATION

Failed intubation is declared when a trained intensivist fails to successfully intubate the within three attempts/one dose of succinylcholine irrespective of the technique(s) used.

If such a thing happens, help should be sought immediately from senior and experienced counterpart. All the while, the focus should be to maintain adequate oxygenation either with a facemask or SAD. The CP should be continued all along.

Flowchart 2 guides for practices during failed attempts.

CANNOT INTUBATE CANNOT OXYGENATE

Cannot intubate cannot oxygenate CICO is a life-threatening emergency. When it occurs, it should be clearly communicated to everyone and help must be sought from senior. Attempts at re-establishing oxygenation and ventilation through FONA should be immediately started. This can be achieved by doing either cannula cricothyroidotomy or by scalpel cricothyroidotomy. Obstetric Anaesthetists' Association (OAA) and Difficult Airway Society (DAS) guidelines advocate the use of scalpel cricothyroidotomy while others support cannula cricothyroidotomy. The equipment and training required for both the techniques is essential and the decision to proceed with either is left to the intensivists' discretion.[5,6]

In case of failure of either or both the mentioned methods, maternal advanced life support should be started. A perimortem cesarean section should be performed in such cases to recover a viable fetus. **Flowchart 3** is useful for such situations.

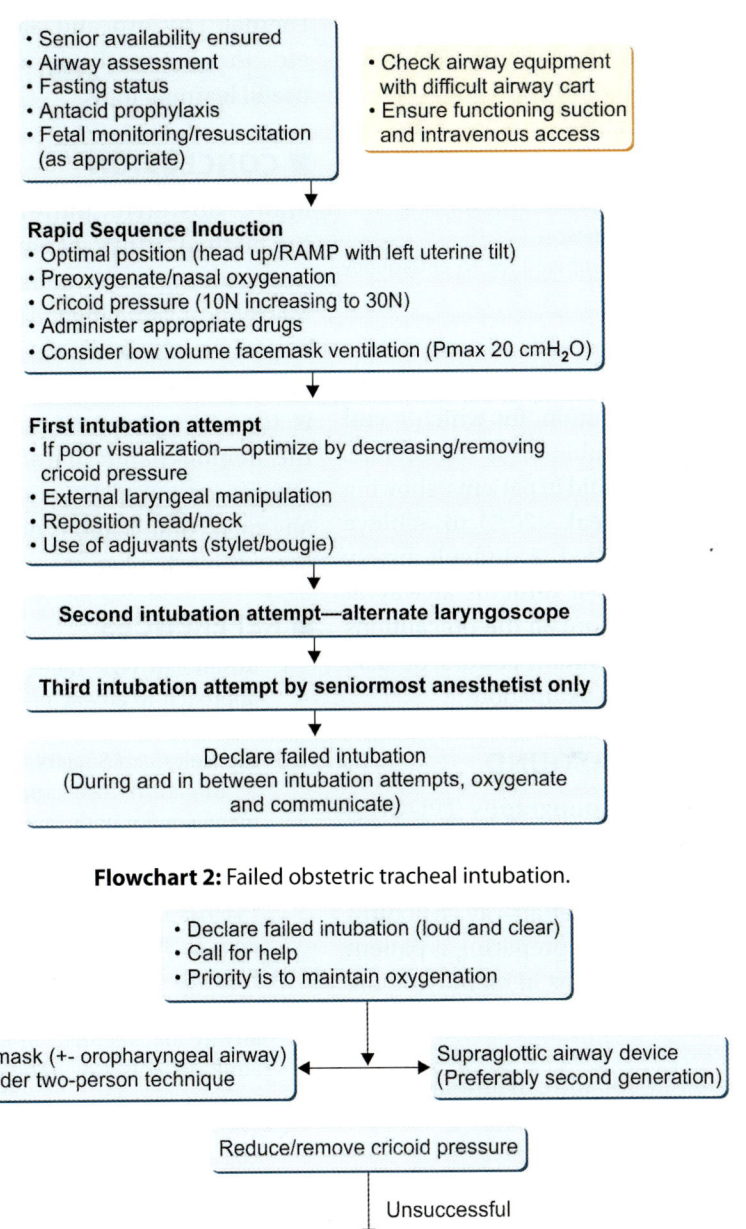

Flowchart 1: Safe obstetric intubation attempt.

Flowchart 2: Failed obstetric tracheal intubation.

■ PLANNING WEANING

It is often said that "intubation is a skill, extubation is an art". Weaning a patient from mechanical ventilation is a challenging task and in an obstetric patient should be performed as expeditiously as intubation.

Flowchart 3: Cannot intubate cannot ventilate.*

- Declare emergency
- Call for help (if not already available)
- Deliver 100 O_2 (facemask or SAD)
- Exclude laryngospasm

↓

Front of neck access

(SAD: supraglottic airway device)
*At any given point be prepared for an emergency cesarean section.

Airway edema of pregnancy can be exaggerated by intubation, for which a cuff leak test prior to extubation is reasonable. Administration of steroid in patients' showing negative leak test (leak <20%) to achieve decongestion is justified. A difficult airway at intubation is also a difficult airway at extubation and therefore all the precautions adopted during intubation should be also followed at the time of extubation.

ROLE OF ULTRASOUND

Point-of-care ultrasonography (POCUS) for airway assessment is a valuable technique for difficult airway management. Ultrasonography of upper airway structures helps in predicting and preparing a patient of difficult airway. It helps in identifying the cricothyroid membrane in case a FONA. Ultrasonography (USG) can also predict postextubation stridor and can be a substitute for cuff leak test.

TRAINING

Despite the availability of various opportunities for training in obstetric difficult airway, simulation seems to be the way forward. Trainees need to be acquainted with the possible difficulties and their management while dealing with this group of patients. There are simulators available from Laerdal, TruCorp, and Global Technologies, etc., that are marketed world over and are useful learning tools.

CONCLUSION

Many obstetric patients are affected by critical illnesses during pregnancy necessitating endotracheal intubation and mechanical ventilation. Airway management in pregnant patients can produce manifold effects on the mother and her fetus. It is therefore essential to closely monitor the hemodynamic parameters to prevent unforeseen complications and to treat early if any such complications occur to prevent any irreversible damage.[7,8]

REFERENCES

1. Rosenblatt WH, Yanez ND. A decision tree approach to airway management pathways in the 2022 difficult airway algorithm of the American Society of Anesthesiologists. A decision-tree approach to airway management pathways in the 2022 difficult airway algorithm of the American Society of Anesthesiologists. Anesth Analg. 2022; 134:910-5.
2. Roth D, Pace NL, Lee A, Hovhannisyan K, Warenits A-M, Arrich J, et al. Airway physical examination tests for detection of difficult airway management in apparently normal adult patients. Cochrane Database Syst Rev. 2018;5:CD008874.
3. Kornas RL, Owyang CG, Sakles JC, Foley LJ, Mosier JM; Society for Airway Management's Special Projects Committee. Evaluation and management of the physiologically difficult airway: consensus recommendations from Society for Airway Management. Anesth Analg. 2021;132:395-405.
4. Roth D, Pace NL, Lee A, Hovhannisyan K, Warenits AM, Arrich J, et al. Bedside tests for predicting difficult airways: an abridged

Cochrane diagnostic test accuracy systematic review. Anaesthesia. 2019;74:915-28.
5. Ahmad I, El-Boghdadly K, Bhagrath R, Hodzovic I, McNarry AF, Mir F, et al. Difficult Airway Society guidelines for Awake Tracheal Intubation (ATI) in adults. Anaesthesia. 2020;75:509-28.
6. Jarraya A, Choura D, Mejdoub Y, Kammoun M, Grati F, Kolsi K. New predictors of difficult intubation in obstetric patients: a prospective observational study. Trends Anaesth Crit Care. 2019;24:22-5.
7. Basaranoglu G, Columb M, Lyons G. Failure to predict difficult tracheal intubation for emergency caesarean section. Eur J Anaesthesiol. 2010;27:947-9.
8. Falcetta S, Cavallo S, Pelaia P, Sorbello M. Ultrasound measurements as predictors of difficult direct laryngoscopy. Trends Anaesth Crit Care. 2017;12:13-6.

CHAPTER 47

Status Epilepticus in Pregnancy

Bhuvna Ahuja, Ahsina Jahan Lopa, Sabina Regmi

INTRODUCTION

Status epilepticus (SE) in pregnancy imposes a therapeutic challenge to the clinicians. While the mother is under high risk of mortality and cognitive sequelae, prolonged seizures and antiepileptic drugs (AEDs) are potentially harmful to developing embryos.[1] In some refractory cases, parturition can be the only therapeutic option. In this chapter we will discuss its implications on maternal health and fetal well-being. Also, the management steps and pharmacological considerations are also discussed.

EPIDEMIOLOGY AND MAGNITUDE OF THE PROBLEM

Status epilepticus in pregnancy is rare, but poses a threat to both mother and fetus. Mortality from SE approaches 20% and convulsive SE accounts for 45–74% of these deaths.[2] The common causes of SE include posterior reversible encephalopathy syndrome (PRES)/reversible cerebral vasoconstriction syndrome (RCVS) spectrum, cortical venous sinus thrombosis (CVT), and autoimmune encephalitis.

IMPLICATIONS FOR MATERNAL HEALTH

The impact of first seizure during pregnancy is different in different trimesters of pregnancy.

TABLE 1: Details of seizure impact in different trimesters of pregnancy.

Trimester	Impacts
First trimester	• Metabolic alterations • Drug and toxic entity assessment (evaluated)
Second trimester	Syncopal episodes occurs due to low blood pressure a dilatation of vascular bed because of normal pregnancy-related physiological changes
Third trimester	Eclampsia, posterior reversible encephalopathy syndrome (PRES), and stroke (possibilities)

Table 1 mentions the details of seizure impact in different trimesters of pregnancy.

Mass lesions, infections, and sudden events due to vascular malformations can occur at any time in pregnancy; hence, appropriate imaging should be performed.

Impact of Seizures in Epileptic Women

In a retrospective study, it was found that frequency of seizures during pregnancy were lower in patients who plan their pregnancy and were receiving monotherapy for seizure control also there was a significantly lower likelihood of altering their AED regime during pregnancy.

Impact of Focal Seizures

It is difficult to measure or observe the effects of focal seizures on fetus, since it is not assessable for studies. It is generally accepted that these types of focal seizures have minimal effect on the fetus. However, where awareness and responsiveness are affected, trauma may occur.

Nei et al.[3] reported a case of febrile seizures in an already diagnosed case of complex partial seizure (CPS) since the age of 5 years. At 39 week of gestation, the estimated fetal weight was below the tenth percentile. At week 42 of the pregnancy, while having uterine contractions every 2–3 minutes, the fetal heart rate fell from 140 to 78 beats per minute.

Impact of Generalized Seizures

Generalized seizures are feared the most. Apart from causing trauma, it can also cause changes in electrolytes, blood pressure, and oxygenation, which may further harm fetus.

Mortality in Pregnant Women with Epilepsy

According to the maternal death registry in United Kingdom, maternal mortality rate was 10 times higher for women with epilepsy. Also reports suggested that seizure occurrence was often associated with stopping AED or with poor compliance.

Delivery

There is an increased risk of complications during delivery with epilepsy. Epilepsy is not considered as a reason for cesarean delivery, unless a seizure occurs during labor or the patient is unable to cooperate.[4]

■ IMPLICATIONS FOR FETAL WELL-BEING

Most epileptic drugs have teratogenic effects. Seizures during pregnancy and delivery affect fetal heart SE is rare, but there are occasional reports of fetal deaths and malformations after SE in AED-treated women.

■ MANAGEMENT

Management of SE in pregnancy is influenced by the etiology of SE and the duration of pregnancy. Etiology can be pregnancy-specific, i.e., SE in eclampsia and pregnancy nonspecific, i.e., convulsive or nonconvulsive SE (NSCE). Pregnancy, a hyperdynamic state, leads to increased volume of distribution, increased hepatic metabolism, and augmented renal excretion.[4] Thus, altered pharmacokinetics of AEDs during pregnancy can result in low plasma concentration and recurrence of SE. There is a paucity of data regarding the exact guidelines for the management of SE in pregnancy.

Diagnostic Workup

Clinical Examination and Laboratory Investigations

A detailed history, a thorough clinical examination, a complete workup, and management should be performed simultaneously on a seizing pregnant patient.

Initial investigations include capillary blood sugar at the bedside, complete blood counts, liver and renal functions tests, electrolytes, coagulation profile, AED levels (in a known case of epilepsy), toxicology screening, and arterial blood gas analysis, and electrocardiogram.

Neuroimaging and Lumbar Puncture

Ideally, a patient with a seizure should be subjected to computed tomography (CT) to look for any structural lesions or acute problems once stabilized. However, radiation exposure is associated with altered organogenesis and fetal growth in pregnancy. Until a CT scan alters the management of

SE, radiation exposure should be avoided in pregnancy.[5] If the history is suggestive of central nervous system (CNS) infections, lumbar puncture should be done at the earliest after completion of CT brain.

Electroencephalography

In case of persistent seizures or inability to regain consciousness, an urgent electroencephalography (EEG) should be ordered. EEG is used for both diagnosis and monitoring the response to treatment. EEG may be of lesser importance in the diagnosis of convulsive SE, as the clinical presentation is clear and movement artifacts will obscure the EEG. However, it may be very helpful in the diagnosis of NCSE and patients with deep coma.

Metabolic Disorder and Autoimmune Workup Whenever Necessary

Testing for the metabolic and mitochondrial disease should be done in young patients with myoclonus, intellectual disability, or unexplained neurologic signs and symptoms.

Autoimmune etiology is to be suspected in cases of new-onset seizures presenting as SE, progression to refractory SE (RSE) or super-refractory SE (SRSE), known history of underlying malignancy, lymphocytic pleocytosis in cerebrospinal fluid (CSF), with prior history, but the abrupt onset and persistent seizures, and new psychiatric symptoms or behavioral changes. After confirmation, early immune modulatory therapy has to be initiated for better outcomes.

Treatment of Status Epilepticus in Pregnancy

A modified figure of the proposed model for management of convulsive SE in pregnancy by Roberti et al.[6] is shown in **Figure 1**.

STATUS EPILEPTICUS IN PREGNANCY (EXCLUDING ECLAMPSIA)

Status epilepticus has been classified into five stages as per timing and approach to management.[7] Stage 1 is the pre-hospital setting and stage 2 is the early in-hospital setting. Benzodiazepines are the preferred drug of choice for both stages. If SE persists despite treatment with benzodiazepines (stage 3), antiepileptics are utilized. SE persisting even after stage 3 management, is termed RSE (stage 4). Anesthetic agents are the treatment options for SE management in stage 4. SE persisting for >24 hours, even after the earlier-mentioned management, is the SRSE (stage 5). The management is summarized in **Figure 1**.

STATUS EPILEPTICUS IN ECLAMPSIA

Eclampsia is a life-threatening hypertensive disorder of pregnancy.[8] It is defined as the occurrence of one or more generalized tonic-clonic seizures not related to any other medical cause other than a hypertensive disorder of pregnancy. Magnesium sulfate either intravenous (IV) or intramuscular (IM) (*see* **Fig. 1**) is the drug of choice for SE in eclampsia as a first-line drug along with management of airway, breathing, and circulation. Fetal monitoring is mandatory whenever SE occurs in pregnancy.

Pregnancy-related concerns with the use of various drugs in the management of SE in pregnant patients are summarized in **Table 2**.

NONCONVULSIVE STATUS EPILEPTICUS IN PREGNANCY

At present, there is no clear consensus on a treatment option for this heterogeneous disorder. Most of the recommendations are extrapolated from the treatment of SE.

CHAPTER 47: Status Epilepticus in Pregnancy

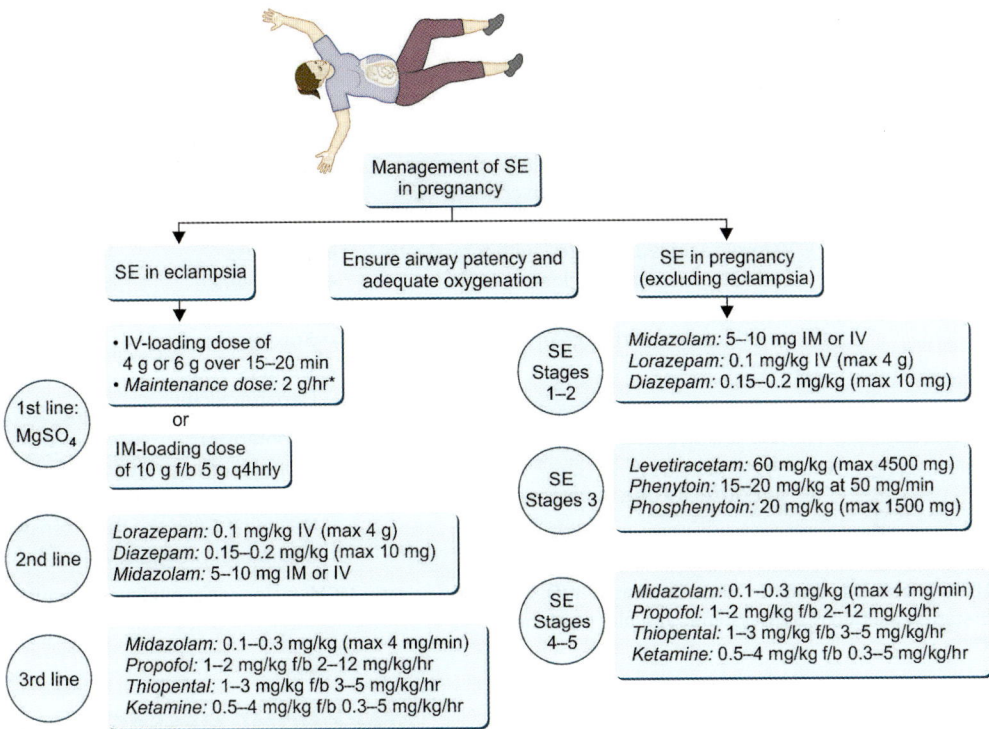

Fig. 1: Proposed management protocol by Roberti et al.[6] for management of convulsive status epilepticus (SE) in pregnancy. After 30 weeks of gestation, labor should be induced when fetomaternal and cervical conditions are favorable and cesarean section should be considered otherwise. Risks and benefits of pregnancy termination should be weighed if SE is not controlled despite multiple antiepileptic measures. Fetal monitoring should be done at all times during SE in pregnancy.

TABLE 2: Fetomaternal concerns for use of various drugs in the management of SE in pregnancy.		
Drugs	**Fetal consideration**	**Maternal consideration**
Benzodiazepines	• High lipid solubility • Rapidly cross the fetoplacental membrane • Reports of miscarriage[9] • Conflicting reports on MCMs[10] • Floppy infant syndrome with high-dose diazepam	• Sedation • Tolerance • Behavioral effects • Reduction in SVR
Magnesium sulfate	• Better APGAR scores • Decreased need for intubation	• Toxicity is rare when carefully administered • Hypotension, tachycardia • Respiratory depression • Headache, dizziness • Dryness, itching, and tingling • Nausea and vomiting

Contd...

Contd...

Drugs	Fetal consideration	Maternal consideration
AEDs	• MCMs with the use of phenobarbital, phenytoin, and valproic acid • Fetal hydantoin syndrome with phenytoin • Lower verbal intelligence in children with phenobarbital use in mothers • Valproic acid is associated with fetal death and IUDs, increased incidence of MCMs, decreased intelligence and cognition • Levetiracetam and lacosamide are relatedly safe	• Hypotension on rapid administration • Nausea • Vomiting • Fatigue • Dizziness • Somnolence • Stevens–Johnson syndrome • Ataxia • Tremors • Hepatotoxicity
Anesthetic agents	• Neonatal depression when administered just before delivery • Neurotoxicity due to ketamine exposure[11]	• Hypotension • Propofol infusion syndrome • Apnea • Ketamine C/I in the hypertensive disorder of pregnancy

(AED: antiepileptic drug; C/I: contraindicated; IUD: intrauterine death; MCM: major congenital malformations; SE: status epilepticus; SVR: systemic vascular resistance)

Antiseizure drugs and IV drugs are the mainstays of treatment. Other alternative treatment modalities include recurrent transcranial magnetic stimulation, immunomodulation, induced hypothermia, ketogenic diet, vagus nerve/deep brain stimulation, and electroconvulsive therapy. Most of these options seem impractical during pregnancy. Immunotherapy has to be considered when the usual treatment fails.

■ CONCLUSION

Status epilepticus is not very common in pregnancy. It holds therapeutic challenge, due to various maternal and fetal implications. Mass lesions, infections, and sudden events due to vascular malformations can occur at any time in pregnancy; hence, appropriate imaging should be performed. Most of antiepileptic drugs have teratogenic effects therefore management and treatment should be implemented as early as possible.

TAKE HOME MESSAGES

- SE is not very common in pregnancy. It holds therapeutic challenge, due to various maternal and fetal implications. The most common cause of SE is PRES/RCVS spectrum followed by CVT and autoimmune encephalitis.
- There can be normal pregnancy-related physiological changes resulting in lower blood pressure and dilatation of vascular spaces. This leads to syncopal events, eclampsia, and PRES and stroke. Mass lesions, infections, and sudden events due to vascular malformations can occur at any time in pregnancy; hence, appropriate imaging should be performed.
- There is increased risk of teratogenic effects due to AEDs prescribed to pregnant females. It may also have effect on neurocognition of the child. There are occasional reports of fetal deaths and malformations after SE in antiepileptic treated women.
- Management should start with clinical examination and laboratory investigations, neuroimaging and lumbar puncture, EEG, metabolic disorder, and autoimmune workup, whenever necessary.

- Treatment in SE in eclampsia includes magnesium sulfate as first-line management. Second-line of treatment includes benzodiazepines such as midazolam, diazepam, and lorazepam and third-line treatment includes midazolam, propofol, thiopental, and ketamine. Whereas in SE in pregnancy excluding eclampsia, in stages 1–2 benzodiazepines is given. Stage 3, levetiracetam, phenytoin, and fosphenytoin and in stages 4–5, midazolam, propofol, thiopental, and ketamine are the treatment options.

REFERENCES

1. Lowenstein DH, Bleck T, Macdonald RL. It's time to revise the definition of status epilepticus. Epilepsia. 1999;40(1):120-2.
2. Betjemann JP, Lowenstein DH. Status Epilepticus in adults. Lancet Neurol. 2015;14(6):615-24.
3. Nei M, Daly S, Liporace J. A maternal complex partial seizure in labour can affect fetal heart rate. Neurology. 1998;51:904-6.
4. Pariente G, Leibson T, Carls A, Adams-Webber T, Ito S, Koren G. Pregnancy-associated changes in pharmacokinetics: a systematic review. PLoS Med. 2016;13(11):e1002160.
5. Yoon I, Slesinger TL. Radiation exposure in pregnancy. Treasure Island (FL): StatPearls Publishing; 2022.
6. Roberti R, Rocca M, Iannone LF, Gasparini S, Pascarella A, Neri S, et al. Status epilepticus in pregnancy: a literature review and a protocol proposal. Expert Rev Neurother. 2022;22(4):301-12.
7. Minicucci F, Ferlisi M, Brigo F, Mecarelli O, Meletti S, Aguglia U, et al. Management of status epilepticus in adults. Position Paper of the Italian League against Epilepsy. Epilepsy Behav. 2020;102:106675.
8. Fishel Bartal M, Sibai BM. Eclampsia in the 21st century. Am J Obstet Gynecol. 2022;226(2):S1237-53.
9. Sheehy O, Zhao JP, Bérard A. Association between incident exposure to benzodiazepines in early pregnancy and risk of spontaneous abortion. JAMA Psychiatry. 2019;76(9):948-57.
10. Ban L, West J, Gibson JE, Fiaschi L, Sokal R, Doyle P, et al. First trimester exposure to anxiolytic and hypnotic drugs and the risks of major congenital anomalies: a United Kingdom population-based cohort study. PloS One. 2014;9(6):e100996.
11. Shi Y, Li J, Chen C, Xia Y, Li Y, Zhang P, et al. Ketamine modulates Zic5 expression via the notch signaling pathway in neural crest induction. Front Mol Neurosci. 2018;11:9.

CHAPTER 48

Pyrexia of Unknown Origin during Pregnancy

Jay Prakash, Tushar Kumar, Bhawesh Upreti

■ INTRODUCTION

Fever during pregnancy not only affects the parturients but also jeopardizes fetal well-being. There is a greater incidence of fetal anomalies, especially defects in the central nervous system, in parturients who witnessed fever during their antenatal period.

In a wide range of animal species, including guinea pigs, rats, mice, pigs, sheep, and monkeys, fever during pregnancy has been identified as a teratogen.[1] Heat shock proteins, which are disrupted by fever, prevent protein synthesis, which can lead to membrane rupture, cell death, vascular disruption, and placental infarction.[2] These all have the potential to result in severe fetal malformations or fetal death.

During the postdelivery period, parturient women are prone to serious infection of the genitourinary tract, which may be life-threatening. Common causes of fever during pregnancy include common cough and cold, flu, bacterial infections, listeriosis, pyelonephritis, tonsillitis, etc. However, when fever occurs without apparent cause, management becomes tough.

Pyrexia of unknown origin (PUO) during pregnancy has its challenges. There is much debate on various investigations, antibiotics, and approaches to the treatment of PUO during pregnancy.

■ EPIDEMIOLOGY AND MAGNITUDE OF PROBLEM

The data on maternal fever and morbidity in India need to be clarified. With the establishment of maternal death surveillance and response (MDSR) guidelines by the Government of India in 2017, more information will be available on morbidity and mortality.[3] The incidence of fever in India is still uncertain; however, "more V in 2017" showed that the incidence is roughly 10.5%, with the majority of cases in the third trimester.[4] There is no recommendation about fever in pregnant women, but usual care for undifferentiated fever can be given. Improving diagnostic techniques to ensure the exact etiology and proper management of fever in pregnant women could modify antibiotic prescriptions and improve maternal-fetal outcomes.[5]

■ IMPLICATION FOR MATERNAL HEALTH

Pyrexia of unknown origin during pregnancy does indeed increase maternal morbidity and mortality. Other consequences of fever of unknown origin during pregnancy include increased hospital stays and financial burden. About 25% of fevers during pregnancy are designated as PUO;[6] 12% of patients need intensive care unit (ICU) admission, and 10% suffer fetal loss.[7] Pregnancy is a state of immunosuppression. Fever during pregnancy is commonly caused by viruses such as varicella-zoster virus, coxsackievirus, human parvovirus B19, Rubella, cytomegalovirus, human immunodeficiency virus (HIV), and herpes simplex virus (HSV); bacteria such as *Listeria*, syphilis, *Borrelia*, group-B *Streptococcus*, coliforms, and protozoa such as toxoplasmosis and malaria. The common infections during pregnancy are urinary tract infections, respiratory tract infections, vaginal infections, typhoid and paratyphoid fever, malaria, dengue, tuberculosis, and chickenpox. Aside from the diseases listed earlier, several other causes of fever go undiagnosed. Some of the causes are osteomyelitis, sinusitis, Epstein–Barr virus, Lyme disease, autoimmune diseases such as systemic lupus erythematosus (SLE), polymyalgia rheumatica, temporal arteritis, rheumatoid arthritis, rheumatoid fever, inflammatory bowel disease, malignancies such as lymphoma, metastatic cancers, renal cell carcinoma, colon carcinoma, hepatoma, and myelodysplastic syndromes, or other causes like drug-induced fever, deep venous thrombosis, sarcoidosis, and factitious fever.[8]

IMPLICATION FOR FETAL WELL-BEING

Fever during pregnancy poses a significant burden to the unborn child. One of the top 20 global causes of disease burden is congenital malformations.[9] Long-term disability brought on by these malformations significantly inhibits personal, familial, and social development. Anomalies are brought on by membrane disruption, cell death, vascular disruption, and placental infarction brought on by maternal fever, which interferes with protein synthesis via heat shock proteins.[2]

Fever during pregnancy, according to numerous studies, can cause renal malformations, oral clefts, cardiac malformations, and neural tube defects.[10] The severity, length, and timing of parturients' fevers appear to affect the nature of the specific malformations. For example, malaria and tuberculosis more commonly cause preterm intrauterine growth restriction (IUGR) and meconium-stained amniotic fluid (MSAF), whereas abortion was more frequent with first trimester fever. Preterm and premature rupture of membranes (PROM) were more frequently associated with third trimester fever.[4] Maternal fever not only causes malformations but also impacts neurodevelopmental aspects. Children born to such patients may develop attention deficit hyperactivity disorder (ADHD) and autism.[11]

Another disease worth mentioning here is Zika virus (ZIKV) infection. Until recently, India remained untouched by the ZIKV, but starting in Gujarat, it has spread to Kerala in mid-2021, Uttar Pradesh, Madhya Pradesh, and other states. Female anopheles mosquito bites spread it. Symptoms include fever, rash, conjunctivitis, muscle and joint pain, and a headache that lasts 2–7 days but goes unnoticed most of the time. ZIKV is diagnosed using real-time reverse transcriptase polymerase chain reaction (rRTPCR).[12] It causes IUGR, fetal microcephaly, and congenital Zika syndrome (CZS), characterized by five distinctive features, namely microcephaly and brain calcifications, ocular manifestations on the retina, and defects on extremities including congenital contractures and hypertonia.[13]

MANAGEMENT AND TREATMENT

Illness during pregnancy is common and so is the pharmacotherapy. Trivial illness often poses no problem but undifferentiated fever

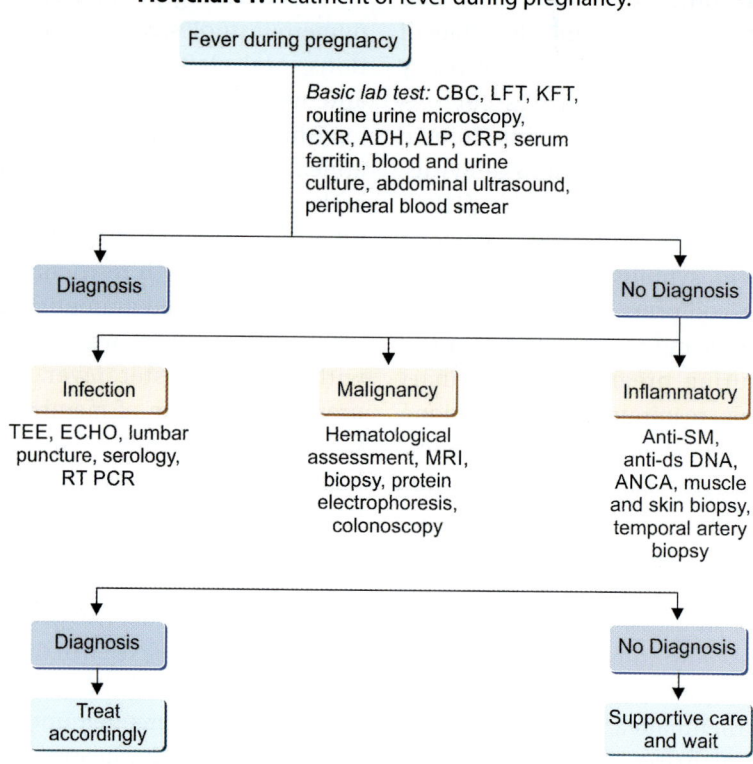

Flowchart 1: Treatment of fever during pregnancy.

(ADH: antidiueretic hormone; ALP: alkaline phosphatase; ANCA: antineutrophil cytoplasmic antibody; CBC: complete blood count; CRP: C-reactive protein; CXR: chest X-ray; DNA: deoxyribonucleic acid; KFT: kidney function test; LFT: liver function test; MRI: magnetic resonance imaging; RT PCR: reverse transcription polymerase chain reaction; TEE: transesophageal echocardiogram)

might warrant treatment. **Flowchart 1**[14] and **Table 1** depicts approach to patient and treatment during pregnancy.

PREVENTING INFECTION IN THE PREGNANCY

Antenatal Screening and Prenatal Counseling

Testing for infections prior to conception should evaluate a woman's immunity to hepatitis B, syphilis, HIV, and rubella. A prepregnancy visit is also an opportunity to provide dietary and other advice on how to lower the risk of contracting listeriosis and toxoplasmosis. For example, avoid eating raw or undercooked meat and meat products, peel or thoroughly wash raw fruit and vegetables to remove contaminating soil, and wash your hands after gardening or disposing of cat litter. The prepregnancy session also gives both partners the chance to receive counseling about avoiding unintentional sexual contact, intravenous drug use, and the ensuing risk of infection. Women who are susceptible to varicella, hepatitis B, or rubella should be encouraged to get immunizations. A minimum of 2 months after the last

TABLE 1: Disease and management.

Disease	Treatment	Do not use
Malaria	Chloroquine, amodiaquine, quinine, azithromycin, sulfadoxine-pyrimethamine, mefloquine, dapsone-chlorproguanil, artemisinin derivatives, atovaquone-proguanil and lumefantrine	Halofantrine, tetracycline/doxycycline, and primaquine
Tuberculosis	Isoniazid, rifampicin, ethambutol and pyrazinamide and ciprofloxacin	• Streptomycin • Kanamycin • Amikacin • Capreomycin • Fluoroquinolones
UTI	Nitrofurantoin, sulfisoxazole or cephalexin	
Q fever	Long-term co-trimoxazole, rifampin	Doxycycline and quinolone
Flu	Oseltamivir (Tamiflu), zanamivir (Relenza) or peramivir (Rapivab)	
STDs like gonorrhea, syphilis, trichomonas	• Doxycycline BD for 7 days—gonorrhea • Metronidazole—2 g orally single dose	
Leptospirosis	Azithromycin, amoxicillin	
Lyme disease (borreliosis)	Oral amoxicillin or oral cefuroxime axetil for 2–3 weeks	
Infective bacterial endocarditis	Emergency surgery	
Herpes zoster	Acyclovir, valacyclovir	
Varicella zoster	• Acyclovir or valacyclovir (best within 24 hours of rash appearance) • Varicella-zoster immunoglobulin (VZIG) on 7th day postexposure	
Herpes simplex	IV acyclovir	
HIV	Dolutegravir (DTG), tenofovir alafenamide (TAF), emtricitabine, efavirenz (after first trimester)	Cabotegravir (CAB), rilpivirine (RPV)
Zika virus	Supportive treatment only, acetaminophen	
Candidiasis, systemic fungal infection	Amphotericin B, topical nystatin	Griseofulvin, ketoconazole, voriconazole, flucytosine and potassium iodide
Dengue, chikungunya	Supportive treatment. Acetaminophen, fluids and rest	
Appendicitis	Surgery	Most common nonobstetric emergency

(HIV: human immunodeficiency virus; IV: intravenous; STDs: sexually transmitted diseases; UTI: urinary tract infection) vaccination should pass before pregnancy. For pregnant women, it is also advised to get tested for *Chlamydia trachomatis*, hepatitis B, syphilis, and HIV. Hepatitis C and *Neisseria gonorrhoeae* screenings for women at risk are recommended.[15]

Vaccination While Pregnant

Live virus vaccines should not be given to pregnant women. Diphtheria, tetanus, influenza, and hepatitis B vaccines are among those that are typically safe to administer during pregnancy. Meningococcal and rabies vaccinations may also be considered. The theoretical risk of fetal transmission makes certain vaccines, such as those for measles, mumps, rubella, varicella, and Bacillus Calmette–Guérin (BCG), contraindicated.

■ CONCLUSION

Pyrexia of unknown origin during pregnancy is often challenging. If left unchecked, may lead to increased maternal and fetal morbidity and mortality (Abortion, neurodevelopmental anomalies, IUGR, MSAF, PROM, etc.). Preconception counseling, timely investigations, and early and appropriate antibiotics may help to prevent the aforementioned manifestations.

TAKE HOME MESSAGES

- Pregnancy is the state of immune compression.
- Detailed history including exposure and travel must be obtained.
- Maternal hyperthermia has implications on fetal development.
- Choose your antibiotics carefully.
- Early intervention and advanced care must not be delayed.

■ REFERENCES

1. Krausova T, Peterka M. Teratogenic and lethal effects of 2–24 h hyperthermia episodes on chick embryos. J Therm Biol. 2007;32(4):193-203.
2. Andersen AM, Vastrup P, Wohlfahrt J, Andersen PK, Olsen J, Melbye M. Fever in pregnancy and risk of fetal death: a cohort study. Lancet. 2002;360(9345):1552-6.
3. Kansal A, Garg S, Sharma M. Moving from maternal death review to surveillance and response: a paradigm shift. Indian J Public Health. 2018;62(4):299-301.
4. More VS. Fever in pregnancy and its maternal and fetal outcomes. Int J Reprod Contracept Obstet Gynecol. 2017;6(12):5523-8.
5. Laxminarayan R, Matsoso P, Pant S, Brower C, Røttingen JA, Klugman K, et al. Access to effective antimicrobials: a worldwide challenge. Lancet. 2016;387(10014):168-75.
6. Charlier C, Perrodeau E, Levallois C, Cachina T, Dommergues M, Salomon LJ, et al. Causes of fever in pregnant women with acute undifferentiated fever: a prospective multicentric study. Eur J Clin Microbiol Infect Dis. 2020;39(5):999-1002.
7. Knowles SJ, O'Sullivan NP, Meenan AM, Hanniffy R, Robson M. Maternal sepsis incidence, aetiology and outcome for mother and fetus: a prospective study. BJOG. 2015;122(5):663-71.
8. Fernandez C, Beeching NJ. Pyrexia of unknown origin. Clin Med (Lond). 2018;18(2):170-4.
9. Murray CJ, Vos T, Lozano R, Naghavi M, Flaxman AD, Michaud C, et al. Disability-adjusted life years (DALYs) for 291 diseases and injuries in 21 regions, 1990-2010: a systematic analysis for the Global Burden of Disease Study 2010. Lancet. 2012;380(9859):2197-223.
10. Sass L, Urhoj SK, Kjærgaard J, Dreier JW, Strandberg-Larsen K, Nybo Andersen AM. Fever in pregnancy and the risk of congenital malformations: a cohort study. BMC Pregnancy Childbirth. 2017;17(1):413.

11. Antoun S, Ellul P, Peyre H, Rosenzwajg M, Gressens P, Klatzmann D, et al. Fever during pregnancy as a risk factor for neurodevelopmental disorders: results from a systematic review and meta-analysis. Mol Autism. 2021;12(1):60.
12. Yadav PD, Niyas VKM, Arjun R, Sahay RR, Shete AM, Sapkal GN, et al. Detection of Zika virus disease in Thiruvananthapuram, Kerala, India 2021 during the second wave of COVID-19 pandemic. J Med Virol. 2022;94(6):2346-9.
13. Zorrilla CD, García García I, García Fragoso L, De La Vega A. Zika virus infection in pregnancy: maternal, fetal, and neonatal considerations. J Infect Dis. 2017;216(suppl_10):S891-6.
14. Roth AR, Basello GM. Approach to the adult patient with fever of unknown origin. Am Fam Physician. 2003;68(11):2223-8.
15. Milne K, Dallard T, Douglas JG. Fever of unknown origin in pregnancy: the need for a full history. BMJ Case Rep. 2012; 2012:bcr2012006307.

CHAPTER 49

Anaphylaxis in Pregnancy

Aklesh Tandekar, Suvadeep Sen, Sachin Narayan Rathore

■ DEFINITION

Anaphylaxis is acute potentially fatal systemic allergic reaction usually triggered by a known allergen.[1] It is a form of immunoglobulin E (IgE) dependent type 1 hypersensitivity reaction mediated by mast cell. In pregnancy, any form of anaphylactic reaction can be life-threatening to both mother and the fetus.

■ EPIDEMIOLOGY

The prevalence of anaphylaxis in general population according to various surveys in United States is 0.05–2%.[2] The data on the prevalence of anaphylaxis in pregnancy is sparse. It is an extremely rare event in pregnant women triggered by similar risk factors as in general population. A population-based descriptive study among UK population found an estimated incidence of 1.6/100,000 pregnant women.

■ RISK FACTORS AND ETIOLOGY

Triggering factor of anaphylaxis in pregnant women is similar to that of general population.[1] The common allergens of specific interest in pregnancy are—antibiotics (penicillin, cephalosporin group of antibiotics), oxytocin, intravenous iron, misoprostol, natural rubber latex, RhD immunoglobulin, breastfeeding, insect bites, and anesthetic agents (local anesthetics, muscle relaxants, and inhalational agents).

■ CLINICAL MANIFESTATIONS

In anaphylactic reaction in pregnant women affects both mother and fetus and may be life-threatening for the both.[3] The common signs and symptoms of anaphylaxis constitute of cutaneous, respiratory, circulatory, and gastrointestinal symptoms. Typical skin feature includes urticarial rash and erythema, flushing, periorbital edema, conjunctival swallowing, and sometimes angioedema. Respiratory symptoms include nasal congestion, hoarseness of voice, laryngeal edema, and in extreme cases stridor and dyspnea. Apart from this in severe form of anaphylaxis, patient develops severe hypotension and circulatory vasodilatory shock. Gastrointestinal symptoms constitute crampy abdominal pain, loose motion, nausea, and vomiting. Specific pregnancy-related symptoms include vulvar edema, vaginal itching, uterine contraction, and commonly lower back pain. These symptoms often accompany systemic symptoms rather than occurring in isolation.

Maternal anaphylaxis can also lead to fetal hypoxia and fetal distress, and sometimes hypoxicischemic encephalopathy in newborn and fetal death.[4]

■ DIFFERENTIAL DIAGNOSIS

Signs and symptoms of anaphylaxis are extremely nonspecific.[5] We need to have high degree of suspicion and rule out other common condition that can mimic this life-threatening condition.[6] Common differential diagnoses are acute fat embolism of pregnancy, acute severe asthma, cardiogenic shock with peripartum cardiomyopathy, vasovagal symptoms, epiglottitis, foreign body aspiration, acute generalized urticaria with angioedema, and laryngopathia gravidarum.[7] The typical dermatological and respiratory feature with cardiovascular collapse following a known trigger should warrant a diagnosis of anaphylaxis.[8]

Diagnosis

Anaphylaxis is a clinical diagnosis as it is precipitated suddenly and carries high mortality unless treated promptly. There is a validated and defined diagnostic criterion for anaphylaxis.[9]

Usually laboratory tests are not required to confirm the diagnosis.[10] In selected cases serum tryptase level can be checked (optimally sample drawn within 15 minute–3 hours of onset of symptoms). Elevated tryptase level point toward mast cell activation and thus supports its diagnosis.[11] However, normal tryptase level does not refute the diagnosis of anaphylaxis.

■ MANAGEMENT

Emergency management of anaphylaxis in pregnant woman is identical to that in general population and it starts with management of airway, breathing, and circulation.[12] All patients with severe anaphylaxis should be admitted in intensive care unit.[13] Adrenaline is mainstay in the therapeutic management of anaphylaxis. Dose and route of administration of adrenaline depend on the clinical situation. In emergency setting, intramuscular (IM) injection of 1 mg of adrenaline is the safest and the most effective way to relieve the crisis. In intraoperative setting, intravenous (IV) bolus in diluted form may be administered. In case of persistent hypotension, continuous infusion may be considered.

Airway management is the crux for successful treatment of anaphylaxis.[14] Most patients with severe form develop laryngeal edema and stridor and they require immediate endotracheal intubation. Fluid resuscitation is also essential as it is a vasodilatory shock. Adequate intravascular volume is essential for maintaining uteroplacental perfusion.[15] Glucose-containing fluid should be avoided as it may cause fetal acidosis and cause neonatal hypoglycemia. Other pregnancy-specific measures such as keeping patient in left side for preventing caval compression, maintaining a minimum systolic blood pressure (SBP) of 90 mm Hg for adequate placental perfusion (as there is no autoregulation in uterine blood flow) and monitoring fetal heart rate throughout the shock period are essential.

In case of severe wheezing and bronchospasm, beta-2 agonist nebulization may be given.[16] H1 antihistaminic may be given for itching and skin rashes. Role of intravenous steroid is unproven but may be used in case of persistent shock or bronchospasm and severe allergic reaction.

Fetal Monitoring

In pregnancy complicated with severe anaphylaxis, continuous fetal heart rate monitoring is indicated.[4] Non-assuring fetal heart rate pattern is an indicator of maternal cardiovascular and respiratory instability during an anaphylactic attack. In that case, after maternal stabilization, cesarean section may be warranted. Any cardiac arrest should be dealt with as per advanced cardiovascular life support (ACLS) guideline with potential need for delivery of the baby as a part of resuscitative process.

Prevention of Anaphylaxis

Strategies to prevent anaphylaxis in pregnancy start with careful history taking during antenatal screening period about specific allergy to any drugs or substances and avoidance of that trigger factor.[17] In case where the specific trigger cannot be avoided, appropriate desensitization should be done. Particularly important and ignored trigger is latex allergy, where complete latex-free environment is required.

CONCLUSION

Anaphylaxis is an uncommon entity during pregnancy. Severe form may be life-threatening for both mother and fetus and may cause permanent brain damage to the neonate. Prevention is the most important strategy to avoid this catastrophic phenomenon. Prompt identification and emergency supportive treatment play pivotal role in patient survival.

REFERENCES

1. Simons FE, Schatz M. Anaphylaxis during pregnancy. J Allergy Clin Immunol. 2012; 130:597-606.
2. Mulla ZD, Ebrahim MS, Gonzalez JL. Anaphylaxis in the obstetric patient: analysis of a statewide hospital discharge database. Ann Allergy Asthma Immunol. 2010;104:55-9.
3. Simons FE. Anaphylaxis. J Allergy Clin Immunol. 2010;125:161-81.
4. Berardi A, Rossi K, Cavalleri F, Simoni A, Aguzzoli L, Masellis G, et al. Maternal anaphylaxis and fetal brain damage after intrapartum chemoprophylaxis. J Perinat Med. 2004;32:375-7.
5. Chaudhuri K, Gonzales J, Jesurun CA, Ambat MT, Mandal-Chaudhuri S. Anaphylactic shock in pregnancy: a case study and review of the literature. Int J Obstet Anesth. 2009;17:350-7.
6. Simons FE, Ardusso LR, Bilò MB, El-Gamal YM, Ledford DK, Ring J, et al. World Allergy Organization anaphylaxis guidelines: summary. J Allergy Clin Immunol. 2011; 127:587-93.
7. Schatz M, Dombrowski MP. Clinical practice. Asthma in pregnancy. N Engl J Med. 2009;360(18):1862-9.
8. Caballero T, Farkas H, Bouillet L, Bowen T, Gompel A, Fagerberg C, et al. International consensus and practical guidelines on the gynecologic and obstetric management of female patients with hereditary angioedema caused by C1 inhibitor deficiency. J Allergy Clin Immunol. 2012;129:308-20.
9. Harper NJ, Dixon T, Dugué P, Edgar DM, Fay A, Gooi HC, et al. Working Party of the Association of Anaesthetists of Great Britain and Ireland. Suspected anaphylactic reactions associated with anaesthesia. Anaesthesia. 2009;64(2):199-211.
10. Braveman FR. Pregnancy-associated diseases. In: Hines RL, Marschall KE (Eds). Stoelting's Anesthesia and Coexisting Diseases, 5th edition, Churchill Livingstone, Philadelphia. 2008;557-80.
11. Berenguer A, Couto A, Brites V, Fernandes R. Anaphylaxis in pregnancy: a rare cause of neonatal mortality. BMJ Case Rep. 2013.
12. ASCIA. Guidelines: Acute Management of Anaphylaxis. In: 2019.
13. Hepner DL, Castells M, Mouton-Faivre C, Dewachter P. Anaphylaxis in the clinical setting of obstetric anesthesia: a literature review. Anesth Analg. 2013;117(6):1357-67.
14. The Australian and New Zealand Committee on Resuscitation (ANZCOR). ANZCOR Guideline 8 – Cardiopulmonary Resuscitation (CPR). In: 2016.
15. Chu J, Johnston T, Geoghegan J; Royal College of Obstetricians and Gynaecologists. Maternal Collapse in Pregnancy and the Puerperium: Green-top Guideline No. 56. BJOG. An International Journal of Obstetrics & Gynaecology. 2019.
16. Simons FE, Ardusso LR, Bilò MB, Cardona V, Ebisawa M, El-Gamal YM, et al. International consensus on (ICON) anaphylaxis. World Allergy Organ J. 2014;7:9.
17. Shank JJ, Olney SC, Lin FL, McNamara MF. Recurrent postpartum anaphylaxis with breast-feeding. Obstet Gynecol. 2009;114(2 Pt 2): 415-6.

Index

Page numbers followed by *b* refer to box, *f* refer to figure, *fc* refer to flowchart, and *t* refer to table.

A

Abortion, septic 321, 352
Abruptio placentae 104
Accelerations 36
Acetaminophen 224
Acetoacetic acid 139
Acetone 139
Acetylcholine receptor 342
Aciclovir 131
Acid–base
  assessment 14
  disorder 16*t*, 17
    mixed 16, 18
    simple 16
  physiology 14
  status 165
Acidity 369
Acidosis 12, 14, 17
  maternal 119
  mechanisms of 17
Activated clotting time 264
Activated partial thromboplastin time 192, 264, 355
Acute disseminated encephalomyelitis 334, 335, 337*b*
  diagnosis 336
  epidemiology 334
  etiology 334
  evaluation 335
  pathophysiology 335
  prognosis 338
  symptomatology 335
  theories 335
  treatment 337
Acute inflammatory demyelinating polyneuropathy 341, 342, 345
Acute kidney injury 104-106, 164, 257*b*, 259, 314
  network 104
  pregnancy-related 104, 257
Acute kidney insufficiency 130

Acute liver diseases, pregnancy-associated 304
Acute liver failure 303, 309
  causes of 312*t*
Acute myocardial infarction, pregnancy-associated 25
Acute pulmonary embolism 64, 64*t*
Acute pyelonephritis 125, 324
  management of 126
Acute respiratory distress syndrome 28, 47, 53-56, 72, 262, 284
Acyclovir 49, 296
Adenosine triphosphate 172
Adrenaline 253
Adrenocorticotropic hormone 162
Adriamycin 362
Adult respiratory distress syndrome 65, 319
Advanced cardiac life support 251, 253, 269
  guidelines 358
Aggressive intensive care unit 135
Air
  ambulance 269
  embolism 71
  large amount of 74
Airway 140, 214
  assessment 369
  edema 10
  management 13, 368, 387
    advanced 252
  obstruction 19
  protection 337
Akinesia 25
Alanine transaminase 308
Albuterol 43
Aldosterone
  antagonistic action 158
  receptor blocker 162
Alkaline phosphatase 382
Alkalosis 161, 163
Allergen immunotherapy 42, 43, 287

Allergic reaction, severe 387
Allograft function 241
Allopurinol 364
Alpha-chains 226
  complete lack of 227
Altered sensorium 291
  causes of 293*t*
Ambu bag 252
American College of Obstetricians and Gynecologists 80, 180, 181
American College of Surgeons Committee on Trauma 353*t*
American Heart Association 97, 250, 358
American Society of Transplantation 239
American Thoracic Society 48
Aminoglycosides 50, 126, 131, 171, 343
Amiodarone 251, 253
Amniotic fluid 33
  embolism 26, 54, 70, 182, 266, 352, 353, 355, 356, 368
  diagnosis of 70
  meconium-stained 381
Amphotericin B 161
Analgesia, postoperative 174
Anaphylactic reaction 386
Anaphylaxis 71
  prevalence of 386
  prevention of 388
Anchoring villi 282
Anemia 119, 129, 132, 260, 368
  acute 72, 223
  dilutional 73
  hemolytic 108
  microangiopathic 206
    hemolytic 108*f*
  mild-to-moderate 231
  physiological 212
Anesthesia, spinal 98
Anesthetic agents 378
Aneuploidies, prenatal screening for 120

Index

Angioedema 386, 387
Angiotensin-converting enzyme
 inhibitor 121, 162, 164,
 241, 261
Angiotensin-receptor
 antagonists 131
 blockers 121, 164, 241, 261
Anion gap 16, 17
Antenatal care 229, 326
 components of 326
Antiarrhythmic agents 343
Antibiotics 111, 125*t*, 126*t*,
 221, 323
 prophylaxis 95, 326
Antibodies 342
Anticardiolipin 205
Anticholinergics 42, 43
Anticoagulants 131, 204, 207
 withdrawal 207
Anticoagulation 94, 237, 265
 long-term 192
Anticonvulsants 131
 therapy, sudden cessation
 of 297
Antidiabetics 131
Antidiuretic hormone 382
 increased levels of 152
Antiepileptic 340
 drugs 374, 378
Antihypertensive agents 182*t*
 first-line 80*t*, 180
Antihypertensive medication 79,
 80, 180, 241, 271
 goal of 180
Antimicrobials 50*t*, 131
 agents 343
Antineutrophil cytoplasmic
 antibody 312, 382
Anti-nuclear antibodies 312
Antiphospholipid antibodies 197,
 198, 203
 levels of 207
Antiphospholipid syndrome 203
Antiseptic solutions 276
Anti-smooth muscle
 antibodies 312
Anti-tubercular treatment 312
Antiviral agents 48, 131
Anxiety 149
Aorta 9
Aortic dilatation 91
Aortic dissection 26, 82, 83
Aortic regurgitation 26, 93
 causes of 93

Aortic stenosis 88, 92
Aortocaval compression 9, 13, 263
Appendicitis 352
Arginine 9
 vasopressin 154*f*, 155*f*
Arrhythmias 47, 89
Arterial blood gas 14, 15*t*, 139, 327
 analysis 15, 375
 interpretation of 16*fc*
Arterial carbon dioxide, lower
 partial pressure of 369
Arterial catheter 15
Arterial oxygen, partial pressure of
 211, 262, 264, 369, 331
Arterial pressure monitoring
 system 28
Arterial puncture 30
Arteriolar tone 261
Arteriovenous oxygen 282
Artificial reproductive
 techniques 291
Aspartate transaminase
 177, 308
Aspiration syndrome 368
Assisted reproductive
 technologies 204, 245
Asthma 41, 42, 54, 287
 acute severe 387
 considerations for 43
 control of 42
 global initiative for 42
 treatment of 42
Atorvastatin 131
Atrial fibrillation 251, 266
Atrioventricular block 174
Atropine 253
Atypical hemolytic uremic
 syndrome 108
Auto positive end expiratory
 pressure 44
Autoantibodies 197
Autoimmune disorders 368
Azathioprine 121, 236, 343

B

Bacteriology 124
Bacteriuria, asymptomatic 124
Bacteroides 320
Bartter syndrome 18, 159
Basal plate 282
Bedside transthoracic
 echocardiography 25*f*
Bell's palsy 345
Benzodiazepines 294, 376, 377

Benzylpenicillin 127
Beta-agonists 43, 161, 172
Beta-blockers 92, 94, 121, 149,
 164, 343
 use of 131
Beta-chains 226
Beta-glycoprotein 205
Beta-human chorionic
 gonadotrophin, renal
 excretion of 243
Beta-hydroxybutyric acid 139
Beta-thalassemia
 intermedia 226
 non-transfusion dependent 226
Bicarbonate
 administration, excessive 18
 ions, increased renal excretion
 of 10
 levels shifts 282
 therapy 141
Bicuspid aortic valve 91, 92
Bilateral parieto-occipital
 region 350*f*
Biophysical profile, components
 of 35
Biparietal diameter 33
Birth
 control pills, estrogen-
 containing 230
 defects, pattern of 240
 weight, low 284
Bisphosphonates 172
Biventricular dysfunction 72
Bladder dysfunction 365
Bleeding issues 254
Bleomycin 362
Blood
 barrier 77
 brain barrier dysfunction 294
 collection 171
 concentration, monitoring
 of 110
 flow
 fetoplacental 54
 velocity, analysis of 34
 loss 353
 pH of 15
 pressure 19, 77-80, 82-84, 97,
 180, 181*t*, 182*t*, 353
 control of 85*t*, 180
 cuffs, automated 24
 diastolic 85, 177
 management 132
 return of 9

systolic 80, 85, 177, 291, 319, 323, 387
sampling of 29
sugar, control of 140, 141
test 65, 203
transfusion 171, 222
urea nitrogen 165
volume 97, 331
Bloodstream infection, catheter-related 274
Body mass index 63, 179, 369
Bone
  density scan 228
  health 132
Botulinum 343
Brachial plexus injury 275
Bradycardia, fetal 82
Brain 76
  computed tomography of 190, 350
  magnetic resonance imaging of 350
  natriuretic peptide 65, 79
Breast
  abscess 321
  enlarged 369
Breastfeeding 243
Breath, shortness of 331
Breathing 140, 214
Bronchial asthma 42
  treatment 45
Bronchospasm 387
Budd–Chiari syndrome 303

C

Cairo–Bishop criteria 363, 363*t*
Calcineurin inhibitor toxicity 240-242
Calcitonin 172
Calcium 171, 363, 169
  channel blockers 131, 343
  chloride 171, 171*t*
  disorders of 169
  elemental 171
  gluconate 171, 171*t*, 174, 253, 363
  intravenous 166
  normal laboratory values of 171*t*
  preparation solution 171
  replacement regimen 171
Campylobacter jejuni 341
Cancers, metastatic 381
Cannula cricothyroidotomy 370

Capillary leak syndrome 24
Carbimazole 149
Carbon dioxide
  low partial pressure of 53
  partial pressure of 55, 56
Carbon monoxide 42
Carboprost 354
Cardiac arrest 358
  maternal 249, 249*t*, 250, 252, 253
  sudden 64
Cardiac arrhythmias 143
Cardiac chamber sizes 97
Cardiac disease 88, 89
Cardiac failure 47
Cardiac insufficiency 89
Cardiac output 261, 331, 355
Cardiac tamponade 26
Cardiogenic pulmonary edema 332, 369
Cardiomyopathy
  diagnosis of 25
  dilated 26*f*
  hypertrophic 91
  peripartum 54, 71, 353, 357, 358, 387
  postpartum 27*f*
  severe 266
Cardiopulmonary stabilization 71
Cardiopulmonary support 72, 365
Cardiotoxicity 130
Cardiovascular collapse, sudden 28
Cardiovascular disease 140
Cardiovascular disorders 76, 287
Cardiovascular symptoms 160
Cardiovascular system 8, 263
  physiology of 97*t*
Carotid artery injury 275
Carpel tunnel syndrome, treatment of 340
Carpreg risk score 89*t*, 90*t*
Catastrophic antiphospholipid syndrome 203, 206*f*
  classification of 203
  development of 205*f*
  differential diagnosis 205
  epidemiology 204
  long-term sequelae of 208
  management 206
  pathophysiology 204
  signs 205
  symptoms 205
  treatment 207

Catecholamines 161
Catheter management 276
Centers for Disease Control and Prevention 46
Central nervous system 196, 206*f*, 336
  disorders 19
  hemorrhage 266
  infection 194
  manifestations 364
Central venous access 273
  use of 273
Central venous catheters 163, 273, 275*t*
Central venous oxygen saturation, monitoring of 29
Central venous pressure
  monitoring 29
  waveforms, relationship of 29*f*
  use of 29
Central venous sinus thrombosis 187, 295
  clinical features 188
  epidemiology 187
  investigations 189
  management 192
  pathogenesis 188
  prognosis 193
  recanalization 194
  recurrence 194
  risk factors 187
Cerebral autoregulation 77
Cerebral microcirculatory dysfunction 364
Cerebral venous sinus 190
  thrombosis 187-189, 191, 193, 292, 293
Cerebral venous thrombosis risk score 194
Cerebrospinal fluid 188, 191, 376
  analysis 335
  pressure, low 187
Cerebrovascular accident 182
Cerebrovascular disease 222
Cervical spine stabilization 214
Cesarean delivery, perimortem 251, 252, 255, 359
Cesarean section 67, 103, 197, 204
  emergency 63
  perimortem 214
Charcot–Marie–Tooth disease 344, 345
Chelation 230

Chemotherapeutic agents cross placenta 361
Chest
  compression 251
    location of 255
  pain 73, 74
  syndrome, acute 222, 223
Chickenpox 381
Chloramphenicol 50, 126
Chlorhexidine-silver sulfadiazine 274
Cholestyramine 150
Chorioamnionitis 321, 352
Chorionic villus sampling 229
Chronic kidney disease 104, 114, 115, 118t, 164, 258
  effect of 116
  staging of 114t
Chvostek's signs 298
Circulation 140, 214
Circulatory collapse 19
Circumoral numbness 19
Cirrhosis 164
Clarithromycin 50
Cleft
  lip 342
  palate 240
Climacteric syndrome 169
Clindamycin 297
Clostridium difficile 107
Coagulation system 11, 258, 263
Coagulopathy 71, 72
Codeine 224
Colloid oncotic pressure 30, 211, 212, 331
Colon carcinoma 381
Complement system activation 107f
Complete blood count 206, 382
Complete heart block, congenital 199
Compression, depth of 251
Compressive nerve 340
Computed tomography 79, 191
  venography 190, 193
Computerized cardiotocography 37
Congestion, pulmonary 64
Conn's syndrome 18
Consciousness, levels of 294, 352
Continuous electronic fetal monitoring 35
Continuous positive airway pressure 53

Continuous renal replacement therapy 111, 259, 295
Continuous waveform capnography, role of 252
Contraception 95, 131, 185, 230, 240
Contraceptive
  long-acting reversible 240
  method 95
Conventional angiography 190
Convulsive status epilepticus, management of 377f
Cord sign 190
Cordocentesis 147
Coronary artery disease 65, 90
Coronavirus disease-2019 4, 9, 46, 187, 264, 334, 369
Cortical venous sinus thrombosis 374
Corticosteroids 58, 121, 343
Corticotrophin-releasing hormone, levels of 41
Cotrimoxazole 131
Cough 74
Coxsackievirus 381
C-reactive protein 382
Creatinine 363
  calculation of 114
Cricoid pressure, application of 369
Cricothyroid membrane 372
Crisis
  abdominal 135
  asthmatic 64
  painful 220
Crystalloid infusion 175
Cushing's disease 18
Cyanide toxicity 83
Cyanosis, peripheral 352
Cyclophosphamide 122, 362
Cyclosporine 121, 240, 343
Cystitis 125
Cytokines, proinflammatory 283
Cytomegalovirus 293, 312, 334, 341, 381
  infection 242, 296
  primary 296
Cytotrophoblasts 282

D

Dacarbazine 362
D-dimer testing 65
Decongestion therapy 94

Deep tendon reflexes, loss of 341
Deep vein thrombosis 62, 73, 381
  assessment for 27
  risk of 127
Deferasirox 228
Deferiprone 228
Defibrillation, role of 251
Dehydration 63, 297
Delavirdine mesylate 131
Dengue 381
Dense triangle sign 190
Deoxycortisone 153
Deoxyribonucleic acid 229, 281, 382
  cell-free fetal fraction of 120
  double-stranded 197, 201
Depot medroxyprogesterone acetate 240
Depression, postpartum 298
Dermatomyositis 344
Desferrioxamine 228
Diabetes mellitus, gestational 132
Diabetic ketoacidosis 135, 138, 139, 142, 292
  euglycemic 143
  hyperglycemic 143
  laboratory diagnosis 138
  occurrence of 298
  pathophysiology of 135, 136f
  signs of 138
  symptoms of 138
Dialysis 120, 167, 363
Diaphoresis 352
Diaphragm
  cephalad
    displacement of 10
    movement of 10
Dicoumarol 130
Didanosine 131
Digital subtraction angiography 191
Digoxin 12
  toxicity 164
Diphtheria 334
Direct thrombin inhibitors 67
Disseminated intravascular coagulation 72, 205, 254, 295, 352, 362
Diuretics 94
Doppler waveform 34f
Dorsal decubitus position 258
Doxorubicin 362
  hydrochloride 362
Dyselectrolytemia 297

Dysglycemia 298
Dyspnea 74, 363
Dysrhythmia, transient 30
Dystrophia myotonica protein kinase gene 344

E

Ebstein's anomaly 94
Echocardiogram 201
Eclampsia 71, 77, 174, 178, 180, 291, 368, 376
  development of 140
  magnesium sulfate regime for 183*f*
  maternal complications of 182
  prevention of 182
  severe 177
Eculizumab 108, 208
Edema 72, 158
  laryngeal 386
  perioperative pulmonary 330
  periorbital 386
  peripartum pulmonary 330
  vulvar 386
Efavirenz 131
Electric vacuum aspiration 326
Electrocardiogram 79, 101
  analysis 37
  changes 161, 165
Electrocardiography 23, 54, 55
  monitoring of 23
Electroencephalography 376
Electrolytes, serum 78
Electrophoresis patterns 228
Elevated alanine
  aminotransferase 177
  transaminase 296
Elevated erythrocyte sedimentation 72
Embolectomy, emergency pulmonary 73
Embolism syndrome 71
Embryo toxicity 130
Emergency medical services 268, 269
Empty delta sign 190
Empyema 47
Encephalitis, autoimmune 374
Encephalopathy 72, 188, 297
  hypoxicischemic 386
Endocarditis 94
  right-sided infective 73
Endocrine changes 11

Endogenous insulin, lack of 135
Endometrial glands 283
Endometritis 321, 324
  postpartum 352
End-organ damage 72, 76, 77
Endoscopic retrograde cholangiopancreatography 63
Endothelial dysfunction 348
Endovascular invasion 283
Endovascular treatment 192
End-tidal carbon dioxide 24, 74, 251
Enzyme
  heme-containing 147
  inosinate pyrophosphorylase 240
Epidural catheter removal 67
Epiglottitis 387
Epilepsy 297, 375
Epinephrine 251, 253
Epstein-Barr virus 312, 334
Ergometrine 354
Ergonovine 354
Ergotrate 354
Erythropoietin 131
  production 11
  stimulating agents 242
Escherichia coli 124, 320
Esmolol 81
Estimated glomerular filtration rate 17
European Stroke Organization guidelines 192
Euthyroid status 228
Everolimus 122
Expiratory reserve volume 54
Extended-spectrum beta-lactamase 324
External fetal heart tracing monitor 271
Extracellular fluid volume 153
Extracorporeal carbon dioxide removal 58
Extracorporeal cardiopulmonary resuscitation 266
Extracorporeal life support 255
  organization 264
Extracorporeal membrane oxygenation 6, 44, 58, 253, 257, 262, 264*b*
  indications of 262*b*
Extracorporeal support systems 315
Eyes 76

F

Facioscapulohumeral muscular dystrophy 344, 345
Fat
  embolism 71, 72
  macroglobulinemia 72
Fatty liver
  acute 106, 108, 109, 112, 206, 292, 293, 295, 303, 308, 308*t*, 310, 314, 368
  disease, nonalcoholic 303
Femoral artery injury 275
Femoral neuropathy 345
Femur length 33
Fetal
  acidosis 10
  assessment 84, 215
  death 47, 184, 208
  distress 156, 386
    mechanisms of 136, 137*f*
  growth 33
    restriction 33, 35*t*, 284
  health 320
    implications for 115, 188, 213
  heart rate 387
    monitoring 260
    recording of 34
    variability 266
  hemoglobin, normal 227
  loss 199
  malformations 361
  management 119
  medicine 223
  monitoring 58, 142, 223, 243, 260, 387
  movements 33
    monitor perception of 32
    protocol 33*fc*
  neuroprotection 174
  outcomes 266
  oxygen level 14
  oxygenation 57
  perfusion 12*fc*
  risks 93, 117
  surveillance 223
  testing 229
    abnormal 184
  weight, estimated 33
  well-being 14, 130, 146
    implications for 47, 73, 74, 89, 170, 178, 199, 220, 227, 255, 309, 375, 381

Fetoplacental system, monitoring of 32
Fetus
　delivery of 357
　development of 152
　growth of 152
Fever 72, 223, 254, 380, 381
　factitious 381
　paratyphoid 381
　syndrome 64
　treatment of 382*fc*
Fibrinogen levels 62, 212
Fibrinolytic pathway 11
Fluconazole 131
Fluid
　attenuated inversion recovery 191, 336
　balance 57, 152
　compartment 152
　management 221
　overload 73
　　chances of 354
　　management of 93
　　restriction, conventional approach of 155
　resuscitation 322
　retention 158
Fluoroquinolones 50, 343
Focal syndrome 188
Fondaparinux 67
Fontan circulation 91
Food and Drug Administration 6, 341
Forced vital capacity 42
Formoterol 43
Fresh frozen plasma 355
Fulminant hepatic failure 303, 312*f*, 314
　medical management of 313*f*
Functional residual capacity 41, 54, 211, 212
Fungal emboli 73
Furosemide 131, 172

G

Gallstones 227
Ganciclovir 131
Gardnerella vaginalis 125
Gas embolism 73
Gastric
　acid aspiration 54
　volume loss 18
Gastrointestinal reflux disease 42
Gastrointestinal symptoms 160, 386

Gastrointestinal tract 293
Gastroparesis 135
Genetic vitamin D resistance syndrome 170
Genitourinary changes, clinical implications of 10
Gentamicin 131
Gitelman syndrome 18, 159
Global end-diastolic volume index 355
Glomerular filtration rate 10, 105*f*, 114-116, 153, 158, 258
Glomerulonephritis
　focal segmental 114
　primary 120
Glucocorticoids 42, 204, 207
Glucose 167
　containing fluid 387
　loading 172
Gordon syndrome 164
Graft biopsy 242
Granulocyte-colony stimulating factor 366
Graves' disease 147
Graves' thyrotoxicosis 149
Gravid uterus
　compresses 9
　effect of 258
Group B streptococcal infection 127
Growth
　fetal 33
　restriction 117
Guillain-Barré syndrome 341
Gurd and Wilson's criteria 72

H

Haemophilus influenzae 46, 107, 222, 228, 236
Hand hygiene 325
Head circumference 33
Headache 79, 188, 291, 364
Head-to-toe examination 215
Heart
　block, congenital 286
　disease 368
　　cyanotic 91
　　valvular 9, 88
　failure 64, 97, 98, 100*t*, 284
　　acute right 64
　　congestive 77, 79, 164
　　diagnosis of 99, 101*t*
　　maternal 100

　　severe right 266
　　treatment of 102, 102*t*
　rate 281, 323, 353
　　baseline 35
　　control 94
　　fetal 387
Heat
　escape lessening posture 370
　intolerance 149
Hematological cancers 360
　diagnosis of 360
　treatment of 360
Hematological malignancies 360, 361, 361*f*, 362*t*
Hematological system 258
Hematology 138
Hematoma, retroplacental 28
Hemodialysis 174, 261, 363
　intermittent 259
Hemodynamic parameters 30*t*
Hemoglobin 228, 229, 284
　abnormal 226
　analysis, maternal 227
Hemoglobinopathies 226, 228*t*
Hemolysis, elevated liver enzymes and low platelets 106, 178, 285, 292, 293, 314
　syndrome 28, 104, 205, 291, 296, 303, 307
　　diagnosis of 308*t*
　　grading of 308*t*
Hemolytic uremic syndrome 104, 107, 107*f*, 205
　diagnosis of 108*f*
Hemorrhage 30, 71, 182, 368
　antepartum 105
　cerebral 76
　control 214
　intracerebral 94, 188, 191, 193
　intraparenchymal 28
　obstetric 111, 268
　postpartum 63, 266, 353
　pulmonary 72, 364
　subarachnoid 191
Hemorrhagic shock 54, 77
　classification of 353*t*
Heparin 66, 171
　intravenous unfractionated 192
　unfractionated 67, 94, 193
　use of 66
Hepatic albumin synthesis 129
Hepatic diseases 303
Hepatic failure 303
　fulminant 303, 312*f*, 314

Hepatic function leading, severe impairment of 303
Hepatic parenchymal infarction 28
Hepatic rupture 28
Hepatitis
  A 334
  autoimmune 310
  B 382
    vaccine 228
    virus 304, 312, 315
  E virus 292, 304, 315
  viral 303, 310
Hepatoma 381
Hepatotoxicity, drug-induced 303
Herpes simplex virus 292, 293, 296, 312, 315, 381
High flux hemodiafiltration 261
High-altitude pulmonary edema 330
High-flow nasal cannula 55
  delivers warm 56
High-performance liquid chromatography 227
Hodgkin's lymphoma 362, 363
Holford method 133
Hormone
  central 153
  counter-regulatory actions of 135
  free forms of 11
Human chorionic gonadotropin 11
Human herpesvirus-6 334
Human immunodeficiency virus 319, 334, 381, 383
Human parvovirus B19 381
Human placental growth factors 282
Hydralazine 80, 81, 83fc, 121, 180, 181, 182
Hydration 172, 221
Hydrazine derived vasodilator 81
Hydrocortisone 172
Hydromorphone 224
Hydroxychloroquine 121, 201
Hydroxydaunorubicin 362
Hydroxyethyl starch 358
Hypercalcemia 170, 172
  familial hypercalciuric 170
  mild 170
  symptomatic 172
Hypercapnia
  permissive 57
  worsening 44

Hypercoagulable states 13, 191, 364
Hyperemesis gravidarum 109, 154, 159, 295, 304, 309
Hyperglycemia 138, 172
Hyperkalemia 111, 138, 163, 164, 363
  causes of 164b, 165fc
  evaluation of 166fc
  medication-induced 164
  severe 165
Hypermagnesemia 169, 174
Hypernatremia 139, 155
Hyperosmolar hyperglycemic syndrome 135, 138, 139
  pathophysiology of 136, 136f
Hyperparathyroidism, primary 170
Hyperphosphatemia 173, 363
Hypertension 80, 117, 140, 179, 180, 241, 260
  acute 80
  chronic 177, 178, 183
  criteria for 291
  gestational 177, 183
  management 118
  mediated end-organ damage 76
  pregnancy-induced 9, 204, 291
  pulmonary 89, 284
  severe 83, 180
Hypertensive disorders 76, 77, 182, 268, 291, 294, 343
  diagnostic criteria of 177
Hypertensive emergency 76, 78, 80t, 85t, 86fc
  diagnosis 78
  epidemiology 76
  management of 78, 80
  maternal complications 76
Hyperthermia, malignant 345
Hyperthyroid 147, 150
  medical management of 149
Hyperthyroidism 73
Hypertonic saline, use of 155
Hyperuricemia 363
Hyperventilation
  maternal 57
  pregnancy-induced 282
Hyperviscosity syndrome 362, 364
Hypoalbuminemia 153, 171
Hypocalcemia 171, 297, 363
  prevalence of 169

Hypocapnia 57
Hypoglycemia 182
  prevention of 141
Hypokalemia 138, 158, 159, 162fc, 163
  causes of 160, 160fc
  evaluation of 162
  persistent 159
  refractory 142
  salmeterol 43
Hypokalemic periodic paralysis, familial 345
Hypokinesia 25
Hypomagnesemia 139, 159, 173
  moderate-to-severe 142
  prevalence of 169
Hyponatremia 154, 182, 297
  acute severe 297
  hypervolemic 155
  iatrogenic 154
  management, standard protocol of 297
Hypoparathyroidism 170
Hypophosphatemia 163, 172
Hypotension 64
  intradialytic 261, 261b
  physiologic 212
  sudden 80
Hypothermia 161, 314
Hypothyroid 12, 148-150
  management of 148f
Hypothyroidism 155
  prevalence of 145
Hypothyroxinemia, isolated 146
Hypotonic solution 154
Hypoxemia 50
  acute 53
  fetal 12
Hypoxia 281, 283, 363
  causes of 281
  maternal 220
  placental 283
  postplacental 286fc
  preplacental 283, 284f
  refractory 44
  uteroplacental 283, 285fc
  fetal 14, 41
Hypoxic placenta 283

I

Ibuprofen 224
Immune thrombocytopenia 236
Immunization 228, 334

Index

Immunoglobulin
  A nephropathy 114
  E 386
  intravascular 204
  intravenous 208, 236, 325, 337, 338
  M 296
Immunosuppressant medications 132*t*
Immunosuppression 240
In vitro fertilization 63, 156, 245
Inappropriate antidiuretic hormone secretion, syndrome of 24, 155
Infarction
  hemorrhagic 190
  pulmonary 30
Infections 111, 296, 324*t*, 334
  clinical manifestations of 321*t*
  endometritis 204
  extra-pulmonary 73
  intrauterine 320
  maternal 320
  nonspecific features of 321
  placental 205
  vaginal 381
Infectious Diseases Society of America guideline 48
Inferior vena cava 9, 311
  compression 323
  filters 67
Inflammation, systemic 172
Inflammatory muscle disease 343, 345
Inflammatory nerve 341
Influenza
  pneumonia 47
  virus 46, 334
Injury severity score 211
Inspired oxygen, fraction of 262, 264
Insulin 161, 167
  infusion 363
  pump failure 135
  strategy 141
Intensive care unit 5, 6, 23, 49, 158, 250, 322*t*, 352
  incidence of 272
Internal jugular vein 272
  anatomy of 274*f*
International Society for Study of Hypertension in Pregnancy 177

Intra-abdominal pressure 355
Intracranial pressure 188
Intrapartum care 230
Intrarenal oncotic pressure 153
Intrauterine contraceptive devices 240
Intrauterine death 378
Intrauterine growth
  restriction 206*f*, 284, 285, 361, 381
  retardation 173
Intravascular volume
  deficit, correction of 140
  loss of 352
Intravenous catheter 272
  flow rates 273*t*
Invasive ventilation 44
Iodide, maternal clearance of 11
Iodine supplementation 147
Ionized calcium 171
Ipratropium bromide 43
Iron
  chelation indications 228
  deficiency 147, 227
    anemia 284
  supplementation 147
Ischemia
  mesenteric 143
  modified albumin level 65
Isolated intracranial hypertension syndrome 188
Isotonic saline 172

J

Jaundice 72, 227
Jugular venous pressure, raised 100

K

Ketoacidosis
  diabetic 135, 138, 139, 142, 292
  monitor resolution of 142
  resolution of 141
Ketorolac 224
Kidney
  disease 140
    chronic 104, 114, 115, 118*t*, 164, 258
    management of 120*t*
  function
    loss of 104
    test 382

injury, acute 104-106, 164, 257*b*, 259, 314
Kissing heart 27
Klebsiella pneumoniae 125, 320

L

Labetalol 80, 121, 132, 180, 181, 182
  reduces blood pressure 81
Labor, stress of 135
Lactate dehydrogenase 11, 78, 295, 308
  levels, raised 363
Lamivudine 131
Lamotrigine 297
Laryngeal mask airway 252
Laryngopathia gravidarum 387
Latex allergy 388
Left ventricular
  dysfunction 83
  ejection fraction 25, 91
  obstruction 89
  outflow tract
    cross-sectional area of 25
    velocity 27*f*
Legionella urinary antigen 48
Leukemia
  acute
    lymphocytic 362, 363
    myeloid 362
    promyelocytic 362
  chronic
    myelogenous 362
    myeloid 361
  increased risk of 58
Leukocytosis 15
Leukopheresis 364
Leukostasis 362, 363, 364*f*
Leukotriene receptor antagonists 43, 287
Levetiracetam 192, 297
Levothyroxine 147
Liddle's syndrome 18
Lidocaine 343
Linezolid 50
Listeria 381
  monocytogenes 320
Lithium 130
Liver
  disease
    acute 303
    autoimmune 303
    characteristics of 305*t*

chronic 156, 303
diagnostic modalities
for 311*t*
differential diagnosis of 305*t*
prevalence of 305*t*
disorders 295
dysfunction 307
enzymes, elevated 156
failure 303, 309, 315*t*
function test 139, 142, 292, 382
abnormal 295, 304
elevated 198
transplantation 244, 295, 316
Long-chain 3-hydroxyacyl-CoA
dehydrogenase, fetal
deficiency of 109
Loop diuretic 167, 172
Low back pain 341
Low lupus disease activity
state 199
Low platelet counts syndrome 295
Low serum
bicarbonate 139
magnesium levels 159
Low-molecular weight heparin
66, 67, 94, 192, 193,
207, 362
Lumbar puncture 190, 375
Lumbosacral radiculopathy 345
Lung 275
cavitation 47
compliance 42
infarction, acute 63
injury, ventilator-induced 56
protective ventilation 10, 56*b*
strategies 56
volumes 9
Lupus
anticoagulant 197, 205
flare 197, 197*t*
signs of 197
symptoms of 197
nephritis 120
Luspatercept 231
Luzius Dettli rule 133
Lymphoma 381

M

Macrolides 343
Magnesium 142, 169, 173, 343
clinical significance of 173
deficiency 173
prevalence of 169

depletion 171
disorders of 169
levels 173
normal laboratory values
of 171*t*
replacement 174
retention test 174
serum 173*t*
level 169
sulfate 182, 183*f*, 294, 376, 377
Magnetic resonance
imaging 101, 311, 336,
350, 382
venography 190, 190*f*, 191, 193
Malaria 297, 321, 381
cerebral 297
Malformations
carries risk of 340
congenital 117, 297
major congenital 297, 378
Malignancy, hypercalcemia
of 170
Mannitol 164
Manual vacuum aspiration 326
Marfan syndrome 91
Massive pulmonary embolism 63
Mastitis 321
Maternal cardiac arrest 249, 249*t*,
250, 252, 253
causes of 254*t*
Maternal cardiopulmonary
cerebral resuscitation,
steps of 250
Maternal critical care units 4*t*
development of 7
Maternal death, causes of 320
Maternal distress, mechanisms of
136, 137*f*
Maternal early warning trigger
78, 79
tool hypertension pathway
79*fc*
Maternal health, implications for
14, 46, 70-72, 74, 88,
115, 129, 146, 169, 178,
188, 198, 211, 220, 227,
255, 304, 320, 330,
374, 380
Maternal monitoring 221, 260
Maternal mortality 177
rate 6, 249
Maternal obstetric early warning
system 5

Maternal resuscitation team
249, 250*b*
Maternal transport system 268
McArdle's disease 345
Mean arterial pressure 30, 85,
254, 264, 322, 355
Mechanical ventilation 56, 369
Melanocyte-stimulating
hormone 153
Membranes
fragment 283
premature rupture of 284,
319, 381
rupture of 37
Mendelson's syndrome 330
Meningitis 47, 321
Mental obtundation 352
Mentzer's index 227
Meralgia paresthetica 345
Metabolic acidosis 17, 18,
111, 141
causes of 17*t*
hyperchloremic 141
Metabolic alkalosis 17, 162*fc*, 304
causes of 18*t*
Metabolic disorders 303, 376
Methyldopa 121, 132, 180, 181
Methylprednisolone 236
Microtia 240
Microvascular thrombosis 208
Midazolam 12
Middle cerebral artery-peak
systolic velocity 229
Midline peripheral catheters 275
Midstream urine 322
Mind mucosal edema 13
Mineral
disorders 169, 170*t*
metabolism, disorders of 169
Mineralocorticoid activity 9
Minimal change disease 114
Minute ventilation 9, 211
Miscarriage 94
carries risk of 340
spontaneous 117
Misoprostol 354
Mitochondrial myopathies
345, 346
Mitral regurgitation 88, 93
moderate 26*f*
significant 25
Mitral stenosis 9, 91
Mitral valve 88

Modified early obstetric warning score 222
Modified sequential organ failure assessment 320*t*
Molecular adsorbent recirculating system 316
Monitoring amniotic fluid index 155
Monoclonal antibodies 208
Mood disorders, postpartum 298
Morbidity, risk of 323*t*
Morphine 224
Motor neuron disease 345, 346
Mucosa, congestion of 42
Multiorgan dysfunction syndrome 47
Multiorgan failure 204, 266
Multiple gestation 63
Multiple myeloma 361
Multiple organ dysfunction syndrome 14
Multivessel fetoplacental Doppler 33
Mural thrombus 30
Murmurs, systolic 100
Muscarinic antagonist, short-acting 43
Muscle
  cramps 18
  specific kinase 342
  weakness 345
Myasthenia gravis 343*b*, 345
Myasthenic crisis 343
Mycophenolate mofetil 122, 240
Mycophenolic acid 240
Mycoplasma pneumoniae 46
Myelodysplastic syndromes 381
Myeloproliferative neoplasms 361
Myocardia infarction 135
Myocardial infarction 65, 71, 82, 143, 352
Myopathies, inherited 344, 345
Myophosphorylase deficiency 345
Myositis, necrotizing 344
Myotonic dystrophies 344, 345

N

Naloxone 253
Nasal congestion 386
Nasogastric suctioning 161
National Institute for Health and Clinical Excellence 181
Necrosis, massive 303

Nelfinavir 131
Neonatal infections, early-onset 321
Neonatal intensive care unit 178, 220
Nephrolithiasis 114, 120
Nephropathy, diabetic 120, 132
Nerve, inherited disorders of 344
Netilmicin 131
Neuraxial technique 67
Neuroendocrine 197
Neurological developmental defects 58
Neuromuscular blocking agents 57, 343
Neuromuscular deformities 287
Neuromuscular disease 19, 345*t*
  treatments 341*t*
Neuromuscular disorders 340, 346
Neuropathy
  autonomic 340
  inflammatory 340
  inherited 344, 345
Neurophysins 153
New York Heart Association 88, 89*t*, 101
Nicardipine 81
Nifedipine 81, 84*fc*, 121, 131, 132, 180-182
Nitric oxide, inhaled 71, 331
Nitrofurantoin 126
Nitrogen production 24
Nitroglycerine 81
Nitrous oxide 74
Nocturnal leg cramps 174
Noncardiogenic pulmonary edema 329, 332, 332*fc*
Non-Hodgkin's lymphoma 362
Non-invasive bilevel positive end expiratory pressure 44
Noninvasive blood pressure monitoring 24
Noninvasive prenatal testing 243
Noninvasive ventilation 19, 55, 332, 369
Nonsteroidal anti-inflammatory drugs 55, 127, 164, 166, 201, 222
Nonstress test 34, 243
Nonthrombotic pulmonary embolism 70, 74

N-terminal pro-brain natriuretic peptide 101
Nuclear deoxyribonucleic acid 346
Nucleic acid metabolism 363

O

Obstetric
  care, emergency 268
  critical care 173
  interventions 251
  management 92, 314, 314*f*
  medicine, advances in 3
  shock 352
    management of 352
    types of 352, 353*t*
Obstructive sleep apnea 287
Olanzapine 298
Oligohydramnios 34, 127, 205, 297
Oliguria 352
Omalizumab 42, 43
Opioids
  overdose of 330
  parenteral 221
Oral ferrous sulfate formulations 231
Oral glucose tolerance test 118, 132
Oral phosphate binders 363
Organ
  adverse effects of physiological changes 319*t*
  dysfunction
    maternal 177
    pathogenesis of 364*f*
  functions 142
Oropharyngeal airway 370
Osmoregulation 153
Osmotic stimulus 153
Osteoporosis 170
  levels of 228
Ovulation induction 245
Oxcarbazepine 297
Oxidative stress 283
  role of 283
Oxygen 282
  consumption 211, 282
  maternal 331
  fetal hemoglobin for 57
  saturation 264, 323, 327
  therapy 222
    modalities 44
Oxytocin 154

P

Pain
  abdominal 79
  management 221, 222*b*
  radicular 365
  stimulating arginine
    vasopressin 297
Pancreas 228
Pancreatitis 171
Pancytopenia 362
Papilledema 364
Paradoxical embolism 74
Paradoxical intracellular
  acidosis 141
Paraplegia 365
Paresthesia 19, 365
Partial thromboplastin time 207
Passive leg raising test 322, 323
Peak expiratory flow rate 42
Peak serum concentrations 13
Pedal edema 198
Pelvic
  thrombophlebitis 352
  thrombosis 205
Penicillin G potassium 164
Pericardial effusion 26, 26*f*
  post-evacuation of 330
Pericardial tamponade 47
Periodontal disease 73
Peripartum chelation
  therapy 230
Peripheral arteries 76
Peripheral blood smear
  examination 234
Peripheral chemoreceptor
  stimulation 19
Peripheral venous access 273
Peritoneal dialysis 259, 260, 261
  catheter placement 168
Permanent atrial fibrillation 92
Peroxynitrite interferes, formation
  of 283
Pertussis 334
Phenytoin 12
Phosphate 142, 172, 363
  correction 142, 172
Phosphorus 169
  homeostasis, disorders of 169
  normal laboratory values of 171*t*
Placenta
  functions 12
  previa 111
  retained 352
Placental abruption 47, 54, 71, 111

Placental development, normal 282
Placental disruption 28
Placental growth factor 106, 120
  low levels of 242
Placental lactogen 153
Placental perfusion 213
Placental trophoblastic
  epithelium, abnormal
  proliferation of 72
Plasma
  albumin 153
  aldosterone 153
  calcium 171
  estrogen 153
  exchange, high-volume 315
  prolactin 153
  protein 179
Plasmapheresis 204, 208, 341
Plasminogen
  activator inhibitor 11
  activator levels 11
Platelet 233
  count 308
Pleocytosis 376
Pleura, puncture of 275
Pleural effusion 47, 64
  post-evacuation of 330
Pneumococcal urinary antigen 48
Pneumococcal vaccine 50
Pneumocystis pneumonia 49
Pneumonia 352
  community acquired 46, 49*t*
  incidence of 46
  morbidity of 46
  mortality of 46
  necrotizing 47
  severity index 48
  varicella zoster immune
    globulin 50
Pneumothorax 30, 47
Point-of-care ultrasound 24, 25,
  28, 34
Poliomyelitis 334
Polycystic kidney disease 114
  autosomal dominant 120
Polycystic ovarian syndrome 330
Polycythemia vera 362
Polymerase chain reaction 297, 312
Polyneuropathy, chronic
  inflammatory
  demyelinating 342, 345
Polytrauma 210
Polyurea 172
Positive end-expiratory pressure
  56, 262

Posterior reversible
  encephalopathy
  syndrome 191, 292-294,
  348, 349, 374
  anatomic distribution 349
  clinical features 349
  diagnosis 349
  etiology of 348, 349*b*
  pathophysiology 348
  prognosis 350
  treatment 350
Postglomerular oncotic
  pressure 153
Posthypercapnia 18
Post-maternal cardiac arrest
  care 253
Postpartum bleeding,
  management of 355*t*
Postpartum foot drop 345
Postpartum hemorrhage 63,
  266, 353
  causes of 354*t*
Postpartum period 8, 76, 150
Post-pneumonectomy 330
Post-thrombotic syndrome 67
Potassium 141, 363
  chloride 163
  disturbances 158
  homeostasis, disorders
    of 158
  sparing diuretics 162
  supplementation, rate
    of 141
Pravastatin 131
Prednisolone 236
  low dose 132
Prednisone 362
Preeclampsia 73, 77, 105, 111,
  112, 117, 156, 174, 177,
  178, 184, 197, 198, 285,
  291, 307, 310, 368
  complicated pregnancy,
    clinical care of 285
  de novo 177
  development of 140
  diagnosis of 242
  early-onset 178
  incidence of 180
  late-onset 178
  management of 179
  preterm 178
  prophylaxis 132
  risk factors for 179, 179*t*
  severe 177, 242
  universal screening for 179

Pregnancy 41, 93, 257, 281
    acute fatty liver of 106, 108,
        109, 112, 206, 292, 293,
        295, 303, 308, 308t, 310,
        314, 368
    airway edema of 372
    anatomic and physiological
        changes of 105f
    cardiomyopathy of 368
    dynamic nature of 114
    ectopic 111
    effect of 115, 241
    embolism of 387
    full-term 318
    hypertensive disorders of 76,
        77, 291, 294, 343
    intrahepatic cholestasis
        of 304, 307, 309
    life-threatening hypertensive
        disorder of 376
    liver in 303
    loss 198
    management of 118t, 200t
    physiology of 41, 272
    problems, intrauterine
        hypoxia-related 285
    result of 8
    thrombotic
        microangiopathies 109f
Premature birth 361
Prepregnancy 118
    care 131
    counseling 241, 244
    planning 199
Preterm birth 198
Preterm labor 197
    management of 159
Procainamide 343
Progesterone 10, 42, 153, 240
    increased levels of 158
    only pill 131, 230
Propylthiouracil 147
Prostacyclin 331
    intravenous 71
Prostaglandins 153, 354
Prosthetic valves 94
Proteinuria 115, 117, 177, 241
    management 118
    severe 180
Proteus 125
Prothrombin time 308, 355
Prothrombotic tendencies 295
Pseudohyperkalemia 163
Pseudohypoparathyroidism 170
Pseudomonas 125

Pseudopneumonia 64
Psychosis, postpartum 298
Pulmonary artery 30, 65
    catheter 29
    occlusion
        pressure 30
        signs of 73
    rupture 30
Pulmonary aspiration,
    complications of 370
Pulmonary capillary wedge
    pressure 30, 332
Pulmonary disease, severe 28
Pulmonary edema 28, 76, 77, 83,
    319, 330
    development of 331
Pulmonary embolism 26, 54, 62,
    65, 66t, 356
    diagnosis of 66b
    life-threatening complications
        of 65b
Pulmonary thromboembolism
    62, 65, 71, 353
    clinical presentation 63
    diagnosis 62
    etiology 62
    management 66
    pregnancy-associated 62
    risk factors for 63b
Pulsatility index 34
Pulse
    oximetry 24
    pressure 353
    pressure variation 355
Pulseless electrical activity 65
Pure non-anion gap metabolic
    acidosis 17
Pyelonephritis 109, 112, 125, 318,
    324, 352
Pyridostigmine, oral 342

Q

Quadriplegia 365
Quetiapine 298
Quick sequential organ failure
    assessment 318
Quinidine 343
Quinine 343
Quinolones 126, 130, 131

R

Radiation, risk of 59t, 62
Radiocontrast-related pulmonary
    edema 330

Radiotherapy 362
Rapamycin, mammalian target
    of 132
Rapid cell lysis 363
Rapid sequence induction 369
Recombinant tissue plasminogen
    activator 294
Red blood cells 11
    number of 282
Red cell mass 97
Reflux nephropathy 114
Regurgitation, acute aortic 94
Rehabilitation 59
    therapy 338
Renal anomalies 240
Renal blood flow 10
Renal cell carcinoma 381
Renal changes 10, 72,
    105t, 213
Renal disease 130
    end-stage 116
    specific 120
Renal failure 77, 129, 171
    end-stage 104
    risk of 104
Renal function
    monitoring of 242
    tests 142
    worsening of 115
Renal impairment 67
    degree of 115t
    moderate-to-severe 116
Renal indications 28
Renal injury, acute 72
Renal insufficiency 83
Renal plasma flow 105f
Renal replacement therapy 111,
    133, 257, 259, 260b
    complications of 261b
    indications of 259b
Renal system 258
Renal transplantation 111, 241
    effects of 241
Renal tubular acidosis 17, 161
Renal ultrasound, baseline 118
Renin-angiotensin-aldosterone
    system 153, 158
Respiration rate 323
Respiratory acidosis 18
    causes of 19t
Respiratory alkalosis 19, 172
    causes of 19t
Respiratory buffer system 14
Respiratory changes 9, 53,
    54b, 211t

Respiratory failure 53, 64, 77, 369
  acute 368
  causes of 54*b*
Respiratory parameters 211
Respiratory rate 79, 211, 319, 353
Respiratory symptoms 160, 223
Respiratory syncytial virus 46
Respiratory syndrome, acute 46
Respiratory system 53, 263
Respiratory tract
  infection 321
  mucosa, capillary engorgement of 211
Resuscitation
  cardiopulmonary 6, 249, 253
  neonatal 270, 271
Resuscitative transesophageal echo, role of 254
Reverse transcription polymerase chain reaction 382
Reversible cerebral vasoconstriction syndrome 191, 374
Rheumatic heart diseases 88
Rhinovirus 46
Rifampicin 131
Ritodrine 131, 159
Ritonavir 131
Rituximab 122, 208
Root disorders 340
Rose approach, phases of 355*t*
Rubella 381

S

Salbutamol 43
  nebulization 363
Salicylate poisoning 330
Saquinavir 131
Sarcoidosis 381
Scalpel cricothyroidotomy 370
Sclerosis, amyotrophic lateral 340, 346
Seizure 72, 188, 294, 297, 364
  disorder 182
  febrile 375
  focal 375
  generalized tonic-clonic 77
  impact of 374, 374*t*
  management of 293
  prolonged 374
  prophylaxis 83
Sensorium 292*fc*

Sepsis 54, 127, 171, 172, 318, 323*t*, 352, 357
  maternal 327*fc*
  neonatal 320
  puerperal 104, 318
  refractory 30
  risk of 319*t*
Septic embolism 73
Sequential organ failure assessment 5, 318
Serum magnesium 173*t*
  concentration 183*t*
Serum placental growth factor 179
Severe hypertension 83, 180
  treatment of 293
Severe maternal morbidity 3, 77, 177
  warning signs 286
Sexually transmitted diseases 383
Sheehan's syndrome 155
Shock 64, 303
  cardiogenic 387
  circulatory vasodilatory 386
  hemorrhagic 54, 77
  identification of 352*t*
  maternal 6
  obstetric 352
  septic 30, 71, 353, 357
  treatment of 355*t*
Short-acting beta agonist 287
Sickle cell
  crisis 219, 224
    epidemiology 219
    investigations 21*b*
    management 220
  disease 219, 220, 284
Sildenafil 71
Simpson biplane method 25
Singleton pregnancy 37
Sinuses, clinical features of 189*f*
Sirolimus 122, 240
Skeletal deformities 227
Smooth muscle cell proliferation 42
Society for Maternal-Fetal Medicine 180
Society of Obstetricians and Gynaecologists 181
Sodium 97, 141, 152
  bicarbonate 10, 155, 167
  excretion 153*t*
  glucose cotransporter-2 inhibitors 140

homeostasis 154, 154*f*, 155*f*
  disorders of 152, 154
  level 156
  nitroprusside 82
Solid organ transplants 244
Somatostatin 164
Speckle tracking echocardiography 25
Spinal cord compression 362, 364
  malignant 364
Spinal deformities 287
Spinal muscular atrophies 340, 345, 346
Spiral artery
  endothelial cells of 283
  remodeling, abnormal 283
Spontaneous circulation, return of 252, 253, 267
Staphylococcus
  aureus 46, 320
    methicillin-resistant 324
    methicillin-susceptible 324
  infection 73
  saprophyticus 125
Status epilepticus 297, 374, 376, 378
  nonconvulsive 376
  treatment of 376
ST-elevation myocardial infarction 23
Stenosis, pulmonary 93
Stenotic lesions 89, 91
Steroids 172, 325
  inhaled 44
  systemic 45
Stomach, cephalad displacement of 10
Streptococcus pneumoniae 46, 49, 107, 222
Stress dose steroids 243
Stroke 76, 294
  acute 223
  incidence of 77
  ischemic 77
  pregnancy-related 187
  risk of 77
  types of 223
  volume 281
Subarachnoid bleed 190
Subclavian artery injury 275
Subclavian vein, anatomy of 274*f*
Succinylcholine 164, 343
Sudden infant death syndrome 174

Sulfa compounds 50
Sulphonamides 126
Superior vena cava
   obstruction of 365
   syndrome 365
Supraglottic airway device 369, 372
Swallowing, conjunctival 386
Syphilis 381, 382
Systemic inflammatory response syndrome, activation of 70
Systemic lupus erythematosus 4, 166, 201, 381
   epidemiology 196
   flare 196
   management 199
Systemic vascular resistance 30, 285, 378

T

Tachycardia 19, 72, 149, 331, 352
   supraventricular 251
   ventricular 65, 165, 251
Tachypnea 74, 352, 363
Tacrolimus 121, 240
Teratogenicity 130
   lithium-induced 130
Terbutaline 131
Tetracyclines 50, 126, 130, 131
Tetraiodotyronine 11
Thalassemia 226, 229, 229*b*, 231
   alpha 226, 227
   beta 226, 227
   diagnosis of 227
Thallium 131
Theophylline 42, 43
Thiazide diuretics 121
Throat swabs 322
Thrombocythemia, essential 362
Thrombocytopenia 106, 108, 108*f*, 178, 233
   acute 72
   causes of 233
   etiology of 234*t*
   evaluation of 234
   gestational 235
   heparin-induced 265
   laboratory tests for 235*t*
   mild 362
   neonatal 237
Thromboelastography 215, 264
Thromboelastometry, rotational 264, 354, 355

Thromboembolic diseases 26
Thromboembolism
   pulmonary 62, 65, 71, 353
   risk of 13
Thrombolytic therapy 357
   role of 67
Thrombopoietin receptor antagonists 237
Thrombosis 64, 182, 189*f*, 275, 362, 366
Thrombotic microangiopathies 85, 104, 106, 112, 114, 237
   pregnancy-associated 104, 109*f*
Thrombotic thrombocytopenic purpura 104, 106, 108, 182, 237
Thyroid 228
   disease 150
   disorder 145, 150
      management of 150*f*
   stimulating hormone levels 11
   supplementation 228
   supplements 148
Thyroiditis, postpartum 149
Thyrotoxicosis 135, 150
   gestational 149
Tissue
   friability 13
   necrosis 204
Tocolytic 131
   therapy 54
Total extracellular fluid volume 152
Total lung capacity 41, 54
Toxic inhalation 330
Toxic shock syndrome 321, 324
Toxicity 183*t*
   signs of 243
   symptoms of 243
Toxoplasma gondii 296
Toxoplasmosis 296
Tranexamic acid 253
Transesophageal echocardiogram 382
Transfusion reaction 71
Transient ischemic attack 89
Transjugular intrahepatic portosystemic shunt 315
Trauma 135, 287
   maternal 211
   mechanisms of 210*f*

Triamterene 131
Tricuspid
   regurgitation 94
   stenosis 93
Tricyclic antidepressant 340
   overdose 330
Tri-iodothyronine levels 11
Trimethoprim 126, 131
Trophoblast stem cells 281
Trophoblastic disease, gestational 72
Trophoblastic embolism 54, 72
Trousseau's signs 298
Tuberculosis 319, 381
Tubulointerstitial diseases 114, 164
Tumor lysis syndrome 362, 363
   diagnosis of 363*t*
Tumor necrosis factor-alpha 283
Twin pregnancy 156
Typhoid fever 381

U

Ultrasonography 308
Ultrasound
   guidance, use of 274
   parameters 33
   role of 372
Upper airway 9
   obstruction 330
Upper extremity, veins of 273
Upper respiratory tract 42
Uremia 108*f*, 363
Ureteral pressure 153
Uric acid 198, 363
Urinary tract
   infection 104, 105*f*, 124, 321, 383
      recurrent 126*b*
      treatment of 110*t*
   obstruction, congenital 120
Urine
   electrolyte 165
   examination 118
   ketones 142
   midstream specimen of 124
   output 24
Ursodeoxycholic acid 315
Urticaria, acute generalized 387
Uterine
   artery pulsatility index 179
   blood flow 12
   contraction 386
   rupture 71
   vessels 357

Uteroplacental blood flow,
  physiology of 12
Uteroplacental Doppler study 34
Uteroplacental dysfunction 178
Uterus
  enlarged 212
  exteriorization of 74

V

Vaginal birth 94
Vaginal examination 215
Valproate 192, 297
Valve
  dysfunction 94
  repair 94
  replacement of 94
Valvular heart disease 91
Vancomycin 50
Varicella 46, 334
  virus immunization 50
  zoster virus 312, 381
Vascular diseases 114
Vascular endothelial growth factor 106, 283
Vasculitis 182
Vasogenic theory 348
Vaso-occlusive crisis 220, 222*b*
Vasopressin production 9
Vasopressors 352, 358*t*

Vasovagal symptoms 387
Vecuronium 343
Vena cava
  inferior 9, 311
  superior 365
Venoarterial extracorporeal
      membrane oxygenation 262, 264
Venous thromboembolism 11, 54, 356
  risk of 11
Venovenous extracorporeal
      membrane oxygenation 262, 264
Ventilation 19, 214, 264
  impaired 19
Ventilator support 149
Ventricular fibrillation 30, 65, 165, 251
Vesico-ureteric reflux
      nephropathy 120
Vinblastine 362
  sulfate oncovin 362
Visual disturbance 74, 79
Visual scotomata,
      persistent 178
Visual semiquantitative
      estimations 25
Vital capacity 42, 54
Vital organs 281

Vitamin
  D
    deficiency 170, 171
    level optimization 228
    physiology, genetic
        disorder of 170
    supplementations 231
  K antagonists 94
Voice, hoarseness of 386
von Willebrand factor 204

W

Warfarin 130
Weaning 59, 264
Weight gain 211, 369
Well-designed anesthetic plan 346
Wernicke's encephalopathy 295
White blood cell 11, 65, 363
Wilson's disease 303

Z

Zahara risk score 90*t*
Zalcitabine 131
Zetachains 226
Zidovudine 131
Zika syndrome 381
Zika virus 341
  infection 381
Zoledronate 172